CORE TOPICS IN GENERAL AND EMERGENCY SURGERY

Seventh Edition

A Companion to Specialist Surgical Practice

Seventh Edition

Series Editors

O. James Garden

Simon Paterson-Brown

CORE TOPICS IN GENERAL AND EMERGENCY SURGERY

Edited by

Hugh M. Paterson, BMedSci, MBChB, MD, FRCS(Ed)

Clinical Senior Lecturer, Coloproctology,
The University of Edinburgh, Edinburgh, UK

Chris Deans, MBChB(Hons), MD, FRCS

Consultant, General and Upper Gastrointestinal Surgeon,
Royal Infirmary of Edinburgh; Senior Lecturer,
The University of Edinburgh, Edinburgh, UK

For additional online content visit eBooks+

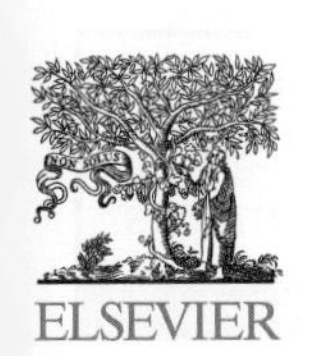

ELSEVIER

First edition 1997
Second edition 2001
Third edition 2005
Fourth edition 2009
Fifth edition 2014
Sixth edition 2019
Seventh edition 2024

ISBN: 978-0-7020-8474-4

Content Strategist: Alexandra Mortimer
Content Project Manager: Arindam Banerjee
Design: Ryan Cook
Art Buyer: Muthukumaran Thangaraj
Marketing Manager: Deborah Watkins

Printed in India

Last digit is the print number: 9 8 7 6 5 4 3 2 1

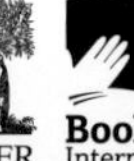

Contents

Series Editors' preface

The *Companion to Specialist Surgical Practice* series has now reached its Seventh Edition and continues to remain popular for both surgeons in training as well as consultant surgeons in independent practice. The strength of this series has always been founded on contemporary, evidence-based information on the subspecialist areas relevant to their general surgical practice and this Seventh Edition has followed this plan.

This Edition continues to keep abreast of increasing subspecialisation in general surgery. The ongoing developments in minimal access and increasingly robotic surgery are discussed, along with the desire of some subspecialities, such as breast and vascular surgery, to separate away from 'general surgery' in some countries. However, all volumes also underline the importance for all surgeons of being aware of current developments in their surgical field. The importance of evidence-based practice and in particular the management of emergency conditions remains throughout, and authors have provided recommendations and highlighted key resources within each chapter. The ebook version of the textbook has also enabled improved access to the reference abstracts and links to video content relevant to many of the chapters.

As in all the previous editions, we are greatly indebted to the volume editors, and contributors, who have all put so much hard work into delivering such a high quality piece of work. We remain grateful for the support and encouragement of the team at Elsevier and we trust that our original vision of delivering an up-to-date, affordable text has been met and that readers, whether in training or independent practice, will find this Seventh Edition an invaluable resource.

We are grateful to Kathryn Rigby and Jonathan Michaels who wrote the guidelines on Evidence-based Practice in Surgery for previous editions of the series. These have been well received and have been retained again for this new edition in order to help guide readers in their assessment of the various levels of evidence discussed in each chapter.

O. James Garden, CBE, BSc, MBChB, MD, DSc(Hon), FRCS (Glas), FRCS(Ed), FRCP(Ed), FRACS(Hon), FRCSC (Hon), FACS(Hon), FCSHK(Hon), FRCSI(Hon), FRCS(Engl) (Hon), FRSE, MAMSE, FFST(RCSEd)
Professor Emeritus, Clinical Surgery, University of Edinburgh, UK

Simon Paterson-Brown, MBBS, MPhil, MS, FRCS(Ed), FRCS(Engl), FCSHK, FFST(RCSEd)
Honorary Senior Lecturer, Clinical Surgery, University of Edinburgh.

Editors' preface

The Seventh Edition of *Core Topics in General and Emergency Surgery* has been extensively revised, incorporating new authors and new chapters. It is been divided into two main sections: the first includes areas of practice we hope will be of interest and relevance to all surgeons, and the second section covers the care of emergency patients with an emphasis on principles for the management of conditions outwith the readers' usual specialist practice, including indications for discussion with or transfer to the care of specialist colleagues. As with previous editions of the Companion series, this volume should be considered complementary to the other specialist volumes, while still encompassing all those emergency areas that remain within the remit of the general surgeon.

ACKNOWLEDGEMENTS

The success of this volume, as with previous editions, very much lies in the quality of the chapters written by our co-authors and we are extremely grateful to all of them for the hard work that went into writing or re-writing each chapter. The additional workload required for the timely delivery of concise, well-referenced and up-to-date chapters for a book such as this, by busy practising surgeons, should never be underestimated. We would also like to recognise the help and support of the whole Elsevier team, particularly given the difficulties encountered during a production period impacted by the global COVID-19 pandemic.

We also acknowledge and offer our grateful thanks for the input of all previous editions' contributors, without whom this new edition would not have been possible.

Hugh M. Paterson
Chris Deans
Edinburgh

Evidence-based practice in surgery

Critical appraisal for developing evidence-based practice can be obtained from a number of sources, the most reliable being randomised controlled clinical trials, systematic literature reviews, meta-analyses and observational studies. For practical purposes three grades of evidence can be used, analogous to the levels of 'proof' required in a court of law:

1. **Beyond all reasonable doubt**. Such evidence is likely to have arisen from high-quality randomised controlled trials, systematic reviews or high-quality synthesised evidence such as decision analysis, cost-effectiveness analysis or large observational datasets. The studies need to be directly applicable to the population of concern and have clear results. The grade is analogous to burden of proof within a criminal court and may be thought of as corresponding to the usual standard of 'proof' within the medical literature (i.e. $P < 0.05$).
2. **On the balance of probabilities**. In many cases a high-quality review of literature may fail to reach firm conclusions due to conflicting or inconclusive results, trials of poor methodological quality or the lack of evidence in the population to which the guidelines apply. In such cases it may still be possible to make a statement as to the best treatment on the 'balance of probabilities'. This is analogous to the decision in a civil court where all the available evidence will be weighed up and the verdict will depend upon the balance of probabilities.
3. **Not proven**. Insufficient evidence upon which to base a decision, or contradictory evidence.

Depending on the information available, three grades of recommendation can be used:

Strong recommendation, which should be followed unless there are compelling reasons to act otherwise.

a. A recommendation based on evidence of effectiveness, but where there may be other factors to take into account in decision-making, for example the user of the guidelines may be expected to take into account patient preferences, local facilities, local audit results or available resources.
b. A recommendation made where there is no adequate evidence as to the most effective practice, although there may be reasons for making a recommendation in order to minimise cost or reduce the chance of error through a locally agreed protocol.

✔✔ Evidence where a conclusion can be reached '**beyond all reasonable doubt'** and therefore where a **strong recommendation** can be given.
This will normally be based on evidence levels:

- Ia. Meta-analysis of randomised controlled trials
- Ib. Evidence from at least one randomised controlled trial
- IIa. Evidence from at least one controlled study without randomisation
- IIb. Evidence from at least one other type of quasi-experimental study.

✔ Evidence where a conclusion might be reached '**on the balance of probabilities'** and where there may be other factors involved which influence the recommendation given. This will normally be based on less conclusive evidence than that represented by the double tick icons:

- III. Evidence from non-experimental descriptive studies, such as comparative studies and case–control studies
- IV. Evidence from expert committee reports or opinions or clinical experience of respected authorities, or both.

Evidence that is associated with either a **strong recommendation** or **expert opinion** is highlighted in the text in panels such as those shown above, and is distinguished by either a double or single tick icon, respectively. The references associated with double-tick evidence are listed as Key References at the end of each chapter, along with a short summary of the paper's conclusions where applicable. The full reference list for each chapter is available in the ebook.

The reader is referred to Chapter 1, 'Evaluation of surgical evidence' in the volume *Core Topics in General and Emergency Surgery* of this series, for a more detailed description of this topic.

Contributors

Iain D. Anderson, MD, FRCS, FRACS(Hon), FFICM(Hon)
Professor
Intestinal Failure Unit
Salford Royal Hospital
Manchester, United Kingdom

Robert Baigrie, BSc, MBChB, FRCS, MD
Adjunct Professor of Surgery
University of Cape Town and Groote Schuur Hospital
Cape Town, Western Cape, South Africa

Andrew C. de Beaux, FRCSEd, MD, MBChB
Consultant General and Upper GI Surgeon
Department of General Surgery
Royal Infirmary of Edinburgh;
Honorary Senior Lecturer
The University of Edinburgh
Edinburgh, United Kingdom

Katherine J. Broughton, MBChB, BHB, FRACS
Department of General Surgery
Fiona Stanley Hospital
Perth, WA, Australia

Kate Carey, MBChB, FRCA
Consultant Anaesthetist
Department of Anaesthesia, Critical Care and Pain Medicine
Royal Infirmary of Edinburgh
Edinburgh, United Kingdom

Maurizio Cecconi, MD, FRCA, FFICM, MD(Res)
Professor
Anesthesia and Intensive Care
Humanitas Research Hospital
Rozzano, Italy

Shannon Melissa Chan, MBChB, FRCS(Gen), FHKAM
Assistant Professor of Surgery
The Chinese University of Hong Kong
HKSAR, China

Saxon Connor, MBChB, FRACS
HPB Surgeon
General Surgery
Te Whatu Ora
Christchurch, New Zealand

Dafydd A. Davies, MD, MPhil, FRCSC
Chief of Surgery
IWK Health Centre;
Associate Professor of Surgery
Dalhousie Medical School
Dalhousie University
Halifax, NS, Canada

Chris Deans, MBChB(Hons), MD, FRCS
Consultant
General and Upper Gastrointestinal Surgery
Royal Infirmary of Edinburgh;
Senior Lecturer
The University of Edinburgh
Edinburgh, United Kingdom

Thomas M. Drake, MBChB, BMedSci
Clinical Research Fellow
University of Edinburgh
Edinburgh, United Kingdom

Barbora East, MD, PhD, FEBS AWS
Doctor
3rd Department of Surgery of 1st Medical Faculty of Charles University
Motol University Hospital
Prague, Czech Republic

Jonathan Epstein, MD, FRCS
Consultant Surgeon
Intestinal Failure Unit
Salford Care Organisation
Northern Care Alliance NHS Foundation Trust
Manchester, United Kingdom

Kirstine Farrer, M.Phil, BSc RD
Consultant Dietitian – Intestinal Failure
Intestinal Failure Unit
Salford Care Organisation
Northern Care Alliance NHS Foundation Trust
Greater Manchester, United Kingdom

Timothy Forgan, BSc(Hons), MBBCh, MMed(Surg), FCS(SA), Cert Gastroenterology(SA) Surg
Colorectal Surgeon
Stellenbosch University
Cape Town, Western Cape, South Africa

Adam Frankel, BSc, MBBS(Hons), PhD, FRACS, FRCSEd
Consultant Surgeon
Upper GI and Soft Tissue Surgery
Princess Alexandra Hospital;
Senior Lecturer
Princess Alexandra Hospital Clinical School
The University of Queensland
Brisbane, Queensland, Australia

Sarah A. Goodbrand, MBChB, BMSc, MD, FRCS
Consultant Colorectal Surgeon
NHS Lothian University of Edinburgh
Edinburgh, United Kingdom

Ewen M. Harrison, MB ChB, MSc, PhD, FRCS, OBE
Professor of Surgery and Data Science
Centre for Medical Informatics
Usher Institute
University of Edinburgh;
Consultant HPB Surgeon
Clinical Surgery
Royal Infirmary of Edinburgh
Edinburgh, United Kingdom

Michael E. Hopkins, MBChB, BSc(Hons), MRCS (ENT), PGCMEd
Ear, Nose and Throat Surgery
NHS Highland
Inverness, United Kingdom

Michael Hughes, MBChB, BMedSci, MD, FRCS
Consultant Surgeon
Department of General Surgery
Royal Infirmary of Edinburgh
Edinburgh, United Kingdom

Scott R. Kelley, MD, FACS, FASCRS
Consultant
Colon and Rectal Surgery
Mayo Clinic
Rochester, Minnesota, United States

Jacob C. Langer, MD
Professor of Surgery
University of Toronto;
Attending Surgeon
Hospital for Sick Children
Toronto, Ontario, Canada;
Visiting Surgeon
Nationwide Children's Hospital
Columbus, Ohio, United States

Kristoffer Lassen, MD, Dr. Med.
GI/HPB surgery
Oslo University Hospital
Oslo, Norway;
Professor
Institute of Clinical Medicine
Arctic University of Norway
Tromsø, Norway

James Lau, MD
Professor of Surgery
The Chinese University Hong Kong
Prince of Wales Hospital
HKSAR, China

Matthew Leeman, MBChB, MSc, FRCS
Upper GI Surgeon
Te Whatu Ora
Christchurch, New Zealand

John A. Livesey, MBBS, MRCP, FRCA, FFICM
Consultant in Intensive Care Medicine and Anaesthesia
Royal Infirmary of Edinburgh
Edinburgh, United Kingdom

Katherine McAndrew, MBChB, MRCP, FRCA
Specialty Registrar
South East Scotland School of Anaesthesia
Edinburgh, United Kingdom

Craig McIlhenny, MBChB, PGCert MEd, FRCS(Urol), FFST(Ed)
Consultant Urological Surgeon
Urology
Forth Valley Royal Hospital
Larbert, United Kingdom

Darek McWhirter, MD, FRCS
Consultant Surgeon
Intestinal Failure Unit
Salford Care Organisation
Northern Care Alliance NHS Foundation Trust
Manchester, United Kingdom

Pradeep H. Navsaria, MBChB, MMed, FCS(SA), FACS
Professor
Department of Trauma
University of Cape Town
Cape Town, South Africa

Valentin Neuhaus, MD
Prof. Dr. med.
Department of Trauma Surgery
University Hospital Zurich
Zurich, Switzerland

Andrew John Nicol, MBChB, FCS(SA), PhD
Director of the Trauma Centre
Groote Schuur Hospital;
Professor of Surgery
University of Cape Town
Cape Town, South Africa

Iain J. Nixon, MBChB, FRCS(ORL-HNS), PhD
Consultant Surgeon
Otolaryngology Head and Neck Surgery
NHS Lothian
Edinburgh, United Kingdom

Gabriel C. Oniscu, MD, FRCS(Ed), FRCS(Glas), KOSM
Professor of Transplantation Surgery
Head of Transplant Division
Department of Clinical Science, Intervention and Technology
Karolinska Institutet
Stockholm, Sweden

Hugh M. Paterson, BMedSci, MBChB, MD, FRCS(Ed)
Clinical Senior Lecturer
Coloproctology
The University of Edinburgh
Edinburgh, United Kingdom

Andrew Rhodes, FCRP, FFICM, FRCA, MD(Res)
Professor
Intensive Care Medicine
St George's University Hospitals NHS Foundation Trust
London, United Kingdom

Richard J.E. Skipworth, BSc(Hons), MBChB, MD, FRCS(Gen Surg), MFSTEd
Consultant General and Upper GI Surgeon
Royal Infirmary of Edinburgh;
Honorary Reader
University of Edinburgh
Edinburgh, United Kingdom

Bruce R. Tulloh, MB, MS, FRACS, FRCS
Consultant Upper GI Surgeon
Upper GI Surgery
Royal Infirmary of Edinburgh
Edinburgh, United Kingdom

Peter G. Vaughan-Shaw, MBChB, PhD, BSc, PGCertEd
Colorectal Surgeon
Western General Hospital
Edinburgh, United Kingdom

Thomas G. Weiser, MD, MPH
Clinical Professor of Surgery
Section of Trauma, Critical Care, and Emergency General Surgery
Stanford University School of Medicine
Stanford, California, United States

Diana A. Wu, MBChB, MRCS, PhD
General Surgery Registrar
Royal Infirmary of Edinburgh
Edinburgh, United Kingdom

Steven Yule, PhD, CPsychol, FRCSEd
Chair of Behavioural Sciences
Clinical Surgery
University of Edinburgh
Edinburgh, United Kingdom

Evaluation of surgical evidence

1

Thomas M. Drake | Ewen M. Harrison

INTRODUCTION TO SURGICAL EVIDENCE

Evidence-based medicine is a relatively recent innovation. It has only been over the past two centuries that scientific methods have become the accepted means of establishing the most effective treatments and tests. Nowhere in medicine has this transformation been more vibrant than in surgical disciplines, where numerous innovations have paved the way for the modern treatments of today.

The generation of high-quality evidence in surgery can be particularly difficult. The reasons underpinning this are four-fold. First, performing surgery is a complex intervention. There are many variables to consider when designing research studies, including postoperative care, variation in surgical techniques and factoring in the natural learning curves required for surgeons to learn new approaches or operative techniques.

Second, surgeons themselves are divided in their attitudes toward research. A survey of Australian surgeons found they believed their own clinical practice was superior to clinical guidelines, that evidence-based surgery adversely affected decision-making for patients and that not using evidence in clinical decision making did not adversely affect patient care. Such attitudes present a large barrier to the uptake of evidence in surgery and require addressing if outcomes and patient care are to be the best they can be.[1]

Third, many operations have historical origins, where an operation was performed for a given indication leading to resolution of the disease process. There may be limited evidence for such procedures as it would be unethical to deny patients an effective and established treatment in the context of a research study.

Finally, a lack of funding and interest has led to research studies becoming the exception rather than the norm. Currently, it is unusual for a patient undergoing surgery to be enrolled in a research study. When these factors are considered together, it is unsurprising that in 1998 surgical research was compared to a "comic opera" by the editor of *The Lancet*.[2]

Over the past 20 years, considerable improvements have been made. Several large initiatives launched by surgical organisations and collaborations have led to new surgery-specific research frameworks being introduced (e.g. IDEAL framework https://www.ideal-collaboration.net). This is proving to be successful, with surgical research increasingly being published in the world's largest medical journals.

CHANGING THE WORLD WITH EVIDENCE

For surgical research to change practice and improve patient care, it must address a new question or an area of genuine clinical uncertainty. The uncertainty around which treatment is best is termed 'clinical equipoise'. A key assumption for the ethical conduct of any interventional research is that equipoise exists; that is, there must be genuine uncertainty around which treatment is best for a given patient group. If clinical equipoise does not exist and it is definitively known that one treatment is better, it is unethical to knowingly expose patients to the inferior treatment.

The research studies listed below can be read, considering the following:

- Who is the patient population or target condition?
- What was the intervention (for interventional research i.e. clinical trials) or exposure (for observational research)?
- What was the comparison (or control group)?
- How was the effect of the intervention measured, and was it measured accurately?
- Are there any sources of bias or confounding present?
- What was the result?
- Is this study relevant to my clinical practice?

Throughout this chapter we will discuss each point in further detail.[3–5]

MRC-CLASICC

This study looked at whether laparoscopic surgery for colorectal cancer was equivalent to open surgery. The study began in 1996 when there was genuine uncertainty as to whether laparoscopic colorectal surgery was safe and effective.[3]

The study demonstrated that for colonic resection for cancer, laparoscopic surgery was as safe as open surgery. The authors went on to publish data on both the short- and long-term outcomes. In conjunction with several other trials, this study paved the way for the implementation of routine laparoscopic colorectal surgery.

FORMULATING A CLINICAL QUESTION

STITCH TRIAL

The small bites suture technique versus large bites for closure of abdominal midline incisions (STITCH) trial was a double-blind, multicentre, randomised controlled trial published in 2015.[4] It compared two different spacings of suture for fascial closure following midline laparotomy—one bite per 1 cm versus one bite per 0.5 cm.

This study demonstrated that with smaller spacing between sutures when closing fascia, there was nearly a 50% reduction in the incidence of incisional hernia in the first year following operation. This trial is an excellent example of how even small technical modifications have the potential to improve patient outcomes if properly evaluated.

PROTECT

This was a study of surgery versus radiotherapy versus surveillance for localised prostate cancer.[5] The use of prostate-specific antigen (PSA) testing for the detection of prostate cancer is controversial. When PSA is elevated and cancer is detected, it is uncertain whether there is benefit to treating tumours detected in this way.

The 10-year results of the ProtecT study found that survival following treatment of PSA-detected local prostate cancer did not differ between treatment groups. Surgery and radiotherapy were found to have lower rates of disease progression; however, these had associated risks. The results of this study pose a dilemma for men with localised prostate cancers in making a choice between surveillance or a radical intervention with urinary, sexual and bowel function complications, both of which have similar long-term survival outcomes.

The first step in the design of a clinical research study is to formulate a study hypothesis or question. Understanding the constituent parts of a clinical hypothesis are key to evaluating the relevance and quality of surgical research studies.

A simple, structured approach can be used to formulate clinical questions. This approach considers several important aspects of a clinical research study:

- 'P'- Population (those patients with the target condition)
- 'I'- Intervention or exposure (the intervention or exposure being studied)
- 'C'- Comparison (the control group that the intervention is being compared to)
- 'O'- Outcomes (what was the outcome of interest and how was it measured)
- 'S'- Study design (how the study was conducted)

This is known as the 'PICOS' approach. We can consider many clinical questions in this way (Box 1.1).

As an example, we can study the use of antibiotics for adults with acute appendicitis. In this situation, antibiotics are used to reduce complications of appendicitis and reduce the necessity for surgical intervention.

Using a PICOS approach:

- P: The population is adults with non-perforated acute appendicitis;
- I: The intervention is use of antibiotics;
- C: The comparison group is that of usual clinical care (appendicectomy);
- O: The primary outcome is complication rate, defined using a validated grading system;
- S: The study design is a randomised control trial.

POPULATION OR TARGET CONDITION

A study population is a group of participants selected from a general population based on specific characteristics. Having a clearly defined study population is key to ensuring research is clinically relevant and can answer a specific question. If a target condition is used as the basis for selecting a population, validated diagnostic criteria should be applied to identify such a population.

The basis for the inclusion of patients in a study should be systematic, to avoid bias. The best way of ensuring a sample is both representative and free from bias is to approach every eligible patient in a consecutive manner. This is often referred to as a consecutive sample.

Specific study populations may have special considerations that must be considered in the study design. An example of this may be an older age group, where visual or hearing impairment may present difficulties with particular data collection methods, such as telephone interviews.

INTERVENTION OR EXPOSURE

The intervention is the main variable changed within the treatment group. In observational research, patients and clinicians decide which treatment will be received. As no direct experimental intervention occurs, the variable is termed the 'exposure'.

When considering an intervention for surgical research, particular care must be given to standardisation between patients and clinicians. Delivering interventions in a standardised manner is essential to ensure patients are comparable. Variation in how a treatment is delivered should be considered during the design process. For example, in a study of a new surgical technique or approach, training in the delivery of the new intervention requires both time and some means of ensuring all patients receive a similar treatment. Standardising the surgical intervention may include an assessment within the research study to determine whether an acceptable level of competence has been achieved. A good study protocol will help to address this (more about Study protocols can be found in the Bias section).

The acceptability of the intervention must also be given due thought. If an intervention is not acceptable to patients, it will be very difficult to convince patients (and research ethics committees) to participate. One means of ensuring interventions are acceptable is to involve patient representatives when designing research studies. These patient representatives are part of the study design team and provide feedback to investigators on the best means of ensuring studies are conducted in a feasible and acceptable manner.

COMPARISON

The comparison describes the control group the intervention or exposure of interest is being evaluated against. This group should be sufficiently comparable to the intervention group to ensure valid conclusions may be drawn about the true effects of the any exposure or intervention.

In controlled trials, the comparison group often uses a *placebo* to reduce bias and maintain blinding. In many studies, the comparison group receives the current gold standard of clinical care, to create a group where the new treatment can be compared directly with the current best or usual therapy.

Box 1.1 Comparison of prospective and retrospective studies

Prospective cohort studies	*Retrospective cohort studies*
Advantages	**Advantages**
• Real-time data collection • Enables investigators to seek missing data as the patient is present during data collection • Allows interventions and changes to the patient pathway to be made (in non-observational studies)	• Faster to conduct • Less expensive
Disadvantages	**Disadvantages**
• Longer time frame • More expensive • Requires more staff time	• Difficult to find missing data • Cases may be missed more frequently • May require case notes to be found • Investigators assessing independent/explanatory variables may already be aware of outcome

If the control group differs from the intervention group, bias may be introduced leading to invalid conclusions. This is of particular concern in observational research, such as case-control studies, where the comparison group is selected by investigators.

OUTCOME

A study outcome is the variable by which the effect of the intervention or exposure of interest is measured. For an outcome to be useful, several properties of the chosen measure should be considered:

- Incidence: The outcome of interest should be sufficiently common. The more common the outcome of interest is, the smaller the sample size required to demonstrate a difference between treatment groups.
- Directness: The outcome of interest should directly measure what the intervention is ultimately intended to achieve. For example, intraoperative warming devices are designed to keep the patient warm, thereby reducing postoperative complications. Therefore, any study investigating the efficacy of intraoperative warming devices should use postoperative complications as a primary outcome rather than looking at differences in temperature (termed a 'surrogate' outcome).
- Definition: All outcomes should be measured using clearly defined criteria. Preferably these criteria would be used widely across the field, so all studies are measuring the same outcome in the same way. One example of such criteria would be the Response Evaluation Criteria In Solid Tumours (RECIST) criteria for the assessment of tumour progression.[6]
- Relevance: Outcomes should be relevant to the research question and to patient care. What may be relevant to clinicians may not also be relevant to patients. To this end, patient representatives should be consulted when selecting study outcomes. Often quality of life and functional outcomes are of primary concern to patients.
- Timing: Outcomes must be measured at appropriate time intervals, which are relevant to the timeframe where the outcome of interest would be expected to occur. For example, measuring an outcome at 72 hours following a procedure may be relevant for postoperative bleeding, but not for surgical site infection.
- Reliability: The chosen outcome measure should be able to reliably detect an event and should be standardised for all patients. This is particularly important for multicentre research, or large-scale trials where multiple observers are judging outcomes. Here having a standardised means of assessing an outcome is important, as it must be ensured that all patients are being assessed in the same way, otherwise the results of the study may be inaccurate.

Patient-reported outcome measures (PROMs) are outcomes which are reported by patients themselves. This contrasts with outcomes where an investigator or clinician reports an outcome. Example of PROMS may include validated general quality of life questionnaires (such as the EQ-5D or HR-QoL). Alternatively, PROMs may focus on specific areas of interest such as sexual function and continence, which are of particular importance in pelvic surgery.[7,8]

Cost-effectiveness is sometimes used as an outcome measure. This is often used by clinical governance bodies to decide whether a treatment represents value for money and should be recommended for use.[9]

Occasionally, different outcomes may be combined to form a single measure. This is known as a composite measure. The use of composite outcome measures can enable researchers to measure two or more outcomes simultaneously and gives better statistical efficiency for the number of patients in a study. An example may be unplanned critical care admission or death, where both represent a major complication, but they are pooled to increase the number of events, which reduces the sample size required for demonstrating the effectiveness of a treatment. While this is beneficial, it can result in outcome measures that prove challenging to interpret.

STUDY DESIGNS

There are many study designs available to answer clinical questions. Study design methodology is constantly evolving; however, all types of study can be broadly divided and subdivided into the following categories:

- Primary research (research at the individual patient level)

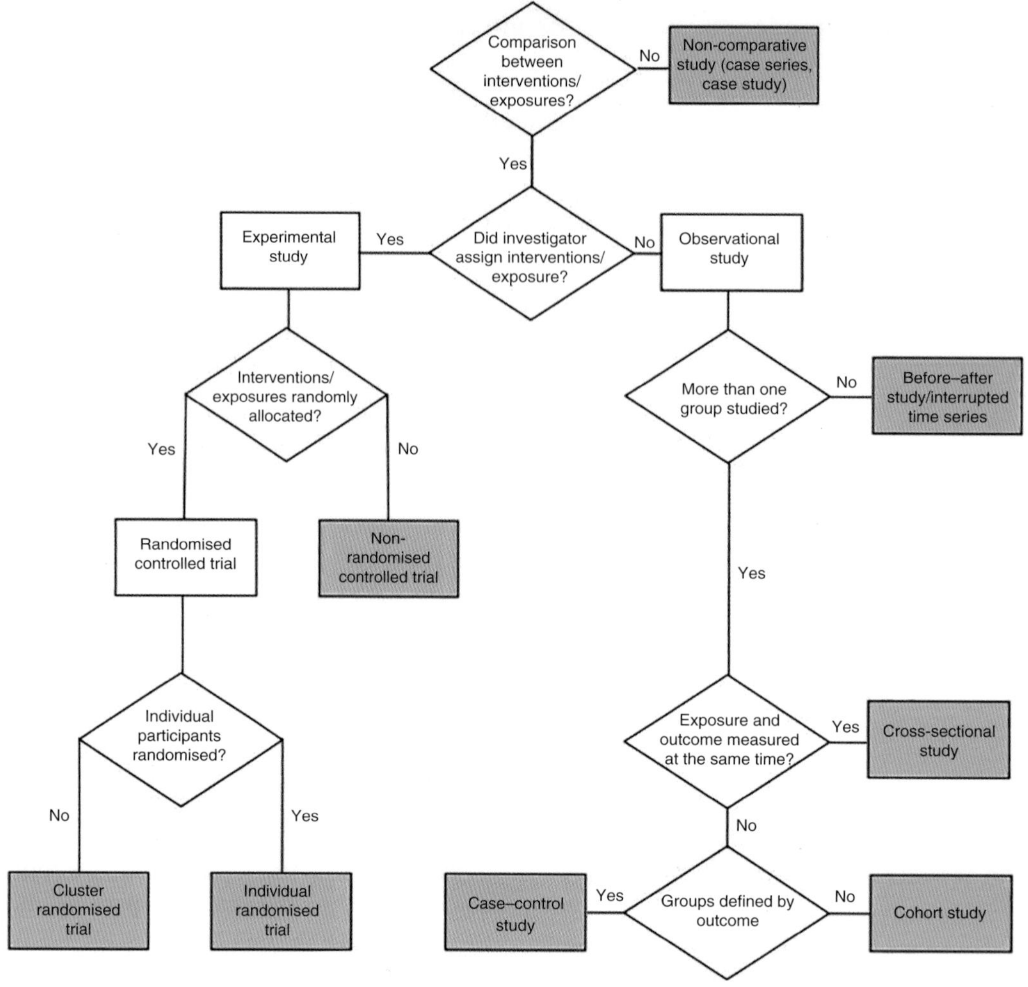

Figure 1.1 Defining study design flowchart.[10] (© NICE [2012] Methods for the development of NICE public health guidance [3rd edition]. Available from https://www.nice.org.uk/process/pmg4/resources/methods-for-the-development-of-nice-public-health-guidance-third-edition-pdf-2007967445701. All rights reserved.)

- Randomised trial
- Prospective cohort study
- Retrospective cohort study
- Cross-sectional study
- Case-control study
- Case series
- Case report

• Secondary research (research that considers multiple sources of primary research)
  - Systematic review
  - Systematic review with meta-analysis

Figure 1.1 below provides a useful means of identifying the type of study where a report may not be explicit as to its design:

Another way of classifying evidence is according to the Oxford Centre of Evidence-based Medicine (CEBM), which divides evidence according to the risk of bias. These are commonly referred to as the 'Level of evidence' (Table 1.1).[11]

One well-known way of classifying these studies is using the 'pyramid of evidence', which provides a simplified means to consider the advantages of one study design over another. This pyramid considers the inherent properties of each study design and classifies them according to how likely the study is to provide a reliable answer to the study question, as close to the 'true value' as possible.

The pyramid of evidence is accompanied by several caveats (Fig. 1.2). First, not all questions can be answered by a randomised controlled trial either due to lack of equipoise (where it would be unethical to conduct a trial) or for logistical reasons (where a trial would be too expensive or simply unfeasible). Second, a poorly conducted study may give an inaccurate, or unreliable answer compared with a well-conducted study of a different design. For example, a small poorly conducted randomised trial may not provide a better answer to a question than a large, well-conducted prospective cohort study. Here is where the Oxford CEBM classification and Grading of Recommendations Assessment, Development and Evaluation (GRADE; discussed later) assessments are useful to help determine whether there can be certainty in the body of evidence for a given research question.[11,12]

SYSTEMATIC REVIEWS AND META-ANALYSIS

At the top of the pyramid are systematic reviews and meta-analyses, which take multiple sources of evidence for a given clinical question. These sources may take the form of randomised trials, cohort studies or even case-control studies (Fig. 1.3). Systematic searching methods are used to attempt to find every possible study which may contain the answer to the clinical question of interest. These methods often

Table 1.1 Oxford CEBM levels of evidence

Level of evidence	Interventional study	Diagnostic accuracy
1a	Systematic review of randomised controlled trials (RCTs)	Systematic review of level 1 diagnostic studies
1b	Individual RCT with narrow confidence interval	Validated cohort study with good reference standards
1c	Where all patients with condition have previously died without fail, but with the intervention tested some survive	Studies with a diagnostic sensitivity or specificity so high the result can rule in or out a diagnosis with very high accuracy
2a	Systematic review of cohort studies	Systematic review of level 2 or higher diagnostic studies
2b	Individual cohort study or low-quality RCT	Exploratory cohort study with good reference standards, or only validated on split sample databases
2c	Ecological studies	
3a	Systematic review of case-control studies	Systematic review of 3b or higher studies
3b	Individual case-control study	Non-consecutive study, or study without consistently applied reference standard
4	Case series and poor-quality cohort and case-control studies	Case series and poor-quality cohort and case-control studies
5	Expert opinion without explicit critical appraisal	Expert opinion without explicit critical appraisal

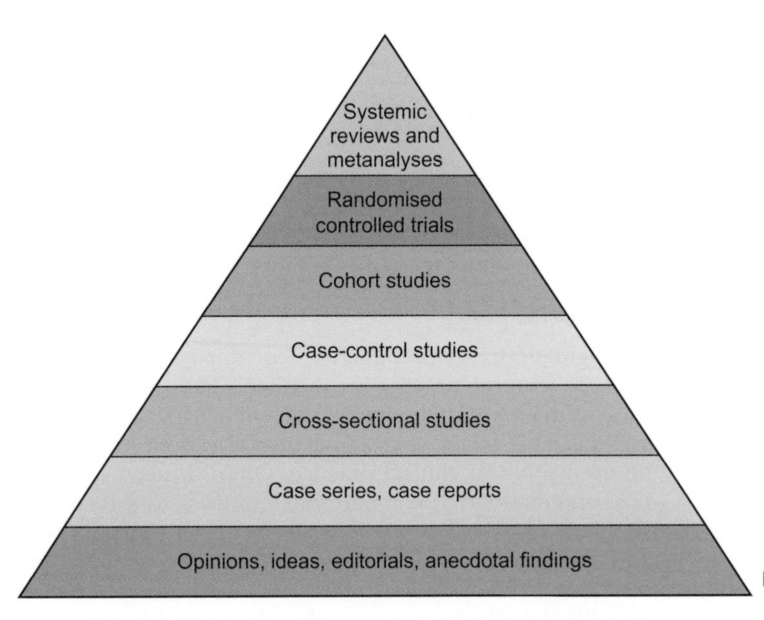

Figure 1.2 The classical pyramid of evidence.

include searching multiple databases, searching the references of key articles in the field and contacting experts to ask if they have suggestions for potential studies to include.[13]

Once all studies that may be eligible are screened, each study is critically appraised individually (see Critical Appraisal). This approach of systematically identifying every possible study, followed by scrutiny of the study methods is then synthesised into the final review, which should present an overarching and balanced view of the evidence for a given clinical question.

Meta-analysis describes the use of statistical methods to combine the numerical results of similar studies in order to derive an estimate of how well the intervention of interest works (i.e. the treatment effect). This is often combined with a systematic review where the results of studies are combined after being screened for inclusion. Combining studies in this manner is referred to as 'pooling'.

An important part of meta-analysis is an assessment of the similarity between different studies of the same clinical question. Variation between studies is termed heterogeneity and takes two forms, clinical and statistical heterogeneity. Clinical heterogeneity concerns how clinically similar a population in one study is to another. It is unlikely to make sense to combine the results of two trials examining the same treatment in two distinct populations, for instance, adults and children. Statistical heterogeneity refers to the differences in the actual results of included studies and whether these are likely to be due to chance (sampling error) or true differences in outcome. This is summarised by the I-squared statistic and is 0% when all included trials provide a similar result. If studies show completely contradicting results, the I-squared statistic is 100% meaning the combined result likely lacks any real meaning.[13] A rule-of-thumb for the interpretation of the I-squared statistic is as follows:

- 0–30%: Low level of statistical heterogeneity
- 30–50%: Moderate level of statistical heterogeneity
- 50–100%: Substantial level of statistical heterogeneity

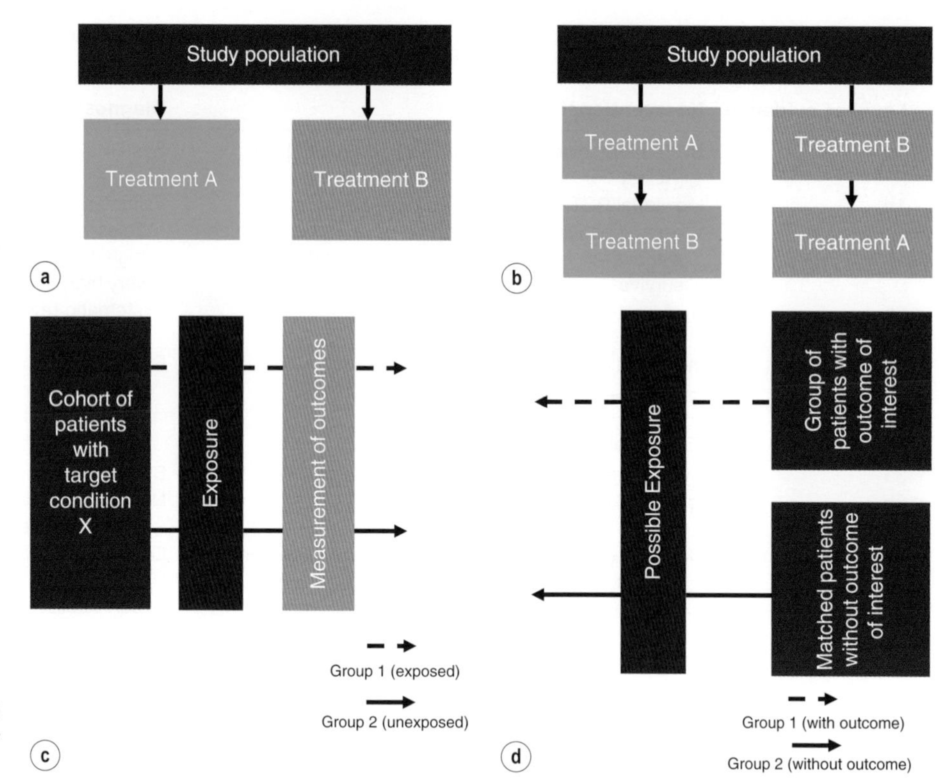

Figure 1.3 (a) Parallel group design. (b) Cross-over group design. (c) Cohort study schematic. (d) Case control schematic.

RANDOMISED CONTROLLED TRIALS

Randomised controlled trials are primary research studies that test the effect of an intervention using experimental methods. After participants are recruited, they are allocated to treatment groups at random, where the choice of treatment is not determined by the patient, clinician or any other person. Removing choice of treatment reduces the risk of selection bias, which is often the largest source of bias in medical research. Selection bias simply refers to how doctors and patients select treatments based upon certain patient characteristics.

The *controlled* part of the name refers to two integral components of high-quality trials. The first is that there is a comparable control group with which to compare the intervention of interest. The second is that the trial is conducted in strict accordance with a pre-defined study protocol.

Study protocols are important and are essentially a detailed instruction manual outlining how a piece of research will be conducted. The main advantages of a study protocol are that it ensures investigators stick to a pre-planned analysis of their data and in the case of multicentre research, promotes standardisation across centres. Study protocols are not unique to randomised controlled trials. It is highly recommended that all clinical research (including systematic reviews and cohort studies) should be conducted according to a pre-defined protocol. Many journals now stipulate this as a requirement for even considering a study for publication.

Randomised controlled trials can be grouped into two categories:

EXPLANATORY TRIALS

An explanatory trial is designed to explain precisely how an intervention may work, in other words, it is designed to elicit mechanisms. To do this, an explanatory trial will find a highly homogenous group of patients to test a hypothesis on. The use of a placebo is common as investigators will attempt to control for as many factors as possible.

PRAGMATIC TRIALS

A pragmatic trial is designed to encompass as much variation in clinical practice as possible. The population of these studies is often highly heterogeneous to make the trial generalizable to the true population the intervention will be used upon in clinical practice. Often, instead of placebos, pragmatic trials compare interventions to the current standard of care. Pragmatic trials are usually large in size and conducted across multiple centres. These trials are intended to determine whether an intervention works in 'real-life' healthcare systems rather than a highly controlled environment.

MONITORING CLINICAL TRIALS

Research studies should ideally capture measures of both effectiveness and safety. A new treatment that is not safe but very effective might not be very useful. The drug thalidomide is an example of why safety monitoring is crucial. Thalidomide was found to be effective in relieving morning sickness in pregnancy and became very popular. However, poor testing and disregard of emerging reports of teratogenicity led to thousands of children being born with severe limb malformations.

Well-conducted clinical trials may identify adverse effects prior to wider uptake of a treatment. However, if an adverse effect is rare, it may only be identified after lots of people have taken the treatment.

Data monitoring committee (DMC) is a team of experts who are independent from the clinical trial investigation team. The DMC looks periodically at data from the clinical trial as it progresses. If a treatment within a trial looks as if it could be causing harm, the DMC should stop the trial to avoid further harm to future participants who might be enrolled. Similarly, if a treatment is shown to be very effective, more so than first thought, the trial can be stopped as it would be unethical to give future participants a less effective control treatment.

LEOPARD-2

This randomised trial compared laparoscopic versus open surgery for removal of pancreas cancer (pancreatoduodenectomy). In other types of surgery, laparoscopic surgery has been shown to reduce complications and shorten the time taken to recover from an operation.[14]

Monitoring of the LEOPARD-2 trial whilst it was ongoing found that 15% of patients who received laparoscopic surgery died within 90 days of surgery compared with none in the open surgery group, prompting discontinuation of the trial.

RANDOMISATION

Randomisation allocates patients to treatment groups without the clinician or patient choosing the treatment.

If done correctly, randomisation aims to ensure treatment groups are equally balanced for confounding factors which may influence outcomes, both observed factors and unobserved factors. This enables us to draw fair comparisons between two treatments.

Randomisation ensures treatment groups are balanced for characteristics and confounding factors, both of which may be observed (data collected upon them) or unobserved (no data collected on or not yet discovered).[15] Randomisation may be performed in two different ways:

Simple randomisation

Simple randomisation methods involve allocating participants to treatment groups using techniques such as coin flipping or rolling a die. These methods do not use any pre-planned methods of allocation. The advantages of these techniques are that they are easy to use and do not require any specialist equipment or planning. The disadvantage is that these methods cannot account for more complex allocation requirements, such as multiple groups or ensuring other factors are accounted for (see 'minimisation' below). With a large enough sample size, simple randomisation methods should result in approximately equally sized groups. However, for small trials, simple randomisation methods can lead to unequally sized treatment groups.

Block randomisation

Block randomisation describes the process of randomising 'blocks' of patients to treatment groups, which may be based upon a specific characteristic (i.e. sex or age). Using blocks theoretically reduces differences across the treatment groups being compared. This is of particular advantage in smaller trials, where unbalanced or unequal groups cause greater problems than in trials with large sample sizes.

A good example of where selection bias may arise would be studying the use of non-steroidal anti-inflammatory drugs (NSAIDs) after surgery. In observational research, it has been found the use of NSAIDs is associated with fewer surgical complications. However, in these studies, where clinicians or patients choose to take NSAIDs, the group of patients who are given NSAIDs are fitter and healthier. Therefore, the observation that patients who take NSAIDs are less likely to suffer complications is confounded. If this was a randomised trial, both treatment groups would have similar baseline characteristics due to the randomisation process, which would reduce or eliminate this confounding.

Randomisation may be stratified, which is a technique that first divides patients into discrete risk groups, or strata, and then randomises a patient within the given stratum to a treatment. This is a straightforward means of ensuring treatment groups are balanced for factors that may result in an increased likelihood of a given outcome occurring. For example, patients with diabetes are more likely to suffer wound infections following surgery. A trial looking at methods to prevent wound infections could use stratified randomisation to first divide patients into 'diabetic' and 'non-diabetic' strata and then randomise these patients to the different treatment arms. This would therefore result in both treatment groups containing a similar number of diabetic patients, thus enabling a fairer comparison.

An extension of stratified randomisation is minimisation. Using sophisticated computer programmes, randomisation procedures can be designed which take into consideration several different patient characteristics, a method known as 'minimisation'. This ensures treatment groups are better balanced.

BLINDING

Blinding is the act of disguising which treatment a participant in a research study has received. Blinding in surgical studies often proves to be difficult, and requires some flair or creativity to identify a suitable strategy for implementing blinding successfully.

There are four main parties which can be blinded to an intervention or an outcome:

- Patients
- Those administering the treatment, i.e. the clinical team
- Those who are measuring the effect of the treatment, i.e. observers
- Those performing the data analysis, i.e. the statistician

In the past, where one of these groups was blinded the study was termed 'single-blind', where two groups were blind 'double-blind' etc. Nowadays it is best practice to specify explicitly who was blinded and what exactly was done rather than use terminology that may be unclear without qualification.

In studies where drug administration is involved, participants and clinicians can be blinded by using placebos (i.e. 'dummy pills'). Where intravenous drugs are used, normal saline could be used in replacement for a drug. Coloured intravenous fluids may be masked by black tubing. If groups are receiving a different surgical procedure altogether, it can be difficult or impossible to blind patients and is impossible to blind the surgeon to the procedure. There are, however, means to address this.

Observers are often used in surgical studies where blinding patients or clinical teams is impossible. These observers measure outcomes but are independent from the clinical team and are blinded to which intervention the patient received.

In all these cases, blinding enables the person who is assessing the outcome to judge it fairly. If the person assessing the study outcome did know which treatment the patient received, they might have preconceptions and judge the outcome in a biased way to favour one treatment over the other.

Finally, it is important to ask patients at the end of the study which treatment group they believe they were allocated to. By asking every patient this question, it enables the adequacy of the blinding to be tested.

OPEN-LABEL STUDIES

An open-label study is one where both the researchers and the patients are aware of which treatment they are receiving. They can be randomised, non-randomised and even omit a control group.

> **FIDELITY**
>
> In Finland, Sihvonen et al.[33] compared arthroscopic surgery versus no surgery for degenerative meniscal tear. The intervention group received arthroscopic surgery and the control group received sham surgery. In the sham surgery group, the patient was exposed to an environment where they believe they were undergoing surgery, but no operation was actually performed. In this trial, participants were taken into the operating theatre, draped and shown a video of arthroscopic surgery. Dressings were then placed to make it difficult to identify whether they underwent operation or not.

Sham surgery is ethically contentious, particularly with regards to procedures that must be conducted under general anaesthesia due to the associated risks of harm.

CLUSTER RANDOMISATION

Some studies may randomise at a group rather than patient level, e.g.by hospital. This can be useful when investigating healthcare processes, public health interventions or complex treatments. Cluster randomised trials (Fig. 1.4) have specific considerations that must be taken on board whilst designing the study and are often more complex to conduct.

Some studies use methods which rely upon factors that appear to be random to allocate patients to treatment groups. These may include birthday, day of the week or even whether the patient's hospital number is odd or even. Although these may appear to be random numbers, they are not. This is called 'pseudo-randomisation' or 'quasi-randomisation' and studies utilising this approach should not be classed as randomised trials.

ALLOCATION CONCEALMENT

Allocation concealment is often confused with blinding. It describes the principle that those determining which treatment a patient receives should not influence the selection process, either consciously or subconsciously. The classical way of addressing this is to use opaque envelopes to disguise which treatment allocation is contained in the envelope. Nowadays, this is more commonly done using a computer.

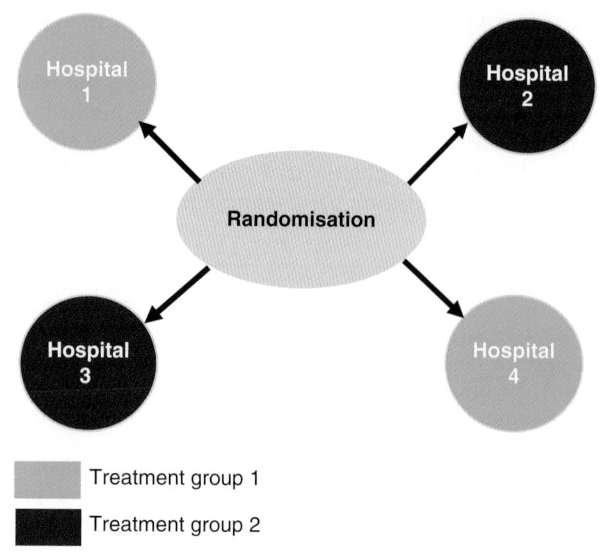

Figure 1.4 Cluster randomisation.

PHASES OF CLINICAL TRIALS

To take a new drug or procedure from concept to clinical practice requires several steps. There are five phases of research trials (Fig. 1.5):

PHASE 0 TRIALS

These trials are 'first-in-man' studies. The compound or procedure has usually only been used in preclinical research (usually in animals or cells) before phase 0 or phase 1 trials. Here, very small quantities of promising new compounds are given to healthy humans in a highly controlled environment. These studies aim to approximate the pharmacokinetic and pharmacodynamic properties of a drug (e.g. half-life, distribution, excretion, absorption, metabolism and potential toxicities).

PHASE I TRIALS

Phase I trials aim to formally assess the **safety** of a treatment. Here a range of doses within the postulated therapeutic range are tested (this is called 'dose ranging') in a larger sample and the side effects of these varying doses assessed. Usually, this sample is of healthy volunteers, but can be those with the target condition. From these studies, the dose with the most acceptable side-effect profile is selected.

PHASE II TRIALS

In phase II trials, a new treatment is administered to patients with the target condition to determine **safety and efficacy**. As these trials are designed to elucidate whether a new treatment works or not, they are usually tightly controlled and may compare the new treatment to a placebo.

PHASE III TRIALS

This is the final stage of testing prior to a new treatment being released on the open market. Phase III trials are the largest trials, where a new treatment is given to patients with the target condition. Large sample sizes are used in order to further identify side effects and to accurately estimate the therapeutic effect of the new intervention. Some phase 3 trials are pragmatic rather than explanatory, and

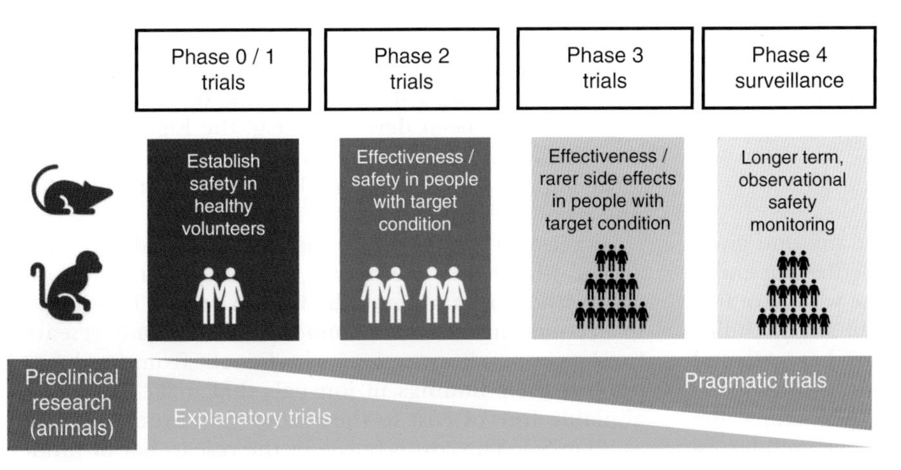

Figure 1.5 Phases and stages of clinical trials.

Table 1.2 The stages of the IDEAL framework

Stage	Innovation	Development	Exploration	Assessment	Long-term monitoring
Description of stage	Proof of principle, typically done in an animal or select patient	Refinement of idea, through practice or laboratory development	Beginning to compare refined idea to current practice to establish feasibility in clinical practice	Compares idea to current practice through well-powered study aimed to show clinical efficacy and safety	Monitors the idea in practice for long-term outcomes, safety and rare events
Type of study	Case report	Case series	Randomised clinical trial/ Prospective study	Randomised clinical trial	Database

seek to confirm that the new treatment will work in the real world.

PHASE IV: POST-MARKETING STUDIES

Once the new treatment has passed national regulatory approvals, it can be sold to healthcare providers. After approval, all drugs undergo monitoring for rare side effects and other harms that may have been missed in the initial studies. This process is called post-marketing surveillance. One well-known approach to post-marketing surveillance in the UK is the 'Yellow-Card Scheme', where clinicians can report adverse events that are suspected to have been due to a specific drug.

IDEAL FRAMEWORK

In surgery, the IDEAL framework (Innovation, Development, Exploration, Assessment, Long-term monitoring) describes how innovations in surgery should be approached to enable direct translation to surgical care (Table 1.2). It describes five stages of development which should be used to guide a new idea from conception to widespread clinical implementation.[16]

COHORT STUDIES

In a cohort study, a defined population with a specific condition or a population undergoing a specific type of surgery is identified and followed over a defined period. Cohort studies are typically observational research, which means instead of patients being allocated to treatment groups, patients and doctors are free to choose. Instead of an 'intervention', which implies allocation to treatment groups, the intervention is often referred to as an 'exposure' (Fig. 1.3c).

As cohort studies are simply observing what happens in clinical practice, they may be conducted looking forwards in time (prospective) or backwards in time (retrospective). There are advantages and disadvantages of each approach are listed in Box 1.1.

CASE-CONTROL STUDIES

In a case-control study, patients are identified who have already experienced a given outcome (cases). They are compared with patients of similar characteristics who have not experienced the outcome in order to identify factors associated with the given outcome (Fig.1. 3d). Case-control studies are always conducted retrospectively and are common in the fields of public health and genetics. They are also useful for the study of rare diseases. The key advantages of case-control studies are that they are relatively fast to perform and inexpensive when compared with other study types. Furthermore, they do not require lengthy follow-up as the outcome of interest has already occurred.

There are several drawbacks to case-control studies. Given that they require a group of participants without the given outcome of interest as a control group, there is a high risk that selection bias could influence the results of the study. Furthermore, the design of case-control studies means that rare exposures can be missed as they lack any kind of consecutive or systematic sampling methods. Furthermore, as the study design starts with a group who already has the outcome of interest, the case-control design makes it impossible to calculate the incidence of that outcome.

CROSS-SECTIONAL STUDIES

Cross-sectional studies take a 'snapshot' at any one given moment in time. These studies aim to describe the entire population of interest rather than just those who have had an outcome of interest as in a case-control study. Unlike cohort studies, all the information is gathered at once and does not necessarily take time into account, with observations being limited to one timepoint. As they sample the entire population, cross-sectional studies can be useful to estimate the point prevalence (existence) or incidence (first occurrence) of a disease. However, as cross-sectional studies collect data at one given time only, they can be susceptible to missing data or data that is unreliable.

CASE SERIES AND CASE REPORTS

A case report is an individual case which may be notable due to a rare condition, or a novel approach to performing a procedure. A case series refers to a collection of individual case reports collated together. In both scenarios, the cases are selected by investigators. Case series and reports are considered low quality evidence and should not be used to draw firm scientific conclusions. They can be used to present key learning points allowing clinicians to improve their own clinical practice based upon the experience of others. As case series and reports neither contain consecutive patients nor are conducted in a scientific manner, they should not be included in systematic reviews or meta-analyses.

SINGLE CENTRE OR MULTICENTRE RESEARCH

A further consideration in study design is whether the study was conducted at a single centre or across many centres. In surgery and other complex interventions, delivery of a surgical intervention and subsequent postoperative care can vary greatly. Conducting a study across multiple centres makes the results more generalisable as variations in practice are accounted for. Conversely, if a study is performed at a single centre, there is less variation and hence the results may be less generalisable to patients elsewhere.

FINDING THE EVIDENCE

Identifying useful studies to answer a clinical query can be difficult. As of 2016, over 26 million scientific papers were contained within the PubMed database alone. Knowing where to start and how evidence is organised can make the process of finding relevant literature more straightforward.

JOURNALS

Journals are the main source of scientific research in medicine. Studies are conducted, written and submitted to journals for peer review. Journals are commonly ranked according to their 'impact factor', calculated by how many times an article published in the journal is cited. Impact factors have received a lot of attention; however, more recently this ranking system has become discredited. Other measures have been developed, e.g. the Eigenfactor metric, which take into account the field of science, longer-term impact and fundamental differences in how disciplines cite previous work.[17]

Increasingly, papers are being published as 'open-access' where they are openly available to anyone to access, without requiring a subscription or fee. This is likely to become increasingly commonplace, as many research funders compel researchers who benefit from funding to publish their findings in journals that make all content available free of cost to the reader (a movement known as 'Plan-S'). The cost is borne by the researcher or funder who wishes to publish their research in the specific journal rather than through subscription payments or fees paid by the reader.

PREPRINT SERVERS

A preprint server is a website that hosts academic papers that have not undergone or are currently undergoing peer review. Papers are often published on preprint servers to make work available at the earliest possible time, as publication of manuscripts often takes several weeks or months from the first point of submission. There are many subject-specific preprint servers, such as bioRxiv (pronounced 'bio archive') for biological sciences and medRxiv for clinical sciences (i.e. surgery and medicine).

BOOKS

Books are another source of scientific information. They are often useful as instructional guides or for educational purposes and enable the authors to spend time developing explanations for complex topics, unlike journal articles which carry a word limit. Often it takes years to put a book together and by the time it is published, the information contained is out of date with contemporary knowledge.

CONFERENCES

Scientific conferences are where recent work is presented to an audience consisting of members of the scientific community who specialise in that field. The latest research is discussed, often before studies are published as papers in journals. This gives investigators the opportunity to obtain peer review prior to submitting for publication. Often conferences are excellent places to network with other people who share similar interests in the field and build collaborative links.

SOCIAL MEDIA

Although not strictly a source of scientific information, social media and blogging have come to the fore in recent years. Informative opinion and debate are increasingly moving to social media platforms such as Twitter. The result is that debate surrounding treatments or medical technologies is becoming increasingly accessible, particularly to patients and the public. This shift is largely positive, helping engage members of the public with healthcare decisions and innovation. Despite this, social media and blogging is somewhat a double-edged sword, as articles are unmoderated and can convey unbalanced opinion, which may be misinterpreted as fact.

MEDICAL LITERATURE DATABASES

At present there are two main databases which contain published medical literature. These databases largely contain journal articles but also contain some articles published in books.

MEDLINE

MEDLINE is a medical literature database curated by the National Library of Medicine in the USA. It covers literature published from 1966 to the present day and contains over 20 million citations. It uses a system called Medical Subject Headings (MeSH) to organise literature in a systematic way that can be easily queried using specific search terms (see 'MeSH Terms' below).

EMBASE

EMBASE is the larger of the two databases and as of 2021, is run by the commercial publisher Elsevier. It contains literature from 1947 through to the present day, but also information that pre-dates this back to 1902. At present, EMBASE contains all of MEDLINE and supplements this with additional literature from across the world. It is the largest medical database in the world, with over 29 million citations. EMBASE specialises in containing detailed literature on pharmacy and drug compounds which may not be contained in MEDLINE. MeSH terms can also be used when searching EMBASE, giving it compatibility with searches designed for use in MEDLINE.

CLINICAL TRIALS DATABASES

According to legislation governing clinical trials, the Declaration of Helsinki, and the policies of many journals, all clinical trials must be registered prior to commencement. The main purpose is to promote the publication of all research trials and reduce wastage, as many trials go unpublished. It also enables researchers and patients to view ongoing studies that may be of interest. For researchers, this might help to avoid duplication of the same study idea. For patients, it may provide information on trials for their condition from which they might benefit. ClinicalTrials.gov is run by the National Library for Medicine in the USA.[18] It was the first and is now the largest clinical trials registry. Trials conducted in any country may be registered on ClinicalTrials.gov, including observational research. EudraCT (European Union Drug Regulating Authorities Clinical Trials Database) is the European database for all interventional clinical trials on medicinal products authorized in the European Union.

SEARCH CLIENTS

Search clients enable researchers to identify evidence contained within medical literature databases. The choice of client often comes down to personal preference.

PUBMED

PubMed is operated by the NCBI and allows searching of the MEDLINE database with additional literature from the NCBI's and National Library of Medicine's own repository of articles. PubMed is a free search client and database service. The NCBI site where PubMed is located also contains a vast collection of other electronic services for conducting research, all of which are free of charge.[34]

OVIDSP

OvidSP is a commercial service operated by Wolters Kluwer and allows the searching of several different medical literature databases at once, where subscribed to, including MEDLINE and EMBASE.

GOOGLE SCHOLAR

Google Scholar is a free-to-use search engine which searches Google's proprietary database, which includes some of MEDLINE amongst other databases. Google does not say how large the scholar database is, but it is estimated to contain over 160 million citations across multiple disciplines. Due to the way the Google search algorithm operates, it can give different results when searched in the same way as other clients.[35]

All of the above search clients allow search results to be exported to reference management software to create bibliographies.

EVIDENCE-BASED MEDICINE ORGANISATIONS

THE COCHRANE LIBRARY

The Cochrane Library is where the systematic reviews and review protocols are published by the Cochrane Collaboration.[19] Cochrane reviews are conducted according to strict standards and have arguably one of the toughest peer-review processes in the world. Protocols and reviews must strictly adhere to specified standards. All reviews undergo at least two rounds of peer review by several experts in the field and methodologists who specialise in Cochrane reviews. In several studies, Cochrane reviews were consistently the highest quality systematic reviews available, hence are often the best source of information for the best evidence for a given intervention. As well as providing information on the clinical utility of a treatment, suggestions are made for future research.

SPECIALIST REGISTERS

Other specialist registers exist, which may encompass literature that cannot be found elsewhere or are of specialist interest. Grey literature, or literature that has not been published as a full paper in a journal, is often found on such specialist registers. One example of a database which includes grey literature is the Web of Science, which catalogues many conference proceedings.[20] Other specialist registers exist for the registration of systematic review protocols.[21]

SEARCHING

To find relevant literature, a good search strategy is required. Often when conducting a search, one of two things may happen. The first is that when a specific query is entered, very few studies are found. The second is the opposite, where thousands of results are generated making it difficult to find the most useful studies. To avoid these situations, a good search strategy should be both sensitive (able to find the right information) and specific (exclude irrelevant studies). Several tools may be used to accomplish a search.

CONSTRUCTING A SYSTEMATIC SEARCH

Care must be taken when constructing a search to ensure it identifies studies within the correct topic. Using the PICOS framework is an excellent place to start.

DEFINING SEARCH TERMS USING PICOS

PICOS allows us to define a research question clearly and build a systematic search that will find relevant studies effectively. Thinking about each element of PICOS allows search terms to be identified. For the following elements of PICOS, we will use the example question 'What is the effect of laparoscopic surgery on wound infection rates after appendicectomy for acute appendicitis?'

Population

Begin by defining the population of interest for your study question. This might be a group of patients with a disease, or patients undergoing a specific operation. In the case of our example, this will be patients undergoing appendicectomy. We would then find keywords related to appendicectomy or acute appendicitis, such as 'appendicectomy', 'appendectomy' (USA spelling) and 'appendicitis'.

Intervention or exposure

Identify the intervention or exposure in your research question. This will be the variable that you wish to know the effect for. In our example, it would be laparoscopic surgery; an example of an exposure might be cigarette smoking. Good keywords to use for laparoscopic surgery searches include 'laparoscopy', 'laparoscopic', 'videoscopic', 'keyhole' and 'endoscopic'.

Comparison

The comparison is the intervention non-exposed group we are interested in studying as a control. In the example of laparoscopic surgery for acute appendicitis, the control group would be open surgery as a contrasting surgical approach. Here, we could use keywords such as 'open', 'laparotomy', 'McBurney's', 'gridiron' or 'Lanz', which describe open incisions. As there are currently only two common approaches for appendicectomy, open or laparoscopic, specifying open surgery may not be required.

Outcomes

Interventions usually influence multiple outcomes. Specifying outcomes in a search can substantially reduce the number of irrelevant studies in the results, although this should be balanced against the likelihood of missing important studies that may not mention outcome measures explicitly in the title or abstract. In our case, we could use terms such as 'wound infection', 'dehiscence', 'surgical site infection' or 'ssi'.

Study design

The study design can also be specified, which is particularly useful in topics with much observational evidence. If we wanted to find randomised trials only, we could use specific terms such as 'randomized', 'randomised', 'trial' or 'randomly'. The Cochrane collaboration has a series of terms which allow these studies to be filtered.[13]

COMBINING TERMS

The first step to a successful search is to use the right types of search terms. Broadly speaking there are three types of search term: text words (.tw), MeSH terms (.sh or [MeSH]) and Boolean operators (usually AND, OR, IF, NOT). Text words are terms which do not correspond to MeSH key terms and describe the study and topic being searched. MeSH terms allow the simultaneous and structured searching of many text words at once. Boolean operators combine text words and MeSH terms together in order to construct searches.[22]

Another consideration is variation in language. Although medical studies are overwhelmingly published in English, they may be written using UK or US English. This is of particular concern when searching for words that can be spelt with a US variation like 'randomised' (which in US English is 'randomized') or appendicectomy ('appendectomy').

Often the most difficult part of searching is to combine all the relevant terms together. Cochrane reviews tend to use numbered lists of keywords, which when combined produce an effective search. Below is an example (Box 1.2) of how this could be laid out, looking to find studies which discuss open versus endovascular aortic aneurysm repair.

Boolean operators

Boolean operators are terms which tell the search engine how to handle search terms. In PubMed, the Boolean operators AND, OR and NOT are used frequently. These are self-explanatory terms, which when used effectively can increase the effectiveness of a search greatly.

An example of Boolean operators:

Appendicitis OR Appendicectomy - to find studies concerning appendicitis or appendicectomy
Appendicitis AND Appendicectomy - to find studies where appendicectomy took place for appendicitis
Appendicectomy NOT Appendicitis - to find studies discussing appendicectomy only, not necessarily relevant to appendicitis

Wildcards

Wildcards enable searches to be performed where the exact spelling of a term is not known, or there are known variations. The symbol denoting a wildcard varies by search client used. In PubMed it is the * symbol. An example would be to find all studies which discuss anything to do with an appendix, appendicectomy or appendicitis, regardless of spelling. To do this, the term 'Append*' would be entered into the search engine. Note this example would also bring up studies to do with anything that began with 'Append'. Nevertheless, wildcards are useful when used in combination with multiple other terms, or for a quick search.

Box 1.2 Building a search strategy for aortic aneurysm repair

Terms	*Rationale*
1. Aortic Aneurysm, Abdominal	MeSH term for abdominal aortic aneurysms
2. AAA.tw	Abdominal Aortic Aneurysm is frequently abbreviated to 'AAA'.
3. Endovascular Procedures	MeSH term for endovascular procedures
4. EVAR.tw	Endovascular aneurysm repair is frequently abbreviated to 'EVAR'
5. Open repair.tw	Open repair is one of the treatments we are interested in; however, there are no specific
6. Vascular Grafting	MeSH terms to describe an open approach!
7. 1 OR 2	MeSH term for vascular surgical procedures involving vessel repair
8. 3 OR 4	Search for either the aortic aneurysm MeSH term or the AAA acronym
9. 5 OR 6	Search for either the Endovascular procedures MeSH term or the EVAR acronym.
10. 7 AND 8 AND 9	Search for either open repair text word or vascular grafting MeSH term.
	Combines all the above terms together.

This search brings up several thousand results. We are only concerned with finding the best randomised controlled trial evidence. To do this, we can add a clinical trials filter (adapted from Cochrane Collaboration) to our search as demonstrated in the next section.

11. randomized controlled trial
12. controlled clinical trial
13. randomized
14. randomly
15. trial
16. groups
17. 11 OR 12 OR 13 OR 14 OR 15 OR 16
18. animals [mh] NOT humans [mh]
19. 18 NOT 19 (N.B. this is a double negative)
20. 10 AND 19

This now gives us a much narrower collection of studies which primarily contain evidence from randomised trials.

CRITICAL APPRAISAL

When reading a clinical research study, the results should not immediately be taken at face value. To understand the results and whether they are valid, we must consider the study and its conduct. To do so, it is useful to have a systematic approach with which to appraise a paper and an understanding of where sources of systematic error commonly arise.

Critical appraisal seeks to clearly determine:

1. Why was the study done?
2. What was done?
3. What was shown?

The most important segments of a research paper are how it was conducted (methods) and the findings. Results should not be interpreted without the study methods. Therefore, applying the 'PICOS' approach at each stage is a useful means of approaching critical appraisal (Fig. 1.6).

Formal critical appraisal tools and learning are readily available as electronic resources on the internet. The Oxford Critical Appraisal Skills Programme and the Cochrane Collaborative's electronic learning packages are useful and provide more details.[23,24]

BIAS

Bias occurs when systematic error is introduced into a study. Bias has the potential to influence the outcomes of a study and produce misleading results (Fig. 1.7). To limit bias, we must understand where it may arise and identify techniques which can reduce the risk from these sources of bias. There are over 30 different types of bias, but the following are the most important to surgical research.

Selection bias arises where individuals are selected to treatment groups based upon their individual or disease characteristics, thus creating systematic differences between groups.[25,26] This may arise either where randomisation has not been performed adequately in interventional studies, or in observational studies where treatment is decided by patients and clinicians. Randomisation is the only method by which selection bias can be reliably eliminated in a study.

SELECTION BIAS

An example of selection bias would be in lung cancer surgery, where there is a choice between keyhole (video-assisted thoracoscopic [VATS]) lobectomy for removing a tumour, or using stereotactic ablative radiotherapy (SABR). As VATS lobectomy is a major operation, those patients who have many comorbidities are likely to have adverse outcomes. Therefore, if we compared VATS lobectomy and SABR in an observational study, there would be a selection bias as the groups would have different clinical characteristics.

Statistical methods, known as 'methods for causal inference', are designed to reduce the effects of selection bias upon an analysis. A popular method for reducing the influence of selection bias in observational studies is regression, where the outcomes are adjusted for important confounding factors. A more recent development gaining popularity is propensity score matching. Here computer algorithms are used to match treated patients to patients in the control group, based upon characteristics that may influence which treatment group they are allocated to. This computer algorithm then weights the analysis towards patients who are

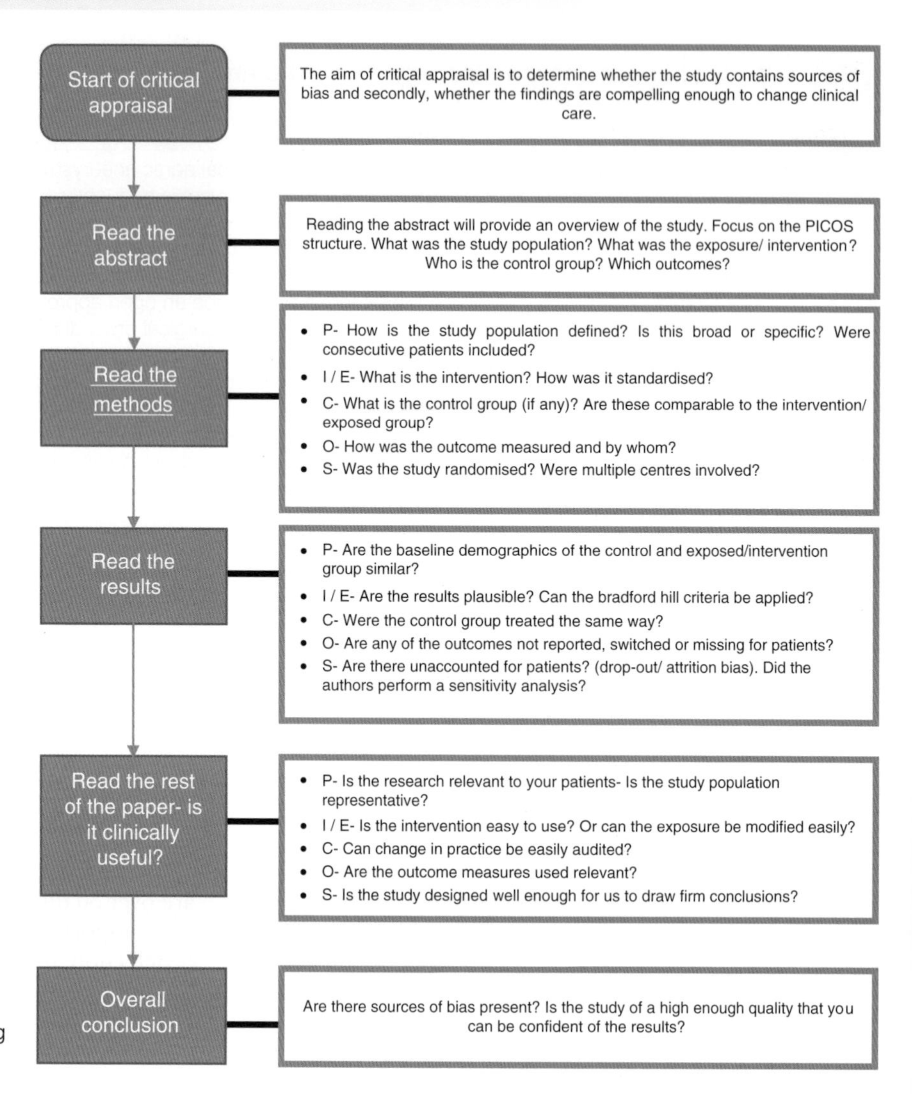

Figure 1.6 Process of critical appraisal using PICOS.

most similar to one another, thereby generating a fairer experiment that compares patients like for like.

RESPONDER BIAS

Responder bias is a broad term which describes situations in which study participants are led toward giving a specific answer. Responder bias affects surveys, questionnaires and interviews. An example of responder bias would be where a surgeon asks a patient 'were you satisfied with the treatment you received?'. In this example, the patient may feel like they have to state they were satisfied in order to be polite towards the surgeon who provided their care. Another example might be the use of leading questions, or multiple-choice answers in interviews or questionnaires. Careful design of studies can eliminate responder bias.

REPORTING BIAS

The selective reporting of all relevant information available in a study is known as reporting bias. Studies may fail to report outcomes if they did not demonstrate findings in keeping with the authors' desired message. Reporting bias is a major issue in medical literature, so much so that a taskforce has been set up to promote improved reporting. The 'Enhancing the QUAlity and Transparency Of health Research' (EQUATOR) network publishes checklists which state specific items that should be reported in scientific papers.[27] Many journals now require adherence to the EQUATOR network guidelines. A reporting checklist exists for nearly every type of study, from randomised trials to studies of diagnostic accuracy. Good reporting permits adequate critical appraisal to be conducted and makes it simpler for subsequent systematic reviews and meta-analyses to be performed (Box 1.3).

These checklists, however, do not eliminate all issues surrounding reporting bias. Studies which fail to incorporate the collection of key outcomes into their design also exhibit a form of reporting bias. To address this, recent work has culminated in the production of 'core outcome datasets'. These datasets, decided on by experts in the given field, consist of important and relevant outcomes which should always be reported.[28–30]

The presence of a study protocol or prior registration of a research study on a registry (such as ClinicalTrials.gov) helps reduce selective reporting. By stating which outcomes will be reported prior to the study, it makes researchers more accountable to do so. Journal editors, reviewers and readers can use the protocol to compare to the final study to identify any deliberate or inadvertent reporting bias.

Reporting bias can also arise from investigators failing to include important outcomes in the initial design of a study.

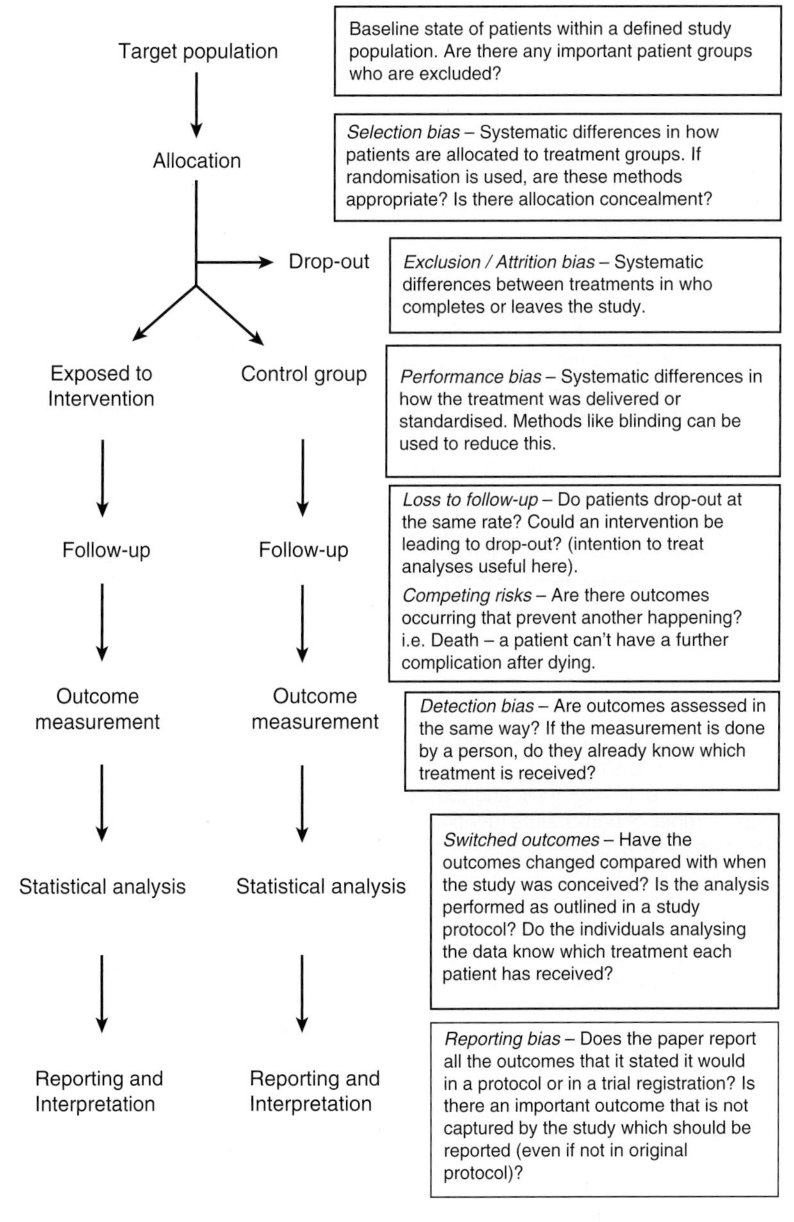

Start / Meta-data
Before reading the main text:
Is the journal reputable? Beware predatory journals!
Has the article been peer-reviewed?
Do the authors have any clear conflict of interest?
How was the study funded? Would the funders have any possible conflict of interest?
In the introduction:
Is the hypothesis clear?
Does the introduction mention already known advantages, and importantly, disadvantages of what is being studied?
During recruitment
Target population
Baseline state of patients within a defined study population. Are there any important patient groups who are excluded?
Allocation
Selection bias – Systematic differences in how patients are allocated to treatment groups. If randomisation is used, are these methods appropriate? Is there allocation concealment?
Drop-out
Exclusion / Attrition bias – Systematic differences between treatments in who completes or leaves the study.
Outcome measurement
Exposed to Intervention
Control group
Performance bias – Systematic differences in how the treatment was delivered or standardised. Methods like blinding can be used to reduce this.
Follow-up
Follow-up
Loss to follow-up – Do patients drop-out at the same rate? Could an intervention be leading to drop-out? (intention to treat analyses useful here).
Competing risks – Are there outcomes occurring that prevent another happening? i.e. Death – a patient can't have a further complication after dying.
Outcome measurement
Outcome measurement
Detection bias – Are outcomes assessed in the same way? If the measurement is done by a person, do they already know which treatment is received?
Analysis and reporting
Statistical analysis
Statistical analysis
Switched outcomes – Have the outcomes changed compared with when the study was conceived? Is the analysis performed as outlined in a study protocol? Do the individuals analysing the data know which treatment each patient has received?
Reporting and Interpretation
Reporting and Interpretation
Reporting bias – Does the paper report all the outcomes that it stated it would in a protocol or in a trial registration? Is there an important outcome that is not captured by the study which should be reported (even if not in original protocol)?

Figure 1.7 Overview of bias.

Omitting an outcome entirely then leads to it not being reported. An example of this could be a study investigating the effect of chemotherapy on breast cancer but failing to collect any data on chemotherapy side effects or tumour recurrence.

ATTRITION BIAS

Attrition bias occurs when there are systematic differences between study groups of withdrawals from research studies. This can be due to missing outcome data from participants withdrawing from the study, or due to the investigators

Box 1.3 The CONSORT checklist for randomised controlled trials[31]

Section/Topic	Item No	Checklist item
Title and abstract		
	1a	Identification as a randomised trial in the title
	1b	Structured summary of trial design, methods, results, and conclusions (for specific guidance see CONSORT for abstracts)
Introduction		
Background and objectives	2a	Scientific background and explanation of rationale
	2b	Specific objectives or hypotheses
Methods		
Trial design	3a	Description of trial design (such as parallel, factorial) including allocation ratio
	3b	Important changes to methods after trial commencement (such as eligibility criteria), with reasons
Participants	4a	Eligibility criteria for participants
	4b	Settings and locations where the data were collected
Interventions	5	The interventions for each group with sufficient details to allow replication, including how and when they were actually administered
Outcomes	6a	Completely defined pre-specified primary and secondary outcome measures, including how and when they were assessed
	6b	Any changes to trial outcomes after the trial commenced, with reasons
Sample size	7a	How sample size was determined
	7b	When applicable, explanation of any interim analyses and stopping guidelines
Randomisation		
Sequence generation	8a	Method used to generate the random allocation sequence
	8b	Type of randomisation; details of any restriction (such as blocking and block size)
Allocation concealment mechanism	9	Mechanism used to implement the random allocation sequence (such as sequentially numbered containers), describing any steps taken to conceal the sequence until interventions were assigned
Implementation	10	Who generated the random allocation sequence, who enrolled participants, and who assigned participants to interventions
Blinding	11a	If done, who was blinded after assignment to interventions (for example, participants, care providers, those assessing outcomes) and how
	11b	If relevant, description of the similarity of interventions
Statistical methods	12a	Statistical methods used to compare groups for primary and secondary outcomes
	12b	Methods for additional analyses, such as subgroup analyses and adjusted analyses
Results		
Participant flow (a diagram is strongly recommended)	13a	For each group, the numbers of participants who were randomly assigned, received intended treatment, and were analysed for the primary outcome
	13b	For each group, losses and exclusions after randomisation, together with reasons
Recruitment	14a	Dates defining the periods of recruitment and follow-up
	14b	Why the trial ended or was stopped
Baseline data	15	A table showing baseline demographic and clinical characteristics for each group
Numbers analysed	16	For each group, number of participants (denominator) included in each analysis and whether the analysis was by original assigned groups
Outcomes and estimation	17a	For each primary and secondary outcome, results for each group, and the estimated effect size and its precision (such as 95% confidence interval)
	17b	For binary outcomes, presentation of both absolute and relative effect sizes is recommended
Ancillary analyses	18	Results of any other analyses performed, including subgroup analyses and adjusted analyses, distinguishing pre-specified from exploratory
Harms	19	All important harms or unintended effects in each group (for specific guidance see CONSORT for harms)
Discussion		
Limitations	20	Trial limitations, addressing sources of potential bias, imprecision, and, if relevant, multiplicity of analyses
Generalisability	21	Generalisability (external validity, applicability) of the trial findings
Interpretation	22	Interpretation consistent with results, balancing benefits and harms, and considering other relevant evidence
Other information		
Registration	23	Registration number and name of trial registry
Protocol	24	Where the full trial protocol can be accessed, if available
Funding	25	Sources of funding and other support (such as supply of drugs), role of funders

excluding cases. In either situation, it must be ensured that there are no underlying reasons for this to occur which may lead to bias. If there are differences between groups with regards to drop-outs or exclusions, there should be a high index of suspicion for attrition bias.

If there are more participants withdrawing from a treatment group, it may indicate that the treatment is causing harm, is ineffective, or is poorly tolerated by the study participants. Performing analyses using an intention-to-treat (ITT) approach addresses this. ITT analyses include all participants who have been allocated to a treatment group, regardless of whether they have withdrawn from or adhered to the intervention. The analysis then will present a more 'real-world' measure of clinical effectiveness.

Per-protocol, or efficacy, analyses look at how effective the treatment was in the patients who completed the treatment course. This provides an estimate as to how effective the treatment is in those patients who adhere to it. Ideally, a study will first perform an ITT analysis, followed by an efficacy analysis. Doing so provides both a measure of real-world clinical effectiveness and a measure of how effective the treatment is for adherent patients.

PERFORMANCE BIAS

Performance bias describes a phenomenon in which those administering an intervention or aftercare are aware of the treatment group the patient is allocated to and consciously or subconsciously alter their behaviour.

An example of this may be where a new surgical operation is being tested. If the staff involved in the postoperative care are aware of the treatment the patient received, they may unknowingly provide different care across groups, thus leading to results which misleadingly favour one treatment over another. Blinding and implementation of clearly defined pathways of care can reduce the risk of performance bias.

RECALL BIAS

Recall bias is systematic error caused by difficulties a patient may have in recalling an event accurately. This is of particular concern in the retrospective determination of a particular outcome.

An example may be conducting a telephone survey of patients who have undergone surgery to ask if they suffered a wound infection. If a study contacted patients at 30 days following surgery, the patient would be likely to recall whether they had a wound issue or not. If the study, however, contacted patients 2 years after the index operation, recalling details would be far more difficult and subject to recall bias.

OBSERVER BIAS

Where an individual determining a study outcome introduces bias, either consciously or subconsciously, by altering their judgements based on knowledge of treatment group allocation. An example is in studies assessing surgical site infection. If the individual assessing the wound is aware of the treatment group allocation of the patient, the assessment of the outcome may be prejudiced and favour one treatment over another.

The only means of adequately addressing observer bias is to use a blinded design, where observers are unaware of the treatment group allocation. In surgical studies, the observer cannot be a member of the surgical team, as they are already aware of the group allocation given they performed the intervention. In this case, an independent blinded observer should assess study outcomes to minimise the influence of observer bias.

PUBLICATION BIAS

Like reporting bias, publication bias involves the selective reporting of research. Publication bias, however, occurs when a study goes unpublished. This may be for many reasons including failure to recruit participants, patients coming to harm leading to the study being terminated early, and results which were not as expected or hoped (i.e. 'negative' results). Studies which show 'positive' results, where there are statistically significant correlations between interventions or exposures are more likely to be published than those which do not.

Thorough systematic reviews attempt to identify publication bias. Investigators of reviews search clinical trials registers, conference abstracts and other sources to ascertain whether additional research studies have been performed but have gone unpublished. Using meta-analysis techniques, it is also possible to determine statistically whether there are likely to be unpublished studies using funnel plots. Funnel plots show the effect size of each study against a measure of precision. Where publication bias exists, the expected distribution of studies showing effects both greater and less than the mean effect is absent, and the plot is asymmetric. This suggests expected 'negative' studies are absent. The use of protocols published prior to a study taking place and registration of studies on clinical trials databases ensure investigators can be held accountable for unpublished work (Fig. 1.8).

JUDGING THE RISK OF BIAS

There are many validated tools to help researchers to systematically assess bias in research studies. These tools ensure that a uniform approach is taken, and studies are directly comparable. One popular tool for appraising the risk of bias in non-randomised research is the Newcastle-Ottawa scale. The Newcastle-Ottawa scale covers the domains of Selection, Comparability, Exposure and Outcome. Using the tool, investigators make judgements as to the quality of the piece of research across these specific domains. Other available tools include the Cochrane Collaboration's tool for appraisal of randomised controlled trials and observational appraisal tool (ROBINS-I).[32]

For making judgements on the overall findings of a systematic review and assessing the strength with which a recommendation can be made, there exist another set of criteria known as 'GRADE'.[12] This set of criteria aims to summarise the findings of a systematic review based upon more than just the quality of evidence contained within the review itself. GRADE considers five domains:

1. Risk of bias: Was there bias across the included studies that may influence the results of the review?
2. Imprecision: If further studies were done, could they plausibly change the results of the review?
3. Indirectness: Are the results of the review applicable to clinical practice?
4. Inconsistency: Were included studies consistent (in agreement) across the review?
5. Publication bias: Was there publication bias present and if this were not present would it change the results of the review?

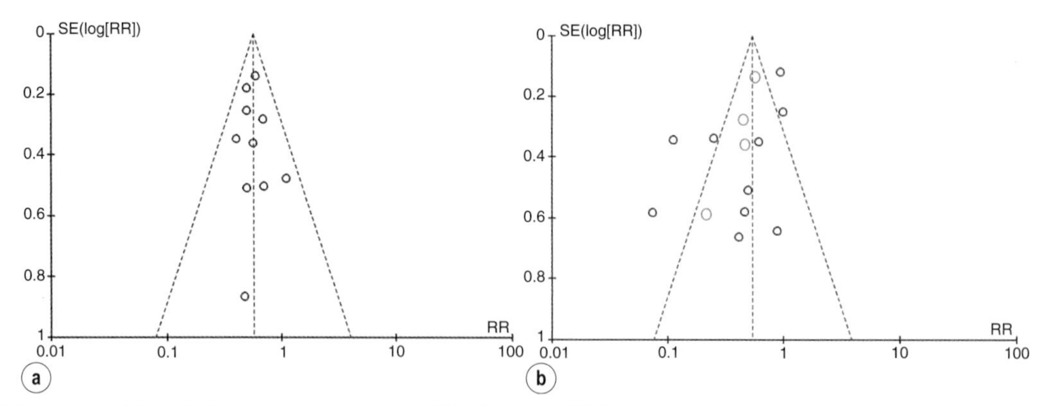

Figure 1.8 (a) Symmetrical funnel plot demonstrating no publication bias. (b) Asymmetrical funnel plot demonstrating the presence of publication bias, with outlying *dots* indicating studies with apparent bias. The *green* dots indicate examples of where we may expect studies to lie (within the dotted funnel).

After analysing the review's findings across the five domains, an overall GRADE rating is awarded. This can be up- or down-graded based on these five domains. There should be one GRADE rating awarded per outcome reported in the review:

- High quality: It is highly likely that the results of the review lie very close to the true value.
- Moderate quality: It is likely that the results of the review lie close to the true value, but further research could alter this.
- Low quality: It is unlikely that the results of the review are close to the true value and are likely to be substantially different.
- Very low quality: It is very unlikely that the results of the review are anywhere near the true value.

SIMPLE STATISTICS

An understanding of basic statistics is crucial to the successful interpretation of research studies. Statistical terms are often confused, and a clear understanding of the definitions and workings of statistics can make a paper clearer to read and interpret. Furthermore, statistics can be used to disguise study results or to claim a treatment effect when one does not truly exist.

In this section, we will provide a brief overview of statistical terms and provide straightforward explanations for frequently used techniques.

SUMMARISING DATA

Often the first table contained in a study summarises the characteristics of the population included in the study. This is useful as it enables the reader to see whether the study is applicable to the population they treat. There are three types of data variable: categorical, ordinal and continuous.

- Categorical data can take one of several defined groups which do not have precedence. Where there are two groups, the data can also be called 'binary'. An example of categorical data is gender which usually takes the value of male or female.
- Ordinal data are similar to categorical data except they have a natural order of precedence. Ordinal data can take only the values of each group, there being no intermediate values possible. An example is the TNM tumour staging system, where there is an order of precedence as to tumour grade, but this cannot be described on a continuous numerical scale.
- Continuous data are numbers which are on a continuous scale. These can be in the form of whole numbers (integers) or be described as parts of a whole using a decimal format (i.e. 12.5).

SUMMARISING ORDINAL OR CATEGORICAL DATA

Summarising ordinal and categorical data is straightforward. Simple counts for each group can be used and percentages calculated.

SUMMARISING CONTINUOUS DATA

Summarising continuous data is less straightforward than categorical or ordinal data. Averages are used instead of simply adding up the number of participants in each group. Continuous data follow a distribution, which describes how the data are spread across study subjects. The data distribution dictates the type of average measure used. An average is also known as a measure of 'central tendency' as it describes the central point around which the data is distributed. The degree to which data is spread around this central point is called 'dispersion'. Where central tendency is measured by using averages, dispersion is measured using values such as standard deviation (SD) or confidence intervals (Cis). When an estimate of the central tendency and dispersion are known, it is possible to interpret using numbers how the distribution of continuous data may look.

Broadly speaking, data can follow a parametric (one with a defined shape) or non-parametric distribution (without an obviously defined shape). In statistics, most parametric data naturally follows a distribution known as the 'normal distribution' (also known as 'Gaussian'). The normal distribution follows a symmetric distribution around a central point. When plotted, the curve generated by this data looks like a bell that might be found in a church (Fig. 1.9).

Not all data follows this exact distribution. One such example is age, where conditions may affect older or younger people disproportionately. If we plotted the distribution of ages of patients at the first diagnosis of Alzheimer's disease, we would see that older patients would be more affected and hence the plot would be moved to the right-hand side. This

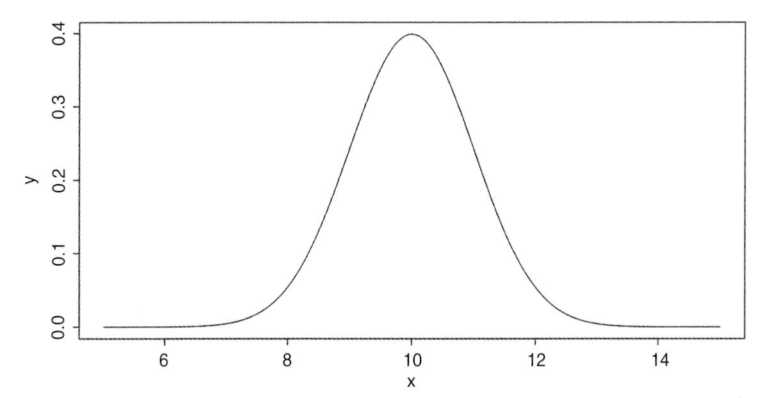

Figure 1.9 The normal, or Gaussian, distribution—an example of a parametric distribution.

effect is known as skew and is important to consider, as highly skewed data will require different measures to assess the central tendency and dispersion of data.

There are three types of average:

- Mean: This is calculated by adding up all the values in the data and dividing by the number of observations. This type of mean is called an arithmetic mean. There are more complex types of mean available, which include geometric and harmonic means, but these are outside the scope of this chapter.
- Median: This is the value of the middle observation when the data are ordered in ascending or descending order. For example, if there were 100 observations made on a continuous scale, the median would be the value of the 50th observation.
- Mode: This is the most common value found within the continuous dataset.

MEASURING DISPERSION

There are five types of measures of dispersion that are important to know about:

STANDARD DEVIATION (SD OR Σ)

$$\sigma = \sqrt{\frac{1}{N}\sum_{i=1}^{N}(x_i - \mu)^2}$$

Where N is the number of observations, μ is the mean of all values and x is the value for each observation. The SD describes the distribution of a continuous variable around a given point. It works well if the data is parametric and is not skewed.

CONFIDENCE INTERVAL (CI)

$$95\%\ CI = x \pm (1.96 \times SE_x)$$

Where x is the effect size, and SE is the standard error of the effect size. A CI describes the certainty of a treatment effect.

INTERQUARTILE RANGE (IQR)

$$IQR = Q3 - Q1$$

Where Q1 is the value of the 25th centile contained within the data and Q3 is the 75th centile. This is a good way to describe non-parametric data (i.e. data that do not follow a normal distribution).

RANGE

$$Range = Maximum\ Value - Minimum\ Value$$

This describes the overall spread of values within a dataset. It is useful for both parametric and non-parametric data.

When a continuous variable is normally distributed (it is always wise to plot it first to check!) and not highly skewed, central tendency can be summarised using the arithmetic mean and dispersion can be summarised using SD or CI.

In the case where a continuous variable does not follow a normal distribution or is highly skewed, the median or the mode can be used in place of the mean. Dispersion is then conventionally presented alongside a measure of dispersion such as the interquartile range or range.

MISSING DATA

Dealing with missing data is important, as missing data may lead to biased results. Missing data on explanatory variables (e.g. age, sex, disease type) should not be simply excluded from an analysis if there is accompanying outcome data present. To do so would be to introduce attrition bias. Data can be missing due to the following reasons:

- Missing not at random (MNAR): Here data are missing for a reason. This may be due to factors which have been collected in the study (observed), or for reasons which have not been collected (unobserved).
- Missing at random (MAR): Here data are missing, but the reason can be fully accounted for using factors which have already been collected (observed).
- Missing completely at random (MCAR): Here data are missing completely independently for no reason at all.

Missing data should never be ignored. There are several means of dealing of missing data, which often include imputing an estimated value for the missing variable.

TREATMENT EFFECT

The treatment effect (also known as effect estimate) describes the influence of the intervention or exposure being studied on the outcome of interest. The treatment effect measures the average difference in outcomes between the group that received the intervention or exposure and the control group. It can be measured using statistical methods and is often presented as either a risk ratio or odds ratio, alongside a CI to demonstrate the level of uncertainty surrounding the estimate. Other measures may also be used, such as absolute risk reduction or number needed to treat.

RISK

Risk is defined as the probability of an outcome occurring in a given population. There are two types of risk measurement used in clinical research—absolute risk and relative risk. Absolute risk measures the actual probability within a population. Relative risk is a measure of the probability of an outcome occurring in one treatment group versus another, sometimes known as a risk ratio. An absolute risk reduction describes how good or bad one treatment is versus another.

$$Absolute\ risk = \frac{Number\ of\ events\ of\ interest}{Number\ of\ participants\ in\ population}$$

$$Absolute\ risk\ reduction(ARR) = \frac{Number\ of\ events\ of\ interest\ in\ exposed\ group}{Number\ of\ participants\ in\ exposed\ group} - \frac{Number\ of\ events\ of\ interest\ in\ unexposed\ group}{Number\ of\ participants\ in\ unexposed\ group}$$

$$Relative\ risk\ (risk\ ratio) = \frac{Absolute\ risk\ of\ an\ event\ occurring\ in\ exposed\ group}{Absolute\ risk\ of\ an\ event\ occurring\ in\ unexposed\ group}$$

ODDS

Odds are defined as the ratio of an event occurring versus an event not occurring in a given population or study group. For example, if in a population of 100 patients undergoing liver surgery, 25 develop complications, the odds of a complication occurring would be 1 to 3.

The 2 × 2 table, risk ratios and odds ratios

For calculating odds and risk, it is useful to consider a 2 × 2 table:

	Exposure Yes	*Exposure No*
Outcome Yes	A	B
Outcome No	C	D

Using the 2 × 2 table, absolute risk can be expressed as:

$$Absolute\ risk\ of\ outcome\ 'Yes'\ in\ exposed\ group = \frac{a}{a+c}$$

$$Absolute\ risk\ of\ outcome\ 'Yes'\ in\ unexposed\ group = \frac{b}{b+d}$$

To calculate a risk ratio, we would calculate the absolute risk for both groups and divide one by the other. Alternatively, based upon the 2 × 2 table, a risk ratio may be expressed as:

$$Risk\ ratio\ of\ outcome\ 'Yes' = \left(\frac{a}{a+c}\right) \div \left(\frac{b}{b+c}\right)$$

Using the 2 x 2 table, the odds of outcome 'Yes' occurring in the exposed group would be expressed as $\frac{a}{c}$ and for outcome 'Yes', in the unexposed group $\frac{b}{d}$.

To calculate an odds ratio, we would calculate this using the following formulae:

$$Odds\ ratio\ (OR) = \frac{a}{c} \div \frac{b}{d}$$

Due to mathematical convention, when two fractions are divided sequentially, this is the same as multiplying them once. Therefore, an odds ratio may be also expressed as:

$$Odds\ ratio\ (OR) = \frac{ad}{bc}$$

If an odds ratio or a risk ratio is greater than 1, the outcome of interest is more likely to occur with the exposure. If the odds ratio or risk ratio takes a value less than 1, the outcome of interest is less likely to occur with the exposure. If the odds or risk ratio is close to one, the outcome of interest does not alter with the exposure.

The difference between the risk ratio and the value 1 is also known as the risk difference. An example of this would be for a risk ratio of 0.8. If we subtract 0.8 from 1, we are left with 0.2. Therefore, we can say there is a 20% relative risk reduction between the treatment groups.

Risk ratio versus odds ratio

Although they may appear similar in numerical format, there are clear distinctions to be made between odds ratios and risks ratios.

Odds can be converted to risks and vice-versa; however, this is not a straightforward process as their relationship depends upon the event rate for the outcome of interest. For common outcomes, odds ratios can be very different from risk ratios and should not be confused. Odds ratios do not translate well to describing risk either as they are not immediately intuitive.

HYPOTHESIS TESTING

Statistical tests are used to reject study hypotheses. There are two types of study hypotheses:

- The null hypothesis is that there is no difference between treatments or exposed groups. It further stipulates that any observed differences may be due to error.
- The alternative hypothesis is that there is a difference between treatments or exposed groups. This is opposite to the null hypothesis.

A hypothesis in this sense can only be rejected or fail to be rejected and never fully accepted, as there is hypothetically always a chance that the observations are due to error.

Statistical testing aims to reject the null hypothesis to demonstrate that there is a significant difference between treatment groups.

ASSOCIATION AND CAUSATION

Perhaps one of the most important skills when interpreting statistics is to discern association from causation. The objective of most medical studies is to identify or postulate as to why a particular result was observed (or in some cases, not observed).

Distinguishing causation from association is particularly important in observational research. If there is a relationship or correlation between two variables, statistically significant or not, these variables are said to be associated. We cannot directly infer that the variables have a cause-and-effect relationship, as the observation may be simply due to chance or bias. Interventional studies, where an experiment is constructed to minimise sources of bias and error are more likely to establish causality. This is a particular strength of the randomised controlled trial design.

According to the Bradford Hill criteria, an observation is likely to be causal if the following are fulfilled:

- Strength of association: The larger the effect size of associated variables, the more likely there is a causal effect present, unless an obvious confounding factor is unaccounted for.
- Consistency: If multiple, independent studies find the same association in different populations, this increases the likelihood of an effect being present.
- Specificity: If there is a very specific association between one group of patients and the exposure of interest, it is likely to be causative.
- Temporality: If the outcome occurs following the exposure within a plausible timeframe, causality is more likely to be present.
- Biological rationale: If there is a 'dose-response' relationship between the exposure and the outcome, this makes causality more likely. For example, the higher the dose of antibiotics a patient receives, the greater the chances of developing *Clostridium difficile* pseudomembranous colitis.
- Plausibility: If there is a clear explanation between a cause and an observed effect, causality is more likely. For example, oranges are high in vitamin C, therefore children who eat more oranges are less likely to suffer from scurvy.
- Coherence: If the observations of a clinical research study tie in with the findings of a laboratory study, causality is more likely.
- Analogy: When a result is observed, other analogous (similar) or confounding factors should be taken into consideration. If when these factors have been taken into consideration, the observed result persists, causality is more likely.

STATISTICAL SIGNIFICANCE

Statistical significance is a concept that is often misunderstood by scientists and clinicians alike. When considering significance, there is one question that should be asked—is the finding clinically significant?

Statistical significance can be described as the level at which the probability of a test reaches an acceptable level at which the null hypothesis can be rejected. Often this is described using a *P* value, which describes the probability of an observation being down to chance (i.e. a *P* value of 0.05 means there is a 1 in 20 probability the observed association is due to chance).

The *P* value has become synonymous with statistical significance over the past hundred years. It was initially invented by Ronald Fisher, an eminent frequentist statistician in the 20th century. Fisher arbitrarily selected 0.05 as an example to illustrate the use of the *P* value and since then it has stuck.

ADJUSTING FOR CONFOUNDING FACTORS

In well-conducted randomised studies, both treatment groups should contain patients with similar characteristics and be reasonably balanced. In observational studies, however, due to a lack of randomisation, patient groups are likely to be unbalanced. To account for this imbalance and address the possible source of selection bias that accompanies this (as imbalance is likely to be due to clinical treatment decisions), these factors can be adjusted for using regression methods.

Key points

- High-quality research can change surgical practice and improve patient care.
- Well-planned, large-scale randomised clinical trials are usually at the lowest risk of bias. Where clinical trials are not possible, high-quality prospective studies can be useful.
- As well as good methods, clear and transparent reporting of research is essential and there are useful tools (EQUATOR checklists) to help with this.
- Understanding how to identify strengths and weaknesses of a study requires practice and is essential to providing good evidence-based surgical care.

MEDICAL RESEARCH AND CHALLENGES

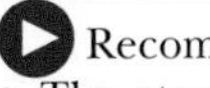

Recommended videos:

- The story of 200 years- how evidence came to the fore- https://www.youtube.com/watch?v=Qxx14RCxblg
- Challenges in surgical research - https://www.youtube.com/watch?v=IeXts3V6Wjo

References available at http://ebooks.health.elsevier.com/

FURTHER READING

Swinscow DV, Campbell MJ. Statistics at square one. 11th ed. BMJ Books; 2002. p. 158. ISBN 0-7279-1552-5.

Greenhalgh T. How to read a paper: the basics of evidence-based medicine. 4th ed. BMJ Books; 2010. ISBN 0-7279-1552-5.

Good Clinical Practice Training Course. Many providers- however, the National Institute for Health Research (NIHR) has a good scheme. https://www.nihr.ac.uk/health-and-care-professionals/learning-and-support/good-clinical-practice.htm.

2 Perioperative care and enhanced recovery

Kristoffer Lassen | Michael Hughes

INTRODUCTION

Updated guidelines focus on comprehensive protocols for each step of the perioperative 'journey' in various abdominal procedures.[1–7] Several reviews confirm an association between the use of an enhanced recovery protocol (ERP) and improved outcomes in abdominal surgery.[8–12] While some results indicate gains from adhering to specific protocols (e.g. Enhanced Recovery After Surgery [ERAS] guidelines) and aiming for an optimal compliance,[13–16] others suggest that it is the use of a protocol in itself that is useful.[8] Comparison with historical controls is the study design used most frequently, but a host of confounding factors exist. As a complex intervention with outdated or contaminated control groups, this is a difficult issue to assess in a controlled manner and poorly suited for randomised design.[17] Nevertheless, the common theme behind these potentially conflicting views is the message that the efforts of the surgeon and anaesthetist do not start and stop solely with the operation itself. Optimal risk reduction through preoperative preparation and prehabilitation as well as structured evidence-based care encompassing every aspect of the postoperative period is crucial to minimise morbidity and mortality following major surgery. The modern surgical intervention begins about 4 weeks prior to the operation and continues for several weeks thereafter.

BEFORE THE OPERATION

The first encounter with the patient is crucial for several reasons. Confidence has to be established; it is the first opportunity to educate the patient for the operation ahead; and it is an opportunity to improve his or her risk profile. For those with cancer, there is often the added consideration of timing of surgery, particularly if neo-adjuvant therapy is required.

PATIENT COUNSELLING

Patient counselling is about more than explaining the operation and the probable outcome, including any risk of complications. It is the key opportunity to make sure the patient realises what the perioperative course will entail and what his/her daily targets should be in terms of mobilisation, drinking, eating and so forth.[1–3,18,19] Counselling should be commenced at the preoperative out-patient clinic, with written or audio-visual information available for patients to review at an early stage to allow adequate familiarisation before surgery. The patient's own part in his or her recovery should be emphasised and is an important factor in achieving compliance. This area is poorly suited for a randomised trial,[17] and it would be unethical to attempt one. It is, however, an intervention with collateral benefits and without known side effects although it requires some extra time.

✔ Preoperative counselling is strongly recommended, and details about risk reduction, the operation and the postoperative course should be covered.

PREOPERATIVE NUTRITION AND IMMUNONUTRITION

Preoperative weight loss is a robust and strong predictor for adverse surgical outcomes. Even as little as 5% weight loss is a significant risk factor.[20] The ESPEN criteria for malnutrition is defined as BMI of < 18.5 kg/m^2 or weight loss $> 10\%$ (or $> 5\%$ over 3 months) and reduced BMI (or a low fat-free mass index).[21] Weighing the patient and comparing the results with patient-reported premorbid weight is sufficient and as a predictor probably as valid as more complex nutritional risk assessment tools. While preoperative dietary interventions can help the patient to regain lost weight before surgery, it is less clear whether this affects postoperative risk or is merely alleviating symptoms.[22] Intravenous nutrition, enteral tube feeding and oral supplements (sip feeds) have all been evaluated as interventions to attenuate patient risk for complications following major surgery and in general they are recommended. Numerous studies suggest a beneficial effect in malnourished patients, but double-blinded trials with adequate control groups are few.[23] Importantly, providing nutrition is a consistent intervention that can be blinded and placebo-controlled in randomised controlled trials (RCTs), and in conditions suitable for optimal design we should accept nothing less.[17] It appears prudent to provide nutritional support to grossly malnourished patients, orally if possible; enteral if oral is not feasible; and parenteral if the gut is not working. For patients with only mild malnutrition, the rationale is mainly supported by uncontrolled or open-labelled trials or trials measuring surrogate endpoints. Weight gain is achieved consistently in these studies, but lowered postoperative risk has not been documented in a reproducible manner.

Additional provision of immune-enhancing formulas like arginine or glutamine has been supported by several trials and international guidelines.[23,24] Immunonutrition (IN) is particularly aimed at reducing infectious complications. However, there are few double-blinded trials with isonitrogenous control groups measuring clinical outcomes. The most recent ERAS guidelines do not recommend the routine use of IN,[2,25] and several recent high-quality trials in high-risk patients have failed to show any benefit.[26–28]

✔✔ There is currently no good evidence to support routine provision of preoperative nutritional support in patients who are not grossly malnourished. Immunonutrition is not recommended.

CESSATION OF SMOKING

Smoking negatively affects oxygen delivery to peripheral tissues, as well as those involved in an anastomosis. While chronic obstructive pulmonary disease (COPD), and risk of bronchial adenocarcinoma and cardiovascular disease will remain unchanged following 3 weeks of cessation from smoking, increasing evidence suggests that both oxygen delivery and pulmonary function can be improved by smoking cessation over as little as 3–4 weeks.[29–31] Even in cancer surgery where delaying the operation will not be done lightly, allowing 4 weeks of complete cessation from smoking is probably wise in high-risk patients or planned high-risk anastomoses, e.g. low rectal, oesophageal or pancreatic head resections. It is a cheap and well-understood intervention, and it places the patient at the centre of the efforts to reduce risk.

✔✔ Patients should stop smoking for at least 3 weeks prior to major surgery.[29,30]

PREHABILITATION

Impaired functional capacity in elderly cancer patients is multifactorial and constitutes a risk during major surgery. Some of the causes are cardiovascular disease, COPD, lean muscle wasting and other elements of cachexia. Prehabilitation, which aims to increase functional capacity in patients with impaired functional capacity, hinges on the issue of whether elderly and frail patients can benefit from short-term exercise to such an extent that risk is reduced. Again, the presence of cancer—as is often the case—will usually not allow for extended periods of intervention. Cardiopulmonary function tests have been shown to correlate closely with risk for major morbidity following surgery[32]; and interestingly, Dunne et al.[33] have shown that a short-term, hospital-based exercise program does indeed improve cardiopulmonary function for patients at risk. However, hospital-based daily training programs may have suboptimal compliance,[33] and may not be feasible to implement.

Over recent years, prehabilitation programmes have become increasingly popular and are becoming a standard component of perioperative care in many countries. A combination of aerobic exercise, nutritional optimisation, inspiratory muscle training and resistance exercises have been shown to improve not only preoperative aerobic threshold as measured by cardiopulmonary exercise testing[34] but also overall and pulmonary postoperative morbidity.[35,36] The precise optimum prehabilitation programme has not been established and heterogeneity exists in current programmes in terms of duration, make up and level of supervision. Additionally, the control groups in several of the recent RCTs include elements of prehabilitation and so overall impact has potentially not clearly been illustrated. It may also be that the real benefit of prehabilitation programs is harvested at a later stage: in the patients' own communities and in the shape of protected physical independence and autonomy. In any case, preoperative programmes are becoming standard of care as the intuitive benefits have become recognised.

✔✔ Prehabilitation programmes should be developed and incorporated into perioperative care pathways.

ANTI-THROMBOEMBOLIC DRUGS IN THE PERIOPERATIVE PERIOD

An increasing number of patients take an increasing variety of anti-thrombotic drugs for primary or secondary prophylaxis. Due to uncertain enteral absorption and risk of intra- or postoperative bleeding, these drugs are transiently withheld during the perioperative period for a duration dependent on the type of surgery. Perioperative prophylaxis with low-molecular-weight heparin (LMWH) or unfractionated heparin (UFH) varies depending on the indication for the patient's use of prophylaxis, the drug in question and the magnitude of increased risk pertaining to the operation. Most departments will have access to local or national guidelines for each drug under several indications, and most cardiology departments will issue additional guidelines for prevention of thromboembolic complications in patients with coronary stents. The following section is intended as an overview and the reader is strongly advised to consult national and local guidelines for details.

VITAMIN K ANTAGONISTS

Warfarin. Antidotes for reversal in the emergency setting include vitamin K, fresh-frozen plasma and prothrombin complex concentrate (PCC). In the elective setting, warfarin is usually withheld for 3–5 days prior to major surgery. Depending on the risk of thromboembolic events balanced against the risk of bleeding during or after surgery, bridging therapy with LMWH/UHF may be indicated. Warfarin is usually resumed the evening after surgery if haemostasis is adequate.

Direct oral anticoagulants (DOACs).[37] Importantly, they have no direct antidote, but PCC will reduce active bleeding. Their half-life increases significantly with impaired renal function and this has clinical implications, as surgery is usually acceptable after a cessation of one half-life. In such cases, it will be important to measure renal function (creatinine and glomerular filtration rate [GFR]) and international normalised ratio/activated partial thromboplastin time (INR/APTT), and identify time of the last dose taken.

Dabigatran. If elevated INR/APTT, consider PCC. Normal APTT suggests low or no drug action. Emergency surgery should be delayed if possible to one half-life from last dose. For scheduled major surgery, there should be a 48 hours suspension period (with normal renal function) and 96 hours if GFR is 30–50 mL/min.[37] Restart dabigatran on postoperative day 1–3 depending on haemostasis and indication. Consider LMWH in the intervening period.

Rivaroxaban. Effect cannot be measured by INR/APTT, consider PCC for reversal. For emergency and scheduled major surgery, as for dabigatran.

Apixaban. Again its effect cannot be measured by INR/APTT, consider PCC for reversal. For emergency and scheduled major surgery, as for dabigatran.

ANTI-PLATELET DRUGS

Acetylsalicylic acid (aspirin). Unless high risk of bleeding is anticipated in areas where surgical control is difficult, aspirin does not need to be discontinued before surgery.[38]

Clopidogrel, ticagrelor, prasugrel. Dual anti-platelet medication (aspirin + clopidogrel, ticagrelor or prasugrel) is prescribed following insertion of coronary artery stents. Duration is usually 6 weeks for bare-metal stents (BMS), and 6–12 months for drug-eluting stents (DES). Abrupt suspension of these represents a significant risk for thrombosis, and replacement therapy (LMWH) must be used in the perioperative period. Clopidogrel should be discontinued at least 5–7 days before any planned, major surgery[39,40]; ticagrelor, somewhat shorter,[41] but prasugrel should be discontinued at least 7 days before.[40] Whether bridging anticoagulants (LMWH/UFH) is indicated must be assessed for individual patients.

IMMEDIATE PREOPERATIVE PERIOD

The patient is usually admitted to the hospital the afternoon before or increasingly on the day of surgery. This is the last opportunity to identify any unforeseen deterioration in the patient that could make surgery hazardous and to check that all preparations to reduce risk are in place as planned.

PREOPERATIVE BOWEL PREPARATION

Traditionally, procedures to empty the large bowel before surgery have been a pillar of preoperative preparation for colorectal procedures with the intention of reducing the bacterial load in the colon and hence risk for infectious complications. Traditional per oral, or mechanical bowel preparation, implies intake of large amounts of fluids together with osmotic and laxative agents that induce diarrhoea. The risk of severe fluid shifts is substantial, especially for elderly and frail patients, and the procedure is quite burdensome. Modern guidelines and reviews have failed to identify significant benefits against the unwanted consequences and have largely advised against it.[1–3,6,19,42–46] Bowel preparation has, however, received some renewed interest in combination with repeated doses of per oral antibiotics aiming at a more complete decontamination of the large bowel. Recent data indicate that such a combination lowers complication rates in colorectal surgery.[47–49] A recent meta-analysis[50] reported benefit of oral antibiotics in combination with bowel preparation compared with bowel preparation alone but no benefit of using bowel preparation with antibiotics compared with antibiotics alone, although randomised prospective data were lacking for this comparison. The most recent ERAS guidelines only recommend bowel preparation for selected rectal surgery.[6]

Mechanical preparation (with or without decontaminating antibiotics) or enemas will be necessary in selected colorectal operations. Identifying small and ill-defined lesions during surgery might require careful palpation or intraoperative colonoscopy, both requiring an empty bowel. Furthermore, the use of diverting ileostomies to protect an ultra-low rectal anastomosis is meaningless if the colon is not emptied preoperatively.

✔✔ There is no strong evidence to support routine preoperative bowel preparation before major colonic or non-rectal abdominal surgery.

PREVENTION OF THROMBOEMBOLIC EVENTS

Patients undergoing major abdominal surgery have a significantly increased risk of venous thromboembolic (VTE) complications, either in the form of deep venous thrombosis (DVT) or pulmonary thromboembolism (PTE). Patients are often elderly, have malignant disease, are immobilised for some time, are exposed to fluid shifts and temporary dehydration and many have co-existent conditions like atrial fibrillation or congestive heart failure. The thromboembolic events may be asymptomatic or symptomatic and this makes interpretation of available data difficult. In addition, many of the earlier trials were conducted in environments where patients were immobilised for many days, limiting the generalisability (external validity) of the results in modern settings. It is a general consensus that patients undergoing major surgery should receive prophylaxis with LMWH for the days they have impaired level of mobility and suffer altered physiology from anaesthesia and surgery.[1–3,19,43,44] There are some other issues that are still under debate. A recent Cochrane review suggests that UFH is equal to LMWH,[51] and UHF has the advantage of not being dependent on renal function.

A large meta-analysis of over 7000 patients, of which 24% underwent general surgery procedures, identified intermittent pneumatic compression (IPC) as being superior to placebo, graded compression stockings and equivalent to pharmacological anticoagulation in terms of preventing thromboembolic events, and a combination of IPC and anticoagulation was superior to IPC alone.[52] A Cochrane review from 2016[53] compared pneumatic compression and anticoagulation with anticoagulation alone and when looking at all studies which included general, orthopaedic and cardiac surgery, the combination intervention was favoured in terms of reduction of PTE incidence postoperatively. This finding was corroborated by a further meta-analysis of 11 RCTs,[54] again including orthopaedic and general surgery cases. This study included a sub-group analysis of four studies assessing abdominal surgery, finding a reduction in DVT rates in the combination group. It is appropriate to comment on the quality of included trials in these analyses being reported as low—mainly related to heterogeneity of surgical procedures, postoperative pathway and pick up sensitivity of thromboembolic outcomes, and the recommendation for combined anticoagulation and IPC was for high-risk patients. However, the risk of adding IPC is low and so is often routinely performed.

Extending thromboembolic prophylaxis beyond the hospital stay has also been advocated, especially in high-risk patients like those undergoing hip replacement surgery.[55] An updated Cochrane review of seven RCTs including 1728 patients reported reduction in all VTE and proximal DVT in the extended treatment group compared with those who had in-hospital anticoagulation only. No increase in bleeding was observed. The included trials were for patients undergoing abdominal and pelvic surgery, including one laparoscopic trial and the review concluded with the recommendation that extended prophylaxis should be provided for such patients at high risk of VTE.[56]

Patients with pancreatic cancer and patients receiving neoadjuvant chemotherapy have been identified at risk for VTE even prior to surgery and a low threshold for deep vein ultrasonography could be considered.[57]

✔✔ VTE prophylaxis using UFH or LMWH is strongly recommended in all patients undergoing major abdominal surgery (whether laparoscopic or open) and should be continued until the patient is mobile. Extended prophylaxis (for 28 days) in high-risk patients (such as after major cancer resections) is also recommended.

PREOPERATIVE FASTING

Following fatal aspirations in the early days of anaesthesia, extensive periods of preoperative fasting has been a part of perioperative care for over a century. Modern evidence-based guidelines now recommend that patients be fasted for 6 hours for solid food and 2 hours for clear drinks before induction of anaesthesia.[1,3,19,42–45]

PREOPERATIVE CARBOHYDRATE LOADING

The theoretical concept of saturating the liver's glycogen storage capacity prior to surgery is appealing, as even overnight fasting will to some extent deplete these stores.[58] Intake of carbohydrate-rich fluids the night before, and on the morning of surgery, has been shown to attenuate postoperative insulin resistance.[59] Being reasonably cheap and safe, they have been recommended in modern guidelines,[6] but significant impact on complications after surgery has not been demonstrated.

ANTIBIOTIC PROPHYLAXIS

In this context, antimicrobial/antibiotic prophylaxis is designating a one-shot, preoperative administration of antibiotics to achieve an appropriate systemic level of drug during surgery and lower the risk of surgical site infections (SSIs). Systemic antibiotic prophylaxis is recommended by a host of perioperative guidelines.[1–3,7,19,43] The magnitude of risk reduction for SSI will depend on the 'a priori' risk of the patient and the type of operation. Patients undergoing contaminated or potentially contaminated operations should receive systemic prophylaxis. The rapidly increasing use of laparoscopy for several types of operations probably lowers the risk of SSI,[60] and extrapolation of evidence from open surgery might not be appropriate. The choice of drugs will vary according to profile of drug resistance and national guidelines should be consulted. Drugs that are recommended for therapeutic settings should not be used as prophylaxis to avoid selection of resistant bacterial strains. Antibiotic prophylaxis in scheduled surgery represents huge numbers of doses provided, and this will spur ecological and economical concerns. Uptake of metronidazole and doxycycline is rapid and adequate for prophylaxis following per oral administration in abdominal surgery patients.[61] As doxycycline is concentrated by the liver and excreted into bile in a biologically active form, it is a useful prophylactic drug in hepatobiliary surgery.

INTRAOPERATIVE CARE

PREVENTING POSTOPERATIVE NAUSEA AND VOMITING

Nausea and vomiting postoperatively are as high a concern as pain for both patients and care providers.[62] Risk factors include female sex, non-smoking status and history of motion sickness (or postoperative nausea and vomiting [PONV]), and scoring systems are available.[63] Patients at risk should receive adequate prophylaxis with dexamethasone and/or serotonin receptor antagonists and/or droperidol.[64,65] Anaesthesia by propofol and remifentanil is probably indicated for high-risk individuals.[64] Several other newer agents are emerging and for individuals at risk, a multimodal approach should be employed.[66]

POSTOPERATIVE ANALGESIA

Pain is an inevitable consequence of surgery, but modern analgesia can attenuate this to a level where most patients can ambulate almost immediately after the operation without too much discomfort. The aim should be complete analgesia at rest and only mild pain upon movement. Aiming for complete analgesia during movement is likely to lead to high doses of drugs that may cause counterproductive sleepiness, nausea and contribute to delayed gut function recovery.

THORACIC EPIDURAL

The thoracic epidural catheter has been the keystone of multimodal pain management after surgery in ERAS for three decades. A functional epidural combining local anaesthetic and opioid provides excellent pain relief and attenuates the physiological stress response to surgical trauma by neuroaxial blockade.[67] A recent meta-analysis suggested a beneficial effect on morbidity and mortality,[68] but most of the included trials were conducted in pre-ERAS environments and the role of epidural analgesia as mainstay today is being disputed.[69–71] While epidural infections or haematomas are rare, they may have disastrous consequences. Almost 30% of epidurals have been documented to have sub-optimal function, even in high-volume centres.[72] Hypotension following vasodilatation and impaired mobility are other undesirable side effects that must be weighed against the perceived benefits. Furthermore, many patients experience some degree of 'withdrawal pain' when weaned from epidural analgesia. This pain may be easily controlled by opiates, but the timing is unfortunate as it hits the patient when on the verge of becoming fully mobilised and increasing to a full solid diet. The increasing use of minimally invasive surgery has further reduced the demand for epidural analgesia.

TRANSVERSE ABDOMINAL PLANE BLOCKS

These blocks can be administered in several fashions, usually by a small-bore catheter positioned just superficially to the external oblique fascia with disposable systems delivering a constant dosage of an anaesthetic. It has some of the benefits of an epidural and fewer side effects, but they must be applied correctly either intraoperatively or guided by ultrasonography. Their benefit has been shown in multiple types of abdominal surgery with comparative analgesic properties to epidural[73] and improvements in functional recovery times compared with other types of analgesia.[74]

INTRAVENOUS ANALGESIA

Patient-controlled intravenous analgesia (PCA) with opioids is the modern modification of the oldest analgesic modality. It provides a baseline infusion rate with a possibility for a patient-activated boost. PCA remains the fallback option for failed peripheral blocks, as it is easy to set up. However, opioid effect may vary, and accumulated doses affect gut motility, mobilisation and appetite. Continuous infusion of the local anaesthetic lidocaine is receiving increasing attention,[75–77] and may attenuate surgical stress besides reducing opiate consumption.[76] Another drug group gaining renewed interest are beta-blockers. Besides their well-established cardiovascular effects, they appear to have an intriguing potential as an adjunct in the treatment of postoperative pain.[78,79]

PER ORAL, NON-OPIOID ANALGESICS

Non-steroidal anti-inflammatory drugs (NSAIDs) provide excellent analgesic effect for moderate pain and have served as valuable opioid-sparing adjuncts for decades. A possible association with increased rates of anastomotic failures has spurred several studies with conflicting results.[80–86] For patients with adequate liver function, paracetamol/acetaminophen is safe and can reduce opioid requirements.

ACCESS AND INCISION

The laparoscopic revolution has significantly impacted on patient recovery, most importantly through attenuated stress response and less pain. While there is an obvious reduction in tissue damage through minimal access surgery, the differences in functional recovery (pain, gut function, mobilisation, length of stay) compared with modern ERAS-era open surgery is much smaller than was previously assumed. Functional recovery is an outcome with high risk of observer bias in open-label trials, but it has received most of the attention. As surgical technique is skill-dependent with a learning curve and hard to blind in trials, this issue is not well suited for randomised trials.[17] Observational data (non-randomised, prospective cohort studies) are weakened by the possibility of selection bias and publication bias.

The modern surgeon should master both techniques and choose the one that is best suited to the patient and the operation. As learning curves have been scaled, for colorectal surgery in particular, minimally invasive surgery has become a standard of care with low conversion rates, established training programmes and good short- and long-term outcomes for cancer surgery. In other surgical disciplines, such as liver resection, the minimally invasive approach can be appropriate in the presence of required skill sets in selected cases, with feasibility and good short-term outcomes reported,[87] but the recommendations are less emphatic. While the standard of care is resection, minimally invasive resection is an accepted treatment option in the appropriate setting.[5]

PERIOPERATIVE FLUID BALANCE, BLOOD PRESSURE, OEDEMA AND DIURESIS

Ensuring adequate oxygen supply to crucial tissues is the core task of intraoperative and immediate postoperative care and is heavily dependent on the patient's fluid balance. The newly created anastomosis is at the periphery of the circulatory bed and has had parts of its natural blood supply severed. Its perfusion is vital to the success of the operation, but at present it is impossible to assess directly. Among the surrogate markers of tissue perfusion used are peripheral oxygen saturation in the capillaries of the fingers, blood pressure, central venous pressure (CVP) and urine output as an assumed reflection of renal perfusion. In the presence of some degree of systemic oedema, which is almost invariably the case, the gut is also likely to be oedematous which in turn will compromise local perfusion and hence oxygen delivery. The challenge is to avoid oedema and optimise stroke volume in the well-oxygenated patient.

INTRAOPERATIVE FLUID BALANCE

In the intraoperative period, it is important that fluid management is appropriate, to ensure optimal organ perfusion, whilst avoiding fluid overload which can lead to gut oedema and contribute to ileus. It is well recognised that traditional pressure monitoring of arterial and central pressures gives a poor indication of intravascular filling.

A number of techniques are now available intraoperatively for estimation of cardiac output (flow) and fluid responsiveness, which provide welcome additional information on which to base intraoperative fluid therapy.

Minimally invasive monitors include arterial pulse contour analysis, which can provide data on stroke volume and variations in pressures and stroke volume when the patient is mechanically ventilated allowing an estimate of intravascular volume status; and oesophageal Doppler, which monitors velocity of blood flow in the descending thoracic aorta from which stroke volume and cardiac output can be calculated.

These are dynamic monitors allowing the anaesthetist to provide a fluid challenge either by placing the patient head down or by infusing a given volume of fluid and assessing the response. Algorithms have been published suggesting goals for fluid therapy intraoperatively based on these measurements of stroke volume. A number of studies suggest that application of these may benefit patients by optimising the volume of intraoperative fluid given.

In the intraoperative period, fluid infusion can be optimised by simple techniques. An arterial cannula showing pulse variation synchronous with the ventilatory cycle (pulsus paradoxus) will allow for assessment of whether infused volumes (preload) will lead to increased stroke volume—i.e. a better positioning along the Starling curve. The absence of pulsus paradoxus indicates that no further increase of stroke volume will result from more infused fluids. The same can be achieved by using a Doppler device. This will help the anaesthetist decide whether fluids will increase cardiac output, but not whether the patient is actually in need of increased output. Interestingly, a recent meta-analysis did not show a benefit of goal-directed fluid therapy guided by oesophageal Doppler in patients undergoing major colorectal surgery. The potential explanations cited were the impact of control groups utilising ERAS protocols of fluid restriction, and the awareness of the negative impact of fluid overload during the intraoperative phase with modern practice advocating against liberal fluid administration intraoperatively.[88]

POSTOPERATIVE FLUID BALANCE

The impact of surgery and anaesthesia has severe effects on most aspects of the patient's physiology. For most of the first day and night, normal homeostatic mechanisms are blocked or overridden; positive pressure ventilation, intravenous infusion of litres of fluids, bleeding and epidural blocking of peripheral regulation of vascular resistance are just a few of the challenges. Unfortunately this often leads to a situation on the first morning after surgery where the patient weighs several kilos more than the morning of surgery, a sure sign of fluid accumulation. Blood pressure is variable or low, or maintained by vasopressors, especially in patients with epidurals. Urine output is poor. All this can and should be avoided by better peri- and immediate postoperative fluid control.

In the immediate postoperative period, fluid status is less well measured than intraoperatively and the result is a tendency to treat hypotension and low urine output with large volumes of fluids.[89] As hypotension is often a side effect of epidural analgesia and low urine output a part of the physiological response to trauma, fluids exceeding maintenance volumes might not be needed at all. At the same time, splanchnic hypovolemia must be avoided. Trials evaluating restrictive fluid regimens or the use of goal-directed therapy have often been compared with obsolete regimens and almost exclusively included ASA I and II patients.[1,43,90] Data for high-risk patients are also lacking in this area. This is an important limitation of these trials, as one must assume that the fittest patients probably have significant safety margins, will probably cope well with quite poor fluid regimens and may not be in need of any optimisation.[91] As emphasised by recent guidelines, it is important to offer ASA III and IV patients a dedicated and optimised fluid guidance led by an experienced anaesthetist to ensure optimal tissue oxygenation.[1,43,92]

Frank postoperative hypotension implies inadequate peripheral perfusion. At what level an individual patient has a clinically significant hypotension is difficult to assess and depends on habitual blood pressure and medication. Significant hypotension must be treated and experimental data indicates that blood pressure should be increased with vasopressors even if these drugs cause some vasoconstriction.[93] If normotension cannot be restored, epidurals should be discontinued and replaced with intravenous analgesics. Fluids should be infused only to patients in need of fluids and not as a reflex manoeuvre to treat hypotension. Cessation of intravenous fluids should be achieved as soon as is possible postoperatively and oral fluids commenced.[94]

Fluids are a medication with side effects. The surgeon prescribing them must know the approximate sodium and chloride content of the formulas prescribed and the daily needs of the patient.[95] Balanced fluids should be used in place of 0.9% saline,[96] and high chloride content is probably not beneficial.[97] It is also worth recalling that infusion of sodium- and chloride-containing fluids is much harder to reverse than judicious use of vasopressors.

Attempts at correcting low urine output with bolus infusions of fluid are unnecessary and probably counterproductive.[98,99] We do not know if the low output is caused by renal hypoperfusion at all—or, if so, whether fluids will increase perfusion. The gain from an additional litre of fluid may be a negligible change in CVP or vasopressor dosage, but the only foreseeable clinical result is over-hydration and oedema.

POSTOPERATIVE CARE

NASOGASTRIC DRAINAGE

The nasogastric (or after gastrectomies, the nasojejunal) drainage tube has been another of the hallmarks of traditional postoperative care. They were believed to be crucial to remove gastrointestinal secretions thereby reducing the risk of aspiration, passage of fluids across a freshly created anastomoses or a paralytic gut. Up to a decade ago, they could be left in for a week following a hemicolectomy.[100] Recent data have shown convincingly that they are unnecessary and even harmful and modern guidelines unanimously advise against routine use.[1–3,7,19,43] A minority of patients will suffer gastric emptying problems following surgery, mostly following Whipple's procedures (pancreatoduodenectomy) where the duodenum is removed. The incidence is lower than previously suggested and they might need a tube on-demand in selected cases. Oesophageal resections pose specific challenges with a positive pressure environment for a denervated gastric conduit frequently resulting in conduit dilatation and risk of aspiration. Decompression tubes should not be removed in these patients without the responsible surgeons being consulted. The default routine in all but oesophageal resections should be to remove the tube before leaving theatre.

GLYCAEMIC CONTROL

The trauma of surgery usually induces a phase of insulin resistance that leads to poorly controlled serum glucose levels. Patients at risk who undergo large operations frequently behave as if having temporary type II diabetes, and an increased susceptibility to infectious complications has been suggested. Reduced rates of infections in critically ill patients intensively treated with insulin was shown in a large trial from 2001,[101] but this has not been reproduced and there are no data to support such treatment outside of the ICU.[102] Modern guidelines suggest glycaemic control well within safety limits to avoid hypoglycaemia.[6]

SURGICAL WOUND DRAINS

This issue is yet another of the traditional pillars being challenged by modern routines.[1–3,19,42–45] A well working drain which drains copious volumes of amylase-rich content following a pancreatic resection will appear as a success when it dries up after a week without any further intervention. This is not often the situation. A variety of drain types and calibres, passive or with suction, all have a tendency to become clogged or dislodged or kinked. A dry drain is either a signal that the patient is doing well, or that the drain is doing badly. There are other and better ways of telling the former. Drains can be painful, prevent mobilisation or even erode into the gut or blood vessels if left for extended periods of time. In the majority of patients, they have no mission as most anastomoses don't leak and most resections don't bleed! Even for pancreatic surgery, where routine use of drains have been studied extensively,[43] robust conclusions are wanting in spite of extensively stratifying patients according to duct calibre and gland texture or volume. The jury is still out regarding the correct cut-off, but pancreatic resections and urology aside,[1,43] the tendency is to use them less and less in straightforward cases. Importantly, the scenario has also changed during recent decades because of modern ultrasound- or CT-guided drainage procedures. Most abscesses, bilomas, haematomas or other fluid accumulations may be drained percutaneously on demand with a small-bore drain that may later be upsized if necessary.

STIMULATION OF BOWEL MOVEMENT

Some degree of gut paralysis will follow any abdominal operation, but the spectrum of clinical presentation is considerable. The small bowel may regain function almost immediately; the remnant stomach after a Whipple's procedure will sometimes need a week or more. Following a large bowel resection, the typical duration is 1–3 days. The symptoms are vomiting or gastric distension needing decompression by NG tube, distended abdomen, nausea and pain. On top of a major operation, it is a very uncomfortable situation. When duration exceeds a few days, the condition impedes mobilisation, halts intake of food and drink and frequently causes anxiety. Stimulating bowel movement after surgery is a key target for perioperative care.

The strategy should be multimodal. Comprehensive protocols within modern enhanced recovery guidelines[1–3,19,42–45] have focused extensively on these strategies. It is likely that the sum of many small adjustments of the perioperative pathway acting in concert will shorten the duration of postoperative gut paralysis to a minimum. Relevant interventions include:

Early oral intake of food and drink is supposed to aid in stimulating bowel movement, but this is hard to prove scientifically as the intervention itself becomes the target. It is however likely that vagal stimulation by smell, taste, chewing and swallowing may stimulate bowel movement.

Chewing gum has been proposed as a cheap and safe way of achieving the same stimulation of vagal reflexes even in patients who do not yet have appetite for eating. A recent meta-analysis of RCTs reported benefit of chewing gum in reducing postoperative ileus in patients undergoing colorectal surgery.[103]

Optimal fluid balance avoiding both hypovolemia and gut oedema is vital.[104]

Epidural analgesia with local anaesthetics in combination with low doses of opioids was for decades a cornerstone of modern regimens.[42,44] The 'opioid-sparing' effect of the epidural was considered a crucial part of the ERP. The increased use of laparoscopy, comprehensive protocols, modern opioids with less motility-blocking effect and other non-opioid analgesic drugs have shifted interest away from the routine use of epidural analgesia.

Minimally invasive surgery (i.e. laparoscopy or robotics) causes less gut manipulation and less tissue trauma and is hence associated with shorter duration of postoperative ileus.

Several pharmaceutical interventions have received considerable attention, but the magic drug remains elusive. Alvimopan is a partial μ-receptor antagonist, i.e. an opioid supposed to induce less gut paralysis. The effect on gut function postoperatively has been evaluated in several studies with conflicting results,[105–108] and additional benefit for patients already treated by modern, enhanced recovery routines is disputed.[109,110] Alvimopan is currently not available for routine use in Europe. Intravenous lidocaine in a recent meta-analysis[111] showed reduced time to gut function and reduced postoperative ileus compared with placebo, representing a further opiate-sparing intervention.

Magnesium oxide was an integral part of the first ERAS guidelines mainly aimed at open colonic surgery.[42] A placebo-controlled trial conducted for colonic surgery in the context of modern enhanced recovery principles failed to confirm a beneficial effect.[112]

✔✔ There is no compelling evidence that any single intervention to stimulate gut activity can be recommended, but a multimodal approach as suggested in ERAS guidelines will reduce time to resumption of gut function.

POSTOPERATIVE ARTIFICIAL NUTRITION

It is important to distinguish oral intake, i.e. eating, which is the volitional and natural intake of ordinary food, from enteral nutrition. Enteral nutrition is a non-volitional, artificial way of providing nutrients through tube or catheter. Nil-by-mouth implies that the patient does not eat or drink, regardless of whether enteral tube feeding is provided or not. The enteral versus parenteral nutrition controversy of the 90s obscured this distinction and wrongly grouped enteral nutrition with natural oral diet.[113]

With the exception—again—for patients undergoing oesophagectomies, all patients should have their NG tubes out and be offered drink and food without delay postoperatively, as soon as they are fully awake and not bothered by nausea. Oral intake at will has been a part of colorectal and liver guidelines for a decade or more.[42,44,45] Oral diet at will is now also recommended for gastrectomies and pancreatoduodenectomies.[2,43] Care is required following the latter as some patients may also have a problem with gastric motility. This means that they need to be well counselled about their altered physiology and digestion. They should be advised to begin carefully and increase according to tolerance.[2,43]

Some patients will need enteral tube feeding or parenteral nutrition, but—save oesophagectomies—these are the exception. Even patients who have undergone emergency surgery for obstruction or perforation will generally tolerate food within 2–4 days. Artificial nutrition becomes an option in a patient who cannot eat. This might be due to rare cases of delayed gastric emptying, long-standing gut paralysis, re-operations, complications, unconscious patients, etc.

Routine provision of hypercaloric supplements to patients who are eating have been evaluated in colorectal surgery. Beneficial effects on surrogate endpoints like hand grip strength or insulin resistance have been demonstrated,[114] but effects on meaningful clinical endpoints have not been shown convincingly. One trial showed an impressive reduction from 9 to 6.5 days length of stay, but without any difference in hand grip strength or time to return of gut function.[115] Such findings must be viewed with caution as bias is highly probably and must be confirmed or refuted by placebo-controlled double-blinded trials with an iso-nitrogenous control. Post-discharge oral supplements were reviewed in 2009 without showing any effect,[116] and neither has intense dietary advice to patients at risk been shown to confer benefit.[117]

✔✔ All patients—save those undergoing oesophagectomies—should as a routine have their NG tube out as they leave theatre and be offered to drink and eat on demand. They should be advised to begin cautiously and to increase according to tolerance.

EARLY AND SCHEDULED MOBILISATION

Mobilisation prevents loss of lean muscle and thromboembolic complications. Being independently mobile is an inherent part of the composite process we call functional recovery. It is probably easier to achieve independent mobilisation if there are set targets to be met and when the patient has a schedule to adhere to.[42,44] There are no RCTs to prove this, but it is a concept that is unsuited for this methodology and probably unethical to attempt!

Key points

- Preoperative care has developed from patient counselling and smoking cessation advice to multifaceted prehabilitation programmes.
- Perioperative analgesia techniques have progressed beyond only thoracic epidural with local anaesthetic wound infiltration devices or intravenous local anaesthesia being increasingly utilised.
- Minimally invasive surgery continues to complement perioperative care pathways and remains a core ERAS principle, and its application is increasingly used in a variety of surgical sub-specialties where appropriate.
- Postoperative care is focused on early intake of normal food and mobilisation. Care pathways should prioritise these care components.

References available at http://ebooks.health.elsevier.com/

KEY REFERENCES

[8] Nicholson A, et al. Systematic review and meta-analysis of enhanced recovery programmes in surgical patients. Br J Surg 2014;101(3):172–88.
Important systematic review identifying the benefits of ERAS protocol on post operative outcomes including length of stay and morbidity.

[33] Dunne DF, et al. Randomized clinical trial of prehabilitation before planned liver resection. Br J Surg 2016;103(5):504–12.
Significant prehabilitation RCT in major abdominal surgery showing benefits of pre operative protocols.

[56] Felder S, et al. Prolonged thromboprophylaxis with low molecular weight heparin for abdominal or pelvic surgery. Cochrane Database Syst Rev 2019;8:CD004318.
Large review identifying benefit of prolonged LMWH administration.

[71] Hughes MJ, et al. Analgesia after open abdominal surgery in the setting of enhanced recovery surgery: a systematic review and meta-analysis. JAMA Surg 2014;149(12):1224–30.
Systematic review illustrating the impact of the analgesic modality within the ERAS protocol.

3 Organisation and quality improvement in emergency general surgery

Thomas G. Weiser | Katherine J. Broughton

INTRODUCTION

Emergency general surgery (EGS) is a core component of general surgical practice. The challenges of caring for such patients include time-sensitive conditions, additional morbidity and mortality commensurate with this particular patient population, frequent diagnostic uncertainty, unpredictability, and the irregular consumption of hospital resources. EGS patients are increasingly managed by a multidisciplinary emergency surgical team requiring appropriate resources. Given the importance of this patient population and the changes to practice in many settings, particularly larger referral and teaching hospitals, emergency and acute care surgery is now being recognised as a distinct specialty by many colleges, professional associations and hospitals. This advance recognises the reality of increasing subspecialisation and the move to provide dedicated care for this patient population, with the resultant growth of emergency and acute care surgery models of care delivery.[1]

EGS services have been shown to improve the timeliness of care and reduce complications, yet postoperative morbidity is still very common.[2,3] Coordination of care, efficient application of resources, access to services and timely intervention are of paramount importance. A study from the USA of 421 476 patients who required EGS between 2008 and 2011 found that the seven most common emergency procedures (partial colectomy, small bowel resection, cholecystectomy, operative management of peptic ulcer disease, lysis of peritoneal adhesions, appendicectomy and laparotomy) accounted for 80% of activity, 80% of mortality, 79% of morbidity and 80% of the costs of the EGS cohort.[4]

The American College of Surgeons' National Surgical Quality Improvement Project (ACS-NSQIP) examined the results of emergency appendicectomy, cholecystectomy and colorectal (CR) resections in 95 hospitals between 2005 and 2008.[5] The risk of severe morbidity or death was 3.7% in the 30 788 appendicectomies performed, 6.37% in 5824 cholecystectomies and 41.56% in 8990 CR resections. High morbidity and mortality is particularly apparent when comparing high-, middle- and low-income countries: in the first GlobalSurg study evaluating outcomes following EGS, mortality was three times higher in low- than in high-income settings.[6]

Given that earlier clinical decision-making and prompt and appropriate surgery reduces length of stay (LoS) and readmissions, improving efficiency is critical. The creation of a dedicated EGS service, separated completely from elective surgical care, has been recommended by a number of professional societies, including the Royal College of Surgeons of England[7]; it is now commonplace in North America, Europe and Australia. Where program certification exists, additional improvements in outcomes have been described.[8]

The variation worldwide in operative experience for trainees in general surgery remains a concern.[9] Providing a dedicated service through which trainees rotate allows for a more concrete and mentored approach to managing these complex conditions, with structured opportunities for training. This also promotes the early assessment of patients by senior surgeons interested and experienced in these conditions coupled with access to radiological investigations and operating theatres for timely surgical intervention.[10,11] The Association of Surgeons of Great Britain and Ireland (ASGBI) conducted a survey of UK consultant surgeons: 55% reported that although they were able to care well for their emergency patients, the workload was increasing while junior support was decreasing; only 19% had comprehensive interventional radiology service out of hours; and 55% felt they had inadequate access to an emergency operating theatre. The results are summarised in Box 3.1. The ASGBI has established an Emergency General Surgery Advisory Board to look specifically at ways of improving the delivery of all aspects of EGS and supporting clinicians who provide this care.[12]

SPECIALISATION IN EMERGENCY AND ACUTE CARE SURGERY

While appropriate support for EGS is critical to improving resources and timeliness of care, such conditions are often best treated by surgeons with a particular interest in and experience with them, and within a surgical team and hospital system organised for this purpose.[13] This mirrors development in other specialty practices, e.g. the regional centralisation of specific high-risk operations.[14] This move to consolidate practices and performance of high-risk operations such as oesophagectomy, gastrectomy, abdominal aortic aneurysm repair, lung lobectomy and colectomy reflects the generally accepted observations of the volume-outcome relationship.[15–19] In addition to surgical volume, institutional and team specialisation also appears to be an important factor.[20–22] Evidence now supports similar improvements in patient outcomes for EGS procedures such as acute gallstone disease, appendicitis, peptic ulcer disease and CR disorders.[23–25] Given the move towards

Box 3.1 A summary of the conclusions of the consensus meeting of the Association of Surgeons of Great Britain and Ireland (ASGBI) in 2006 on emergency general surgery

1. There is wide variation in the quality of emergency general surgery (EGS).
2. EGS is a huge clinical service with approximately 1000 finished consultant episodes per 100 000 population per year.
3. All hospitals should have a named surgeon responsible for the clinical leadership of EGS.
4. Emergency admissions must have dedicated resources and senior surgical personnel readily available.
5. There must be a clear and identifiable separation of delivery of emergency and elective care.
6. Local circumstances will determine the model of delivery.

subspecialisation that has occurred in general surgery over the last several decades, dedicated emergency surgery teams lead by consultant surgeons may be best placed to manage such conditions.[26]

In the USA and Canada, there is now a specialist association of Acute Care Surgery (http://www.aast.org/AcuteCareSurgery) that exists within the American Association for the Surgery of Trauma (AAST). This professional organisation is for surgeons specialising in the care of the injured and critically ill surgical patients, as well as for the organisation and management of EGS. Beyond general surgery, board certification by the American Board of Surgery is awarded in Surgical Critical Care and allows surgeons to manage and provide comprehensive care for surgical patients in the intensive care unit. The fellowship is one year long, with the option to engage in a second year of acute care surgery, typically as a junior faculty member with oversight and guidance provided by more experienced acute care and critical care surgeons. This service has been demonstrated to reduce hospital LoS, costs, and increase efficiency. In a study of 1363 emergency surgery patients comparing management between trauma and critical care-trained surgeons versus general surgeons and subspecialists, trauma and critical care-trained surgeons saw 61% of the patients, and while there was no difference in operative management between the two groups, patients cared for by trauma and critical care-trained surgeons spent significantly less time waiting for an operation (7 vs 13 hours). Patients with acute appendicitis and acute cholecystitis also had shorter hospital stay (2.5 vs 2.8 days), and lower emergency department costs ($822 vs $876).[27]

There is, however, wide variation in how EGS services are organised and implemented.[28] In structured interviews with leaders of acute care surgery in the USA, respondents noted variability in whether services included trauma, elective general surgery, scheduled operating room time, and the sharing of responsibilities with other specialist surgeons. Other variations included whether formal sign out was performed, prospective data collection and the use of evidence-based protocols. The biggest concern was that this service might become a 'wastebasket for everything that happens at inconvenient times'.

ORGANISATION OF ELECTIVE AND EMERGENCY SURGERY CARE

Over the past decades, many large medical centres have rearranged services to separate emergency and elective general surgery, with the goal of providing a dedicated acute surgical team to provide continuity for these high-risk patients. This separation is typically provided in one of two ways: a 'surgeon-of-the-day' rota with a dedicated consultant on call without conflicting clinical duties, or an Acute Surgical Unit (ASU) where all emergency patients are managed by a single team, typically with oversight by a consultant providing Monday–Friday continuity. ASUs now exist to manage such patients throughout the USA, Australia, New Zealand, the UK and Asia. The division between teams performing elective and EGS creates a dedicated surgical unit typically consisting of a consultant, trainee surgeons and junior doctors who can assess, investigate and manage EGS patients efficiently (Box 3.2). In comparison to a surgeon/general surgical team having simultaneous elective and emergency responsibilities, this achieves improved ED assessment times, earlier investigations, 24/7 access to an emergency operating theatre and greater familiarity with acute general surgical conditions.

There is evidence that the ASU approach reduces mortality and morbidity. The ACS-NSQIP data from the USA demonstrated a reduced 30-day mortality in EGS patients treated in hospitals with an ASU model for EGS, especially in patients undergoing intestinal resections (30-day mortality 8.5% in ASU hospitals compared with 11.6% for all patients).[29] This evidence has been reproduced in Australia, with higher index admission operation rates, shorter LoS, and reduced morbidity in patients requiring acute cholecystectomy.[30] Most Australian units have embraced the ASU model and the General Surgeon Association (GSA) published a 12-point plan for EGS.[31] In Singapore, which has more recently introduced the ASU model, data further confirmed reduced LoS and mortality (reduction in mean LoS from 4.5 to 3.5 days and mortality from 1.9% to 0.9%).[32]

The separation of elective and emergency services was adopted in many UK hospitals in the late 1990s and typically consists of the Emergency Surgical Consultant (ESC) rather than the ASU model more commonly observed elsewhere. The ASGBI published a joint document with CR and upper gastrointestinal (UGI) subspeciality associations in 2015, making clear recommendations for the management of EGS including many of the key tenets mentioned above.[33]

While having a dedicated surgical team to manage EGS patients reduces mortality and morbidity, the organisation of services may include a surgical assessment unit (SAU) to facilitate assessment and admission, timely access to investigations (notably radiology), and a dedicated emergency operating theatre. Depending on the size of a hospital and the number of EGS patients, the details of this set-up may differ.

For example, the Edinburgh, UK, experience with consultant-staffed 'hot' clinics reduced the need for inpatient admissions (85.0% vs 78.2% vs 54.4% before, 4 weeks and 6 months after clinic introduction, respectively) and shorter mean inpatient admission (64 vs 49 hours).[34] Such a clinic allows general practitioners to refer directly to a consultant surgeon for rapid assessment, a quicker review

Box 3.2 Summary of recommendations for separation of emergency and elective surgical care[7]

1. A physical separation of services, facilities and rotas works best, although a separate unit on the same site is preferable to a completely separate location.
2. The presence of senior surgeons for both elective and emergency work will enhance patient safety and the quality of care, and ensure that training opportunities are maximised.
3. The separation of emergency and elective surgical care can facilitate protected and concentrated training for junior surgeons providing consultants are available to supervise their work.
4. Creating an 'emergency team', linked with a 'surgeon of the week', is a good method of providing dedicated and supervised training in all aspects of emergency and elective care.
5. Separating emergency and elective services can prevent the admission of emergency patients (both medical and surgical) from disrupting planned activity and vice versa, thus minimising patient inconvenience and maximising productivity for the hospital. The success of this will largely depend on having sufficient beds and resources for each service.
6. Hospital-acquired infections can be reduced by the provision of protected elective wards and avoiding admissions from the emergency department and transfers from within/outside the hospital.
7. The improved use of information technology (IT) solutions can assist with separating workloads (e.g. scheduling systems for appointments and theatres, telemedicine, picture archiving and communication systems), although it is recognised that developments in IT for the NHS are generally behind schedule.
8. High-volume specialities are particularly suited to separating two strands of work. Other specialities can also benefit by having emergencies seen by senior surgeons—this can help to reduce unnecessary admissions, deal with ward emergencies and facilitate rapid discharge.

of patients with acute abdominal pain in the emergency department, and in-person senior review of patients sent home after hours. Such a clinic must have ready access to radiological investigations (ultrasound [US], computed tomography [CT] and magnetic resonance cholangiopancreatography [MRCP] as required), bed space for short-term observation and review, as well as nursing and trainee doctors' support.

OUTCOMES OF SUBSPECIALITY CARE IN EMERGENCY GENERAL SURGERY

While some countries such as the USA have moved to an Acute Care Surgery specialty model for managing EGS, many have shifted towards acute general surgery being undertaken by subspecialty upper and lower GI surgeons, or having on-call rosters of such surgeons to allow speciality care for hepatobiliary, oesophagogastric or CR emergencies. There is some evidence for improved outcomes when emergency laparotomies are undertaken by GI surgeons, in particular when CR emergencies are treated by specialist CR surgeons. National Emergency Laparotomy Audit (NELA, see below) data from nearly 38 000 patients indicated a higher 30-day mortality rate in both CR and gastroduodenal procedures undertaken by non-CR and non-UGI surgeons, respectively (all-cause risk-adjusted OR 1.23 [95% CI 1.13–1.33] and 1.24 [95% CI 1.02–1.53], respectively). LoS and returns to theatre were also lower in CR operations performed by CR surgeons.[35] A Spanish observational study examined CR patients between 1993 and 2006 and assessed rates of primary anastomosis and stoma formation in emergency colectomies performed by CR or General Surgeons. The primary anastomosis rate was significantly higher, 30-day mortality (17.9% vs 28.3%), morbidity (52.2% vs 60.5%) and anastomotic leak rate (6.2% vs 12.1%) were lower in the procedures performed by a CR surgeon.[36]

Edinburgh, UK, has a long-established subspecialty service for upper and lower GI emergencies. A comparison of emergency left-sided large bowel resections by CR and UGI surgeons found that two-thirds of the resections were undertaken by CR surgeons with the primary anastomosis rate higher (64.3% vs 36.5%) and mortality rate (10.4% vs 17.4%) lower than UGI surgeons; anastomotic leak rate did not differ between the surgeon types.[37] A subsequent publication highlighted the differences brought about by separation of UGI and CR units across two hospital sites, providing 24-hour subspeciality surgical care in the city: primary anastomosis rates increased (50.3% vs 77.9%) and stoma formation decreased (46.6% vs. 27.7%) in colonic resections for diverticular disease, accompanied by a corresponding fall in mortality from 3.3% to 1.5%.[25]

Outside of the UK and Europe, similar findings have been noted in Australia and the USA. In 196 consecutive left-sided emergency CR resections from a single institution in Australia, resections performed by a subspeciality CR surgeon noted higher primary anastomosis rates (85.5% vs 28.7%) and lower stoma formation rates (40.4% vs 88.8%) without significant differences in 30-day mortality, anastomotic dehiscence or LoS.[38] In a retrospective study from New York State involving 10 780 patients undergoing urgent/emergency colectomy for diverticulitis between 2000 and 2014, operation by a CR surgeon was associated with a significantly lower odds of death (OR 0.66, 95% CI 0.46–0.96), but no difference in morbidity or LoS.[39]

Subspecialist care of EGS is not suitable for provincial or small hospitals where general, breast and/or endocrine surgeons still service an EGS on-call roster. NELA reported that 40% of CR resections were performed by non-CR surgeons, while in the New York State study 94% of cases were performed by non-CR surgeons; this sizable workload is not likely amenable to care exclusively by subspecialists. Removing other specialist surgeons from on-call rosters may substantially increase the burden of out of hours work on subspecialty CR and UGI surgeons, and further contribute to the de-skilling of the surgeon workforce. Furthermore, the ASU model provides training and experience in emergency general surgical procedures including the majority of CR and UGI emergency conditions. A UK study from 2006 looked at the discrepancy between subspecialisation of the consultant surgeon providing after-hours care and the surgical condition: 30% of the high-complexity cases did not match the surgeon's subspecialty interest, of which the majority occurred after-hours; most of these were complex CR conditions.[40] The size, location and staffing of a unit will ultimately dictate the specific arrangement of a general surgical unit and the provision of on-call surgeons. However, particularly in the setting of complex CR emergencies, patients appear to have better outcomes when operated on by a CR surgeon.

Notably, none of the studies cited above controlled for provider experience even though surgeon factors are known to contribute to variability in outcomes.[41] In one of the few studies evaluating this issue in EGS, investigators assessed the impact of surgeon experience on outcomes of care in 772 patients undergoing emergency surgery (defined as going directly to the operating theatre from the emergency room, excluding appendicectomy, cholecystectomy, and simple incision and drainage procedures) for trauma (51.3%) or other acute surgical conditions (48.7%) from five USA academic trauma centres.[42] They divided consultant surgeons by years of experience and noted that the vast majority of patients (83%) underwent an operation by a surgeon with 10 or less years of experience. Mortality, complications and LoS were similar between surgeon experience groups, but patients undergoing surgery by early-career surgeons had higher rates of unplanned return to the operating theatre. Surgeons with less than 3 years of experience had similar mortality rates compared with the rest of the cohort (OR = 1.97, 95% CI 0.85–4.57) but higher rates of complications (OR = 2.07, 95% CI 1.05–4.07). Surgeon experience and hospital volume matter across a host of surgical conditions; given that matching specific subspecialisation to specific surgical conditions is impractical, these attributes could likely be leveraged to improve EGS outcomes across a health system.

FACILITIES AND RESOURCES

The resources available in all hospitals providing emergency surgical care and the subsequent outcomes are clearly important issues. The results of an audit of 367 796 emergency general surgical operations for higher-risk surgical conditions (average national 30-day mortality rate > 5%) in 145 hospitals in England between 2000 and 2009 demonstrated an overall 30-day mortality of 15.6% (range 9.2–18.2%).[43] Independent risk factors distinguishing low- and high-performing hospitals included access to critical care beds and early use of CT. Another study, undertaken during a similar time period (2005–2010) evaluated higher-risk EGS patients and reported mortality of between 1.6% and 8% for all patients admitted (not just undergoing emergency surgery), again demonstrating a significant difference between hospitals, based on their staffing and infrastructure.[44] The lowest mortality rates were observed in hospitals with higher levels of medical and nursing staffing, and a greater number of operating theatres and critical care beds relative to provider size. Further studies indicates that the higher the complexity of care managed by an organisation, the better the outcomes.[45] In a study of patients undergoing one of five high-risk operations—above-knee amputation, abdominal aortic aneurysm repair, coronary artery bypass graft, colon resection and small bowel resection—in 2691 hospitals in the USA, hospitals that were identified as 'complex' (as defined by the number of unique primary diagnoses admitted to each hospital) had lower surgical mortality rates even after adjusting for surgical volume. Patients receiving care at the hospitals in the lowest quintile of complexity had a 27% higher risk of death than those in the highest quintile.

For an emergency team system to work efficiently, patients must have rapid access to diagnostic blood tests, appropriate imaging, including plain and contrast radiographs interventional radiology (including percutaneous drainage and angiography, US and CT. There is increasing use of interventional radiology networks as not all hospitals receiving emergencies have this expertise. In addition, it is not always advisable to delay transfer for life-saving therapy in order to fully deploy the diagnostic investigations available at local facilities, and clinical judgement must be balanced with potential delays in urgently needed care.

There remains some controversy as to whether admission during the week or at weekends alters risk of mortality in surgical patients. One very large study that retrospectively examined 14 217 640 patients admitted to NHS England hospitals as an emergency between 2009 and 2010 observed 187 337 in-hospital deaths within 30 days.[46] This study included all patients from all specialities and noted the risk of death was higher following admission at the weekend. There has been some disagreement in these findings: a study looking at 50 844 general surgical patients in Scotland who underwent emergency surgery between 2005 and 2007 failed to demonstrate any difference in either short- or long-term mortality according to whether the surgery took place during the week or at the weekend,[47] although a recent meta-analysis of over 1.4 million patients did indicate an increased odds of death on the weekend relative to weekday admissions (OR = 1.27; 95% CI = 1.08–1.49).[48] Resources, staffing and management capabilities are undoubtedly relevant issues, and where similar structures and standards exist between midweek and weekend care, mortality appears to be lower.

Another important consideration in survival pertains to the important role the hospital system plays in the ability to 'rescue' patients following complications, and its role in hospital mortality and quality initiatives. This concept, called 'failure to rescue' or more recently 'capacity to rescue', has led to studies demonstrating that infrastructure, organisation and management characteristics play important roles in improving outcomes.[49,50] Failure to rescue has been proposed as a measure of the overall standard of care of a facility.[51] Given the complexity of management, hospitals require supportive infrastructure and appropriate human and technical resources to deliver optimum care, including appropriate oversight and staffing. The Academy of Medical Royal Colleges[52] provides clear standards for consultant-delivered care in all specialities, not just surgery:

1. *Standard 1*: Hospital inpatients should be reviewed by an on-site consultant at least once every 24 hours, 7 days a week, unless it has been determined that this would not affect the patient's care pathway.
2. *Standard 2*: Consultant-supervised interventions and investigations along with reports should be provided 7 days a week if the results will change the outcome or status of the patient's care pathway before the next 'normal' working

day. This should include interventions which will enable immediate discharge or a shortened length of hospital stay.
3. *Standard 3*: Support services both in hospitals and in the primary care setting in the community should be available 7 days a week to ensure that the next steps in the patient's care pathway, as determined by the daily consultant-led review, can be taken.

QUALITY IMPROVEMENT INITIATIVES

Between 2007 and 2015, the Royal College of Surgeons of England and the National Confidential Enquiry into Patient Outcome and Death (NCEPOD)[53] produced several reports around the management of high-risk, elderly and emergency non-cardiac surgical patients, with a particular focus on EGS patients.

A major advance in the understanding of the variability in care and management was produced by the UK NELA.[54] Given that these patients are at particularly high risk, the Royal College of Anaesthetists undertook this work and published the first-year results in 2015. The aim of the audit was to examine how many patients received what was considered to be the recommended standard of care based on accepted guidelines (Box 3.3).

The group collected detailed data on over 20 000 emergency laparotomies (representing approximately 83% of all emergency laparotomies performed in the UK) across 192 NHS hospitals in England and Wales, comparing care of these patients to standard of care guidelines. The first report noted an11.7% in-hospital mortality with wide variation amongst hospitals. The second NELA report measured similar but more refined standards of care noted in Box 3.4 in 186 hospitals and 23 000 patients, noting a slightly lower mortality of 11.1%.[55]

These studies prompted further attempts to improve outcomes for emergency abdominal surgery. The implementation of an acute high-risk abdominal surgery (AHA) protocol—including continuous staff education, consultant-led care, early resuscitation and high-dose antibiotics, surgery within 6 hours, perioperative stroke volume-guided haemodynamic optimisation, intermediate level of care for the first 24 hours after surgery, standardised analgesic treatment, early postoperative ambulation and early enteral nutrition—in 600 patients resulted in a significantly lower postoperative mortality rate compared with 600 historic controls (unadjusted 30-day mortality rate was 15.5% vs 21.8% in the control cohort).[56] This improvement was still significant at 180 days (22.2% vs 29.5%). Another improvement study involved the introduction of an emergency laparotomy pathway quality improvement care (ELPQuiC) bundle into four hospitals in England.[57] The care bundle consisted of: initial assessment with early warning scores, early antibiotics, interval between decision and operation of less than 6 hours, goal-directed fluid therapy and postoperative intensive care. There was an associated increase in the number of lives saved per 100 patients treated in all hospitals, from 6.5 in the baseline interval (299 patients) to 12.4 after implementation (427 patients), with risk of death reduced from 15.6% to 9.6%. The Emergency Laparotomy Collaborative (ELC) similarly assessed the impact of an evidence-based care bundle in 28 hospitals in the south of England, again with reduced mortality (unadjusted mortality 9.8% to 8.3%) and mean LoS (20.1 to 18.9 days) associated with implementation of a standardised care bundle.[58]

Box 3.3 Recommended standards for managing emergency general surgical patients who require laparotomy based on the first NELA report

1. **Before surgery**
   - Clinical review and formulation of a care plan by a consultant surgeon soon after admission to hospital.
   - Ready availability of diagnostic investigations to help define the need for and type of surgery.
   - Formal assessment of a patient's risk of death and complications.
   - Prompt administration of antibiotics where there is evidence of infection.
   - Prompt access to an operating theatre.
2. **During surgery**
   - Direct care by a consultant surgeon and consultant anaesthetist.
3. **After surgery**
   - Planned admission to critical care for patients when the estimated risk of death exceeds 5%.
   - Review of patients older than 70 years by specialists in Medicine for Care of the Older Person.

Box 3.4 Revised standards of care for managing emergency general surgical patients who require laparotomy as defined in the second NELA report

1. **Timeliness of care**
   - Review by a consultant surgeon within 14 hours of admission.
   - Prompt administration of antibiotics (when indicated).
   - CT scans reported by a consultant radiologist before surgery.
   - Access to theatres without delay.
2. **Appropriate level of care guided by assessment of risks of complications and death**
   - Documented assessment, before surgery, of the risks of surgery.
   - Review before surgery by consultant surgeon and anaesthetist for high-risk patients.
   - Presence of consultant surgeon and anaesthetist in theatre for high-risk patients.
   - Admission to critical care after surgery for high-risk patients.
   - Input from Elderly Medicine specialists in the care of older patient.

NELA published its sixth report in 2020, noting a reduction in 30-day mortality to 9.3% over the previous 5 years with reduced LoS and increased consultant presence in preoperative decision-making and intraoperative attendance.[59] The improvement in outcomes was attributed to improved compliance with a care bundle similar to that in the ELPQuiC study, notably risk assessment, critical care admissions and reduced delay to definitive surgical intervention.[57]

Other national programs have evaluated mortality in these high-risk patients. In the USA, the ACS-NSQIP collects data to predict outcomes and risk. The published 30-day mortality following emergency laparotomy is 14%, comparable to that reported in the UK.[60] In Australasia, the college's ANZELA-QI (Australian and New Zealand Emergency Laparotomy Audit-Quality Improvement) is underway in pilot form in its third year since its inception in 2018. In-hospital mortality has been comparatively low at 7.1% when benchmarking against international standards.[61–64] Widespread variation between units has been demonstrated. The reasons behind the lower mortality are still unclear without higher-quality nation-wide data but may be associated with avoiding operating on the highest risk patients in whom survival is unlikely, and the geographic arrangement of EGS resulting in a larger proportion of cases being performed in tertiary centres despite relatively low compliance with evidence-based standards of care.[61,62]

Since the introduction of emergency surgery audits, overall compliance with evidence-based practices has improved and most studies have demonstrated a reduction in mortality following intervention. Between years 1 and 6, NELA demonstrated a 20% reduction in 30-day mortality. NELA and similar improvement projects in EGS patients have spurred other countries to assess their outcomes and gather data in order to understand practices and opportunities for improved quality. Changes have been instigated at government level, within the structure of acute general surgical units and by treating clinicians themselves. In the UK, Best Practice Tariffs (BPTs) provide increased funding to NHS trusts for achieving evidence-based care. The current BPT for an emergency laparotomy patient requires the presence of a consultant surgeon and anaesthetist, and direct admission to critical care, in at least 80% of high-risk patients.

However, implementation still faces challenges, exemplified by the EPOCH study (Enhanced PeriOperative Care for the High-Risk surgical patients), a multicentre stepped-wedge cluster randomised trial over a 85-week period across 90 NHS hospitals with over 8000 emergency laparotomy patients.[65] In this study, a quality improvement bundle was introduced to units based on geographical clusters, but no reductions in 90-day mortality were noted on an intention-to-treat analysis. Implementation struggles, diverted resources and slow rates of uptake were cited as potential reasons for the lack of improvement.

SUMMARY

There is no doubt that the delivery of emergency general surgical care has improved, concurrent with support by the colleges, associations and individual hospitals. The use of specific services and the identification of cohorts of emergency surgery patients can allow for the benchmarking of specific quality metrics, as even the use of a small subset of common emergency procedures represents the vast majority of emergency laparotomies while also accounting for the vast majority of costs, morbidity and mortality.[4] Quality indicators can be identified and used to improve care practices and routines[66] and leverage experience, hospital capabilities and service organisation to obtain improvements in decision-making, care and outcomes.[65] In addition, the concepts of 'hot-spotting' and deviant outlier assessments can help improve underperforming facilities.[67]

Efficiencies in delivery have been assisted by regional reorganisation of services, separation of elective and emergency surgical services and, in some units, dividing upper and lower GI care. Specialist care in particular has helped drive this improvement, using consultants with particular interest in emergency surgical care.[35] Provision of acute receiving wards and observation facilities greatly helps such service delivery along with senior surgeon-delivered 'Hot Clinics'. Resources in each hospital must be put in place to facilitate the optimum management of emergency general surgical patients and should include: care protocols; early consultant assessment and decision-making, and direct involvement in emergency surgery; ready access to appropriate investigations including CT with consultant radiologist reporting; appropriate use of, and access to, critical care beds; and clear lines of communication across the institution. Service models are continually in development as the nature of surgical care changes, but many units are now supporting improved practices and demonstrating models of how these services can evolve.

Key points

- Regular reassessment of patients admitted with acute abdominal pain is essential and facilities should be provided so that emergency patients are kept in an area of the hospital where regular review is facilitated. Introduction of a consultant-led 'Hot Clinic' further facilitates this process, reduces hospital admissions and speeds up decision-making.
- The ability to provide adequate emergency surgical care, with careful observation, reassessment and early access to the operating theatre, is best provided by dedicated emergency surgical teams without elective commitments.
- Swift access to investigations and an emergency theatre is an essential requisite for the appropriate management of patients with acute abdominal pain.
- Although emergency subspecialisation has great attractions for the overall care of the emergency patient with complex problems, this area of development will depend very much on local resources and workload.

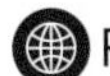 References available at http://ebooks.health.elsevier.com/

KEY REFERENCES

[4] Scott JW, Olufago OA, Brat GA, et al. Use of national burden to define operative emergency general surgery. JAMA Surg 2016;151(6):e160480. PMID: 27120712.

This study from the USA of 421 476 patients who required emergency general surgery between 2008 and 2011 found that the seven most common emergency procedures (partial colectomy, small bowel resection, cholecystectomy, operative management of peptic ulcer disease, lysis of peritoneal adhesions, appendicectomy and laparotomy) accounted for 80% of activity, 80% of mortality, 79% of morbidity and 80% of the costs of the EGS cohort.

[45] McCrum ML, Lipsitz SR, Berry WR, Jha AK, Gawande AA. An analysis of inpatient surgical mortality in the United States. Med Care 2014;52:235–42.

This study evaluated patients undergoing one of five high-risk operations—above-knee amputation, abdominal aortic aneurysm repair, coronary artery bypass graft, colon resection and small bowel resection—in 2691 hospitals in the USA. Hospitals that were identified as 'complex', defined by the number of unique primary diagnoses admitted to each hospital, had lower surgical mortality rates even after adjusting for surgical volume. Patients receiving care at the hospitals in the lowest quintile of complexity had a 27% higher risk of death than those in the highest quintile.

SUGGESTED READING

National Emergency Laparotomy Audit (UK). Available at: http://www.nela.org.

The most recent NELA report noted a reduction in both mortality and length of stay over the prior 5 years of reporting, for an overall mortality rate of 9.3%, down from 11.7% during the initial audit.

4 Patient assessment and surgical risk

Kate Carey | John A. Livesey

INTRODUCTION

Few patients do not survive an operation, but many will incur significant morbidity around the time of surgery. These adverse outcomes are considered together as ***perioperative risk.*** ***Patient assessment*** is the process of gathering information to determine the particular risk for a given individual undergoing an operation, which carries distinct ***procedural risks.*** Care of the patient is also dependent on the system in which that care is being delivered. Managing these ***system risks*** is key, and one of the most important functions of multidisciplinary preoperative risk assessment is to inform perioperative care planning for the patient.

WHY IS ASSESSING RISK IMPORTANT?

Informed consent cannot be obtained without an estimation and communication of risk.[1] This must include both the risk of the procedure itself and the competing risk of non-intervention. Conveying risk should also help the patient to form reasonable expectations for the perioperative and recovery process. Assessment of risk helps clinicians, in discussion with patients, to make better decisions when considering if a surgical procedure or intervention is appropriate for a given patient with a particular clinical need. Surgical technique has advanced significantly resulting in shorter and less invasive procedures, allowing patients with higher levels of comorbidity to be considered for surgery. However, it is important to remember that surgery is not always appropriate for all patients.

Despite improvements in surgical tools and technique, complications remain common. Planning the patient's journey through the hospital to allow timely recognition and management of these complications will reduce resulting morbidity. The best performing high-volume centres often have similar complication rates to low-volume centres, but achieve better outcomes due to robust early warning systems when a patient deteriorates triggering prompt clinical action, i.e. a low rate of 'failure to rescue'. Risk assessment informs pre-planned perioperative management strategies, e.g. provision of postoperative critical care resources. As part of this process, identification of specific risks may also allow for pre-optimisation (also known as pre-habilitation) covered elsewhere in this book.

Adjusting for the level of risk present within a case-mix also allows for a fairer comparison of local or individual surgical outcomes against national standards.

It is therefore essential that clinicians endeavour to accurately estimate risk on an individual patient basis for every patient, particularly for those patients who are either comorbid and/or undergoing a major surgical intervention and are therefore considered to be high risk.

WHAT ARE WE AIMING TO IDENTIFY IN RISK ASSESSMENT?

Our aim is to identify the higher-risk patient, generally accepted to be any patient who has an estimated perioperative 30-day mortality of greater than 5%.[2] Perioperative risk is a broad term which can be thought of as a combination of:

- *Patient risks*: not related to the surgery per se, but specific to that individual patient
- *Procedural risks*: related to the surgery itself and the anaesthesia required, and which would apply to any patient undergoing that procedure
- *Systems risks*: quality of preoperative investigation/optimisation and perioperative care

Procedure-related risks are generally easier to identify and communicate. The development of surgical quality improvement programmes has allowed a more accurate appreciation of procedural complications and the rate at which they are encountered on a national, local or even individual surgeon level. Examples include rates of haemorrhage, infection, nerve damage or anastomotic leak. These procedure-related risks are also dependent on other factors, such as urgency and duration of the procedure, volume of blood loss and type of surgery undertaken. The National Institute for Health and Care Excellence (NICE) has attempted to stratify surgical procedures into different grades of severity to provide guidance on the use of preoperative investigations and estimate perioperative risk (Table 4.1).[3]

Patient-related risks are more complex, and thus more challenging to identify and communicate, as they are usually due to individual disorders of physiology. This may lead to an increased risk of a complication less commonly observed in the healthy population. For example, patients with chronic obstructive lung disease (COPD) could reasonably be expected to encounter postoperative pulmonary complications (PPCs) more frequently. Alternatively, it may lead to a decreased ability to tolerate a known complication of a specific procedure, e.g. a patient with significant cardiac disease may fail to tolerate the expected degree of haemorrhage, even if relatively moderate. Patient-related risks may be broadly classified as:

Table 4.1 Examples of surgical procedures by severity grading (NICE)

Grade 1	Grade 2	Grade 3	Grade 4
Upper gastrointestinal endoscopy	Haemorrhoidectomy	Amputation	Gastrectomy
Vasectomy	Varicose vein surgery	Mastectomy	Colectomy
Tooth extraction	Adenoidectomy	Thyroidectomy	Renal transplant
Excision skin lesion	Reduction of dislocated joint	Prostatectomy	Hip replacement

- Major adverse cardiac events (MACEs)
- PPCs
- Perioperative acute kidney injury (AKI)
- Perioperative cerebrovascular events and cognitive dysfunction
- Other morbidities such as urinary tract infection, surgical site infection (SSI) and venous thromboembolism
- Other risks related to an individual's other underlying disease processes, functional status or nutritional status

Systems-related risks include seniority/experience of clinicians, availability of diagnostic investigations such at CT imaging, rapid access to emergency operating theatre, and provision of perioperative critical care. These risks are modifiable and many healthcare systems now have robust standards and quality improvement projects to assess compliance with accepted standards of best practice. Examples include the UK National Confidential Enquiry into Patient Outcome and Death (NCEPOD), and more recently the National Emergency Laparotomy Audit (NELA). This subject is discussed in detail in Chapter 3.

HOW DO WE ASSESS RISK IN THE ELECTIVE SETTING?

The timescale of non-urgent operating allows for robust risk calculation. For many patients, the process can be completed at the initial clinic consultation, based on an accurate history and examination augmented with basic point of care, laboratory and radiological investigations. The majority of low-risk patients will not require more than this and can be quoted the usual procedural risks. Although there is evidence that the gut instinct of an experienced surgeon may be more effective than risk modelling tools,[4,5] modelling has become more sophisticated since these studies were undertaken and many tools are now used routinely to help predict risk for patients with chronic conditions undergoing major complex procedures.

It is important to remember that most available tools predict risk as a 28-day or 30-day mortality and/or morbidity figure. This is an accepted standard within surgical practice and is useful for quality improvement work, but most patients will expect to survive for more than 28 days after their operation and will expect to return to at least their preoperative quality of life. The risk of longer term or permanent impairment to quality of life is a key consideration in undertaking the process of informed consent, particularly after the landmark *Montgomery vs. Lanarkshire Health Board* UK Supreme Court decision.[6] This ruling has changed the requirements of the process of informed consent, such that it must now include communication of all risks, no matter how small, if they could be deemed to be of significance to the patient.

RISK PREDICTION MODELS AND SCORING SYSTEMS

Risk assessment is often subjective, leading to significant variation in the prediction and interpretation of risk. Risk prediction models have been created to reduce this subjectivity. These range from the most basic which define population-level risk for a given severity of concurrent disease, to vastly more complex risk models which account for individual variation in risk. The reality is that quoting a patient a numerical risk is often unhelpful as few patients ever truly believe they may be one of those who contribute to mortality statistics. These models are therefore more useful to the operating surgeon when deciding if offering surgery is appropriate, and clinical experience must be used in conjunction with the numbers produced by these tools. Nevertheless, their use is widespread and has value, so some of the more commonly used tools are described in the following text. This review is by no means exhaustive and many other models are in use. When evaluating accuracy of risk prediction models, we present statistical data where available. The median value for concordance statistic (c-statistic) or area under the receiver operating characteristic curve (AUROC) value is used to compare discrimination of outcomes, with 95% confidence intervals (95% CIs) where available. For these tests, a value of 1.0 would represent perfect performance and a value of 0.5 reflects the score performing no better than random chance. When describing calibration, an observed/expected ratio (O:E) is provided, with a value of less than 1.0 representing overestimation of the predicted outcome and greater than 1.0 underestimation.

GENERAL SCORING TOOLS

AMERICAN SOCIETY OF ANESTHESIOLOGISTS CLASSIFICATION

This five-point classification system for assessing the fitness of a patient prior to elective surgery was developed by the American Society of Anesthesiologists (ASA) in 1963 and is used worldwide. The five grades each represent an increasing level of comorbidity and physiological derangement (Table 4.2). A sixth category was later added to encompass the patient who has had death diagnosed by neurological criteria and is brought to theatre for heart beating organ donation. The tool correlates with in-hospital mortality but predicts an average risk defined from population level data rather than individual risk, and does not account for the severity

Table 4.2 American Society of Anesthesiologists grades

I	Healthy
II	Mild to moderate systemic disease caused by the surgical condition or other comorbidity, but medically well controlled and not affecting daily life
III	Severe disease process which limits activity but is not incapacitating
IV	Severe incapacitating disease process which is a constant threat to life
V	Moribund patient not expected to survive with or without the operation
VI	Patient diagnosed dead by neurological criteria and whose organs are being removed for donation

of the operative procedure planned. It has been validated in several studies across multiple surgical specialties,[7–17] which report a c-statistic for accuracy of 0.77 (95% CI 0.59–0.93) and a calibration O:E ratio of 1.08. However, ASA scoring is a markedly subjective assessment; one study reported such marked variation in inter-individual assessment that the authors concluded that ASA score alone should not be used to predict risk.[18] Although of limited use as a risk prediction tool, ASA score does have value as a simple, easy-to-use and easy-to-understand measure to convey a patient's degree of preoperative ill health to the wider theatre team at the beginning of an operation.

✔ The ASA classification remains a quick, simple, widely used and reasonably accurate assessment of surgical risk in both the elective and emergency settings.

SURGICAL OUTCOME RISK TOOL – SORT (v2)

The original Surgical Outcome Risk Tool (SORT) was a collaboration between researchers at NCEPOD and the University College London Surgical Outcomes Research Centre in the UK. It was developed from analysis of 19 000 patient outcomes, estimating risk of 30-day mortality from six variables: ASA, complexity of procedure, urgency, patient age, surgical risk specialty (gastrointestinal, thoracic or vascular surgery) and the anticipated presence of malignancy. The original version demonstrated a c-statistic of 0.8[19] for accuracy when discriminating for prediction of mortality. The latest update of the score in 2020 to SORT version 2 (SORTv2)[20] has been validated in patients from the UK, Australia and New Zealand, updated to take account of the experienced physician's estimation of risk and to include surgery on all parts of the body. The newer model outperforms the older version with an AUROC value of 0.91, and is accurate in predicting outcomes in neurological and cardiothoracic surgery.

SURGICAL RISK SCALE

The Surgical Risk Scale (SRS) identifies three factors as the main determinants of surgical outcome prediction: complexity of procedure (minor, intermediate, major and major-complex), urgency of procedure (elective, urgent, emergency) and ASA grade.[21] It is simple to use, requiring only these three variables, but predicts average population outcome rather than individual risk. For mortality, it has a c-statistic of 0.85 (95% CI 0.66–0.95) and O:E of 0.81. Most of the more complex models are built on the three variables used in the SRS.

PHYSIOLOGICAL AND OPERATIVE SEVERITY SCORE FOR THE ENUMERATION OF MORTALITY MODELS

The original Physiological and Operative Severity Score for enUmeration of Mortality (POSSUM) score was developed in 1991 through multivariate analysis of 62 parameters from a heterogenous general surgical population, from which the most statistically powerful outcome predictors were selected. It uses 6 operative variables to estimate the risk of both mortality and morbidity following a specific surgical procedure, with adjustment for the individual patient by the inclusion of 12 physiological parameters (Table 4.3). Values for each variable are bracketed and given a weighting of 1, 2, 4 or 8 to calculate an Operative Severity Score and a Physiological Score. The use of additional operative variables such as blood loss and the presence of peritoneal soiling mean that these must be predicted by the surgeon if the score is to be used preoperatively, but despite this limitation it has been one of the most commonly used risk scoring tools and has been extensively validated.[22] It demonstrates a c-statistic of 0.82 (95% CI 0.47–0.95) and calibration O:E of 0.86 (95% CI 0–1.73) for mortality. For morbidity, the c-statistic is 0.75 (95% CI 0.56–0.84) and calibration O:E 1.0 (95% CI 0.8–1.44).

PORTSMOUTH POSSUM

The original POSSUM model was found to overpredict mortality significantly, particularly in the lowest risk groups, and was revised by Whiteley et al.[23] from Portsmouth, UK, to produce an amended predictor calculation termed Portsmouth Physiological and Operative Severity Score for the enUmeration of Mortality (P-POSSUM) with a closer fit to observed in-hospital mortality.

The P-POSSUM model has been extensively validated in many large cohorts[8,24–29] and demonstrates a c-statistic for mortality of 0.81 (95% CI 0.56–0.94), calibration O:E for mortality of 1.03 (95% CI 0.56–15.87), and a c-statistic for morbidity of 0.61. Despite this improved fit, the score still overestimates mortality in the elderly, and in lower-risk groups, e.g. elective surgery. It also overestimates mortality in certain surgical subspecialties,[30] which has prompted development of specialty-specific POSSUM-based scores for major elective colorectal (CR-POSSUM), oesophagogastric (O-POSSUM) and vascular (V-POSSUM) surgery.

Colorectal POSSUM

Minimally invasive laparoscopic techniques and Enhanced Recovery After Surgery (ERAS) protocols have changed the risk profile of major elective colorectal surgery, widening consideration of surgery in an older population, and are increasingly applied to emergency work.

POSSUM and P-POSSUM models underpredict mortality in emergency CR surgery and lack calibration at the extremes of age in elective work.[31] CR-POSSUM was developed to include elective and emergency procedures. CR-POSSUM was superior to P-POSSUM when predicting perioperative mortality in index and validation cohorts of almost 23 000 UK patients[32,33] across a variety of emergency and elective colorectal procedures, but a subsequent systematic review of

Table 4.3 Variables used for the calculation of the Physiological and Operative Severity Score for enUmeration of Mortality (POSSUM) score and its derivatives

Operative variables	Physiological variables
Operation severity class	Age
Number of procedures	Cardiac disease
Blood loss	Respiratory disease
Peritoneal contamination	Electrocardiogram
Malignancy status	Systolic blood pressure
Urgency	Pulse rate
	Haemoglobin concentration
	White cell count
	Serum urea concentration
	Serum sodium concentration
	Serum potassium concentration
	Glasgow coma scale score

18 studies comparing POSSUM, P-POSSUM and CR-POSSUM in surgery for colorectal malignancy found P-POSSUM to have the greatest predictive accuracy for mortality.[34] A study of patients undergoing elective sigmoid resection for either carcinoma or diverticular disease found that CR-POSSUM overpredicted mortality for malignant disease and underpredicted in benign disease, despite good accuracy for the group as a whole.[35]

Risk prediction for emergency laparotomy is a unique challenge and is covered in greater detail later in the chapter.

Oesophagogastric POSSUM

There has been significant interest in developing a risk prediction model specific to oesophagogastric surgery, particularly in oesophagectomy where the rates of both perioperative mortality (5%) and major morbidity (~60%) remain high.

The original POSSUM model discriminates poorly for morbidity or mortality in patients undergoing oesophagectomy[36] and an adjusted O-POSSUM model (which includes age, physiological status, mode of surgery, type of surgery and histological stage) was developed, demonstrating improved accuracy for risk-adjusted prediction of death in the index cohort.[37] However, a systematic review of further studies found that O-POSSUM overpredicted in-hospital mortality and did not identify patients at higher risk.[38]

Several other models have been proposed, but a systematic review of the evidence for all these scores, including O-POSSUM, has concluded that no currently available model can be applied to clinical practice with any confidence.[39]

Vascular POSSUM

For patients undergoing arterial surgery, 'extra items' were added to the original POSSUM dataset; however, this did not significantly improve the accuracy of prediction.[40] The score has been shown to perform poorly in elective abdominal aortic aneurysm repair,[41] and neither P-POSSUM nor V-POSSUM appear accurate in the setting of ruptured abdominal aortic aneurysm.[40]

CR-POSSUM, O-POSSUM and V-POSSUM each illustrate limitations of adjusting existing risk prediction tools for differing populations. The original POSSUM model is 'data driven', based on logistic regression and goodness of fit modelling applied to data collected in a mixed emergency and elective population. Weighting of haematological, biochemical and clinical parameters values significantly outside the normal range is of less relevance when calculations are revised to fit a purely elective population. For example, a patient with an abnormal Glasgow Coma Scale score would be highly unlikely to be considered for oesophagectomy, yet it remains within POSSUM-based scores.

Large, prospectively collected datasets for each subspecialty will be required to develop risk prediction models which can be reliably applied to clinical practice, but this is challenging in lower-volume specialties.

AMERICAN COLLEGE OF SURGEONS NATIONAL SURGICAL QUALITY IMPROVEMENT PROJECT RISK CALCULATION TOOL

The American College of Surgeons (ACS) have used the data from over 5 000 000 procedures across 855 hospitals collected as part of the National Surgical Quality Improvement Project (NSQIP) from 2015 to 2019 to develop a risk prediction tool. The tool takes account of 20 patient variables and the specific planned procedure, to provide risk of mortality. It also predicts the risk of a number of morbidities such as renal failure, pneumonia, cardiac events and SSI, which makes it unique amongst the risk prediction tools available.

Performance of the tool has been assessed in a number of large cohorts,[42–46] and whilst it has a reasonable degree of accuracy for mortality, it performs much less well for composite morbidity (c-statistic for mortality 0.83 [95% CI 0.62–0.97] and for composite morbidity 0.625 [95% CI 0.55–0.88]; calibration for mortality 1.23 [95% CI 0.64–1.28] and morbidity 1.06 [95% CI 0.76–1.84]).

SUMMARY OF THE GENERAL RISK SCORING TOOLS

The recent guideline from the National Institute of Health and Care Excellence (NICE) which describes ***perioperative care in adults*** looks in detail at risk stratification tools in Evidence Review C of NICE Guideline 180 on preoperative risk scoring.[47] The committee discussed the results and utility of the risk tools reviewed and agreed that a c-statistic of >80% represents a good level of predictive accuracy, with results of >90% demonstrating an excellent test. The committee added that a test yielding <70% accuracy would be considered poor. The committee also noted that calibration data showing a test O:E ratio of 0.9–1.1 would be considered a fair level of accuracy, adding that it would be better to overestimate the event rate than to underestimate morbidity or mortality.

The committee agreed that tools such as POSSUM, P-POSSUM, NSQIP, E-PASS and SRS showed a fair level of overall performance for mortality (Table 4.4) as evidenced by a median c-statistic of ~85%. The committee highlighted

Table 4.4 A summary of available data to assess performance of the most widely used risk prediction tools

	Mortality		Morbidity	
	Discrimination concordance statistic median (95% CI)	**Calibration observed:expected median (95% CI)**	**Discrimination concordance statistic median (95% CI)**	**Calibration observed:expected median (95% CI)**
ASA	0.77 (0.59–0.93)	1.08	0.69 (0.52–0.78)	–
SORT	0.80	–	–	–
SRS	0.85 (0.66–0.95)	0.81	–	–
POSSUM	0.82 (0.47–0.95)	0.86 (0–1.73)	0.75 (0.56–0.84)	1.00 (0.8–1.44)
P-POSSUM	0.81 (0.56–0.94)	1.03 (0.56–15.87)	0.61	–
NSQIP	0.83 (0.62–0.97)	1.23 (0.64–1.28)	0.625 (0.55–0.88)	1.06 (0.76–1.84)

ASA, American Society of Anesthesiologists; *95% CI*, 95% confidence interval; *NSQIP*, National Surgical Quality Improvement Project; *POSSUM*, Physiological and Operative Severity Scoring for the enUmeration of Mortality; *P-POSSUM*, Portsmouth POSSUM; *SORT*, Surgical Outcome Risk Tool; *SRS*, Surgical Risk Scale.
(Based on UK National Institute for Health and Care Excellence NG180.)

that there was notable inconsistency (~60% to ~90% accuracy) in the individual studies for predicting mortality, which are generally of low to very low quality on the GRADE scale. All tools performed less well for morbidity.

No one tool can be recommended. Both under- and over-prediction of risk can result in harm, and these tools should be used as part of a wider clinical judgement by a multidisciplinary team.

✔ Accurate risk prediction tools provide benefit by informing surgeons when planning surgery. Prediction of mortality and morbidity risk can inform decisions on proceeding with surgery, or selecting an alternative surgical or non-surgical treatment. Prediction of morbidity allows selection of an appropriate postoperative care destination. P-POSSUM, NSQIP and SRS all show a fair level of accuracy for mortality. P-POSSUM and NSQIP perform less well for morbidity than mortality.

No one tool outperforms the others to a point where a particular tool can be recommended.

SCORING SYSTEMS TO PREDICT CARDIAC RISK IN NON-CARDIAC SURGERY

LEE'S REVISED CARDIAC RISK INDEX

The Revised Cardiac Risk Index (RCRI) was developed to predict risk of cardiac complications in non-cardiac surgery. It was derived from a cohort of 2893 patients aged > 50 years undergoing major non-cardiac surgery, and validated in a cohort of 1422 patients.[48] The risk of a MACE, defined as cardiac death, non-fatal myocardial infarction and non-fatal cardiac arrest can be calculated from the presence of a number of risk factors as described in Table 4.5.

ACS-NSQIP

In addition to mortality, the ACS-NSQIP tool calculates predicted risk of a MACE in non-cardiac surgery (see above); however, when assessing composite morbidity, this tool performs relatively poorly.

SCORING SYSTEMS TO PREDICT RISK OF POSTOPERATIVE PULMONARY COMPLICATIONS

The incidence of PPCs after major surgery is estimated to be 1–23%.[49] This wide variation is likely due to inconsistent definitions, worldwide differences in healthcare setting and population health (e.g. obesity and smoking prevalence), but two large European studies estimated the incidence at 5%[50] and 7.9%[51] for patients undergoing non-cardiac surgery. PPCs prolong hospital stay adding to healthcare burden[52] and adversely affect patient outcomes[53]; a 20% risk of mortality in those developing a PPC was reported in one large study.[50] This has led to recent interest in predicting and preventing PPCs.

ASSESSMENT OF RESPIRATORY RISK IN SURGICAL PATIENTS IN CATALONIA SCORE

The Assessment of Respiratory Risk in Surgical Patients in Catalonia (ARISCAT) score was developed in 2010 from an index cohort of 2464 patients[50] to predict the risk of PPCs, defined as: respiratory failure, respiratory infection, pleural effusion, atelectasis, pneumothorax, bronchospasm and aspiration pneumonitis. The score has been externally validated in two further cohorts.[51,54]

The study identified seven variables through multivariate analysis, each assigned a score (described in Table 4.6). Patients were stratified into three groups based on total score: low risk (score < 26) associated with a 1.6% risk of PPCs, intermediate risk (score 26–44) associated with a 13.3% risk of PPCs, and high risk (score > 44) associated with a 42.1% risk of PPCs.

NSQIP

The ACS-NSQIP tool calculates predicted risk of postoperative pneumonia in addition to mortality as previously described. When assessing composite morbidity, this tool performs poorly and this should be taken into account.

Table 4.5 Lee's Revised Cardiac Risk Index

Risk factor	Number of risk factors	Risk of major adverse cardiac event
Ischaemic heart disease	0	0.4%
Congestive cardiac failure	1	0.9%
Cerebrovascular disease	2	6.6%
Diabetes requiring insulin use preoperatively	3+	>11%
Chronic kidney disease (creatinine > 176.8 μmol/L)		
Supra-inguinal vascular, intraperitoneal or intrathoracic surgery		

Table 4.6 Variables involved in calculation of Assessment of Respiratory Risk in Surgical Patients in Catalonia (ARISCAT) score and breakdown of risk by score group

ARISCAT score variable	Answer options	Points
Patient age	<50	0
	50–80	3
	>80	16
Preoperative SpO_2	>=96%	0
	91–95%	8
	<=90%	24
Respiratory infection in the past month (upper or lower respiratory symptoms with fever and antibiotic use)	No	0
	Yes	17
Preoperative anaemia (Hb <= 10 g/dL)	No	0
	Yes	11
Surgical incision	Peripheral	0
	Upper abdominal	15
	Intrathoracic	24
Duration of surgery	<2 hours	0
	2–3 hours	16
	>3 hours	23
Emergency procedure	No	0
	Yes	8

ARISCAT score	Risk group	Risk of in-hospital postoperative pulmonary complications
<26	Low	1.6%
26–44	Intermediate	13.3%
>44	High	42.1%

SCORING SYSTEMS TO PREDICT PERIOPERATIVE ACUTE KIDNEY INJURY

Perioperative AKI of any stage, defined by KDIGO criteria,[55] is a common complication occurring in up to 50% of patients undergoing major surgery.[56,57] It is directly associated with increased mortality, morbidity and an increased risk of developing chronic kidney disease. Despite this, no robust risk prediction score exists. Several specific scores have been designed but performed poorly in validation cohorts and are not worth further discussion here.

Even tools developed from large datasets such as the NSQIP perform poorly when assessing risk of AKI, but there is hope that with more sophisticated large volume data capture from perioperative monitoring, and the use of machine learning, it may be possible to develop a more accurate risk prediction model.

SCORING SYSTEMS TO PREDICT PERIOPERATIVE CEREBROVASCULAR EVENTS OR COGNITIVE DECLINE

Postoperative cognitive dysfunction (POCD) is a medical complication of surgery that is increasingly common in an aging population. It usually manifests as a self-limiting delirium in the postoperative period[58] but can persist in to a more permanent cognitive decline.[59] Aetiology is multifactorial and includes primary neurodegenerative change and systemic inflammatory states such as diabetes.

Current risk prediction is based on clinical parameters including age and duration of surgical procedure, but is relatively crude. Pre-existing cognitive dysfunction may be identified through the use of scoring tools such as the Montreal Cognitive Assessment (MOCA) tool, and if present should prompt discussion of the risk of longer lasting or permanent POCD, as well as the associated increased risk of mortality.[60] The European Union–funded BioCog project[61] aims to

Table 4.7 Clinical Frailty Scale

1 – Very fit	Robust, active, energetic and motivated. These people are amongst the fittest for their age.
2 – Well	No active disease symptoms but less fit than category 1. They exercise or are very active occasionally.
3 – Managing well	Medical problems are well controlled but are not regularly active beyond routine walking.
4 – Vulnerable	Not dependent on others for daily help, but their symptoms limit activities. A common complaint is being 'slowed up' or tired during the day.
5 – Mildly frail	More evident slowing. Need help with high-order activities of daily living (finances, heavy housework, transportation). Typically mild frailty progressively impairs shopping and walking outside alone, meal preparation and housework.
6 – Moderately frail	Need help with all outside activities and with keeping house. Inside, they may struggle with stairs or require assistance bathing.
7 – Severely frail	Completely dependent for personal care from physical or cognitive cause. Even so they may appear stable and not at high risk of dying within 6 months.
8 – Very severely frail	Completely dependent and approaching the end of their life. May not fully recover from even a minor illness.
9 – Terminally ill	Approaching the end of life. This category applies if life expectancy < 6 months, even if not otherwise appearing to be frail.

deliver a multivariate risk prediction model for perioperative cognitive decline but remains in its early stages.

SCORING SYSTEMS TO ASSESS FRAILTY

Frailty is a well-established condition. It is a state in which an individual has limited physiological reserve to cope with the stress of acute medical illness, trauma or surgery, and can exist in the absence of significant organ dysfunction on preoperative examination and static diagnostic testing. The presence of frailty is associated with higher mortality and morbidity after surgery in the elective and emergency setting,[62–66] and is predictive of increased duration of hospital stay and institutionalisation. Frailty is often assessed subjectively, but tools are available to assist in its diagnosis. It is not specifically accounted for by any of the existing risk prediction tools at present. Future work will inform adjustment of these scoring tools to account for the impact of frailty on surgical risk.

CLINICAL FRAILTY SCALE

The latest version of the Clinical Frailty Scale from Rockwood et al.[67] is a simple nine-point scale (Table 4.7). It has been validated in general surgery to predict increased mortality and length of stay when used as a binary measure of 'frail' (score 5 or greater) or 'not frail' (score 4 or less).[68] Notably, the association of frailty with increased mortality was independent of age in a general surgical cohort[66] where the prevalence of frailty was 25%.

✔ Frailty is common, affecting up to one in four general surgical patients, and is associated with increased mortality and morbidity regardless of age.

Screening for frailty using validated tools such as the Clinical Frailty Scale is quick and easy to perform. Existing scoring tools may significantly underpredict morbidity and mortality where significant frailty is present.

NUTRITIONAL STATE, SARCOPENIA AND BODY COMPOSITION ANALYSIS

The surgical stress response induces various metabolic changes, including catabolism. Therefore, nutritional status of the patient is a very important part of the preoperative assessment of risk in order to assess nutritional reserve for recovery and healing.[69]

Sarcopenia is a clinical syndrome characterised by the loss of lean body mass as a result of ageing. The reduction in skeletal muscle is associated with loss of strength and functional capacity. Cachexia is a similar syndrome also associated with loss of skeletal body mass that is associated with disease states (most notably cancer) but has different pathophysiology. Both syndromes are refractory to conventional treatments such as nutritional supplementation, may lead to progressive functional decline and are associated with poor treatment outcomes and prognosis. Both conditions may be difficult to recognise in obese patients who may nonetheless meet the criteria for sarcopenia or cachexia despite a high body mass index (sarcopenic obesity).

Sarcopenia is identified through measurement of muscle mass and by assessing muscle strength and function. Muscle strength is most commonly measured using hand-grip strength, and functional performance is determined by methods already described in this chapter, such as timed stair climb. Morphometric parameters may be measured from routine computed tomography (CT) or magnetic resonance imaging (MRI) using computer software programs to calculate lean body mass and visceral adipose tissue from cross-sectional images at the level of the third lumbar vertebra. A standardised lumbar skeletal muscle index (LSMI) is generated following adjustment for patient height. Studies have demonstrated association of sarcopenia with increased risk of postoperative complications in patients undergoing oesophagogastric surgery and colorectal surgery.[70–73] The strongest associations were between reduced lean body mass and increased rates of pulmonary complications and wound infections. A systematic review of patient outcomes following gastrointestinal surgery identified that sarcopenia was associated with increased rates of immediate postoperative complications as well as adverse longer-term prognosis and outcomes.[74] This information is clearly important in selecting treatment options for patients with confirmed sarcopenia.

Although the syndrome of sarcopenia is not fully reversible, there is some evidence to suggest that early identification of these patients with focused attention on nutritional and functional (physical) support may reduce mortality

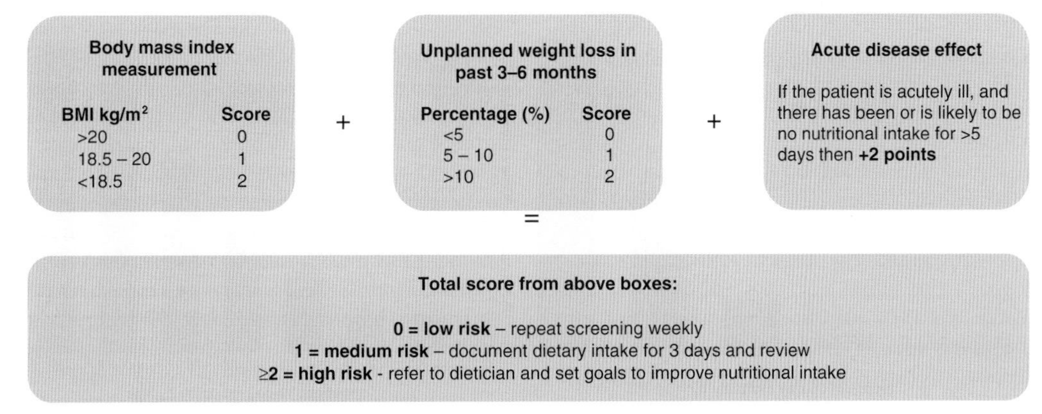

Figure 4.1 Malnutrition Universal Screening Tool.

rates and length of stay following surgery.[75] Trials adopting a multimodal approach addressing exercise, nutrition and anti-inflammatory treatment strategies (MENAC Trial) are ongoing.[76]

Preoperative assessment of nutrition may be achieved with various screening tools, such as the MUST (malnutrition universal screening tool) as depicted in Fig. 4.1, MST (malnutrition screening tool) or the PG-SGA (Patient-Generated Subjective Global Assessment), as well as in-person dietician assessment. A comparison of these assessment tools is beyond the scope of this book. Whichever tool is used, it is imperative that nutritional assessment occurs preoperatively (where possible), and continues during the patient's journey so that interventions are timely.

Sarcopenia is associated with postoperative complications, particularly SSI and pulmonary complications, but also mortality. This risk is partially reversible. Repeated assessment throughout the perioperative period and a multimodal approach including tailored nutritional support is essential.

FUNCTIONAL ASSESSMENT

Surviving any operation requires the patient to respond to the surgical stress by increasing tissue oxygen delivery. Comparison to exercise tolerance is a useful analogy, although in reality it is much more complex. When exercising, at the point at which the heart and lungs cannot increase cardiac output and/or ventilation any further, the patient will experience feelings of exhaustion and muscular discomfort and will slow down or stop to reduce tissue oxygen consumption and anaerobic metabolism. If this point is reached when under anaesthesia during an operation, then the patient cannot stop the increased oxygen demand and organ dysfunction will occur as a result.

Assessing a patient's ability to cope with the demands of exercise is a widely used method of predicting ability to cope with a surgical procedure, and this can be done in a number of ways.

METABOLIC EQUIVALENTS

The simplest way to assess exercise capacity is to ask the patient what they are able to do. This can then be equated to a number of metabolic equivalents (METs), where 1 MET (also the resting metabolic rate) approximates consumption of 3.5 O_2 mL/kg/min. Common questions to do this include: 'How far can you walk on the flat?' (representative of 2–3 METs for whatever time/distance they can achieve), 'Can you climb two flights of stairs without stopping?' (4 METs), 'Can you manage brisk swimming?' (6 METs), or 'Can you manage brisk running?' (10 METs). Clearly this is subjective, and many patients overestimate their capacity.

Patient-reported inability to achieve 4 METs (14 O_2 mL/kg/min) has a positive predictive value of 82% for the development of cardiopulmonary complications in major abdominal or thoracic surgery[77] and correlates with data derived from cardiopulmonary exercise testing (CPET).

CARDIOPULMONARY EXERCISE TESTING

CPET has been part of perioperative practice since an index study defining its predictive value in 1993,[78] but its use has rapidly expanded in the last decade, particularly in the UK.[79] It provides an objective measure of exercise capacity by evaluating the integrated physiological response, and where limitation is observed it allows identification of the cause. A full review of the practicalities of CPET is beyond the scope of this chapter, and covered in existing consensus guidelines,[80] but most commonly it is performed on a cycle-ergometer measuring power (Watts), breath-by-breath spirometry, measurement of inspired and expired O_2 and CO_2 fractions, continuous electrocardiogram, oxygen saturation and regular non-invasive blood pressure measurement. This data is reported in a nine-panel plot, which can be used to derive several values.

The $\dot{V}O_2$ peak is the maximum oxygen delivery achieved by the patient during the test. A $\dot{V}O_2$ peak of less than 15 O_2 mL/kg/min is predictive of greater risk of postoperative complications.[81]

The anaerobic threshold (AT) is an index of submaximal sustainable exercise capacity and is defined as the $\dot{V}O_2$ at which arterial lactate begins to increase in response to incremental exercise. This measure predicts postoperative mortality and complications with the greatest accuracy of the CPET variables.[82] Where AT occurs at a $\dot{V}O_2$ of less than 10.2 O_2 mL/kg/min, the risk of complications increases significantly.[83] AT is predictive of postoperative outcomes for intra-abdominal procedures,[81] with studies supporting its use in colorectal,[84] urological,[85] hepatobiliary,[86] liver transplantation,[87] bariatric,[88] and vascular[89] surgery. So far, it appears less useful in oesophagogastric surgery.[90]

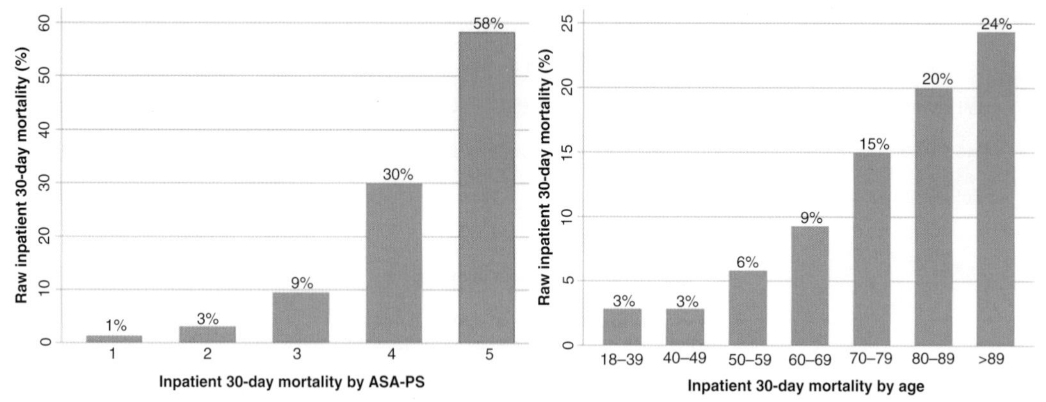

Figure 4.2 30-day inpatient mortality by American Society of Anesthesiologists performance score (ASA-PS) and age.

✔ CPET is used increasingly commonly and is supported by evidence across a number of surgical sub-specialties. A VO_2 peak of < 15 O_2 mL/kg/min and an AT of < 10.2 O_2 mL/kg/min are strongly associated with increased risk of postoperative morbidity and mortality.

OTHER OBJECTIVE MEASURES OF EXERCISE CAPACITY

CPET is not available in many centres, and even where it is available it is not practical to perform this expensive and time-consuming test on every patient presenting for consideration of surgery. An alternative objective functional assessment tool is the incremental shuttle walk test (ISWT). The ISWT involves repeatedly walking between two markers set 10 metres apart within a set time period, which gets shorter as the test progresses. It has been shown to correlate with measured oxygen consumption in surgical patients with cardiac and chronic lung disease[91] and in one study, all patients who managed more than 360 metres distance had ATs above 10.2 O_2 mL/kg/min.[92]

A different tool, the 6-minute walk test has been validated to screen patients for referral to formal CPET testing, where walking a distance of 563 metres during the 6-minute window was universally associated with an AT of > 11 O_2 mL/kg/min and did not require CPET.[93]

HOW CAN WE ASSESS RISK IN THE EMERGENCY SETTING?

Clearly it is not possible to undertake complex, time-consuming and invasive investigations in the emergency setting with an acutely unwell patient. In this setting, we must rely on an accurate history and focused clinical examination to identify organ dysfunction, the patient's reporting of their functional ability, and any investigations that may have been undertaken in the recent past. Whilst this is mainly a subjective assessment, senior surgeons will bring accurate insight into assessing the perioperative risk of these patients from their own extensive experience. This clinical acumen and the patient-specific clinical examination, augmented by the use of the scoring systems already described, offer the best opportunity to accurately inform the patient of the potential outcomes from proceeding with emergency surgery. Multidisciplinary discussion with the surgeon, anaesthetist and intensivist, in conjunction with the patient or their representative, is paramount.

Appreciation of the higher level of risk involved in emergency abdominal surgery is important for all clinicians involved. There has been increased scrutiny of this patient group in the last two decades, most recently with the UK NELA.[94] This large, contemporaneous audit collects data on patients requiring an emergency laparotomy. The data are designed to focus primarily on patients with intestinal pathology within the stomach, small and large bowel, excluding patients with vascular conditions and abdominal trauma (a comprehensive list of inclusions and exclusions is available at https://www.nela.org.uk).

The first report from NELA in 2015 provided specific detail about the risk patients are exposed to when undergoing an emergency laparotomy.[95] Raw inpatient 30-day mortality increased with age, from 3% for adults aged 18–39 years, to 24% for adults aged 90 years and over. Similarly, raw 30-day inpatient mortality increased exponentially with ASA grade, from 1% in ASA 1 patients to 30% and 58% in ASA 4 and 5 patients, respectively (Fig. 4.2). This hugely important audit programme has prompted a significant improvement initiative whereby clinicians are able to use contemporaneous data collection to assess changes in their care that they are delivering, and in the systems in which they work, in order to improve patient outcome (see Chapter 3).

Successive annual reports from NELA have had different areas of focus. For instance, in the most recent Sixth Patient Report in 2020[96] (available at https://www.nela.org.uk/All-Patient-Reports#pt.), the authors highlight the higher risks for the patient who has come from outside the surgical ward or emergency department. The common theme running through all the reports is the high-risk nature of emergency laparotomy, particularly in older, frail patients, and that accurate risk prediction is essential to achieving the best possible outcomes for these patients.

Recently, as part of its ongoing quality improvement remit, the NELA has developed a scoring system specific to emergency abdominal surgery.

RISK SCORING TOOLS IN THE EMERGENCY SURGICAL PATIENT

NELA SCORE

The development of the NELA score,[97] validated using data collected as part of the NELA (over 38 000 patients), was launched in July 2017 and has provided a useful additional tool for understanding patient risk. A further development of the P-POSSUM calculation, this risk prediction model specifically for emergency laparotomy uses information about individual patient physiological status, combined with anticipated operative findings, to provide clear information about perioperative risk. The NELA score now forms the basis of preoperative multidisciplinary decision-making and postoperative care planning in many UK centres. The NELA score can be calculated online from https://www.nela.org.uk. Note that this tool has only been validated in patients undergoing emergency laparotomy for surgical problems as included in the audit (i.e. pathology of the stomach, small and large bowel). It does not include patients with pathology of the appendix, gall bladder, pancreas, liver, spleen, gynaecological or bladder issues, or injury secondary to trauma (Box 4.1).

SURGICAL OUTCOME RISK TOOL v2

The updated SORTv2 can be used in both the elective and emergency setting. Where the NELA score is not applicable, it is useful to have this as an alternative means for mortality prediction.

> ✔ Emergency laparotomy is associated with significantly increased risk, particularly where the patient presents from outside the emergency department or surgical ward. Increasing age and worsening ASA grade are associated with exponential increases in risk.

Senior clinician opinions from surgery, anaesthesia and critical care, together with use of a risk scoring tool validated in the emergency setting are essential to inform discussion of risk with the patient.

FRAILTY IN THE EMERGENCY SURGICAL PATIENT

The recent observational study from the ELF trial group[98] looked at the incidence of frailty, and the relationship between frailty and mortality in the emergency surgical patient. This UK multicentre study found that 20% of patients requiring emergency laparotomy were frail, and that increasing frailty has a direct association with increasing mortality even when adjusted for age and sex. Increasing frailty was also associated with increased risk of complications, length of ICU stay and overall hospital stay.

Box 4.1 Links for online access to freely available risk models

- National Emergency Laparotomy Audit http://www.nela.org.uk
- P-POSSUM/O-POSSUM/CR-POSSUM/V-POSSUM http://www.riskprediction.org.uk
- Surgical Risk Calculator http://riskcalculator.facs.org/RiskCalculator/PatientInfo.jsp
- Surgical Outcome Risk Tool v2 http://sortsurgery.com
- Revised Cardiac Risk Index http://www.mdcalc.com/revised-cardiac-index-pre-operative-risk

SUMMARY

An accurate estimate of perioperative risk is imperative for both informed decision-making by the patient and their team, and also for the optimal perioperative planning for patient care, particularly in the emergency setting.

Senior clinician experience and clinical opinion are invaluable. Increasingly, objective measures of risk, including risk scoring tools, are able to provide accurate information derived from outcomes in large, relevant patient cohorts. All components of risk should be considered, including patient, surgical and system factors. In particular, frailty and nutritional status should be included in the routine multisystem assessment of the patient and re-examined throughout the patient's journey. Thorough communication of risks involved must be communicated to the patient at the earliest opportunity, to maximise informed patient consent, including the risk of not proceeding or following a different treatment pathway. In the emergency setting, the majority of patients fall into the high-risk (>5% mortality) category, many at significantly higher risk, and should be treated as such, with decision-making and procedures being led and delivered by senior clinicians.

Key points

- Thorough assessment of patient risk is dependent on individual patient characteristics, the procedural risk and the systems risk.
- A variety of procedure- and complication-specific risk scores are available to augment the opinions of senior, experienced clinicians.
- Accurate risk prediction enables patients and their families to plan for their procedure. In addition, multidisciplinary teams can prepare together to maximise outcomes, and this is particularly important in the emergency setting.
- All patients with an estimated perioperative mortality of > 5% are high risk, and adequate perioperative support is essential, including access to critical care.
- Functional status, including frailty and nutritional status, require particular attention, in addition to documented comorbidities.

References available at http://ebooks.health.elsevier.com/

KEY REFERENCES

[16] Moonesinghe SR, Mythen MG, Das P, Rowan KM, Grocott MP. Risk stratification tools for predicting morbidity and mortality in adult patients undergoing major surgery: qualitative systematic review. Anesthesiology 2013;119(4):959–81.

[47] Excellence NIfHaC. [C] Evidence review for preoperative risk stratification tools NICE guideline NG180. Evidence reviews underpinning recommendations 1.3.1 and 1.3.2 in the NICE guideline 2020 [Available from: www.nice.org.uk/guidance/ng180.

[97] Eugene N, Oliver CM, Bassett MG, Poulton TE, Kuryba A, Johnston C, et al. Development and internal validation of a novel risk adjustment model for adult patients undergoing emergency laparotomy surgery: the National Emergency Laparotomy Audit risk model. Br J Anaesth 2018;121(4):739–48.

[98] Parmar KL, Law J, Carter B, Hewitt J, Boyle JM, Casey P, et al. Frailty in older patients undergoing emergency laparotomy: results from the UK Observational Emergency Laparotomy and Frailty (ELF) study. Ann Surg 2021;273(4):709–18.

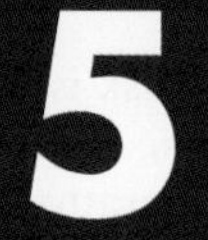

5 Perioperative and intensive care management of the surgical patient

Katherine McAndrew | Maurizio Cecconi | Andrew Rhodes

INTRODUCTION

The incidence of death directly attributable to anaesthesia has decreased significantly over the last 60 years. In the 1950s, several studies demonstrated that the postoperative mortality solely associated with anaesthesia was approximately 1 in 2500,[1–3] but by 1987, in the UK Confidential Enquiry into Perioperative Death (CEPOD), this had decreased to an estimate of 1:185000.[4] Whilst anaesthetic practice has continued to evolve over the subsequent 30 years, the marginal improvements in mortality have been likely offset by an increasingly fragile and elderly group of patients who are now operated on, leaving the underlying rate of death attributable to anaesthesia much the same.[5]

Although deaths as a direct consequence of anaesthesia are relatively rare, the rate of morbidity and mortality following major surgery remains much higher. The European Surgical Outcomes Study in 2012 (EuSOS) found an overall mortality rate of 4% in patients undergoing non-cardiac surgery throughout Europe.[6] These findings have been replicated globally, highlighting the need for safe perioperative care.[7] This chapter deals with the perioperative and intensive care management of these patients with a specific focus on how to ensure that each patient has adequate cardiovascular performance for their needs during the perioperative period, in order to reduce their risk of complications and death.

Postoperative critical care is a key factor in the improvement of outcome for surgical patients, particularly those who are at high risk of postoperative morbidity and mortality. Thus, postoperative critical care admission should always be considered when the preoperative physiological condition of the patient in tandem with the planned complexity of the surgical procedure suggests that there is a reasonable risk of postoperative complications and organ dysfunction. In order to provide this postoperative critical care, it is necessary to be able to identify these high-risk patients preoperatively.

HOW BIG IS THE PROBLEM?

It is estimated that over 300 million operations take place globally per year and these growing numbers of patients need to be cared for in an appropriate setting.[8] A high-risk group of patients was identified from the UK population who accounted for over 80% of all deaths but only 12.5% of procedures. Despite high mortality rates, fewer than 15% of these patients were admitted to the intensive care unit (ICU), and the highest mortality rate (39%) was found in patients who required ICU admission following initial care in a ward environment.[9] These findings have been confirmed, with only 5% of all patients being admitted to ICU electively after their procedure.[6] Unplanned admissions were associated with higher mortality, and 73% of those who died were not admitted to ICU at any stage. Admission to critical care following surgery is most common in patients who are elderly, have a high body mass index, have comorbid clinical conditions or require emergency surgery.[10]

Despite this, there continues to be a problem with the allocation of critical care resources to those most in need following elective surgery. However, as also exposed by the 2020 SARS-CoV2 pandemic, the availability of critical care beds remains limited, with an average of 2.8 critical care beds per 100 acute care beds across Europe.[11] This varies considerably between countries, with Germany having 6.9 times the number of critical care beds per head of population that Portugal has. Studies have demonstrated the paucity of both ICU and high-dependency unit (HDU) beds in the UK and found that patients were often admitted later and with worse severity of illness.[12–14] This mismatch between the need/demand for postoperative critical care and the capacity to deliver it has been recently exposed during the COVID-19 pandemic with the shutting down of surgical services to prioritise the urgent and emergency care pathways resulting in a very significant surgical backlog on the waiting list.[15]

Repeated publications by the NCEPOD have cited inadequate preoperative preparation, inappropriate intraoperative monitoring and poor postoperative care as contributing causes of perioperative mortality.[4,16,17] The NCEPOD report (*Knowing the Risk*) suggests that patients in the UK often die after surgery because they are not given the level of care they are entitled to or could reasonably expect.[16] In this report, less than half of the patients received the care that the advisors felt was the minimally acceptable standard. Predicting which patients will most likely benefit from admission to intensive care is hugely complex and is fraught with difficulties. The significant variation in these patients' underlying pathology and premorbid physiology makes it very difficult to provide hard-and-fast rules as to which patients will benefit from perioperative admission to either ICUs or HDUs.[18]

WHY DO PATIENTS DIE AFTER SURGERY?

Major surgery is associated with a significant stress response[19] vital for the body to recover and heal from the surgical trauma. This response manifests in many different ways, but a typical delineating pattern is hyperdynamic circulation with increased oxygen requirements postoperatively.[20] If the body is unable to increase the cardiac output in response to the surgical stress, then the increased need for oxygen cannot be met, and the patient develops tissue dysoxia and cellular dysfunction. This has been described by some authors as an acquired oxygen debt[21] which if left, results in organ failure and death. The important point to recognise is that the normal response to surgery is to increase the cardiac output and the delivery of oxygen to the tissues. Any patient who, for whatever reason, is unable to develop this response is at higher risk of subsequent complications.

WHAT IS A HIGH-RISK SURGICAL PATIENT?

The challenge is the early identification of patients who are at a high risk of postoperative complications and death, and this is vital to ensure that correct care and therapy are initiated at an optimal time. Patients admitted to ICU following a postoperative complication tend to experience worse outcomes. A recent systematic review has identified that age, anaemia, American Society of Anesthesiologists (ASA) grade, body mass index, extent of comorbidity, emergency and high-risk surgery, male sex, sleep apnoea, increased blood loss and operative duration are all independent risk factors for unplanned critical care admission. Given these are mostly known preoperatively, resource planning should be done in a pre-emptive manner.[10]

Overall, this patient group is characterised by undergoing major surgery whilst having concurrent medical illnesses that limit their physiological reserve to compensate for the stressful situation. Patient assessment of surgical risk is discussed in detail in Chapter 4.

Individualised clinical risk interpretation is challenging, although the use of well-validated risk assessment scores such as P-POSSUM is commonly used to mediate this variability, inform shared decision-making with patients, and guide further preoperative assessment.[22] It has been suggested that elective surgical patients can be assessed by cardiopulmonary exercise testing,[20,23,24] in which a strong correlation has been demonstrated between anaerobic threshold and postoperative outcome. The anaerobic threshold is the point where aerobic metabolism fails to provide adequate adenosine triphosphate and anaerobic metabolism starts to reduce the resultant deficit. The threshold is determined by monitoring inhaled and exhaled levels of oxygen and carbon dioxide during escalating levels of exercise. This provides an objective measure of physiological reserve. However, it must be remembered that complex cardiopulmonary testing in patients who have established poor cardiorespiratory reserve is only of use if used to target preoperative preparation and these patients must have specific optimisation of their comorbidities prior to surgery whenever possible. This requires that patients booked for elective surgery have all their comorbidities treated and investigated to ensure best possible physiological status prior to surgery. This is also the opportunity to consider if surgical intervention is the best course of action in view of the risk of the potential adverse outcomes. A complete and truthful risk assessment should be undertaken and the patient fully involved in the decision to proceed to surgery. A national report published in 2011 suggested that only 7.5% of patients at high risk of death or severe complications were given any indication of their risks of mortality and morbidity prior to surgery.[16] It is now regarded as a minimum standard of care to provide each patient with an individualised risk estimation and document this clearly in the clinical records.

✔ Risk assessment scores such as P-POSSUM can assist in shared decision-making and preoperative assessment.[22]

VARIABLES ASSOCIATED WITH POSTOPERATIVE COMPLICATIONS AND DEATH

Several authors[24,25] have examined the prognostic ability of many of the variables that can be monitored in the postoperative setting. One group found that none of the routinely measured variables such as heart rate, blood pressure, central venous pressure, urine output or any marker of acid–base status could predict subsequent postoperative complications.[26] The variables independently associated with subsequent significant complications were the central venous oxygen saturation and cardiac index. This association between oxygen flux in the perioperative period and subsequent complications is not new and is essentially the same as work published by Shoemaker et al.[21] in 1992, when they identified the key variables as being cardiac index, oxygen delivery and oxygen consumption. It was from this body of work that the theories surrounding the targeting of oxygen delivery to values of over 600 mL/min/m^2 in the perioperative period to improve patient outcome originated.

THE ROLE OF THE SPLANCHNIC CIRCULATION

There is some evidence that splanchnic circulation has a role in the pathogenesis of postoperative morbidity and mortality. It has been shown that increasing global tissue oxygen delivery increases splanchnic oxygen delivery,[27–29] and in the early stages of shock any inadequacy of tissue oxygen delivery predominantly affects the splanchnic circulation.[30] The splanchnic circulation is particularly sensitive to hypoperfusion states, and the reduction in flow to the splanchnic bed is out of proportion to the overall reduction in cardiac output and is usually the last major system blood flow to recover when the hypoperfusion state improves.[31,32] It is thought that this splanchnic hypoperfusion leads to disruption of the enteric mucosal barrier with translocation of endotoxins and microorganisms into the systemic circulation.[33–36] This translocation initiates a cytokine pathway, increasing the risk of sepsis and organ failure. This risk of splanchnic hypoperfusion and translocation increases with age, the urgency of the surgery and the preoperative presence of bowel obstruction. The translocation of bacteria and endotoxins induces cytokine release by tissue macrophages, activates the complement and coagulation systems, and produces a proinflammatory state. These cytokines themselves can impair oxygen delivery to the splanchnic circulation, further increasing translocation.

STRATEGIES TO IMPROVE OUTCOMES

The overall postoperative standard of care has improved significantly through the use of education and quality improvement initiatives, such as the National Emergency Laparotomy Audit (NELA)[37] and the Surviving Sepsis Campaign.[38] Evidence-based guidance is now available for emergency surgery to support clinicians in navigating this difficult area from the Enhanced Recovery After Surgery (ERAS) group.[39] These recommendations cover the early identification of physiological derangement and intervention, screening for sepsis, imaging and source control of sepsis, risk assessment and the age-related evaluation of frailty.

The concept of augmenting cardiac output in the perioperative period to improve the outcome of surgical patients has been described by many authors as 'optimisation' or 'goal-directed therapy'. The main aim of all optimisation strategies for high-risk patients has been to ensure that the circulatory status is adequate for the patient's needs in the perioperative period. This has been achieved with a number of differing protocols utilising different time periods, resuscitation endpoints and pharmacological agents. Recent systematic review and meta-analysis have described a reduction in postoperative complications.[40,41]

The OPTIMISE trial, published in 2014, attempted to determine whether overall benefits could be reproduced on a large scale. Initial analysis found no apparent reduction in complications or mortality. However, after incorporating the results into an updated systematic review and meta-analysis, there remains evidence of clinically significant reductions in both these outcomes. The OPTIMISE II trial should provide further clarity on the benefits of cardiac output-guided haemodynamic therapy treatment algorithms.[42]

✔✔ The OPTIMISE trial demonstrated that algorithm-based goal-directed therapy probably reduces the risk of postoperative morbidity and mortality. The OPTIMISE II trial will provide more information on the potential benefits.[42]

OXYGEN DELIVERY

To understand the rationale behind many of the protocols that have been utilised in the perioperative setting, it is vital to appreciate the important variables that determine oxygen delivery: haemoglobin (Hb) concentration, arterial oxygen saturation (SaO_2) and cardiac output. It, therefore, becomes clear that to ensure that an adequate volume of oxygen is delivered to the body's vital organs, Hb concentration (Hb), SaO_2 and the cardiac index must all be at a satisfactory level. Maximising all three of these variables to clinically acceptable levels is the aim of resuscitation in any given patient, although not always achievable. The Hb level is governed by the clinical situation and the underlying pathophysiological process, but many experts aim to keep the Hb level above 7–8 g/dL in a stable perioperative setting.[43–46] Frail and vulnerable patients are often anaemic. It had been recommended to actively manage preoperative iron deficiency with intravenous iron therapy, hoping to avoid the complications associated with blood transfusion such as increased hospital stay and infection rate.[47–49] However, the PREVENTT trial has added weight to the argument that intravenous iron therapy does not necessarily benefit patient outcomes.[50]

The SaO_2 is usually targeted to be 94–98% (or 88–92% in those at risk of type 2 respiratory failure)[51] with increased inspired oxygen and/or continuous positive airway pressure (CPAP) if necessary. Postoperative pulmonary complications such as pneumonia and acute respiratory distress syndrome are rare but associated with significant morbidity and mortality. Expert opinion supports intraoperative lung protection strategies such as low tidal ventilation (6–8 mL/kg) and positive end-expiratory pressure (5 cm H_2O) to minimise the impact of perioperative lung injury. Atelectasis is common in the postoperative period, and there is a growing understanding that it is not just associated with hypoxaemia but also with a proinflammatory response that potentiates tissue injury. As a result, the use of CPAP, or other non-invasive positive pressure ventilation (NIPPV) therapy, has the potential to improve many physiological parameters without serious side effects in certain high-risk groups of patients.

Postoperatively, studies suggest that NIPPV can reduce pneumonia and the need for intubation.[52,53] High-flow nasal oxygen therapy has similar efficacy to NIPPV in preventing postoperative atelectasis and may be more comfortable to some patients.[54]

Cardiac output can be increased with several easy-to-use protocols. The targeting of the cardiac index does necessitate the measurement and monitoring of this variable, which can be done relatively non-invasively. Once measured, if the cardiac output is perceived to be too low, then it is increased with intravenous volume therapy and then, if it has still not improved sufficiently, pharmacologically, using appropriate cardiovascular pharmaceutical agents that will improve cardiac output.[55]

✔ NIPPV and high-flow nasal oxygen therapy postoperatively have been shown to reduce postoperative pulmonary complications.[52–54]

MEASUREMENT AND MONITORING OF CARDIAC OUTPUT

There are a variety of technologies available to monitor cardiac output. In the past, pulmonary artery catheters were used, which enabled a thermodilution curve to be constructed across the right ventricle, thus enabling cardiac output to be calculated from the Stewart–Hamilton equation. In recent times, this tool is rarely used due to a lack of evidence demonstrating a beneficial effect on outcome and the perceived invasiveness of its approach. Many devices and techniques are now available that can provide the same information in a less invasive fashion.[56] The National Institute for Health and Care Excellence (NICE) in the UK, in their appraisal of the evidence noted that the approaches to monitoring fluid management have developed in tandem with surgical approaches and management. The benefits seen in the early studies now seem to be less, but this may be that many of the underlying principles of pre-emptive monitoring of perfusion and resuscitation have been taken on board by practising clinicians. Although cardiac output monitoring is not a standard practice for most surgical interventions, it does have a place in complex and emergency patients.[56]

FLUID RESUSCITATION

It is important to recognise that the aim of management is to give the right amount of fluid at the right time. There is evidence that excessive fluid administration is detrimental in critically ill and postoperative patients, but it is also suspected that a very restrictive regime can also cause harm.[57] The 2011 NCEPOD report shows that mortality is related to fluid management, with mortality being only 4.7% in patients receiving adequate preoperative fluids compared with 20.5% and 33.3%, respectively, in those patients receiving either inadequate or excessive preoperative intravenous fluid.[16] This mandates the need to monitor very carefully fluid administration in critically ill or high-risk patients where simple measures or markers of preload status are often inadequate. Clinical examination and cardiac monitoring can guide the clinician in predicting whether a fluid challenge will be effective; however, defining the endpoint at which filling is optimal and the need for inotropic therapy begins is difficult. A plateau in the stroke volume, the flow correction time as determined by oesophageal Doppler and the stroke volume variation (with the pulse pressure analysis) can all be used to define the endpoint.

DELIRIUM AS A POSTOPERATIVE COMPLICATION

High-risk surgical patients are more likely to develop postoperative delirium, and it has been demonstrated that 54% of patients undergoing major elective non-cardiac surgery will develop this fluctuation in cognition.[58] Elderly patients are at a particularly high risk. It has been suggested that prophylactic low-dose dexmedetomidine significantly decreases the occurrence of delirium during the first 7 days after surgery in those aged over 65 years.[59] Whilst this is not routine practice, it highlights the ongoing area of research aimed at improving overall post-surgical outcomes in the high-risk surgical patient.

ROYAL COLLEGE OF SURGEONS RECOMMENDATIONS

The Royal College of Surgeons of England have considered the high-risk surgical patient and have made a series of key suggestions for improvement in care and outcomes.[60] These include: recommendations that all hospitals should formalise their pathways for unscheduled adult surgical care; that there should be prompt recognition and treatment of emergencies and complications to improve outcomes and reduce costs; hospitals should match theatre access to patient needs; every patient should have his/her expected risk of death estimated and documented; high-risk patients are those at greater risk of death than 5% and all should have active consultant input and be admitted to a critical care area postoperatively for at least 12 hours; surgical procedures with a risk of death greater than 10% should only be conducted under the direct supervision of a consultant surgeon and consultant anaesthetist.

✓✓ Decision-making regarding high-risk surgical patients should be made at consultant level.[60]

Key points

This overview of the literature relating to the high-risk surgical patient and current improvements associated with goal-directed therapy leads to some inevitable conclusions:

- There is good evidence to suggest that patients with poor cardiorespiratory reserve have a higher mortality and complication rate when undergoing major surgery. Most of these patients can be identified by simple clinical methods before surgery.
- It is likely that there are significant numbers of patients undergoing different types of surgery who may be at substantial risk of developing major complications or death.
- There is some evidence that targeted protocolised treatment for this group can improve outcome, but this is becoming less certain with improving basic standards of care.
- It is apparent that optimising the circulation can be carried out using several different techniques and at different times (i.e. preoperatively, intraoperatively and postoperatively).
- Goal-directed therapy aims to ensure that tissue oxygen delivery is enhanced to levels shown to confer survival without postoperative complications.
- The decision to operate on high-risk patients should be made at consultant level and should involve surgeons as well as those who will provide the intraoperative and postoperative care (anaesthetists and critical care consultants).
- An assessment of mortality risk should be made explicit to the patient and recorded clearly on the consent form and in the medical notes.
- All hospitals undertaking surgery for high-risk patients should have facilities to provide perioperative goal-directed monitoring and therapy and the hospital should analyse the volume of work they undertake to ensure they have sufficient capacity of facilities to be able to accommodate all the patients they treat. This should be assessed annually.

References available at http://ebooks.health.elsevier.com/

KEY REFERENCES

[7] International Surgical Outcomes Study g. Global patient outcomes after elective surgery: prospective cohort study in 27 low-, middle- and high-income countries. Br J Anaesth 2016;117(5):601–9.

[10] Onwochei DN, Fabes J, Walker D, et al. Critical care after major surgery: a systematic review of risk factors for unplanned admission. Anaesthesia 2020;75(Suppl.1):e62–74.

[16] Cain D, Ackland G. Knowing the risk? NCEPOD 2011: a wake-up call for perioperative practice. Br J Hosp Med 2012;73(5):262–4.

[42] Pearse RM, Harrison DA, MacDonald N, et al. Effect of a perioperative, cardiac output-guided hemodynamic therapy algorithm on outcomes following major gastrointestinal surgery: a randomized clinical trial and systematic review. JAMA 2014;311(21):2181–90.

6 Surgical nutrition

Kirstine Farrer | Derek McWhirter | Jonathan Epstein

INTRODUCTION

Perioperative nutrition is a critical aspect of surgical care. Surgical teams should screen elective patients for existing malnutrition or risk of developing malnutrition postoperatively. Optimising macronutrient anabolism and correcting micronutrient deficiencies are important goals for elective and emergency surgical patients. In this chapter, we will describe:

- Preoperative screening for malnourished patients or patients at risk of malnutrition
- How to optimise nutritional support during hospital admission
- Strategies to achieve the optimal nutritional recovery in the postoperative period

DEFINING MALNUTRITION

A definition of malnutrition for the surgical patient is: 'a nutritional state in which nutrient intake does not match nutrient needs—due to underlying disease(s), the surgical stress response, chronic or acute inflammation, intestinal malabsorption (e.g. diarrhoea) and/or patient-related factors (e.g. socioeconomic status)—leading to losses in lean tissue and diminished function'.[1]

The key nutrition goals before elective surgery are to evaluate the patient for pre-existing malnutrition, treat any malnutrition to optimise readiness for surgery, prevent predictable postoperative malnutrition and support anabolism for rehabilitation.

The Global Leadership Initiative on Malnutrition (GLIM) was convened in January 2016 to standardise clinical practice in malnutrition diagnosis and management.[2] A two-step approach for malnutrition diagnosis was developed: first, screening to identify 'at-risk' status by the use of a validated screening tool; and second, assessment to diagnose and grade the severity of malnutrition. Criteria for malnutrition were retrieved from existing approaches and ranked by consensus expert opinion. The top five ranked criteria comprised three phenotypic criteria (non-volitional weight loss, low body mass index [BMI], and reduced muscle mass) and two aetiologic criteria (reduced food intake or assimilation, and inflammation or disease burden). Diagnosis of malnutrition required at least one phenotypic criterion and one aetiologic criterion. Phenotypic metrics for grading severity as stage 1 (moderate) and stage 2 (severe) malnutrition were proposed. It was recommended that the aetiologic criteria be used to guide intervention and anticipated outcomes.

CONSEQUENCES AND SIGNIFICANCE OF MALNUTRITION

The clinical significance of malnutrition in surgical patients is profound. Patients with low skeletal muscle mass (*sarcopenia*) have limited reserve to respond to surgical stress (see below).[3] Malnourished patients have disturbances in function at the organ and cellular level with the following physiological consequences:

- Impaired normal homeostatic mechanisms[4]
- Muscle wasting and impairment of skeletal muscle function[5]
- Impaired respiratory muscle function[6]
- Impaired cardiac muscle function[6]
- Impaired immune function[4]
- Impaired wound healing and increased anastomotic leak rate[4]

Prospective cohort studies from around the world confirm that malnourished surgical patients have significantly poorer clinical outcomes, including as much as fourfold greater risk of mortality, greater risk of complications, more frequent re-admissions, prolonged hospitalisation and increased healthcare costs.[7–9]

Fortunately, malnutrition is a modifiable risk factor. A meta-analysis of 15 randomised controlled trials (RCTs) including 3831 malnourished patients undergoing a range of surgical procedures identified that perioperative nutritional support led to decreased infectious and non-infectious complications and was associated with a 2-day shorter length of hospital stay.[10] A Cochrane review of 13 RCTs (548 patients) assessing the effect of preoperative nutritional therapy in gastrointestinal surgery found that preoperative immune-enhancing nutrition significantly reduced total postoperative complications compared with no nutrition or standard nutrition.[11] This review also included 260 malnourished patients, in whom parenteral nutrition (PN) compared with no nutritional support was beneficial in reducing major complications. Collectively these studies indicate that nutritional optimisation can have an impact on surgical recovery.

Maintaining muscle mass is imperative to facilitate wound healing and immunity.[12,13] Computed tomography scanning can identify body composition profiles, including sarcopenia, that predict surgical risk. Low muscle mass before surgery was an independent predictor of reduced overall survival in patients with colorectal cancer. Furthermore, the presence of myosteatosis (fatty infiltration, an indicator of muscle quality) was associated with prolonged hospital stay. Thus, obese patients with low muscle mass were most likely to suffer from morbidity and mortality at 30 days.[13] These findings suggest that specific body composition profiles predict different surgical risks.

NUTRITION SCREENING: PREOP CLINIC

Nutritional screening aims to detect patients who are at risk of becoming malnourished and should be part of standard preoperative assessment.[11] Malnutrition remains highly prevalent: in 2018, the British Association of Parenteral and Enteral Nutrition (BAPEN) documented that 30% of patients admitted to hospital in the UK and 15% attending outpatient clinics were malnourished or at risk of malnutrition.[14] Trauma, sepsis and inflammation accelerate loss of tissue mass and reduce appetite. Such patients may also find it difficult to meet their nutritional needs through food intake due to pathology–related gut obstruction or malabsorption.

NUTRITION SCREENING

Validated screening tools[15–18] and surgical nutrition guidelines are produced by the European Society for Clinical Nutrition and Metabolism,[6] the American Society of Parenteral Enteral Nutrition[19] and the American Society for Enhanced Recovery with Perioperative Quality Initiative.[20] All provide details on selecting nutrition screening tools, malnutrition assessment tools, and treatment for malnourished and at–risk patients. All recommend routine screening for malnutrition and subsequent nutrition assessment with a validated malnutrition assessment tool or a comprehensive nutrition assessment by a registered dietician if the nutrition screen is positive.

In 2006, the BAPEN developed the Malnutrition Universal Screening Tool ('MUST') and this has gained widespread acceptance in UK practice.[18]

MUST SCREENING TOOL

Step 1 Calculate patient's body mass index (weight in kg/height in m^2)
If BMI >20, score 0
If BMI is 18.5–20, score 1
If BMI is < 18.5, score 2

Step 2 Percentage weight loss
If unplanned weight loss <5%, score 0
If unplanned weight loss is 5–10%, score 1
If unplanned weight loss >10%, score 2

Step 3 If a patient is acutely ill and there has or is likely to be no nutritional intake for >5 days, score 2

If a patient scores 2 or above, they are classified at high risk of developing malnutrition or have pre-existing malnutrition. Many UK hospitals have treatment plans or community dietetic referral criteria based on 'MUST' scores.

The Mini Nutritional Assessment (MNA) includes more information than 'MUST' and is often used in older adults. In addition to percentage weight loss and BMI, the short form MNA includes food intake, mobility, neuropsychological status and a measurement of calf circumference.[17]

Duke University preoperative nutrition score (PONS) utilises questions from the validated MUST to assess for malnutrition risk in perioperative patients. A score ≥ 1 signifies malnutrition risk, and the authors recommend that such patients should be considered for preoperative nutrition therapy.[18,19]

Whichever tool is used, the next step is to intervene for patients identified as being at risk.

NUTRITIONAL ASSESSMENT

Nutritional assessment involves a more detailed evaluation of a patient's nutritional status than the screening instruments described above and is conventionally conducted by a dietitian. The assessment of nutritional status is essential for determining energy and protein requirements for nutritional support, which may require multi-professional discussion with the surgical team, especially if commencing perioperative enteral nutrition or PN.[21]

Nutritional assessment includes a detailed dietary history, anthropometric measurements, body composition measurements, biomarkers and functional measurements. Anthropometric measurements include weight, height, BMI, trunk measurements (e.g. waist and hip circumferences), sagittal abdominal diameter, limb measurements (mid-upper arm and calf circumferences) and skinfold thickness.[22] Functional measurements aim to determine muscle strength as a potential indicator of body muscle status or function.

Body composition measurements aim to assess individual components of the human body including fat, muscle, bone and water content. In clinical practice, dietitians routinely measure mid-upper arm muscle circumference, triceps skinfold thickness and grip strength. Reference tables are available, but they have significant limitations as many are based on a male Italian military population,[23] and White males and females participating in the 1971–1974 United States Health and Nutrition Survey.[24]

Biomarkers used in nutritional assessment seek to assess nutritional status from the measurement of serum, plasma or urine levels. It is a commonly held surgical myth that a low albumin is a marker of malnutrition. Albumin is an acute-phase protein and is reduced in the setting of inflammation. A low albumin does not necessarily represent malnutrition, and although patients with chronic inflammation may have concomitant malnutrition, it is perfectly possible for a patient to have massive weight loss and significant malnutrition with an entirely normal albumin.[25]

METABOLIC RESPONSE TO FEEDING, TRAUMA AND SEPSIS

In order to maintain the health of cells, tissues and organs, metabolism must adapt to changes in nutritional intake, trauma and sepsis. While a detailed knowledge of complex biochemical pathways is not necessary, it is important to understand the principles of these metabolic and biochemical changes, and the metabolic response when a patient experiences trauma, undergoes surgery or develops sepsis. This underpins nutrition and nutritional support in critically ill patients.

TRAUMA

A major advance in understanding occurred more than 80 years ago when Sir David Cuthbertson described the loss of nitrogen from skeletal muscle that occurred following trauma.[26] Cuthbertson concluded that the response to injury could be considered as occurring in two phases:

1. The 'ebb' phase, which is a short-lived response associated with hypovolaemic shock, increased sympathetic nervous system activity and reduced metabolic rate.
2. The 'flow' phase, which is associated with a loss of body nitrogen and resultant negative nitrogen balance.

These changes result in the following:

Ebb phase
- Decreased resting energy expenditure
- Increased glycogen breakdown
- Increased gluconeogenesis

Flow phase
- Increased resting energy expenditure
- Increased heat production, pyrexia
- Increased muscle catabolism and wasting, and loss of body nitrogen
- Increased breakdown of fat and reduced fat synthesis
- Increased gluconeogenesis and impairment of glucose tolerance

If the changes of the 'ebb phase' are not replaced by the 'flow phase', then despite any advances in surgery, anaesthesia and intensive care support, death of the patient is the inevitable outcome.

The central nervous system and the neurohypophyseal axis play key roles in regulating these metabolic changes via a range of hormones and cytokines. Afferent nerve impulses stimulate the hypothalamus to secrete hypothalamic releasing factors that, in turn, stimulate the pituitary gland to release prolactin, arginine vasopressin (antidiuretic hormone [ADH]), growth hormone and adrenocorticotrophic hormone.

SEPSIS

The metabolic response to sepsis is also characterised by alterations in protein, carbohydrate and fat metabolism, with the following key differences:[27]

- The breakdown of skeletal muscle and nitrogen losses can be substantial (more than 15–20 g/day).
- There is increased production of glucose by the liver (both gluconeogenesis and glycogenolysis), resulting in an elevated plasma glucose.
- In contrast to the situation following trauma, there is an increased rate of glucose uptake and oxidation by peripheral tissues.
- Decrease in the peripheral uptake of triglyceride and defective ketogenesis in the presence of sepsis leads to hypertriglyceridaemia.

A significant abnormality in the patient with sepsis is the disruption of the microstructure of the hepatocyte mitochondria, particularly of the inner membrane. There is a block in energy transduction pathways, with consequent reduction in the aerobic metabolism of both glucose and fatty acids. The body therefore depends on *anaerobic* metabolism of glucose, which results in lactate production. An adequate supply of glucose is therefore essential. If gluconeogenesis is impaired or inadequate, then hypoglycaemia may ensue. Hypoglycaemia during sepsis indicates an extremely poor prognosis and is frequently associated with mortality.

NUTRITION AFTER SURGERY

In addition to the response to trauma and/or sepsis, general surgery patients may face multiple barriers to adequate food intake including gut obstruction or paralysis and organisational barriers in hospital (e.g. missed meals or tube feeds withheld due to scheduled clinical investigations). Nutritional monitoring and review should continue postoperatively. Patients identified as malnourished, or at risk, require individualised treatment plans that may include therapeutic diets (e.g. high protein), fortified foods, high-protein oral nutrition supplements, enteral nutrition and/or PN.[28]

EVIDENCE FOR MICRONUTRIENTS IN SURGERY

Additional nutrients may complement the protein anabolic response. Corn oil supplementation for 8 weeks had no effect on muscle protein synthesis rate, whereas omega–3 fatty acid supplementation was found to augment muscle protein synthesis.[29] A meta–analysis of 13 RCTs of supplemental vitamin D in adults aged > 60 years compared with placebo or standard treatment on muscle function found that supplementation with at least 800 IU of vitamin D decreased postural sway, reduced time to complete the 'Timed Up and Go Test', and marginally increased lower extremity strength.[30] However, these findings have no implications for surgical care currently.

ROUTES OF ACCESS FOR ENTERAL NUTRITIONAL SUPPORT

ENFit® is the global enteral feeding device connector designed to reduce the likelihood of tubing misconnections that complies with the new International Standard (ISO 80369-3). All enteral feeding tubes, devices and associated equipment are required to be compatible.[31]

NASOGASTRIC TUBES

Nasogastric (NG) feeding via fine-bore tubes (polyvinyl chloride or polyurethane) may be used in patients with a functioning gut who require nutritional support for a short period of time. The fine-bore tube may be manipulated through the pylorus into the duodenum to reduce the risk of gastric aspiration. In patients with delayed gastric emptying, double-lumen tubes may be useful: one lumen resides in the stomach and is used to aspirate gastric contents while the more distal lumen is placed in the jejunum for feeding. Regardless of initial position, it is common for NG tubes to become misplaced, with a potential for pulmonary aspiration. In the UK, the National Patient Safety Agency produces reports on incidents (including a number of fatalities) related to NG feeding tubes and issues advice on reducing potential harm. Radiographic confirmation should be obtained if NG feeding tube placement cannot be confirmed by pH monitoring (pH < 5.5 indicates gastric placement); individual hospitals often have their own governance protocols.[32]

Other complications associated with the use of nasoenteric tubes include:

- Pulmonary atelectasis
- Oesophageal necrosis, stricture formation
- Tracheo-oesophageal fistulas
- Sinusitis, post-cricoid ulceration

GASTROSTOMY TUBES

Gastrostomy tube placement should be considered if enteral feeding will be required for 4–6 weeks. A gastrostomy tube can be placed into the stomach at laparotomy although percutaneous endoscopic or radiologic techniques are more common. A radiological inserted gastrostomy should be considered in patients where access for an endoscope is difficult e.g. oesophageal cancer, head and neck cancer.

The establishment and use of a gastrostomy has certain disadvantages and there is a recognised morbidity:

- Infection of the skin at the puncture site
- Necrotising fasciitis or deeper-sited sepsis
- Damage to adjacent intra-abdominal viscera
- Leakage of gastric contents into the peritoneal cavity
- Haemorrhage from the stomach
- Blockage, fracture and displacement
- Persistent gastrocutaneous fistula following removal of the feeding tube

The overall mortality rate for a gastrostomy is 1–2%[33] with major and minor complications occurring in up to 15% of patients.[34]

JEJUNOSTOMY TUBES

A feeding jejunostomy is often inserted at the time of laparotomy if it is envisaged that a patient will need prolonged nutritional support, particularly after oesophagogastric or pancreatic resections. Details of the operative technique are found in standard operative texts and the smaller needle-catheter tubes are to be preferred. Advantages of a feeding jejunostomy compared with a gastrostomy are:

- Less stomal leakage
- Gastric and pancreatic secretions are reduced because the stomach is bypassed
- Less nausea, vomiting or bloating
- Reduced risk of pulmonary aspiration

NUTRIENT SOLUTIONS AVAILABLE FOR ENTERAL NUTRITION

A range of nutrient solutions is available for use in enteral nutritional support and examples can be found in specialised texts. There are four main categories of enteral diet.

POLYMERIC FEEDS

Polymeric diets are 'nutritionally complete' diets and provided to patients with inadequate oral intake, but whose intestinal function is good. They contain whole protein as the source of nitrogen, and energy is provided as complex carbohydrates and fat in a range of concentrations from (1 kcal/mL to 2 kcal/mL). They also contain vitamins, trace elements and electrolytes in standard amounts.

SEMI-ELEMENTAL FEEDS

The main difference between an elemental and a semi-elemental diet is in the protein structure. The semi-elemental diet provides protein that is hydrolysed into peptides (short chains of amino acids), which are more readily absorbed than individual amino acids or whole proteins.

Semi-elemental diets also contain fats in the form of medium-chain triglycerides (MCTs). MCTs are found in coconut oil and are more easily digestible than other types of fats because of their shorter length. Unlike other fats, MCTs go straight from the gut to the liver, where they are converted into energy or turned into ketones. MCT fat is also partially water-soluble and therefore can aid energy absorption in the colon.

ELEMENTAL FEEDS

Elemental diets are required if the patient is unable to produce an adequate amount of digestive enzymes or has a reduced area for absorption (e.g. severe pancreatic insufficiency). Elemental diets contain nitrogen as oligopeptides (free amino acids are not as easily absorbed as dipeptide and tripeptide mixtures). The energy source is provided as glucose polymers and MCTs. Each oligopeptide molecule contributes as much to the osmolarity of the solution as one molecule of intact protein, and it can be difficult to meet total nutritional requirements without producing side effects associated with an osmotic load, for example 'dumping' and diarrhoea.

MODULAR PRODUCTS

Modular dietary products can be helpful to boost the energy content of the oral diet and fortify food. For example, the diet may be enriched in protein in the post-bariatric surgery phase if the patient is protein-deficient, or carbohydrate maltodextrins used in Enhanced Recovery After Surgery (ERAS) programme as part of carbohydrate loading before surgery. Modular diets can also be used to supplement other enteral regimens or oral intake.

ENTERAL NUTRITION DELIVERY AND COMPLICATIONS

Enteral feeding regimens are commenced on a reduced rate of infusion for the first 2 or 3 days to reduce gastrointestinal complications. Feeding may be cyclical (e.g. 16 hours feeding with a post-absorptive period of 8 hours) or continuous.

Enteral nutrition should be administered through a volumetric enteral feeding pump. Volume-based feeding approaches are preferable to an hourly target rate of infusion, allowing nursing staff to calculate the remaining daily feed volumes to be delivered and to adjust the rate to accommodate time lost due to investigations or other interventions (e.g. airway management).[21]

Metabolic disturbances (e.g. re-feeding syndrome [RFS], see below) are less likely with enteral feeding. The other complications of enteral nutrition are those associated with the route of access to the gastrointestinal tract.

PARENTERAL NUTRITIONAL SUPPORT

Patients who require nutritional support when enteral feeding is inadequate or contraindicated will require PN. For optimal provision of nutritional support, a multidisciplinary nutritional support team is required. This often comprises a clinician with a special interest in nutritional support and understanding of metabolic pathways, a biochemist, a pharmacist, a dietitian and a nutrition nurse specialist. The provision of nutritional support by such a team results in the most cost-effective use of nutritional support and the least risk of infective, metabolic and feeding-line complications.[35]

INDICATIONS FOR PARENTERAL NUTRITION

- Patients with a non-functioning or inaccessible gastrointestinal tract
- High-output enteric fistulas (enteral nutrition may stimulate gastrointestinal secretion—discussed further later)
- Insufficient enteral absorption (e.g. short gut, malabsorption)

PARENTERAL ROUTES OF ACCESS

CENTRAL VENOUS ACCESS

A central venous access device (CVAD) is usually placed into the superior vena cava through subclavian or internal jugular veins. The catheter either emerges through the skin (usually after being tunnelled in the subcutaneous layers) or is connected to a port placed in the subcutaneous tissue of the anterior chest wall. Catheters may be introduced into the internal jugular or subclavian vein directly by 'blind' percutaneous puncture, using small hand-held ultrasound imaging, by 'cut-down' techniques utilising the cephalic vein to access the subclavian vein, or under fluoroscopic control. Details of these techniques and their advantages/disadvantages can be found elsewhere; however, it is important that whoever inserts a central venous line is expert, well-practised and does so under full aseptic conditions.

TECHNICAL ASPECTS OF FEEDING LINES

CVADs are manufactured from polyurethane or silicone. Both materials are tolerated well, with low thrombogenic potential. However, polyurethane does have advantages:

- It is stiffer than silicone at room temperature, but at body temperature is pliable
- It has a higher tensile strength than silicone and is less likely to fracture
- Polyurethane catheters have smaller outside diameters, making cannulation easier, as well as a greater resistance to thrombus development on their surfaces

Following insertion, a semi-permeable dressing, a transparent polyurethane dressing and/or the use of gauze and tape may be used to secure and protect the catheter. Transparent dressings allow for continuous visual inspection of the exit site and all exit site dressings are recommended to be changed every 7 days unless the dressing becomes damp, loose, or visibly soiled.[36]

CARE OF PARENTERAL NUTRITION CATHETERS

Prevention of catheter-related bloodstream infections (CRBSIs) is vital to maintaining long-term venous access.[37] All healthcare professionals, patients and/or their caregivers must be educated appropriately regarding the management of CVADs based on stringent aseptic catheter care (aseptic non-touch technique).[38] The British Intestinal Failure Alliance (BIFA) published guidelines for safe catheter care management for patients with long-term feeding CVADs in 2018.[39] The guidelines are applicable to both adults and children commencing home parenteral nutrition (HPN).

Key points when handling HPN catheter:

- A full effective hand washing technique is essential, paying attention to in between fingers, thumbs, rubbing the palms and above the wrists.
- Ensure all equipment required is present, and that there is a clean area in which to carry out the procedure.
- Open all sterile packs carefully to prevent contamination of the contents.
- Ensure only sterile items come into contact with the catheter, and that sterile items do not come into contact with non-sterile objects.
- Do not touch key parts at any time.
- The wearing of gloves is not a substitute for hand washing.
- Needle-free connectors should be disinfected using pressure and friction for a minimum of 15 seconds each time they are accessed.

CRBSI is characterised by systemic signs of sepsis and high pyrexia, often most prominent just after each PN bag is commenced. Paired blood cultures should be obtained from both peripheral venepuncture and via the CVAD. Coagulase-negative staphylococcus remains the primary cause of CRBSI and can be successfully salvaged with antibiotic therapy in some cases; however, the CVAD may have to be removed to eradicate the infection.[40] Infection may also occur in the skin at the exit site of the catheter. This is recognised by skin erythema, possibly associated with fluid exudate and pus, and is usually treatable with antibiotics.

PERIPHERAL VENOUS ACCESS

Peripheral venous cannulation may be used to supply nutrients intravenously to avoid complications associated with central venous catheters. Peripheral intravenous nutrition is likely to be used in patients who do not require nutritional support for long enough to justify risks of central vein cannulation or in whom central vein cannulation is contraindicated (e.g. central line insertion sites are traumatised, increased risks of infective complications, thrombosis of the central veins or significant clotting defects).

Problems associated with the delivery of intravenous nutrition using the peripheral route include:

- A limit to nutrient quantity deliverable—this is not the route of choice in those with high requirements for protein or energy
- A high incidence of complications, particularly phlebitis (occurs in up to 45% of patients)

The lifespan of a peripheral intravenous cannula can be prolonged by rigorous aseptic care and by using a narrow-gauge cannula. The risk of phlebitis can be reduced by frequent changes of infusion site, ultrafine-bore catheters or using a vasodilator patch over the cannulation site (e.g. transdermal glyceryl trinitrate). Peripheral intravenous nutrition should only be used with fat emulsion as part of the single-phase administration of nutrients to avoid thrombophlebitis.

NUTRIENTS USED IN PARENTERAL FEEDING SOLUTIONS

Various nutrient solutions (amino acids, glucose and fat) are available and a complete list is available in the British National Formulary (www.bnf.org/bnf). A variety of multi-chamber bags containing various concentrations of amino acids and glucose, with or without fat are available. They may or may not contain electrolytes depending on the clinical situations. These mixtures do not usually contain vitamins or trace elements, which must be given additionally to avoid development of metabolic complications. It is important to be aware of the volume and sodium contribution from other intravenous fluids and medications given in parallel.

NITROGEN SOURCES

Nitrogen sources are solutions of crystalline L-amino acids containing all essential and a balanced mixture of non-essential amino acids. Amino acids that are relatively insoluble (e.g. L-glutamine, L-arginine, L-taurine, L-tyrosine, L-methionine) may be absent or present in inadequate amounts. Solutions are available which provide 5–25 g nitrogen. One gram of nitrogen equates to 6.25 g protein and contributes 25 kcal/g of nitrogen to the PN regimen. Nitrogen requirements range 0.17–0.3 g/kg/day.[21]

ENERGY SOURCES

Energy is supplied as a balanced combination of dextrose and fat. Glucose is the primary carbohydrate source and the main form of energy supply to the majority of tissues. During critical illness, the body's preferred calorie source is fat (fasted or fed states). For critical care ventilated patients, it should be noted that propofol contains 1 kcal/mL. Energy requirements vary dependent on the assessment of nutritional status and are reliant on the measurement of actual body weight or fat free mass in kg. Considerations must include re-feeding risk, age, diagnosis, degree of metabolic stress and enteral intake. For a surgical patient with a BMI of 18.5–30 kg/m^2, a range of 20–25 kcal/kg is appropriate.[21]

Glucose utilisation may be impaired in certain patients and glucose is then metabolised through other pathways. This results in increased production and oxidation of fatty acids, resulting in increased carbon dioxide (excreted through the lungs). In addition, if glucose is the only energy source, patients may develop essential fatty acid (linolenic, linoleic) deficiency.

Lipid (e.g. soyabean oil, egg phospholipids, olive oil, fish oil emulsions) provides a more concentrated energy source. Aim to give < 50% of the total calories as lipid, aiming not to exceed 1.5 g/kg/day. The provision of exogenous lipids has also been associated with problems. Intravenous fat emulsions can impair lung function, inhibit the reticuloendothelial system and modulate neutrophil function. European Society of Parenteral and Enteral Nutrition (ESPEN) recommendations include the use of fish oils in postoperative surgical patients as a source of fat rich in omega-3 polyunsaturated fatty acids, as this appears to be associated with reduced incidence of hepatic dysfunction.[41]

OTHER NUTRIENTS

Commercially available preparations of trace elements (e.g. Nutryelt® Decan, Cernevit) and vitamins, water-soluble (e.g. Solivito®) and fat-soluble (e.g. Vitlipid®), must be added on a daily basis to the PN regimen. Larger amounts, particularly of the water-soluble vitamins, may be required initially if recent nutritional intake has been inadequate. Additionally, total fluid volume and amounts of electrolytes can be modified daily to meet particular requirements e.g. in renal and cardiac patients.

DELIVERY AND ADMINISTRATION OF PARENTERAL NUTRITION

It is possible to give individual components, but in practice it is safer and more convenient to use compounded bags. Compatibility between different prescribed constituents must be ensured before the parenteral infusion is compounded under sterile conditions in laminar flow facilities. No additions of drugs should be made as this could make the emulsion unstable, affect the bioavailability of the drug or compromise sterility.

Advantages of pre-mixed bags include:

- Cost-effectiveness
- Reduced infective risks
- More uniform administration of a balanced solution over a prolonged period
- Decreased lipid toxicity as a result of the greater dilution of the lipid emulsion and longer duration of infusion
- Ease of delivery and storage and reduced long-term accumulation of triglycerides (occurs with glucose-based PN)

'Off the shelf' PN including PN with supplemented micronutrients is now available covering a range of nutritional requirements, as many hospitals have limited on-site compounding capacity. A bag is chosen which approximates to anticipated nitrogen and calorie requirements. Nothing should be added to these bags–extra fluid, electrolyte and minerals can be given by separate infusion if required.[21]

COMPLICATIONS OF PARENTERAL NUTRITIONAL SUPPORT

Instant availability of nutrients via the intravenous route can lead to metabolic complications if the composition or flow rate is inappropriate. Rapid infusion of high concentrations of glucose can precipitate hyperglycaemia, which may be further complicated by lactic acidosis. Electrolyte disturbances may develop, not least because the intravenous feeding regimen is usually prescribed 24 hours in advance. Prediction of the patient's nutrient requirements must be complemented by frequent monitoring. The provision of nutrients may lead to further electrolyte abnormalities when potassium, magnesium and phosphate enter the intracellular compartment. This is particularly noticeable in patients whose previous nutrient intake was poor.

RE-FEEDING SYNDROME

RFS is not a single condition but a group of biochemical shifts and clinical symptoms that can occur in a malnourished or starved patient upon the re-introduction of oral, enteral tube feeding or PN.[26] When commencing nutritional support in the malnourished surgical patient, an awareness of the potential for RFS is essential as significant complications can result (see Box). Patients are at risk if they have not fed for over 7–10 days. This is not an unusual period of time in a surgical patient if they have presented with conditions such as oesophageal cancer or bowel obstruction.

During periods of starvation, insulin levels decrease while glucagon levels rise. This leads to the conversion of glycogen stores to glucose along with gluconeogenesis (the generation of glucose from non-carbohydrate sources—lipid and protein). Glycogen stores will be depleted by 48–72 hours. Breakdown of adipose tissue releases large volumes of fatty acids and ketone bodies, and free fatty acids become a major energy source. Catabolism of adipose tissue and muscle leads to weight loss.[21,26]

When feeding is re-introduced, there is a shift from fat to carbohydrate metabolism. This results in a surge of insulin release leading to increased cellular uptake of glucose, phosphate, potassium, magnesium and water. This may result in hypophosphataemia, hypokalaemia and hypomagnesaemia which in turn can cause cardiac arrhythmias, muscle weakness, neurological impairment, seizure and death.[21,26]

Identification of patients at risk of RFS is essential so that safe feeding may be introduced. Any electrolyte abnormalities should be identified and corrected, feeding should be started at a reduced rate and built up gradually, and electrolyte levels should be monitored daily and corrected as required.

It is imperative to consider whether a patient is at risk of RFS. Biochemical markers may be normal, and so the possibility of re-feeding must be anticipated on history alone. The other essential nutrient liable to become depleted in this situation is thiamine, a cofactor of pyruvate kinase, which is required for glucose to undergo oxidative phosphorylation, and without which glucose is metabolised to lactic acid. Thiamine must therefore be replenished before feeding is commenced in the starved patient to prevent development of Wernicke–Korsakoff syndrome. The potential for this is considerably higher in patients with a history of chronic excessive alcohol intake where even greater caution is required.[21] Thiamine deficiency must always be considered in patients who have had no nutritional intake for more than 1 week, who have a history of excessive alcohol intake or in the presence of an unexplained metabolic acidosis.

MONITORING PATIENTS RECEIVING NUTRITIONAL SUPPORT

Patients receiving nutritional support should be monitored by accurate recording of fluid balance and regular weighing. Daily intake of calories and nitrogen should be documented. Biochemical assessments include daily measurements of renal and liver function, with twice-weekly checks of phosphate, calcium, magnesium, albumin and protein concentrations, and haematological indices (haemoglobin, white blood cell count, haematocrit) until the patient is stabilised. Thereafter, weekly or fortnightly measurements are adequate. Patients starting PN require urinalysis daily in case glycosuria occurs, as this induces further fluid and electrolyte losses. If glycosuria occurs, it may be necessary to commence intravenous insulin on a sliding scale with blood glucose monitoring.

Routes of access should be regularly examined to ensure that the catheter remains correctly positioned and mechanically satisfactory.

When feeding is prolonged, other assessments, such as muscle function, nitrogen balance, measurement of trace elements and vitamins, may be performed regularly to ascertain patient progress (see Nutritional Assessment section above).

NUTRITIONAL SUPPORT IN THE PERIOPERATIVE PERIOD

PARENTERAL NUTRITION

Debate continues as to which patients require preoperative and/or postoperative nutritional support. Many studies have evaluated nutritional support in the perioperative period; no consistent clinical benefit has been found. This may be because studies were small, with many different end points (e.g. morbidity, mortality), poorly designed or failed to stratify for pre-existing malnutrition. Any benefit is dependent on the nature of surgery required; ESPEN guidance is available for a number of specific situations.[2,36,41]

ESPEN guidance is summarised as follows:

Patients who should receive perioperative nutritional support:
- Those expected not to eat for > 7 days perioperatively
- Those unable to have an oral intake > 60% of their recommended intake for > 10 days

Patients who should receive preoperative enteral nutritional support:
- Preoperative nutritional support should be considered in specific situations, e.g. significant weight loss in Crohn's disease

Patients who should receive postoperative nutritional support:
- Early enteral feeding (i.e. < 24 hours after surgery) should be considered for patients who have undergone upper gastrointestinal anastomosis with the tip of a feeding tube placed distal to the anastomosis

In conclusion, avoiding malnutrition and supporting anabolism are basic surgical nutritional goals. Before surgery, these goals can be met through nutrition screening and assessment to diagnose, treat and prevent malnutrition. Preoperative nutritional interventions, such as nutritional prehabilitation, aim to optimise overall nutritional status and support protein anabolism aiming for earlier recovery after surgery with reduced complications.

Key points

- ADH is released as a normal part of the stress response to surgery. This results in an anti-diuresis and the re-absorption of water from the collecting tubules of the kidney. It is therefore expected that patients may have a urine output at the lower end of normal in the hours following a major operation. Chasing this low urine output with fluid resuscitation will lead to fluid overload.
- Biochemical markers are unreliable, and so the possibility of re-feeding must be anticipated from history alone.

 References available at http://ebooks.health.elsevier.com/

KEY REFERENCES

[6] Weimann A, Braga M, Carli F, et al. ESPEN guideline: clinical nutrition in surgery. Clin Nutr 2017;36:623–50.
Authoritative overview from this highly regarded nutritional group.

[19] Wischmeyer PE, Carli F, Evans DC, et al. American society for enhanced recovery and perioperative quality initiative joint consensus statement on nutrition screening and therapy within a surgical enhanced recovery pathway. Anesthesia and Analgesia 2018;126:1883–95.
Expands on nutritional screening and optimisation within ERAS pathways.

7 Abdominal hernias

Barbora East | Andrew C. de Beaux

INTRODUCTION

A hernia is defined as an abnormal protrusion of a cavity's contents through a weakness in the wall of the cavity, taking with it all the linings of the cavity, although these may be markedly attenuated. With any definition, there will be exceptions to the rule—is a lipoma of the cord a hernia? A hernia can be described as reducible, incarcerated or strangulated. A reducible hernia is one in which the contents of the hernial sac can be manually introduced back into the abdomen; conversely, an irreducible or incarcerated hernia cannot be manipulated back into the abdomen. A strangulated hernia occurs when the vascular supply to the contents contained within the hernia is compromised, resulting in tissue ischaemia.

AETIOLOGY

Multiple factors contribute to the development of hernias. Hernias are associated with a number of medical conditions, including connective tissue disorders such as Ehlers–Danlos syndrome, as well as a number of abnormal collagen-related disorders such as varicose veins and arterial aneurysm. In essence, hernias can be considered design faults, either anatomical or through inherited collagen disorders, although these two aetiological factors probably work together in the majority of patients. Anatomical design faults can be considered at any site where structures within the cavity exit through an opening in the wall of the cavity, such as blood vessels, bowel or the spermatic cord. This is typical, for example around the oesophagus and in the groin. However, not everyone develops a groin hernia, so other factors must be important in its aetiology. The fascia and surrounding tissues that cover muscle, acting to hold the muscle bundles together, may appear relatively avascular, but it remains a complex and living structure. The genetic code for fascia is coded on DNA, and within fibroblasts the sequence is messenger RNA, transfer RNA, peptide formation, with fusion of peptides into approximately 1000 amino acid polypeptides called alpha chains. The endoplasmic reticulum converts these to procollagen. Procollagen is the large building block of collagen, comprising triple-helix strands, stabilised by hydroxylation of proline and lysine, which is vitamin C dependent. These triple-helix strands form microfibrils, then fibrils, then fibres and finally bundles. These collagen bundles surrounded by extracellular matrix comprise fascia. The control of this process is mediated through matrix metalloproteinases, which in turn are controlled by tissue inhibitory metalloproteinases. If this is not complex enough, there is also control by collagen-interacting proteins and receptors such as fibronectin, tenasin and collagen receptor discoidin domain receptor 2. Fascia and tendon are made up of type I and type III collagen (type II is found in cartilage and type IV in the basement membrane of cells). In cross-section, there is a bimodal distribution of bundle size with the fibres orientated in the line of pull. The larger bundles are type I collagen, imparting the strength to the fascia or tendon. The type III collagen bundles are smaller and are thought to provide elastic recoil following stretch when the tissues have been loaded. The type I to III collagen ratio varies between individuals but is constant in all the fascia of a particular individual.

A clinical observation was made by surgeons in the late 1960s that the anterior rectus sheath some distance from the hernial defect was thinner than normal, especially in those patients with direct hernias.[1] Since then, research has demonstrated a variety of defects in collagen synthesis in such patients.[2] The current notion is that the majority of hernias are a disease of collagen metabolism. One of the key factors in this is the type I to III collagen ratio. The lower this ratio, from an average of around 5, the more likely the individual is to develop a hernia. Currently, collagen typing is not used in clinical practice to help decide perhaps which patients merit a mesh as opposed to a suture repair, but this may well be a development in the near future.

✔ Hernias are a collagen disease, with reduced collagen type I to III ratio.[2]

CLASSIFICATION OF HERNIAS

A number of hernia classifications exist, both for the description of hernia characteristics such as size and location and also hernia surgery-related complications. The use of such classifications aids the reporting of hernia series, reducing the risk of comparing 'apples with oranges'. For example, the use of mesh in the repair of small hernias in general does not have such a marked benefit in terms of reducing hernia recurrence compared to larger hernia defects. Classifications based on size and location allow the surgeon to think more about tailored surgery, as one operation technique does not always fit all. The European Hernia Society inguinal hernia classification[3] and the EuraHS ventral hernia classification[4] are two such useful pragmatic classifications.

MESH

Much will be mentioned about mesh repairs of hernias in the remainder of this chapter, but this section gives a brief overview of mesh and its science. Many companies produce a variety of mesh for hernia repair. These are either synthetic (man-made) or biological (preparations from animal or human tissue). The majority of synthetic meshes are woven from either polypropylene (monofilament) or polyester (multi- and monofilament), but new polymers continue to be developed. Biological meshes are typically animal collagen, either from skin or bowel, but there are also human preparations. Biological meshes tend to be much more expensive and should be reserved for specialist use.

It goes without saying that any mesh should have the usual properties of any implant, including being non-allergenic, non-carcinogenic, have good incorporation into tissue and mimic the tissue it is replacing or reinforcing. The abdominal wall is not a rigid structure, but regularly copes with increases in abdominal pressure on coughing and sneezing, etc. of up to 200 mmHg. The abdominal wall elasticity is greater in women than in men and is greater in the craniocaudal direction than transversely or obliquely. The traditional standard weight polypropylene mesh, of around 100 g/m^2, is significantly over-engineered, with a burst strength at least an order of magnitude greater than the anterior abdominal wall and an elasticity of much less. As a result, there are now many polypropylene meshes on the market of lighter weight. However, 'lightweight' is a misnomer. Some heavyweight meshes behave in a 'lightweight' fashion and vice versa, as it is not just the weight of the mesh that imparts mesh elasticity and flexibility. The weave of the strands in the mesh may impart varying flexibility or elasticity to the mesh in different directions of pull, so-called anisotropy. Pore size or the size of the large holes in the mesh is also important. Mesh has a volume with length, breadth and thickness. The amount of empty space within the 'volume' of the mesh is the porosity and the effective porosity is the amount of empty space within the volume of the mesh made up of holes that are bigger than 1 mm diameter. It has been proposed that an effective porosity of a mesh for hernia repair should be at least 60%.[5] Fibrosis will occur around each strand of the mesh. If the strands are close together, the fibrosis around each strand will coalesce, forming a solid scar plate. As the scar plate matures, it will shrink, reducing the overall size of the mesh. The minimum pore size should be about 1 mm^2, but many meshes have pore sizes around 3–5 mm. Increasing the macroporosity of the mesh produces a scar net, rather than a scar plate, with normal tissue in between the fibre/scar complex, reducing mesh/scar shrinkage and improving flexibility (Fig. 7.1). Furthermore, increasing the macropore size reduces the bulk of the foreign body implant, and their use in contaminated fields, due to reduced bacterial adherence and increased bacterial clearance, is becoming acceptable practice. In addition to the macropore size, mesh also has micropores within the mesh material itself. These should be at least 10 μm in size. If the micropore size is smaller, bacteria can harbour in the pores out of reach of the larger inflammatory cells.

The majority of synthetic meshes in the UK are polypropylene. Gore-Tex and other polytetrafluoroethylene (PTFE)-based meshes also have some popularity. PTFE has no macropores so will be encapsulated by fibrous tissue with minimal tissue ingrowth. Polyester-based meshes are gaining popularity and have some advantages over polyproplyene but are mostly multifilament rather than monofilament. The multifilament arrangement increases the developed surface of the mesh (around 10-fold) and thus improves

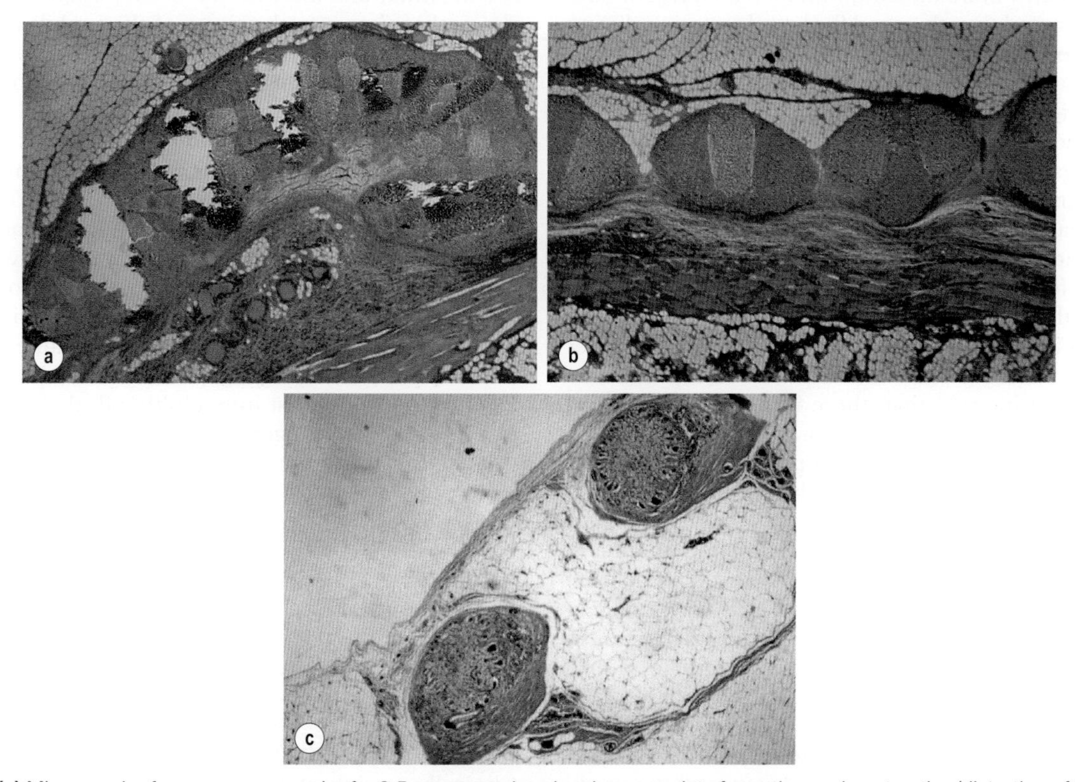

Figure 7.1 **(a)** Micrograph of a macropore mesh of < 0.5 mm pore size showing scar plate formation and contraction/distortion of the mesh. **(b)** Micrograph of a macropore mesh of 0.8 mm pore size showing minimal scar bridging and no distortion of the mesh. **(c)** Micrograph of a macropore mesh of 3 mm pore size showing scar net formation and no contraction/distortion of the mesh. (Micrographs used by permission of Medtronic.)

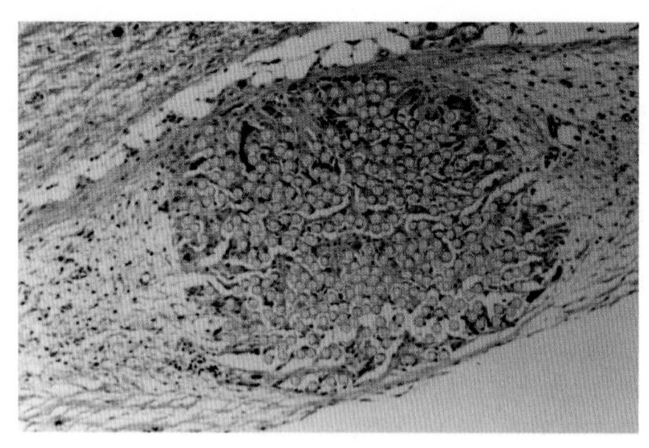

Figure 7.2 Micrograph of a polyester mesh fibre. There is evidence of fibrosis around the fibre bundle as well as fibrous ingrowth around each strand. (Micrograph used by permission of Covidien UK.)

tissue incorporation. As a result, the peel strength (the effort required to separate the mesh from the tissues once it is incorporated) is greater (Fig. 7.2).

The latest mesh category is slowly resorbable synthetic mesh, with resorption taking many months to years. It is hoped that such meshes will reduce the sensation of mesh, or the risk of problems from mesh infection, but there are no long-term data available to comment on hernia recurrence risk, for example.

✔ Preferred mesh should be 'lightweight' (<80 g/m^2), large pore (>1 mm) and macroporous (>10 µm).

Traditional meshes placed within the abdominal cavity have a high rate of adhesions of the omentum and bowel to the mesh. This can result in bowel fistulation or make subsequent laparotomy more difficult, with increased risk of bowel perforation and thus the need for bowel resection during the process of re-entering the abdominal cavity.[6] A number of tissue-separating meshes are available, where the intra-abdominal side of the mesh is coated with a product to minimise adhesion formation. It would be fair to say that while such coatings do reduce adhesion formation, in the majority of patients significant adhesion to such coatings still occurs. The main points of adhesion appear to be the edge of the mesh and to the points of fixation, either sutures, tacks or staples. Nevertheless, it is likely that these products will improve in the future, as meshes become more physiological, perhaps impregnated with growth hormones and other biologically active molecules to improve the mesh/tissue integration. Having said that, there is an increasing trend amongst hernia surgeons to perform minimally invasive hernia surgery using techniques to place mesh within the layers of the abdominal wall, rather than intra-peritoneal.

Biological mesh (a slight misnomer as most biological meshes are really sheets of collagen) has gained popularity in hernia repair. It is, however, disappointing that from the thousands of biological meshes that have been implanted worldwide (often at great expense as biological mesh is 10–100 times more expensive than polypropylene mesh), follow-up data on only a few thousand patients have been published. What is becoming evident though is that biological meshes are not all the same. The major difference, in addition to the animal and anatomical source of the mesh, is the degree of chemical processing, or cross-linking, of the biological product. The more the collagen is cross-linked, the more resistant it is to bacterial collagenase breakdown in the presence of infection. The downside to cross-linking is that the more the collagen is cross-linked, the less tissue ingrowth and integration occurs, with reduction in potential strength to the repair. It is becoming evident that most biological meshes have no role in dirty wounds, acting as little more than a very expensive dressing. They are too expensive for use in clean wounds as any benefit is not worth the huge price difference, and using them for bridging (mesh spanning the fascial gap as opposed to augmentation, where the mesh reinforces or augments the fascial closure) also results in a high percentage of failure. The author's opinion is that there is no good evidence available to suggest that biological mesh is superior or even as good as polypropylene in clean/contaminated operations, or in patients with significant medical comorbidity. Similarly, there is a lack of comparative evidence in contaminated operations, although fortunately this is a very small part of hernia surgery.

PRIMARY VENTRAL HERNIAS

UMBILICAL HERNIAS

There are several distinct types of hernia that occur around the umbilicus: congenital (omphalocele), infantile and adult umbilical hernias. The term 'para-umbilical' is suggested as an obsolete term in the current primary ventral hernia guidelines.[7]

CONGENITAL AND INFANTILE UMBILICAL HERNIAS

A congenital umbilical hernia occurs when the abdominal viscera herniate into the tissue of the umbilical cord. Normally, the gut returns to the abdominal cavity at 10 weeks of gestation. If this fails to occur, normal rotation and fixation of the intestine are prevented, the umbilicus is absent and a funnel-shaped defect in the abdominal wall is present through which viscera protrude into the umbilical cord. The abdominal wall defect may vary in size from no larger than an umbilical stump to a defect that appears to involve the entire abdominal wall. Congenital umbilical hernia occurs in 1 in 5000 births and is associated with other serious congenital anomalies. Congenital and infantile umbilical hernias are discussed in more detail in Chapter 18 and will not be dealt with further here. While some infantile umbilical hernias will persist into adulthood, their management can be considered together with umbilical hernias even if their aetiology is different.

ADULT UMBILICAL HERNIAS

Adult umbilical hernias are acquired hernias and occur in all age groups. They occur secondary to disruption of the linea alba in the region of the umbilical cicatrix. Aetiological factors include stretching of the abdominal wall by obesity, multiple pregnancy and ascites.

CLINICAL PRESENTATION

Clinically, umbilical hernias are frequently symptomatic. Patients complain of intermittent abdominal pain (possibly caused by dragging on the fat and peritoneum of the

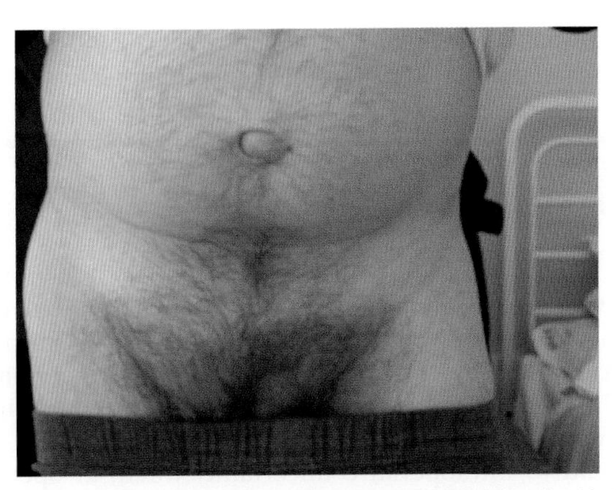

Figure 7.3 Clinical photograph of a para-umbilical hernia. Note the swelling of the right groin of an associated right inguinal hernia – a common finding consistent with a generalised collagen disorder.

falciform ligament) and, when the hernial sac contains bowel, colic resulting from intermittent intestinal obstruction. The hernia tends to progress over time and both intertrigo and necrosis of the skin may occur in patients with large dependent hernias. Such symptoms are a good indication for surgery.

MANAGEMENT

The diagnosis of an umbilical hernia is usually obvious on clinical examination (Fig. 7.3). However, occasionally ultrasound or cross-sectional imaging is necessary when there is diagnostic uncertainty. The majority of umbilical hernias will become symptomatic with time. The small ones often contain pre-peritoneal fat only, so incarceration and strangulation of these, while painful, is of little risk to the patient. But as they become bigger, a true peritoneal sac develops with risk of omental and bowel incarceration and strangulation. Thus, discussion around watch-and-wait versus surgical correction is part of informed consent. Small umbilical hernias in young women are best repaired once their family is complete, unless symptomatic, as subsequent pregnancy does increase the recurrence rate. An important assessment of the patient with a primary midline ventral hernia is to look for divarication of the recti. This patient group has a much higher rate of hernia recurrence from simple suture repair.

Umbilical hernias can occur in patients with ascites from cirrhosis or congestive cardiac failure and patients undergoing peritoneal dialysis. Management should be non-operative where possible, as the majority of these patients have serious underlying comorbidity. Operative repair is not indicated unless the hernia incarcerates or becomes extremely large and the overlying skin is thinned down to such an extent that spontaneous rupture is possible. Careful selection and pre-optimisation of any liver or cardiac failure is important, due to the real risk of mortality in this group from elective surgery.

OPERATIVE DETAILS

For solitary hernias around the umbilicus, a transverse incision or curved incision just below the umbilicus produces the best exposure. If multiple fascial defects in the midline are present or there is concern about the integrity of visceral contents of the sac, a vertical incision may be better employed. If the defect simply contains pre-peritoneal fat, this may be reduced. In patients with strangulated or ischaemic pre-peritoneal fat, it is best excised. If there is a sac present, it should be dissected free from the fascial edges, opened and the contents examined. Once the contents have been dealt with appropriately, they may be reduced and redundant sac excised. Repair is performed by fascial apposition either transversely or longitudinally, depending on the defect and the direction of least tension. As this is an acquired defect, non-absorbable sutures are recommended. Indeed, the author usually creates a pre-peritoneal pocket, inserting a 5 cm × 5 cm square (minimum size—bigger if necessary) mesh and closing the fascia over this. Again, the higher recurrence rate for suture repair over mesh repair for small hernias is noted.[7] For larger umbilical hernias, with a neck size > 2 cm (or smaller hernias in an obese patient), it is the author's preference to repair these laparoscopically and very large hernias with a neck size > 6 cm by an open sublay technique (described later). Newer techniques such as eTEP and TARUP are minimially invasive techniques that allow mesh to be placed in the retromuscular position.

The overlying umbilical skin need not be excised unless it is macerated or infected, although the cosmetic appearance is often enhanced by judicious removal of excess skin and subcutaneous fat. Patients should be warned that it might be necessary to excise the umbilicus.

COMPLICATIONS

Complications include the development of seromas, haematomas and infection. Sealed suction drains may be employed in the retromuscular and subcutaneous planes to help avoid the development of large seromas. In addition to local problems, these patients may have respiratory and cardiovascular complications.

EPIGASTRIC HERNIA

An epigastric hernia is defined as a fascial defect in the linea alba between the xiphoid process and the umbilicus.

AETIOLOGY

The aetiology is related to the functional anatomy of the abdominal wall. The anterior abdominal wall aponeurosis consists of tendinous fibres that lie obliquely in aponeurotic sheets, allowing for changes in the shape of the abdominal wall, for example during respiration, or distension. Such abdominal wall movement/change may result in tearing of fibres leading to the development of an epigastric hernia.

CLINICAL PRESENTATION

The majority of epigastric hernias (probably 75%) are asymptomatic. Typical symptoms, if present, include vague upper abdominal pain and nausea associated with epigastric tenderness. The symptoms can be more severe when the patient is lying down (usually the opposite if the pain is caused by a hernia), attributed to traction on the hernial contents. Pain on exertion localised to the epigastrium is also a common symptom. Incarceration is frequent, and strangulation of pre-peritoneal fat or omentum results in localised pain and tenderness. Incarceration or strangulation of intra-abdominal viscera is rare, the symptoms obviously depending on the incarcerated organ.

The presence of a midline mass on physical examination usually confirms the diagnosis. In obese patients, palpation of the mass may be difficult and confirmation of the diagnosis by ultrasound or cross sectional imaging may be helpful.

MANAGEMENT

Epigastric hernias are rare in infants and children, and asymptomatic hernias in children under the age of 10 years may resolve spontaneously. The decision for surgical intervention depends on the presence and severity of symptoms.

OPERATIVE DETAILS

Small solitary defects may be approached with either a vertical or transverse (better cosmesis) incision in the midline, centred over the hernia. For larger hernias, if the defects are multiple or in the emergency setting when a strangulated viscus is suspected, a vertical incision is preferred. The hernia and its contents are dissected free of the surrounding tissues and, if present, the hernial contents examined and dealt with appropriately. If the defect is small (<2 cm), repair by primary suture closure using non-absorbable material may be sufficient. The orientation of the suture closure remains controversial, some surgeons preferring a vertical closure and others a horizontal orientation. There are few data to support one technique over the other and probably the direction resulting in the least tension is the most appropriate. If the defect is large (>2 cm), or occurs within a divarification of the recti, the hernia should be repaired with prosthetic mesh. This technique is described later in the chapter when considering incisional hernias. The technique applied to intermediate-sized hernias is controversial and suture or mesh techniques are both currently deemed acceptable. Laparoscopic repair of epigastric hernias has grown in popularity. The author prefers an open technique under local anaesthetic whenever possible for smaller hernias (defect < 2 cm), suture or mesh depending on the quality of the tissues, and the laparoscopic approach for larger, multiple, recurrent hernias, or hernias in the obese. At laparoscopic repair, it is important to take down the falciform ligament and remove any pre-peritoneal fat above the linea alba, otherwise the 'hernia' may still be palpable following the alleged repair. Again, newer techniques such as eTEP and TARUP are minimially invasive techniques that allow mesh to be placed in the retromuscular position.

COMPLICATIONS

Complication rates are low and most are the usual complications associated with abdominal wall incisions (haematoma, infection). There are few data on recurrence rates, but a recent study supports mesh repair for even small hernias.[7] In a number of patients, however, the recurrence probably represents the persistence of a second hernia or area of weakness overlooked at the initial procedure, or a new hernia nearby. The laparoscopic technique avoids this problem because all fascial defects are visible laparoscopically if adequate dissection is carried out, and the mesh will re-enforce a large part of the midline at risk of hernia formation.

SPIGELIAN, LUMBAR AND OTHER PRIMARY VENTRAL HERNIAS

Away from the midline, there are a number of anatomical sites where abdominal wall hernia is possible. Sometimes the hernia that develops is called an interstitial hernia—when the hernia protrudes through transversus abdominis and internal oblique, but external oblique remains intact although it may become stretched over the hernia. This can lead to intraoperative uncertainty when, at open surgery, the external oblique is exposed but no hernia is found. Careful marking of the bulge preoperation, and then incising external oblique at this site will uncover the underlying interstitial hernia. The occasional misdignosis of a subcutaneous lipoma as a Spigelian hernia is recognised but is usually obvious at the time of surgery.

As for midline ventral hernias, there are various open and laparoscopic operations for repair, with the type of operation chosen following discussion with the patient taking into account surgeon and patient factors.[8]

INGUINAL HERNIAS

ANATOMY

The inguinal canal is approximately 4 cm in length and is located just above the inguinal ligament between the internal and external rings. The inguinal canal allows passage of the spermatic cord into the scrotum, along with the testicular, deferential and cremasteric vessels. The superficial ring is a triangular aperture in the aponeurosis of the external oblique and lies about 1 cm above the pubic tubercle. Normally, the ring will not admit the tip of the little finger. The deep ring is a U-shaped condensation of the transversalis fascia and it lies about 1–2 cm above the inguinal ligament, midway between the pubic tubercle and the anterior superior iliac spine. The transversalis fascia is the fascial envelope of the abdomen and the competency of the deep inguinal ring depends on the integrity of this fascia.

The anterior boundary of the inguinal canal comprises mainly the external oblique aponeurosis with the conjoined muscle laterally. The posterior boundary is formed by the fascia transversalis and the conjoined tendon (internal oblique and transversus abdominus medially). The inferior epigastric vessels lie posteriorly and medially to the deep inguinal ring. The superior boundary is formed by the conjoined muscles (internal oblique and transversus) and the inferior boundary by the inguinal ligament.

DEFINITION

An indirect hernia travels down the canal on the outer (lateral and anterior) side of the spermatic cord. A direct inguinal hernia comes out directly forward through the posterior wall of the inguinal canal. While the neck of an indirect hernia is lateral to the epigastric vessels, the direct hernia

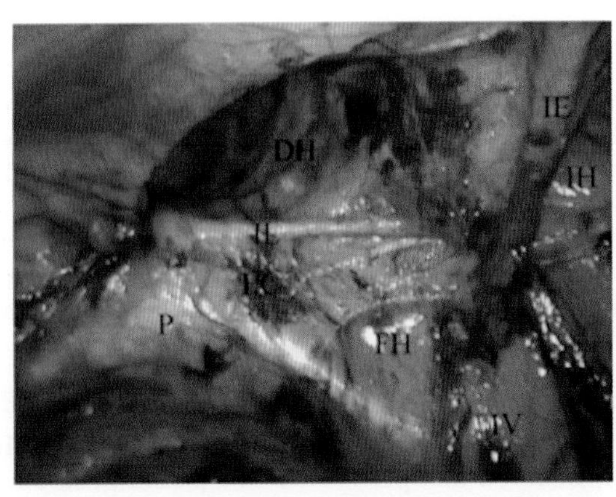

Figure 7.4 Laparoscopic totally extraperitoneal (TEP) view of the right groin with a direct inguinal hernia (*DH*) lying medial to the inferior epigastric vessels (*IE*), above the inguinal (*IL*) and lacunar (*LC*) ligaments. The pubic bone (*P*), iliac vessels (*IV*), vas and vessels (*VV*) are also seen. The positions of a femoral hernia (*FH*) and indirect inguinal hernia (*IH*) are also marked.

usually emerges medial to these vessels, except in the saddlebag or pantaloon type, which has both a lateral and a medial component (Fig. 7.4).

INGUINAL HERNIA IN INFANTS AND CHILDREN (SEE CHAPTER 18)

Repair of congenital inguinal hernia is the most frequently performed operation in the paediatric age group. Although inguinal hernias can present at any age, the peak incidence is during infancy and childhood. About 3–5% of full-term infants may be born with a clinical inguinal hernia, with prematurity increasing the incidence, as does male sex. Congenital inguinal hernias have a 15% bilateral presentation.

CLINICAL PRESENTATION

Examination of the inguinal area for a hernia may show an obvious bulge at the site of the external ring or within the scrotum that can often be gently reduced. However, the bulge may only be seen during severe straining, such as with crying or defaecation. If the infant is old enough to stand, he or she should be examined in both the supine and standing positions. If not, the parent can hold the infant upright so that the surgeon can closely observe the inguinoscrotal area. Sometimes, photographs taken by the parent when a swelling appears can aid in the diagnosis in the difficult case. It is essential to make sure that the testis is within the scrotal sac to avoid mistaking a retractile testis for a hernial bulge. The presence of an empty scrotum should alert the examining surgeon to a possible undescended or ectopic testis, which is associated with an inguinal hernia in more than 90% of patients. Although routine orchidopexy is usually delayed until the child is 1 year of age, a coexisting symptomatic hernia should be promptly repaired and orchidopexy accomplished at the same time.

Inguinal hernias in infants and children are prone to incarcerate, with the overall rate being around 10%. Incarceration is most common in the first 6 months of life, when more than half of all instances are observed. An incarcerated hernia usually presents as an acute tender mass in the inguinal canal. The mass may protrude beyond the external inguinal ring or into the scrotum. The skin over the mass may be discoloured, oedematous, erythematous or blue. Strangulation, characterised by abdominal distension, vomiting, failure to pass faecal material, tachycardia and radiological evidence of small-bowel obstruction, demands emergency operative intervention for relief of obstruction, intestinal salvage and hernia repair. In contrast to the adult with an incarcerated hernia, in children testicular ischaemia is far more common than intestinal ischaemia, and it is therefore appropriate to be aggressive about early reduction and surgery to the hernia (see Chapter 18).

MANAGEMENT

In general, hernias in children and particularly infants should be managed by experienced paediatric surgeons (see Chapter 18). However, this is not always possible depending on geography and availability. In these circumstances, the general surgeon on call may be required to manage these patients. As most (80%) incarcerated hernias in children may be managed initially by non-operative measures, which include sedation, and then gentle reduction when the baby is quiet, exploration may be safely delayed for about 24–48 hours, allowing, if possible, a more experienced paediatric surgeon to become involved. However, if the hernia remains irreducible at this stage, emergency repair is indicated, accepting that the complications rate of emergency surgery is much greater than that of elective surgery. This is covered in more detail in Chapter 18.

OPERATIVE DETAILS

Surgical access is achieved through a short (2–3 cm) transverse incision in the lowest inguinal skin crease. The superficial fascia (Scarpa's fascia) is incised and the external oblique fascia identified. The aponeurosis is traced inferiorly and laterally to identify the inguinal ligament and the exact location of the external inguinal ring. The hernial sac is always located in an anteromedial position in relation to the cord and gentle blunt dissection of the cremasteric fibres usually brings the sac into view. The sac is elevated with a haemostat and the cremasteric fibres carefully freed from the anterior and lateral aspects. Retraction of the sac medially allows identification of the spermatic vessels and vas deferens, and these structures may be carefully teased away from the sac in a posterolateral direction. Injection of 1–2 mL of saline into the cord may help to define the planes of separation. The vas itself should not be grasped and the floor of the canal not disturbed. Once the end of the sac has been freed, the dissection of the sac is carried superiorly to the level of the deep inguinal ring. If the sac extends down into the scrotum, it may be divided once the cord structures are identified and protected. The base of the sac may then be gently twisted to reduce any fluid or viscera into the peritoneal cavity. The base of the sac should be suture ligated with an absorbable suture and, once the suture is cut, the peritoneal stump should retract proximally through the deep inguinal ring. Free ties should not be used because of the risk of them becoming dislodged if abdominal distension occurs. Absolute haemostasis is essential to prevent postoperative haematoma formation. The position of the testis within the scrotum should be confirmed to avoid iatrogenic entrapment within the inguinal canal. There is an increasing role for laparoscopic hernia repair in infants and young children. An emergency operation is required for patients with an incarcerated hernia, with toxicity and obvious intestinal obstruction or after failed attempts at reduction. As previously mentioned, a paediatric surgeon should be involved in all cases if possible as this can be a difficult undertaking. After appropriate resuscitation, prophylactic antibiotics and insertion of a nasogastric tube, the operation begins with preparation of the whole abdomen in case laparotomy is required. An inguinal incision is utilised and the incarcerated intestine carefully inspected for viability once the obstruction at the internal ring is relieved. A rapid return of pink colour, sheen, peristalsis and palpable or visible pulsations at the mesenteric border should be observed. If there is any question regarding intestinal viability, resection and anastomosis should be carried out and hernial repair accomplished.

In certain circumstances, the incarcerated intestine may reduce during surgical manipulation, before the intestine has been visualised. However, such spontaneous reduction of infarcted bowel is very rare. Laparoscopy through the hernial sac can be undertaken if there are serious concerns regarding bowel viability. Surgery for incarcerated hernia may be difficult because of oedema, tissue friability and the presence of the mass, which may obscure the anatomy. The gonad should be carefully inspected because it may become infarcted by vascular compression caused by the incarcerated intestine. The undescended testis is more vulnerable to this complication in the presence of incarcerated intestine.

COMPLICATIONS

Complications may be divided into intraoperative and postoperative categories. Intraoperative complications include: division of the ilioinguinal nerve, which can be avoided if the external oblique fascia is elevated before incision; division of the vas deferens, which should be repaired with interrupted 7/0 monofilament sutures; and bleeding, which can usually be controlled with the application of pressure and cautious diathermy.

Postoperative complications include wound infection, scrotal haematoma, postoperative hydroceles and recurrence. The wound infection rate is low (1–2%) and recurrence rates of less than 1% are reported, 80% of recurrences being noted within the first postoperative year. The major causes of recurrence in infants and children include: (i) a missed hernial sac or an unrecognised tear in the peritoneum; (ii) a broken suture ligature at the neck of the sac; (iii) injury to the floor of the inguinal canal, resulting in the development of a direct inguinal hernia; (iv) severe infection in the inguinal canal; and (v) increased intra-abdominal pressure, as is noted in patients with ascites after ventriculoperitoneal shunts, in children with cystic fibrosis, after previous operation for incarceration and in patients with connective tissue disorders. Although failure to repair a large internal inguinal ring is a possible (and very occasional) cause of recurrence, attempts to tighten the internal ring at the time of the first repair by approximating the transversalis fascia medial to the inferior epigastric vessels risk compromises the blood supply to the testicle and should be avoided where possible. Simple excision of the sac is all that is required in most patients. Re-operations for recurrent inguinal hernia may be a technical challenge and a preperitoneal approach is a useful alternative for recurrent hernias.

ADULT INGUINAL HERNIAS

Inguinal hernias are more frequent in males (1 in 4 males will develop an inguinal hernia in their lifetime), with a male-to-female ratio of 12:1. Around two-thirds are indirect, and a right-sided hernia is slightly more common than a left-sided hernia. Bilateral hernias are four times more common in direct than indirect forms (1 in 2 males who develop an inguinal hernia will present with bilateral hernia or develop a contralateral hernia).

AETIOLOGY

The pathogenesis of groin hernias is multifactorial. It was initially believed that persistence of a patent processus vaginalis into adult life was the predisposing factor for indirect inguinal hernia formation. However, postmortem studies have shown that up to one-third of adult males without a clinically apparent inguinal hernia have a patent processus vaginalis. Similarly, review of the contralateral side in infantile inguinal hernias reveals a patent processus vaginalis in 60% of neonates and a contralateral hernia in 10–20%. During 20 years of follow-up after infantile hernia repair, only 20% of men will develop a contralateral hernia.

It is therefore apparent that the problem of indirect inguinal hernia is not simply one of a congenital defect. The high frequency of indirect inguinal hernia in middle-aged and older people suggests a pathological change in connective tissue of the abdominal wall to be a contributory factor, as discussed earlier.

DIAGNOSIS

The diagnosis of an inguinal hernia is usually straightforward. The patient presents with a swelling in their groin, which is often associated with discomfort on activity, coughing and sneezing. On lying down, the swelling often disappears. On examination, asymmetry between the two groins is often obvious (Fig. 7.5), even with bilateral presentation. Where there is diagnostic doubt, a dynamic ultrasound scan may help, but a word of warning: a small hernia evident on ultrasound which is not clinically detectable is rarely the cause of the patient's symptoms! Many clinical tests have been described to determine between a direct and indirect hernia and indeed a femoral hernia, but in practice, they perform no better than tossing a coin!

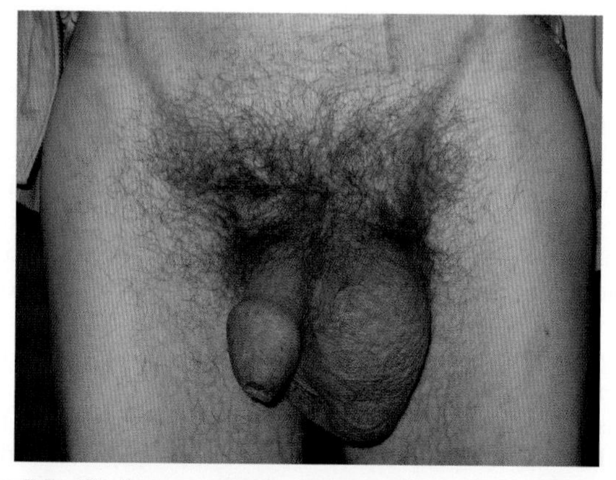

Figure 7.5 Obvious asymmetry between the normal right side and small inguinoscrotal hernia on the left side.

MANAGEMENT

The goal of hernia repair is to restore the functional integrity of the groin. It is beyond the scope of this chapter to review the history of the various repair techniques that have been previously employed and are now mainly historical. Only the latest techniques (i.e. prosthetic repairs) will be considered here.

'Tension-free' open mesh repair

Lichtenstein first described the technique of tension-free repair of groin hernia, which now bears his name.[9] 'Tension-free' repair of primary groin hernias may be performed as an outpatient procedure under local anaesthesia, although in the UK open mesh repair is still more commonly performed under general anaesthetic.

Once the local anaesthesia has been administered (typically a mixture of 0.5% bupivacaine and 1% lignocaine) along the line of the proposed incision, an incision is made in the groin crease through the skin and subcutaneous tissues including Scarpa's fascia exposing the external oblique aponeurosis (from just lateral to the deep ring to close to the midline). Additional anaesthetic is then injected under the external oblique aponeurosis, following which a small incision is made in the external oblique along the line of the fibres, to the superficial ring. The edges are lifted with haemostatic forceps avoiding damage to the ilioinguinal nerve. After the contents of the inguinal canal have been gently separated from the external oblique aponeurosis, a self-retaining retractor is inserted under its edges. The spermatic cord is then mobilised utilising the avascular space between the pubic tubercle and the cord itself to avoid damage to the floor of the canal, injury to the testicular blood flow and crushing of the genital nerve, which always lies in juxtaposition to the external spermatic vessels (Fig. 7.6).

In order to thin out the spermatic cord and remove any lipoma present, the cremaster fibres are incised longitudinally at the level of the mid-canal. Complete excision of the cremaster fibres from the spermatic cord is unnecessary and may result in damage to the vas deferens, increasing the likelihood of postoperative neuralgia and ischaemic orchitis. Indirect hernial sacs are opened and digital exploration performed to detect any other defects or the presence of a femoral hernia. The sac can be suture-ligated at the deep ring, but Lichtenstein states that the sac may be simply inverted into the abdomen without excision, suture or ligation, which he feels is unnecessary and may contribute to postoperative discomfort.[9] To minimise trauma to the cord structures and prevent postoperative hydrocele formation, inguino-scrotal sacs are transected at the midpoint of the canal, with the distal section left open and *in situ*. If performing the procedure under local anaesthetic, handling of the sac at this stage can cause pain and often further local anaesthetic to the sac area in the region of the deep ring is required.

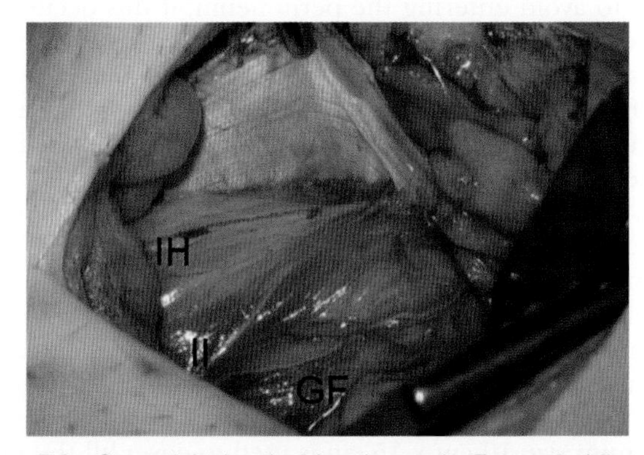

Figure 7.6 Open right inguinal hernia repair. External oblique has been opened. Medial is to the right of the picture with superior at the top. Note the iliohypogastric (*IH*), ilioinguinal (*II*) that splits into two branches, and the small genitofemoral nerve (*GF*) lying inferiorly. (Clinical photograph used with permission of Mr Martin Kurzer, London, UK.)

In the event of a large direct hernia, the sac (transversalis fascia) is invaginated with an imbricating suture to achieve a flat surface over which to lay the prosthetic mesh. The external oblique aponeurosis is separated from the underlying internal oblique muscle at a point high enough to accommodate a mesh measuring around 12 cm × 7 cm. This size will vary depending on the size of the patient and the size of the hernial defect.

The mesh is trimmed as appropriate so that the patch overlaps the internal oblique muscle and aponeurosis by at least 2 cm above the border of the Hesselbach's triangle. The medial portion of the mesh is rounded to the shape of the medial corner of the inguinal canal. The mesh is sutured to the aponeurotic tissue over the pubic bone, overlapping the bone to prevent any tension or weakness at this critical point, but ensuring the periosteum is not caught in the suture as this is believed to be a source of chronic pain. The medial part of the mesh should extend at least 2 cm medial to the pubic tubercle to reduce the risk of medial recurrence. The same suture is continued along the lower edge, attaching the mesh to the shelving portion of the inguinal ligament to a point just lateral to the deep ring.

A slit is made at the lateral end of the mesh, creating a wider tail above the cord and a narrower one below the cord. This manoeuvre positions the cord between the two tails of the mesh and avoids the keyhole opening, which is less effective at preventing recurrence. The upper edge of the patch is sutured to the internal oblique aponeurosis using a few interrupted sutures or widely spaced continuous suture. Retraction of the upper leaf of the external oblique aponeurosis from the internal oblique muscle is important because it provides the appropriate amount of laxity for the patch. When the retraction is released, a 'tension-free' repair is taken up when the patient strains on command during the operation (if under local anaesthetic) or resumes an upright position afterwards. Using a single non-absorbable monofilament suture, the edges of the two tails are re-approximated snugly around the cord structures creating a new deep ring of mesh (Fig. 7.7).

The excess patch is trimmed on the lateral side, leaving 3–4 cm beyond the deep ring. This is tucked underneath the external oblique aponeurosis and the external oblique aponeurosis closed with a continuous suture. Unrestricted activity is encouraged and patients are expected to return to their normal activity 2–7 days after surgery.

In the past few years, there has been an explosion in different mesh types for the open repair of inguinal hernias. The plug and patch utilises a cone-shaped mass of mesh that can be inserted, tip side inwards, into either the deep or superficial rings, depending on the type of hernia. A flat mesh is then placed over the plug akin to the Lichtenstein

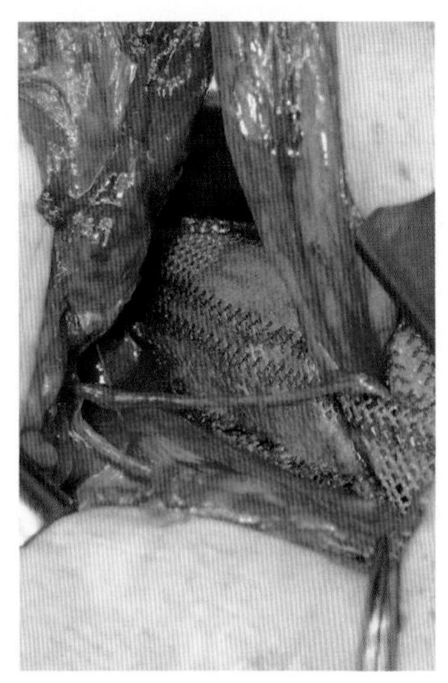

Figure 7.7 Left inguinal hernia repair. Mesh in place. Note continuous suture attaching inferior edge of mesh to inguinal ligament and mesh fish-tailed laterally to create a new deep ring. Cord structures and ilioinguinal nerve are intact. The mesh is lying flat and 'tension' free.

technique. The prolene hernia system is two flat meshes secured together by a small cylinder of mesh. The aim is to insert one mesh into the preperitoneal space and the other is secured akin to the Lichtenstein technique. These techniques are not recommended by international groin hernia guidelines. There is also the open preperitoneal approach. All these alternatives report good results in the hands of experts, but the open flat mesh technique in its various forms, akin to the Lichtenstein technique, remains the commonest technique in Western countries to date. It is also the author's prejudice that if a mesh is to be inserted into the preperitoneal space, it makes sense to do this under direct vision using a laparoscope rather than using a largely blind, blunt finger dissection technique.

Laparoscopic repair

The alternative to an open operation is a laparoscopic approach. Since the early 1990s, laparoscopic hernia repair has evolved from simple closure of a small indirect hernia, through the placement of mesh plugs and a small mesh patch over the internal ring, to the current use of large pieces of prosthetic mesh to reinforce the lower abdominal wall. Although a variety of laparoscopic repairs have been described, they can be categorised in general according to the approach used to expose the defect. Three exposures are used: the intraperitoneal approach, in which the prosthesis is placed as an onlay graft over the peritoneum; the transabdominal preperitoneal (TAPP) repair; and the totally extraperitoneal (TEP) repair.

Intraperitoneal prosthetic repair

In the intraperitoneal repair with an onlay graft, the prosthesis is placed within the peritoneal cavity. Compared with the TAPP and TEP approaches, it has the advantages of being less time-consuming to perform and requires no dissection of the preperitoneal space. It has the disadvantage of leaving the prosthetic material exposed within the peritoneal cavity and has a higher recurrence rate. It is the author's view that this operation is very much an operation of last resort, when other open or laparoscopic techniques have failed.

Transabdominal preperitoneal prosthetic repair

TAPP repair is one of the most popular approaches used for laparoscopic herniorrhaphy, particularly in Europe. The abdomen is insufflated with carbon dioxide and the laparoscope introduced through an umbilical incision. Two accessory trocars, placed above and slightly medial to the anterior superior iliac spines, are used to provide access for the dissecting instruments. After both groins have been inspected, an incision is made in the pelvic peritoneum several centimetres above the hernia defect and the peritoneum then peeled away to expose the hernia defect. The peritoneum is dissected (with a combination of blunt and scissor dissection) away from the abdominal wall, allowing the hernia sac to be inverted and dissected free of adherent tissue, with sufficient mobilisation to create a large enough pocket for the mesh. A mesh of approximately 10 cm × 15 cm is inserted and manipulated into position so that it covers the entire myopectineal orifice. Some surgeons fix the mesh in place with staples, sutures or glue, although there is little evidence to support such practices (except in larger direct hernias).[10] The peritoneum is closed over the mesh with staples/sutures/glue. This approach has the advantage of permitting inspection of the abdominal cavity in general, and of the opposite side in particular, enabling bilateral repairs to be performed if necessary. In addition, exposure is usually excellent. The disadvantage is that the intra-abdominal instruments present the possibility of injury to intraperitoneal structures and the peritoneal incision in the groin increases the potential for adhesion formation and late bowel obstruction. Furthermore, port site hernia at the umbilicus is recognised.

Totally extraperitoneal prosthetic repair

TEP repair is a laparoscopic adaptation of the open posterior preperitoneal approach first described by Annandale.[11] The laparoscope is introduced into the preperitoneal space through an infra-umbilical incision. The preperitoneal space is dissected towards the symphysis pubis, Cooper's ligament and the iliac vessels with a blunt instrument or space-making balloon. Carbon dioxide is insufflated into the preperitoneal space to maintain exposure. Care must be taken to avoid entering the peritoneum; if this occurs, loss of pressure in the preperitoneal space can result, making exposure more difficult. A venting Verres needle in the right iliac fossa will usually resolve this problem, or alternatively a structural balloon attached to the umbilical port will help to keep the preperitoneal space open. Two additional 5-mm ports are inserted, either in the right and left iliac fossa, after extending the dissection laterally or in the midline below the umbilicus. Direct hernial sacs usually reduce with ease, but an indirect hernial sac may need more work. The key landmark here is the vas. The indirect hernial sac lies above and lateral to the vas, taking the dissection away from the iliac vessels, preventing their inadvertent injury. A mesh of minimum size 10 cm × 15 cm is used to cover all the inguinal and femoral myopectineal orifices, ensuring good cover laterally and superiomedially. As with TAPP repairs, there is now good evidence that suturing, tacking or stapling of mesh does not reduce the risk of hernia recurrence but is a cause of postoperative chronic pain.[10] The author does occasionally tack the mesh, confined mainly to the patient with a very large direct hernial defect or when there has been more bleeding than usual, especially patients on aspirin. In all circumstances, tacks are placed medial to the inferior epigastric vessels and superior to the pubic bone only. The TEP approach avoids the risks of entering the peritoneal cavity and subsequent intraperitoneal adhesion formation as well as minimising port site hernias.

There is little evidence to support TEP versus TAPP, and the technique used is largely down to the individual surgeon.[10]

Single-incision laparoscopic surgery and robotic surgery

Single-port hernia surgery for both the TEP and TAPP approach is described. There is also increasing use of robots in laparoscopic hernia surgery. At present, these should be considered an alternative surgical approach, with little proven benefit to either the surgeon or the patient—and in the case of the robot, a significant increase in both cost and time of the surgery. However, as robot-assisted hernia surgery develops, robot-assisted groin hernia repair will likely become a good training operation for the more complex cases, to no detriment of the patient.

✔✔ Laparoscopic repair of inguinal hernias causes less acute and chronic pain, thus earlier return to work, less wound and mesh infection, fewer wound complications and less numbness than the open operation. Where expertise in laparoscopic inguinal hernia surgery is present, it is now the preferred technique suggested for primary unilateral inguinal hernia and recommended for recurrent inguinal hernias after anterior open repair, bilateral primary inguinal hernias, and groin hernia in women.[10]

COMPLICATIONS

Complications of herniorrhaphy include recurrence, urinary retention, ischaemic orchitis and testicular atrophy, wound infection and nerve injuries. A wide variation in recurrence rates is reported in the literature, depending on both the surgical technique employed and the method and length of follow-up (questionnaire, physical examination, etc.). In general, studies comparing mesh with suture repair note lower recurrence rates in the mesh group.[10] Furthermore, direct inguinal hernias are more likely to recur than indirect inguinal hernias.[10] Nevertheless, the percentage of recurrent to primary hernia repair has remained largely constant in industrialised countries over the past 30 years at around 10%. Perhaps the only role for suture repair remains in the adolescent age group, where perhaps a herniotomy alone is insufficient and the risks of mesh insertion not merited.[10] There has been a suggestion that mesh repairs in the groin can affect fertility in males. This is a very controversial area, as the occurrence of a hernia per se in the young is associated with reduced fertility. There is no convincing evidence to support the view that a mesh repair affects fertility except when there is obviously direct trauma to the vas or vessels to the testicle.[10]

The complication that is becoming the benchmark for comparing hernia repairs is the incidence of chronic pain rather than recurrence rate. Risk factors for chronic pain include nerve damage, preoperative pain in the hernia, young age, male sex, chronic pain syndromes at other sites of the body, postoperative complications and psychosocial features.[10] Pain response to a standardised heat stimulus appears to be a useful tool in assessing risk of postoperative chronic pain.[12]

OPEN SUTURE, OPEN MESH OR LAPAROSCOPIC REPAIR?

Which technique is performed on a particular inguinal hernia will depend on a number of factors, and it is true that no one technique fits all. The concept of 'tailoring' surgery to the patient is important.[10] The skills and resources of the local surgical team, applied to the variation in hernia size and type as well as the comorbidity and previous abdominal surgery present in the patient will all play a part in the decision for which operation for a particular patient. The process of informed consent with the patient will also help decide the operative technique. In general, there are few patients with a hernia that are not suitable for a general anaesthetic, which would exclude the laparoscopic approach. (There are reports of laparoscopic repairs undertaken under local anesthetic with sedation but these are on ASA 1 and 2 patients with no generalisability to the comorbid patient.) The laparoscopic repair, as opposed to the open repair, is associated with less acute pain and thus a quicker return to daily activities and work, fewer wound complications such as haematoma, seroma and infection, and less risk of chronic pain. There is a similar recurrence rate (in experienced hands accepting a longer learning curve), and a similar risk of major vessel, bowel or bladder injury. The disadvantage of a laparoscopic approach has traditionally been along the lines that surgery takes longer and is more expensive. Current studies would now support the laparoscopic repair being just as quick if not quicker, especially with bilateral hernia repair.[10] Costs can be minimised by avoiding disposable equipment and unnecessary fixation devices, and the use of standard synthetic flat mesh. The cost of open surgery has to be set against the price of open surgery for the patient and society, namely more acute and chronic pain, more time off work and more wound complications. Indeed, for laparoscopic surgery, current guidelines propose that patients can return to all activities as soon as they want, within their level of discomfort, without any increased risk of hernia recurrence.[10] Nevertheless, a caution about widespread laparoscopic repair is the increased complication rate over open surgery in national registry studies.[13]

CONTRALATERAL REPAIR

Inguinal hernia arises as a design fault, both anatomically and at the level of collagen metabolism, so there is every reason why it should be a bilateral disease. Furthermore, clinical assessment of bilateral or unilateral hernia has a false-positive and false-negative rate of around 10%. The rate of development of a contralateral inguinal hernia following open repair is around 25% at 10 years,[10] with up to a 50% life-time risk. Bilateral repair as a routine is not recommended, but in skilled laparoscopic hands, bilateral exploration at TEP with prophylactic mesh inserted even if no contralateral hernia is found is suggested.[10] At TAPP, the contralateral side is more easily examined, but will miss cases of lipoma of the cord. Again, bilateral repair is suggested with appropriate informed consent, especially when the finding is of a direct hernia in a younger patient.[10]

RECURRENT INGUINAL HERNIAS

The repair of recurrent inguinal hernia remains a common operation and there is now some evidence to suggest that the increasing use of mesh may be having a small effect in reducing the number of recurrent hernia repairs[14] (see section on prophylactic hernia repair at the end of this chapter). As a result, there is little role now for suture repair of recurrent inguinal hernias, except in centres where mesh is unavailable or too expensive for routine use. As a general rule, the anterior approach should be used for recurrent posterior/laparoscopic repairs, and a laparoscopic repair for previous anterior repairs.[10] Thus repair techniques that involve both the anterior and posterior planes at the first operation are to be avoided as they make revisional surgery much more difficult.[10] However, redo laparoscopic surgery is possible in experienced hands, and allows assessment as to why the first laparoscopic repair failed. The TAPP approach is likely safer than redo TEP surgery, and the dissection plane is to take down the peritoneum along with the original mesh. But again, a tailored approach is necessary. It is possible that the first anterior approach was because the laparosopic route was contraindicated. And the laparoscopic route may again not be possible for the recurrent operation.

OPEN MESH REPAIR OF RECURRENT INGUINAL HERNIAS

The Lichtenstein repair remains the commonest open operation for recurrent inguinal hernias. Rate of re-recurrence depends to an extent on the length of follow-up, but is typically around 10%. When a Lichtenstein repair is performed for a recurrent hernia after a previous laparoscopic repair, the complication rate is similar to that of a primary repair. However, when a redo Lichtenstein is performed, the risk of testicular ischaemia rises dramatically from around 0.1% to as high as 5%. This obviously has more major implications for a man with only one testicle on the recurrence hernia side.

LAPAROSCOPIC REPAIR OF RECURRENT INGUINAL HERNIAS

The advantages of the laparoscopic approach include: elimination of one of the commonest causes of recurrence—the missed hernia (hernia present but not detected by the operating surgeon). In addition, the laparoscopic approach allows the surgeon to identify those patients with complex hernias (inguinal and femoral/obturator); and to cover the entire myopectineal orifice with mesh, buttressing the intrinsic collagen deficit, thereby overcoming one of the causes of late recurrence. The complication rate is low, and the majority of such repairs are as easy as primary laparoscopic repair. The data from the Swedish Hernia Registry would support the benefit of a preperitoneal repair (open or laparoscopic) for recurrent inguinal hernia following a previous open non-peritoneal repair.[15]

THE ASYMPTOMATIC HERNIA

Traditional teaching used to suggest that once an inguinal hernia was detected, it merited repair to prevent hernia-related complications unless the patient was not fit for such surgery. However, increasing awareness of complications following hernia repair, particularly chronic pain, has questioned this approach. Two randomised trials have reported similar results.[10] In essence, chronic pain on follow-up is similar between the operation group and the watchful waiting group. Significant numbers in the watchful waiting group will crossover to the surgery arm because of increasing symptoms (at a rate of around 10% a year).[10] These trials also noted that the risk of incarceration or strangulation is much lower than previously thought, about 1% risk per year.[16] Thus, following informed consent, surgery or watchful waiting for an asymptomatic hernia is an acceptable management strategy. The younger the patient, or less fit the patient on presentation, then perhaps the earlier surgery should be offered, with suitable informed consent of the risks, benefits and alternatives to the proposed surgery.

✔✔ Repair of an asymptomatic hernia does not increase the incidence of chronic pain as compared to a wait-and-see policy. Either treatment option is acceptable with appropriate informed consent.[10,16] The majority of wait-and-see patients will crossover to surgery with time as their hernia increases in size and/or becomes more symptomatic. The risk of an acute hernia event is about 1% per year.

FEMORAL HERNIA

Femoral hernia represents the third most common type of primary hernia. It accounts for approximately 20% of hernias in women and 5% in men, strangulation being the initial presentation in 40%. Its incidence increases with age.

ANATOMY

The femoral canal occupies the most medial compartment of the femoral sheath, extending from the femoral ring above to the saphenous opening below. It contains fat, lymphatic vessels and the lymph node of Cloquet. The femoral ring is bounded anteriorly by the inguinal ligament and posteriorly by the iliopectineal (Cooper) ligament, the pubic bone and the fascia over the pectineus muscle. Medially, the boundary is the edge of the lacunar ligament, while laterally it is separated from the femoral vein by a thin septum (see Fig. 7.4).

AETIOLOGY

Femoral hernias are likely to have an aetiology similar to inguinal hernias. The multifactorial factors will include a significant component related to an underlying collagen disorder.

MANAGEMENT

The treatment of femoral hernia is surgical repair due to the high risk of incarceration and the associated risk of strangulation. Several operative approaches have been described: the low approach, the high approach and the inguinal approach. To these can now be added the laparoscopic or robot-assisted approach.

OPERATIVE DETAILS

Low approach (Lockwood)

The low approach is based on a groin crease incision and dissection of the femoral hernia sac below the inguinal ligament. The anatomical layers covering the sac should be peeled away and the sac opened to inspect its contents. Once empty, the neck of the sac is pulled down, suture-ligated as high as possible and redundant sac excised. The neck then retracts through the femoral canal and the canal is closed with a plug or cylinder of polypropylene mesh, anchored to the inguinal ligament and iliopectineal ligament with non-absorbable sutures.[10] Suturing of the iliopectineal ligament to the inguinal ligament may result in tension due to the rigidity of these structures and may predispose to recurrence.

Transinguinal approach (Lotheissen)

Techniques of femoral hernia repair that open the posterior inguinal wall for exposure and repair should rarely be used, except at open inguinal hernia surgery when no inguinal hernia is found (and a missed femoral hernia is suspected). This technique usually involves ligation and division of the inferior epigastric vessels at the medial border of the internal inguinal ring followed by incision of the transversalis fascia to expose the extraperitoneal space and the femoral hernia sac. This is reduced and the defect closed by either suture (as in the original description) or, increasingly, with mesh. However, the need to incise the natural fascial barrier in Hesselbach's triangle for exposure results in this technique being inferior to either the low or high approach, both of which leave the inguinal floor intact.

High approach (McEvedy)

The high approach was classically based on a vertical incision made over the femoral canal and continued upwards above the inguinal ligament. This has now been replaced with a lateral transverse incision on the affected side. The dissection is continued through the subcutaneous tissue to the anterior rectus sheath, which is divided transversely. The rectus muscle is retracted laterally and the preperitoneal space entered (or sometimes with a low arcuate line, anterior to the posterior rectus sheath). The femoral hernia sac is identified medial to the iliac vessels and reduced by traction. If the hernia is incarcerated, the sac may be released by incising the insertion of the iliopubic tract into Cooper's ligament at the medial margin of the femoral ring. The sac is then opened, the contents dealt with appropriately and the sac ligated at its neck. The hernioplasty may then be completed by either suturing the iliopubic tract to the posterior margin of Cooper's ligament or by insertion of a flat mesh, covering the whole of the myopectineal openings. The wound is closed in layers. This technique is particularly useful in the presence of a strangulated femoral hernia as it is easy to convert to laparotomy for bowel resection.

Laparoscopic approach

The laparoscopic approach is the same as for inguinal hernias and may employ the TAPP or TEP technique. The femoral ring is easily seen during either of these approaches and, indeed, visualisation of the whole of the myopectineal opening is frequently quoted as one of the advantages of laparoscopic herniorrhaphy. Furthermore, the laparoscopic repair appears to reduce the risk of re-operation for recurrence.[10] However, there appears to be little difference in short-term quality of life between open and laparoscopic surgical approaches for femoral hernia.[10]

INCISIONAL HERNIA

AETIOLOGY

Incisional hernias are unique in that they are the only hernia to be considered iatrogenic and constitute the commonest complication of a laparotomy. The cause of wound complications after laparotomy is multifactorial, influenced by local and systemic factors and by preoperative, perioperative and postoperative factors. Again, inherited collagen-type abnormalities have a significant role to play.[17] In addition, several factors including smoking, advanced age, pulmonary disease, morbid obesity, malignancy and intra-abdominal infection are associated with impaired wound healing and predispose patients to serious wound complications such as wound dehiscence, wound infection and incisional herniation. It is always easy to blame the patient for complications, but surgeon or technical factors influencing wound complications include surgical technique and suture material choices.

What is the best way to close the abdominal wall? It is amazing that today we still do not know for sure. A recent review[18] proposed mass closure (compared with layered closure), continuous (compared with interrupted sutures), slowly absorbable monofilament (compared with non-absorbable monofilament and absorbable multifilament), with a suture length-to-wound length ratio of at least 4:1. Controversy over the 4:1 ratio also exists. This ratio can be achieved by big bites far apart or small bites close together. The first small-bite small-stitch randomised controlled trial (RCT)[19] reported a 50% reduction in wound infection and a 67% reduction in incisional hernia rates in the 2/0 polydioxanone 20-mm needle small-bite arm compared with more conventional closure techniques. Using such a suture technique, suture-to-wound length ratios greater than 4:1 were not associated with increasing wound complications.[20] A further RCT[21] of small-bite small-stitch midline closure recently reported a reduction in incisional hernia rate from 21% to 13% at 1-year follow-up, although in this trial there was no significant difference in wound infection or burst abdomen (sometimes called an acute hernia or deep wound dehiscence). However, patients who were obese and undergoing emergency laparotomy were excluded from these trials, so the generalisability of the small-bite small-stitch closure to all laparotomy wounds is not known. Nevertheless, the development of an incisional hernia is inevitable if there is separation of the fascia by 12 mm at 12 weeks, so it is not difficult to see that the events that lead to an incisional hernia are determined early in the healing phase, and technical issues are likely to have a significant part to play.

✔✔ Closure of a laparotomy wound to minimise incisional hernia formation includes:[18]

Avoid the midline
Mass closure
Simple running technique
Absorbable monofilament
Suture length-to-wound length ratio of at least 4:1
Small-stitch small-bite technique[19,21]

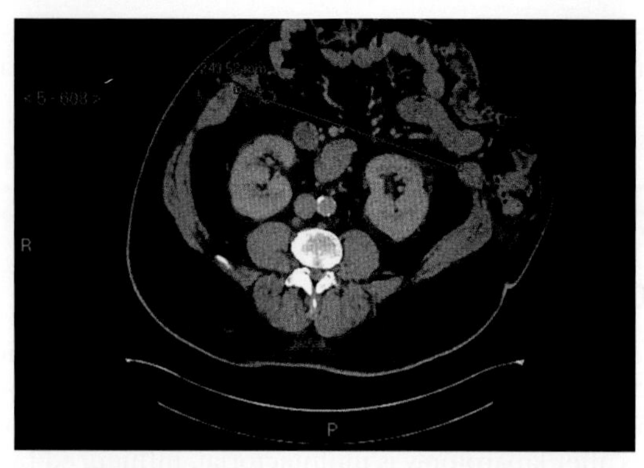

Figure 7.8 CT scan of a large incisional hernia demonstrating loss of domain. The gap between the medial ends of the left and right recti muscles on this slice is 25 cm.

MANAGEMENT

The diagnosis of an incisional hernia is usually easy, except in the very obese. However, CT is helpful to identify the size of the defect and the state of the abdominal wall muscles (Fig. 7.8). Part of the CT assessment is considering the degree of 'loss of domain'—the percentage of the abdominal cavity contents that lie within the hernia sac. When these contents are returned within the confines of the abdominal wall, they will increase the dimensions of the hernial defect. Restoring integrity of the abdominal wall with significant loss of domain will require a variety of ways to elongate the abdominal wall musculature, such as Botox injections into the lateral muscles 1 month prior to surgery,[22] progressive pneumoperitoneum[23] or component separation techniques (described below). Sometimes excision of abdominal cavity contents such as omentectomy or right hemicolectomy may be necessary. Occasionally, bridging the gap in the abdominal wall muscles (as opposed to mesh augmentation of the primary closure) with mesh is necessary. Weight loss prior to surgery is to be encouraged, especially for larger hernias. As a rough rule of thumb, for every 3 kg of weight loss, about 1 litre of abdominal volume is gained, which is very helpful when there is loss of domain.

The large number of surgical procedures described in the literature to repair incisional hernias illustrates that no single technique has stood out as being effective. While 50% of incisional hernias occur within 1 year after the primary operation, 20% are diagnosed more than 5 years later. Any study reporting re-recurrence rates following incisional hernia repair should therefore ideally have at least 5 years of follow-up data for analysis. Unfortunately, prospective randomised trials comparing different types of incisional hernia repair are lacking and the majority of studies are retrospective.

As a consequence of the disappointing data on mesh-free repair of incisional hernias, including the Mayo ('vest-over-pants') procedure, meshes were introduced to strengthen the abdominal wall repair. Several different techniques were developed: inlay, onlay and sublay (Fig. 7.9). Mesh implantation as an inlay does not achieve any strengthening of the abdominal wall and is essentially a suture repair at the muscle/fascia mesh interface. It has the highest recurrence rate of the three techniques. The results of randomised trials comparing mesh repair with suture repair demonstrate a clear advantage for mesh repair, even for small hernias.[24] However, incisional hernia should be considered an

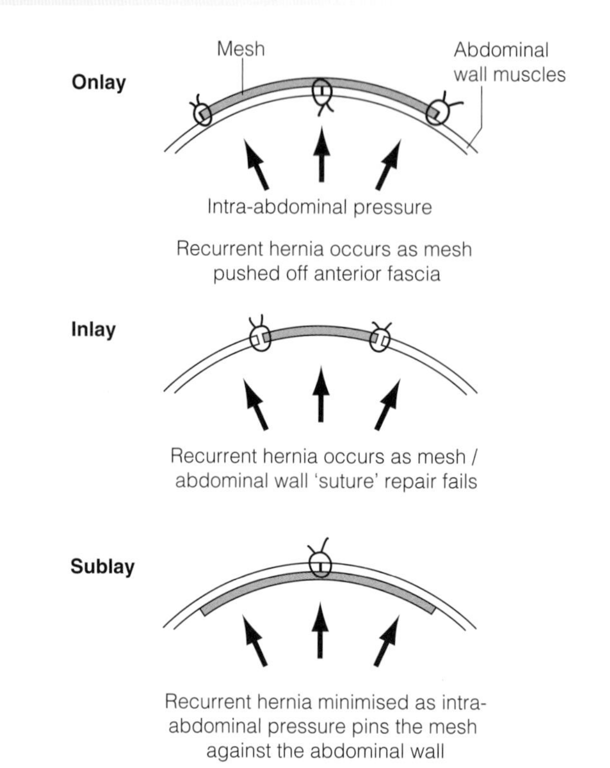

Figure 7.9 Cross-sectional appearance of mesh position in incisional hernia repair. (Reproduced from Schumpelick V, Klinge V. Immediate follow-up results of sublay polypropylene repair in primary or recurrent incisional hernias. In: Schumpelick V, Kingsnorth AN, editors. Incisional hernia. Berlin: Springer-Verlag; 1999. p. 312–26. With kind permission of Springer Science + Business Media.)

incurable disease, mesh just increasing the time from repair to recurrence. Although suture repair is now rarely indicated, it might still have a role in young women who wish repair of an incisional hernia but are also contemplating further pregnancy.

✔✔ Mesh repair of incisional hernia reduces the recurrence rate, even for small hernias.[24]

MESH REPAIR

The onlay technique remains a common technique, largely because it is relatively easy to perform. The technique is dependent on closure of the anterior abdominal wall and adequate fixation of the mesh to the fascia, and a minimum overlap of 5–8 cm is recommended. If the connection between the mesh and the fascia is lost, a buttonhole hernia develops at the edge of the mesh. Good results can be reported with attention to detail, namely wide overlap of the mesh and obliteration of large skin flaps with fibrin glue.[25] However, for many surgeons, the relatively high rate of hernia recurrence, seroma formation, mesh infection and skin flap complications make this operation a poor option for the patient.

The sublay technique is the procedure favoured by the author. A mesh in the sublay position is not only sutured into position but is also held in place by the intra-abdominal pressure. Mesh in this position is therefore able to strengthen the abdominal wall both by mechanical sealing and by the induction of strong scar tissue. The sublay operation is effective for both midline and transverse wounds. Mesh

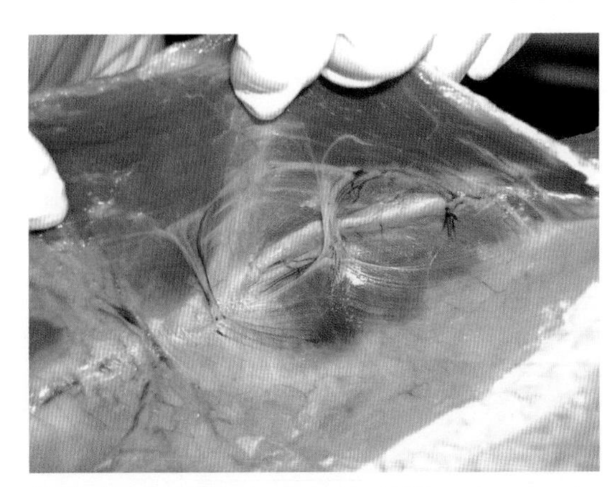

Figure 7.10 Fresh cadaveric dissection of the retromuscular space for sublay incisional hernia. (Courtesy of Dr J Conze, Berlin, Germany.)

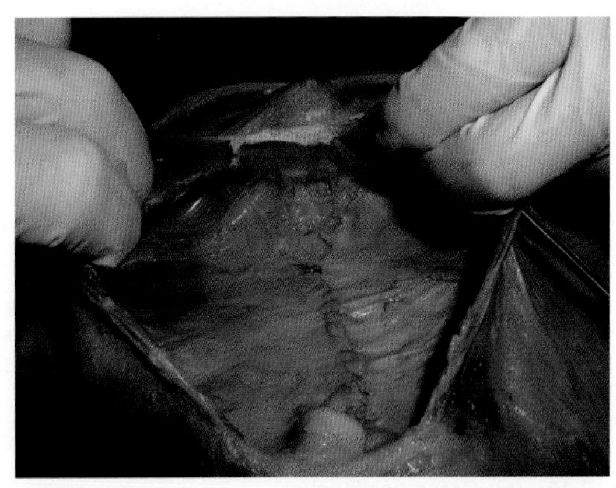

Figure 7.11 Fresh cadaveric dissection demonstrating the fatty triangle by division of the posterior rectus sheath as it attaches to the linea alba. This allows development of the sublay space behind the xiphisternum. (Courtesy of Dr J Conze, Berlin, Germany.)

placement in the preperitoneal space as opposed to the retro-rectus position is also described. However, the peritoneum is often thin and/or difficult to dissect intact in the region of the hernia making this a less effective technique compared with midline primary ventral hernias.

Open, intraperitoneal onlay mesh is also described. It is a useful technique when the abdominal wall is very scarred from previous surgery or when the abdominal wall is very attenuated. However, placing a large mesh in the abdominal cavity has a significant adhesion risk, and the open technique is still associated with significant wound complications, in effect combining the worst of the open and laparoscopic techniques.

Open sublay repair

The sublay operation begins by excising the old scar in the skin and performing a laparotomy. Adhesions tend to be maximal at the neck of the sac, so entering the abdominal cavity through the hernia sac is usually straightforward. It is helpful to mobilise adhesions off the underside of the anterior abdominal wall. It is not the author's routine practice to mobilise all the bowel adhesions unless there is a good history of recurrent episodes of bowel obstruction. The sublay space is then developed, which is the space anterior to the posterior rectus sheath, although this becomes preperitoneal below the semi-arcuate line. Care should be taken to mobilise the inferior epigastric vessels up with the belly of the rectus muscle to minimise bleeding. It is also important to preserve as many of the intercostal nerves as possible to minimise muscle denervation (Fig. 7.10). The preperitoneal space can be developed behind the pelvis, akin to a TEP repair, especially if the hernia arises in a Pfannenstiel incision. Superiorly, the sublay space can be developed behind the xiphisternum if necessary. The posterior rectus sheath is divided on either side close to the linea alba to expose the area known as the fatty triangle (Fig. 7.11). The posterior rectus sheath is approximated with an absorbable suture. The mesh is cut to size, aiming to have at least a 6-cm overlap in all directions. This mesh is sutured to the posterior rectus sheath with interrupted absorbable sutures, avoiding any obvious nerves. These sutures are purely to hold the mesh flat until it is encased in fibrous tissue. A suction drain is often left anterior to the mesh. Any further redundant skin and hernial sac is excised and the anterior rectus sheath closed with an absorbable suture, as is the skin, minimising any subcutaneous dead space. The cross-sectional appearance is illustrated in Fig. 7.12. If an abdominoplasty is performed at the same time, then further drains are placed to the subcutaneous space. In larger incisional hernias, the peritoneal flaps can be used to aid anterior and posterior fascial closure.[26]

Component separation techniques to allow midline closure for large ventral hernias are described. The anterior technique involves dividing the tendon of the external oblique as it attaches to the anterior rectus sheath from above the costal margin to close to the inguinal ligament, followed by mobilisation of this muscle off the internal oblique. The posterior approach involves mobilising the transversus muscle in a similar manner but from the inside, avoiding the larger skin flaps created by the open anterior approach and the risk of seroma, skin necrosis and wound breakdown. (The anterior release can also be undertaken using endoscopic techniques.) Both these techniques rob Peter to pay Paul and weaken the abdominal wall at these sites, which in some cases results in lateral bulging in the longer term. Use of the peritoneal flap technique[26] avoids the need for component separation in the majority of cases.

✔ The open sublay technique for incisional hernia repair has a lower recurrence rate and wound complication rate than onlay or inlay repair techniques. Randomised trials comparing the three mesh position techniques, however, are lacking.

Laparoscopic repair

The laparoscopic (intraperitoneal) approach has also been applied to incisional hernias. The laparoscopic approach has the advantages of shorter hospital stay, lower analgesic requirements, fewer wound complications and an earlier return to normal activities over open surgery. However, while the complication rate is lower overall when compared with open surgery, there is concern that when complications do arise with the laparoscopic approach, they are more likely to be life-threatening or require further surgery to deal with compared with open surgery.[27] Furthermore, the cosmetic result for larger hernias may not be as good, as there is no abdominoplasty component to the laparoscopic approach. Remember, the majority of patients wish surgery for their incisional hernia because of the cosmetic deformity rather

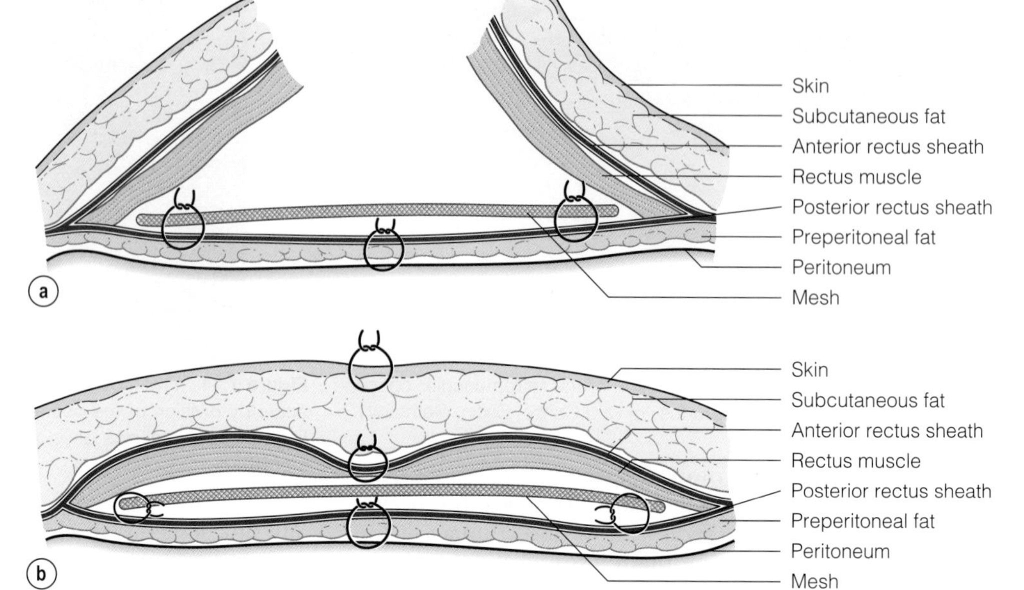

Figure 7.12 **(a)** Cross-sectional appearance of posterior fascia/peritoneum closure showing the sublay position of the mesh, which is fixed to the posterior sheath of the rectus muscle with an interrupted absorbable suture. **(b)** The anterior and posterior rectus sheath is closed continuously.

than symptoms related to the hernia. The laparoscopic approach works well for smaller incisional hernias, with a hernia neck size less than 7 cm and when cosmesis is not a significant concern. A number of controversies exist in the technique, related to (i) the method of fixation of the mesh, (ii) whether the hernia defect should be closed or not and (iii) the size of the mesh overlap. The method of mesh fixation divides surgeons between those who believe transfascial sutures to be essential to prevent hernia recurrence and those who believe such sutures cause chronic pain post surgery and their use should be avoided. The author prefers a double-crown tack technique (two rings of tacks around the hernia defect), although there is a lack of quality studies to make this an evidence-based decision. The recent introduction of absorbable tacks may reduce the risk of chronic pain and bowel adhesion to the tacks. Centring the mesh over the hernial defect is important to minimise hernia recurrence. The mesh can be centred with a central stitch, although two or four corner sutures are probably more accurate.

What about closure of the defect? Bridging of the defect is recognised to be a problem at open surgery, so why bridge with laparoscopic surgery? It is clear that once adhesions to the abdominal wall are taken down, inserting a mesh and tacking it in place is usually quick and easy. Closing the defect is thus not attractive to the majority of laparoscopic surgeons, introducing tension and perhaps increasing postoperative pain. However, many groups are talking about pseudo-recurrence[28]—the redevelopment of a bulge at the hernia site several years after laparoscopic repair as the mesh slides into the hernia sac. Thus closing the defect, the so-called IPOM-plus, does appear to reduce recurrence and pseudo-recurrence.[29] The size of the mesh overlap in a bridged repair and the mesh size when the defect is closed are still controversial.

One of the main long-term risks of the laparoscopic repair of incisional hernias is the placement of the mesh in direct contact with the intra-abdominal structures. As mentioned earlier, the use of meshes that have one side coated with a relatively non-adhesive material will help reduce (but not abolish) adhesion formation to the mesh. The other main risk is infection of the mesh, which is nearly always due to contamination from a bowel injury. Care should be taken with any adhesiolysis to minimise bowel injury, with thermal sources such as diathermy dissection kept to a minimum. The current consensus is that if the colon is injured, then it should be repaired, laparoscopically or open, according to the skills of the surgeon and no mesh inserted at this time. The patient can return in a number of months for a further attempt at repair. If the small bowel is injured with minimal contamination, then laparoscopic repair of the injury, washout and mesh insertion, is acceptable. If there is significant small-bowel injury and risk of failure of the bowel repair, then no mesh should be inserted. The patient should be observed in hospital and if they remain well 4–5 days later, then it is appropriate to re-laparoscope the patient and if no continuing contamination/infection is observed, the laparoscopic mesh repair can be completed. The use of antibiotic-impregnated mesh may allow a change to this policy with placement of such a mesh at the same time as bowel injury and repair.

PARASTOMAL HERNIA

Parastomal hernias occur at the site of an abdominal wall stoma. Indeed, the majority of patients with a stoma will develop such a hernia. Techniques to fashion a stoma to minimise parastomal hernia are beyond the scope of this chapter. However, many patients with a parastomal hernia will seek repair because of pain, cosmetic deformity and poor-fitting stoma appliances. Localised suture repair always fails. Moving the stoma to another location will have short-term benefit until a new hernia develops, and perhaps a hernia at the original site! Mesh can be inserted in the onlay, sublay and intraperitoneal positions. Traditionally this mesh is keyholed around the stoma, not too tight to cause ischaemia and not too loose for early failure. In practice, this is easier said than done. More durable results are being reported for the laparoscopic Sugarbaker technique, especially if performed with a keyhole mesh at the same time. However, lateralisation of the colon is usually straightforward, but for small-bowel stomas this is often more difficult, and can result in kinking of the bowel as it passes over the mesh, with resultant bowel obstruction.

EMERGENCY HERNIA SURGERY

Much of what has been mentioned above is applicable to hernia repair in the emergency situation. However, there are a few dilemmas that occur more frequently in the emergency setting. Patients who present as an emergency but have no bowel compromise can be treated as per elective hernia surgery. When bowel is compromised, especially when there has been significant contamination, current opinion is that synthetic mesh should not be used. However, there is little in the way of evidence apart from anecdote to support such a view, and this view has been challenged.[30] The case for biological mesh in such scenarios is also lacking in evidence.[31] For those who support the laparoscopic approach, it is not unreasonable to offer this in the emergency setting and laparoscope the patient with an irreducible groin hernia. If the bowel can be reduced and is viable, then convert the operation to a TEP/TAPP and place mesh as usual. If the bowel is compromised, then resect the bowel through a small incision and return 6 weeks later for a TEP. In the emergency incisional/ventral hernia setting, if the hernia is large, then proceed directly to open sublay mesh repair. If the hernia is smaller, then laparoscopy and intra-abdominal mesh are appropriate if there is no bowel compromise. If there is bowel ischaemia, then convert to the open sublay repair. The use of mesh in the sublay space in the emergency setting should not be associated with an increase in mesh infection as it lies external to the peritoneal cavity, but clearly each case will need to be assessed individually.

Emergency hernia surgery remains a high-risk surgical procedure, with the main risk factor for postoperative mortality being infarcted bowel.[32,33] Such operations should not be left to junior members of the surgical and anaesthetic teams. Appropriate resuscitation, followed by timely and appropriate surgery, may save lives. Occasionally, the techniques of damage limitation surgery (see Chapter 19) may be appropriate.

✓ Bowel infarction is the main risk factor for mortality in emergency hernia surgery.[32,33]

PORT SITE HERNIA

This is a hernia with an increasing incidence associated with the increase in laparoscopic surgery. Insertion of larger ports through the midline as opposed to more laterally appears to be a significant risk factor.[18] This is especially true in the presence of a divarification of the recti or an unrecognised umbilical hernia. There is little evidence to support closure of the fascia, except when a cut-down is performed for the first port. The use of dilating rather than cutting trocar tips may reduce the incidence of port site hernia formation. However, the risk of port site hernia at the umbilicus with larger ports such as the single-incision laparoscopic surgery technique is associated with an increased port site hernia risk.

ANTIBIOTIC PROPHYLAXIS IN HERNIA SURGERY

In general, elective hernia surgery to the groin and ventral regions does not require antibiotic prophylaxis.[10] However, as the risk of bowel injury is always present in incisional hernia surgery, it would be reasonable to give routine antibiotic prophylaxis for such surgery. Patients at increased risk of infection, including the immunocompromised, skin conditions with higher bacterial carriage such as psoriasis and in the emergency setting, all merit antibiotic prophylaxis.

All theatres have bacteria (called colony-forming units) in the circulating theatre air. It therefore makes sense to open the mesh just before it is required during the operation. Changing to fresh gloves before the handling of the mesh, minimising mesh contact with the skin and inserting the mesh deep to the subcutaneous tissues may all help reduce the risk of mesh contamination. The author uses a gentamicin solution (160 mg gentamicin in 100 mL normal saline) to irrigate larger meshes following insertion, although there is no evidence-based medicine to support this manoeuvre. Methicillin-resistant *Staphylococcus aureus* (MRSA) bacteria have been found on mesh several years after insertion, so prophylaxis to MRSA is appropriate if a previous repair has been complicated by MRSA infection.

✓✓ Antibiotic prophylaxis is unnecessary for uncomplicated elective hernia surgery to the groin and ventral regions.[10] However, antibiotic prophylaxis is appropriate for the majority of incisional hernia repairs.

'PROPHYLACTIC' HERNIA SURGERY

The topic of prophylactic mesh insertion to minimise subsequent incisional hernia formation in high-risk groups of patients remains controversial but is an active area of surgical research. High-risk patients, such as the obese, aneurysm surgery and the creation of a permanent stoma are all under study.[18,34,35] These studies report significantly reduced incisional or parastomal hernia rates at the same time point, with no increase in morbidity related to the prophylactic mesh, even in clean-contaminated situations. It is likely that prophylactic mesh to minimise subsequent hernia formation will become more mainstream practice, but there are many unanswered questions, including mesh type, mesh size and position of the mesh within the abdominal wall. The selective use of prophylactic mesh may be supported by preoperative collagen type I/III ratio typing to identify patients more at risk. This concept of collagen disease is important and introduces the notion that hernia repair of any type will fail if the patient lives long enough. It is true that some surgeons' repairs last longer than others, so technical factors remain important, and mesh repairs at any time point are more likely to be intact compared with a suture repair. (Re-operation rates are a surrogate for recurrence

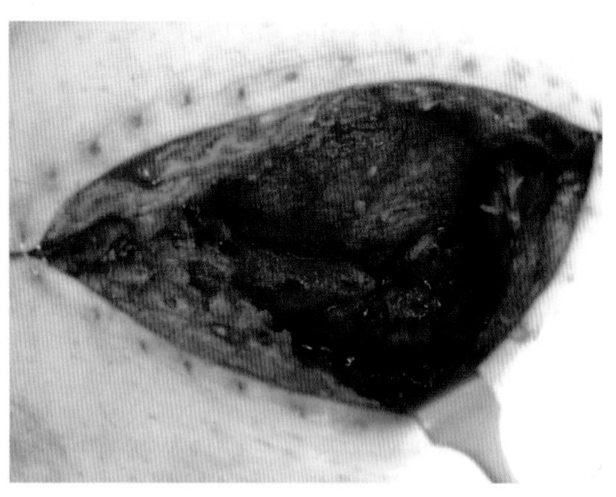

Figure 7.13 Early wound infection following onlay large pore mesh repair of incisional hernia. There is good granulation tissue through the mesh pores already. Opening the wound, washout and negative-pressure therapy salvaged this mesh repair.

rates, although re-operation will underestimate the true recurrence rate.) However, a hernia repair at present is a patch-up job, and will probably fail eventually (if the patient lives long enough). Nevertheless, randomised trials of prophylactic mesh use in patients at high risk of developing incisional hernia are ongoing.

MANAGEMENT OF AN INFECTED MESH

In general, an infected mesh has to be removed or exposed to the surface. If the mesh is lying in a pool of pus with no adherence to the patient, then the only real option is removal of the mesh. This is the more likely scenario with early infection in the first week or so following repair. If the mesh is partly embedded in tissue, then if there is adequate drainage through an open wound (or a laparoscopically placed drain for meshes in the preperitoneal space), many infected meshes will slowly granulate over and remain sound (Fig. 7.13). The exposure of the mesh to the skin surface, aided with negative pressure therapy,[36] will salvage the majority of meshes, especially those placed in the sublay position. However, sometimes chronic sinuses will develop and the only option is excision of these along with as much of the visible mesh as possible. Not all patients who require mesh removal will develop a hernia recurrence, although the majority probably will at some stage in the future on longer follow-up.[37] If mesh has to be removed/excised, it is best to remove as much of the mesh foreign body material as possible, control the sepsis and return at a later date for further hernia repair. The use of biological mesh in such a contaminated field is rarely indicated. The use of vacuum-assisted dressing to control the fluid exudates from the wound may aid wound care in such patients.

Key points

- Herniorrhaphy is one of the commonest operations performed.
- Techniques advanced considerably during the 1990s.
- The use of prosthetic mesh should now be considered for the repair of all hernias.
- The laparoscopic approach may be more appropriate than a traditional open approach.
- Recurrent hernias may be best managed in specialist centres or by surgeons with a specialist interest in hernia surgery who are technically competent to perform both open and laparoscopic procedures.
- A multidisciplinary approach, including plastic surgeons, may be appropriate for complex, multiply recurrent hernias.

 References available at http://ebooks.health.elsevier.com/

RECOMMENDED VIDEOS

- https://websurg.com/en/herniabc/. Users have to register with Websurg the first time to use the learning platform, but this is free. Then there is a large library of video lectures, operations etc on all things hernia.

KEY REFERENCES

[3] Miserez M, Alexandre JH, Campanelli G, et al. The European Hernia society groin hernia classification: simple and easy to remember. Hernia 2007;11:113–6. PMID: 17353992.
Pragmatic, easy to remember and use classification.

[7] Henriksen NA, Montgomery A, Kaufmann R, et al. Guidelines for treatment of umbilical and epigastric hernias from the European hernia society and Americas hernia society. Brit J Surg 2020;107:171–90.
Important guidelines from the EHS/AHS.

[9] Lichtenstein IL, Shulman AG, Amid PK, et al. The tension-free hernioplasty. Am J Surg 1989;157:188–93. PMID: 2916733.
The original description of an operation that has been considered the gold standard repair of inguinal hernia.

[10] HerniaSurge Group. International guidelines for groin hernia management. Hernia 2018;22:1–165. PMID: 29330835.
The first world inguinal hernia guidelines! They are undergoing refresh due out in 2022.

[12] Aasvang EK, Gmaehle E, Hansen JB, et al. Predictive risk factors for persistent postherniotomy pain. Anaesthesiology 2010;112:957–69. PMID: 20234307.
Chronic pain can be predicted prior to surgery with simple bedside tests.

[18] Muysoms FE, Antoniou SA, Bury K, et al. European Hernia Society guidelines on the closure of abdominal wall incisions. Hernia 2015;1–24. PMID: 25618025.
Excellent review of key step of every laparotomy.

[24] Luijendijk RW, Hop WC, van den Tol MP, et al. A comparison of suture repair with mesh repair for incisional hernia. N Engl J Med 2000;343:392–8. PMID: 10933738.
The first randomised trial to demonstrate the benefit of mesh in reducing recurrence in incisional hernia repair.

Neck surgery for the general surgeon

8

Iain J. Nixon | Michael E. Hopkins

INTRODUCTION

A neck mass is a common clinical presentation. Surgeons should be familiar with common causes, red flag symptoms and characteristic examination findings. A wide range of conditions can present with a neck mass and an exhaustive explanation of investigation and management of all such conditions is beyond the scope of this text. Instead, the aim of this chapter is to review the surgical investigation of a neck mass and to outline the surgical approach to managing common conditions which may face general surgeons as well as those with an interest in diseases of the head and neck.

DIAGNOSTIC APPROACH TO NECK MASSES

INITIAL ASSESSMENT (BOX 8.1)

A full clinical history is critical and should include not only features relating to the mass (site, duration, tenderness, growth, overlying skin changes) but also associated features which may point to the underlying diagnosis such as fevers, hoarseness, dysphagia, upper airway sounds and weight loss. Patient features including smoking, alcohol consumption and comorbidities may be critical in overall case management. On occasion, family history may be of interest, particularly in thyroid and parathyroid conditions which can be familial as in familial thyroid cancer and multiple endocrine neoplasia. Likewise, a brief occupational history may provide some clues such as a link between textiles industry workers and some head and neck malignancies. Establishing a previous medical history, specifically any previous malignancies or HPV and EBV exposure is useful.

The majority of neck masses requiring investigation arise within lymph nodes. However, salivary and thyroid masses are also common. Although vascular and neurogenic tumours are uncommon, an appreciation of such conditions is useful for forming a differential diagnosis (Table 8.1).

In areas of the world where tuberculosis is endemic, tuberculous cervical lymphadenopathy is common. Patients present with cold collar and stud abscesses and may have systemic features of the infection. Such patients require an accurate diagnosis, and will often benefit from aspiration of pus in order to target antibiotic therapy. Open incision and drainage should be avoided as this often results in an unsightly chronic sinus.

Malignancy should always be considered when investigating a neck mass, and a full head and neck examination is indicated to screen for an upper aerodigestive tract primary lesion. When considering the high-risk sites for primary disease, an understanding of lymphatic drainage from the head and neck is critical. Malignancy from the oral cavity will tend to drain to the submental or submandibular (level I) nodal basin. Lesions more posterior in the throat (the oropharynx) will more commonly metastasize to the jugular nodal chain (level II/III/IV). Laryngeal and thyroid cancers spread first to nodes in the central (level VI) or low lateral (level III/IV) neck (Fig. 8.1). When metastatic nodes are encountered in the posterior triangle (level V), primary disease may be present in the nasopharynx, scalp (skin cancer) or sites below the clavicle (lung, breast or gastrointestinal metastases to Virchow's node). Lymphoma commonly presents with cervical nodal enlargement, and can affect any or all lymph node groups.

In order to assess all at-risk sites appropriately, visualisation of the mucosal surfaces of the upper

Box 8.1 Approach to assessing a neck mass

Modality	Specific technique	Advantages/ Disadvantages
Clinical history		
Examination		
Imaging	Chest X-ray	Identification of primary lung disease or metastases
	Ultrasound	Cheap and no ionising radiation. Facilitates tissue sampling
	CT scan	Quick, readily available but exposure to radiation
	MRI scan	Slow leading to claustrophobia and swallow artefact but no radiation
Biopsy	Fine-needle aspiration	Minimally invasive but small number of cells
	Core	More invasive but provides greater cell number, useful for immunohistochemistry and also provides cellular architecture
	Open (avoid where possible)	Large number of cells but potential for seeding

aerodigestive tract is required. Although the oral cavity can be adequately assessed using a light, further examination requires mirror (indirect) or endoscopic (direct) assessment.

Having completed an examination, basic investigations including full blood count, erythrocyte sedimentation rate, glandular fever screen and chest X-ray will be considered on a case-by-case basis.

Following a full history and examination, some patients will require further investigation for an overt primary malignancy. However, a large percentage of patients will require further consideration of the neck mass without evidence of primary disease elsewhere.

IMAGING

Ultrasound (US) has become widely accepted as routine in assessment of the neck mass. This non-invasive investigation provides an accurate assessment of the neck and allows targeted tissue sampling where appropriate. However, it has limitations. The accuracy of findings are operator dependent and the images produced are less useful for surgical planning than those from cross-sectional imaging. Certain areas of the neck including the parapharyngeal space and the central neck are poorly visualised on US. Despite this, the majority of neck masses which require further assessment should be considered for US.

Computed tomography (CT) scans have become increasingly available in modern clinical practice. When contrast enhanced, CT scans allow assessment of potential malignant features and accurately display the relationship of the mass to the great vessels of the neck. In addition, CT provides valuable information about the mucosal surfaces of the head and neck. When extended to the thorax, the mediastinal nodes and lungs can be assessed for metastatic disease and possible synchronous primary lesions. CT scans are performed rapidly, which limits movement artefact due to swallowing and breathing during the examination. However, dental amalgam produces significant artefact which may obscure the structures within the oral cavity and oropharynx.

Magnetic resonance imaging (MRI) has the advantage of not involving ionising radiation. In addition, dental amalgam is less of an issue than for CT. However, images take longer to capture which makes movement artefact more of an issue. Improved soft tissue definition and increasing availability has led some groups to adopt MRI routinely in preference to CT for assessment of the neck. For staging of certain mucosal head and neck malignancies in the nasopharynx, oropharynx and hypopharynx, it is now considered a gold standard approach to use MRI alongside CT.

Positron emission tomography (PET) scanning involves the use of a radiolabelled tracer (most commonly FDG-18F) to provide functional imaging. In head and neck surgery, it tends to be used for identification of unknown primary disease in the setting of squamous cell carcinoma within a neck node, and for detection of recurrent or residual disease following treatment.

BIOPSY

Many neck masses will require a tissue diagnosis in order to plan treatment. In most situations, fine-needle aspiration (FNA) is the method of choice. Ideally, this should be US-guided in order to sample the area of highest suspicion, but free-hand biopsy is used by many groups who do not have access to US. The samples obtained on FNA allow cytologists to assess cell groups in order to guide diagnosis. There is minimal bleeding, and tumour seeding is not an issue with this technique.

In order to achieve increased cell number and in particular to demonstrate tissue architecture, core biopsy may be used. This technique removes a core of the neck mass (again ideally US-guided) which can be used for histological analysis. Although core biopsy is slightly more invasive than FNA, complication rates are low and tumour seeding is not considered a practical issue.

If a diagnosis cannot be reached using FNA or core techniques, open biopsy may be required. Although appropriate for certain conditions (e.g. salivary tumours and lymphoma), surgeons have been warned against this approach if squamous cell carcinoma is in the differential diagnosis. This caution stems from early 20th century evidence that open biopsy was associated with seeding of tumour, recurrence within the skin and compromised outcomes. However, surgical and radiotherapy techniques have improved significantly, hence this concept is increasingly considered outdated. In any case, the vast majority of patients can be diagnosed by accurate assessment and appropriate tissue sampling without proceeding to open biopsy.

Table 8.1 Differential diagnosis of neck mass

Lymphadenopathy	Salivary	Thyroid	Congenital	Vascular	Granulomatous	Neurogenic
Infective	Infective (sialadenitis)	Neoplastic (benign goitre or malignant)	Thyroglossal duct cyst	Carotid artery ectasia	Sarcoidosis	Neuroma
Malignant	Neoplastic (benign or malignant)	Inflammatory (Graves' disease)	Branchial arch anomalies	Carotid body tumour		
	Inflammatory (Sjögren's syndrome)	Infective (thyroiditis)		Lymphovascular abnormality		

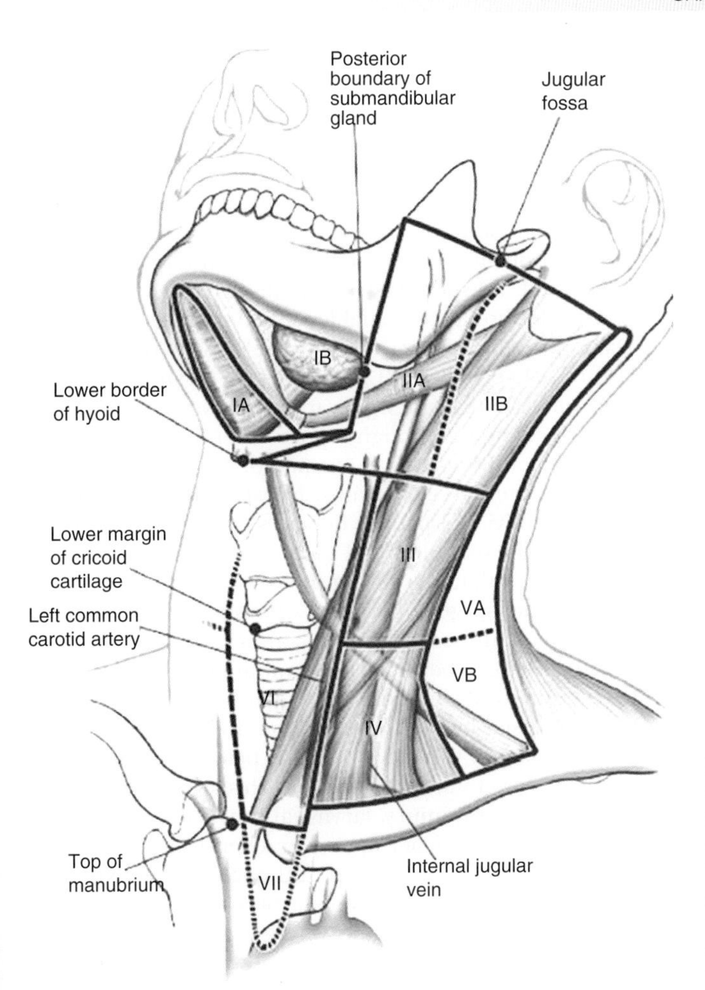

Figure 8.1 Diagram outlining cervical node levels in relation to neck anatomy. This figure shows American Joint Committee on Cancer classification of cervical lymph nodes (LN). Level 1 LN are sub-mental and sub-mandibular; level 2 LN are upper internal jugular chain nodes; level 3 LN are middle internal jugular chain nodes; level 4 LN are lower internal jugular chain nodes; level 5 LN are spinal accessory chain nodes and transverse cervical chain nodes; and level 6 LN are anterior cervical nodes (From Lorrie L. Kelley, Connie M. Petersen. Sectional Anatomy for Imaging Professionals. ed 3. St Louis: Elsevier; 2013).

THYROID MASS

Thyroid disease is common and as our population is increasingly screened with modern imaging techniques, the number of thyroid nodules presenting to surgeons is increasing.[1] For this reason, an appreciation of the investigation and management of thyroid masses is important for the surgeon.

The main indications for thyroid surgery are malignancy, pressure symptoms, hyperthyroidism and cosmesis. With this in mind, the approach to a thyroid mass should include a clinical history, examination, blood work, imaging and biopsy as indicated.[2,3] Risks of thyroid surgery include damage to the recurrent laryngeal nerve (RLN).[4] As such, all patients considered for surgery should undergo dynamic assessment of the recurrent nerve using direct endoscopic or indirect mirror assessment of the larynx. This is of particular importance in the setting of preoperative voice change, previous neck surgery or when there is suspicion of thyroid cancer with extra thyroidal extension which places the RLN at increased risk.[2,3]

✔ Where there is suspicion of involvement of the RLN in the setting of thyroid malignancy, the dynamic function of the larynx should be assessed with laryngoscopy.[2,3]

In almost all circumstances, US will be the first investigation for thyroid masses. Not only does this give information about the size and number of nodules present, but features such as the shape and structure of the nodule allows accurate prediction of risk of malignancy. These features have been standardised in the 'U' staging system (1–5), which groups nodules in ascending order of risk of malignancy.[2] In those patients with a thyroid that extends behind the sternum, or in the setting of malignant disease with nodal metastases, cross-sectional imaging (normally CT) may be a useful adjunct to assist surgical planning.[5]

Complications from thyroid surgery range from minor to life-threatening (Box 8.2). All patients require an incision

Box 8.2 Complications from thyroid surgery

Thyroid lobectomy	Scar Haemorrhage/neck haematoma Unilateral nerve injury (recurrent laryngeal and external branch of superior laryngeal)
Total thyroidectomy	Late hypothyroidism Hypocalcaemia (early and late) Bilateral recurrent laryngeal nerve injury (requires tracheostomy)

and therefore a scar. For most, an incision in a skin crease around the level of the cricoid will afford excellent access and minimal cosmetic impact.

In some cultures however, a neck scar is associated with significant negative connotations. In response, groups in the Far East are using a transaxillary approach to the neck using endoscopes or robotic techniques.[6] Such procedures involve wide-field dissection, high levels of expense and significant operative time. An alternative is the 'minimally invasive' endoscopic technique.[7] With this approach, a small (<2 cm) incision is placed in the central neck and with video endoscopic assistance, adequate exposure can be achieved to allow thyroid surgery.

Such modern techniques of thyroidectomy have potential advantages. The cosmetic outcome from surgery is superior due to the absence or reduction of a cervical incision. As experience is gained, groups are reporting favourable outcomes and expanded indications.[8,9] However, there are significant limitations. Large goitres cannot be removed through small incisions; therefore, such 'minimally invasive' approaches are not suitable for the majority of patients who undergo thyroid surgery for compressive symptoms. In addition, these techniques do not allow lymphadenectomy or wide-field thyroidectomy to address extra thyroidal extension. In particular, techniques which approach the thyroid from a lateral position (transaxillary approach) prevent access to the contralateral lobe and hence are not appropriate for total thyroidectomy. In addition, the oncological safety of opening a wide field in the setting of malignancy has been questioned, with reports of recurrence within the dissection field.[10] Another significant limitation is cost. Increased duration of surgery and the cost of consumables make such procedures extremely expensive and at a time of global healthcare rationing this has prevented widespread adoption of these approaches.[11] Furthermore, reducing the size of neck incision may not convey improvement in patient satisfaction scores postoperatively.[12]

The most serious complication from thyroidectomy is bleeding. Around 1.5–2% of patients suffer postoperative haemorrhage.[13] For this reason in the UK, most thyroid surgeries are performed with an overnight stay[14] in order to allow patients to be regularly assessed and dealt with promptly in the event of haemorrhage. Some groups have found that modern electrosurgical devices are associated with lower rates of haemorrhage[15] and as such some surgeons now advocate day-case surgery. UK National Institute for Health and Care Excellence (NICE) guidance now states that same day discharge may be considered in hemithyroidectomy; however, patients undergoing total thyroidectomy should be observed overnight due to the increased risk of haemorrhage and hypocalcaemia.[16] Despite all efforts, the risk of haemorrhage cannot be completely avoided.[17]

✔ Total thyroidectomy requires an overnight postoperative stay to monitor for complications including haemorrhage and hypocalcaemia. The risk is much lower in hemithyroidectomy and therefore these cases can be considered for day-case admission.[14,16]

Increasing neck swelling in a postoperative patient requires urgent intervention. With delay, arterial bleeding increases the pressure in the central neck compartment until it exceeds venous pressure. This leads to venous oedema of the larynx causing swelling, progressive stridor and asphyxiation. Immediate action is required. An anaesthetist should be alerted and early intubation with haematoma evacuation and haemorrhage control under general anaesthesia is preferred. If there is audible airway compromise (stridor), the incision line should be opened on the ward to allow a temporary reduction in pressure and buy time while the airway is secured. Ideally both the skin incision and deeper sutures are removed. As such, instrumentation to allow suture or clip removal should be available at the bedside.

Damage to the nerves supplying the muscles of the larynx is also of concern. The RLN supplies all laryngeal muscles apart from cricothyroid. Injury to this nerve leads to significant voice change. Although reported nerve injury rates depend on when the larynx is examined, permanent damage occurs in around 1–2% of most major series.[4] The precise risk to an individual patient depends on the nature of the disease and the experience of the surgeon.[18] Previously, surgeons believed that identifying the RLN was not mandatory during thyroid surgery, provided an intracapsular operative approach was utilised. However, contemporary practice requires the nerve to be visualised to minimise the risk of inadvertent injury while mobilising the gland.[19–24] This approach is now endorsed by both American and British guidelines.[2] Clearly, unilateral thyroid lobectomy places only one nerve at risk, whereas total thyroidectomy threatens both. In the event of a bilateral injury, laryngeal function is significantly compromised and permanent tracheostomy may be required to secure a safe airway. Although this is extremely rare (around 0.02% of all cases), rates are higher in total thyroidectomy than lobectomy where it is only encountered if a pre-existing contralateral vocal cord palsy is present.[18]

It is now common practice to use a nerve monitor during the procedure to assist in identification of both the vagus and RLN. By first identifying the vagus on the side of initial lobectomy, integrity and function of the nerve monitor and nerve can be confirmed. This can be re-confirmed on completion of the first side to ensure that the nerves remain functional. This is especially important in total thyroidectomy: if the RLN is damaged on one side, proceeding to excising the contralateral lobe may have to be reconsidered.

The external branch of the superior laryngeal nerve approaches the larynx from above to innervate the cricothyroid muscle. It has a variable position in relation to the superior thyroid artery and its branches. Most authors do not advocate specific identification during thyroidectomy but recommend taking branches of the artery low in order to minimise the risk of injury.[3] Permanent injury leads to a loss of high-pitch voice, most evident during singing.

✔ The recurrent laryngeal nerve should be identified in all thyroidectomy procedures. Steps should be taken to minimise the risk to the external branch of the superior laryngeal nerve during dissection.[3,19–24]

The parathyroid glands are small structures on the posterior surface of the thyroid and have a role in calcium homeostasis. During thyroidectomy, these glands should be identified and protected. Following thyroid lobectomy, up to 11–25% of specimens will be found to contain parathyroid tissue on histological analysis.[25,26] Both removal and devascularisation of the glands will interfere with function. Around 20% of patients suffer temporary hypocalcaemia following total thyroidectomy, but only 1–2% will have long-term problems.[4] This complication is almost never seen after thyroid lobectomy and is more common when a central neck dissection is performed along with total thyroidectomy.

If half of the thyroid is removed (thyroid lobectomy), less than one-third of patients will become hypothyroid.[27] This is more likely if there is a background of Hashimoto's thyroiditis (such patients are at risk of becoming hypothyroid even without surgery). Clearly if the entire gland is removed, the patient will require lifelong thyroxine therapy.

The surgical approach depends on the indication for the procedure, and as such each scenario will be considered individually.

SURGERY FOR MALIGNANCY

A spectrum of malignancies affects the thyroid gland. However, differentiated thyroid cancer is most common (90%) and within that group, papillary cancer is the most common subtype. Medullary[28] and anaplastic[29] thyroid cancers are uncommon, and thyroid lymphoma and metastases to the thyroid are rare.[30]

Most thyroid cancers present either with a palpable mass, or as an incidental finding on imaging.[31] Assessment of the regional nodes with US is critical. Assuming there are suspicious findings on US, biopsy will be indicated to confirm the diagnosis.

For differentiated thyroid cancer (papillary and follicular), FNA is considered the gold standard and ideally should be US-guided. The results can be stratified by the 'THY' staging system (1–5) in order to allow cytologists to communicate effectively with surgical colleagues (Box 8.3).[2]

✔ Patients considered at risk of thyroid malignancy should have fine needle aspiration biopsy.[2,3]

In patients with malignant lesions (THY 5), therapeutic surgery will be indicated. In those with lesions not confirmed as malignant (THY 3f or THY 4), diagnostic surgery is indicated. Generally THY3a lesions will be re-biopsied unless clinical concern exists in which case surgery will be indicated. If cytology indicates benign disease (THY 2), the patient may be suitable for discharge, unless there is significant concern from the US scan images, in which case a further biopsy may be indicated.[2]

The details of surgical procedure in each case are beyond the scope of this chapter. However, broadly speaking, for differentiated thyroid cancer with significant extra thyroidal extension, regional nodal or distant metastases, total thyroidectomy is indicated (Box 8.4). This procedure removes disease and renders the patient suitable for adjuvant radioactive iodine (RAI) therapy which would otherwise be absorbed by the remnant thyroid lobe. If residual normal thyroid tissue remains present in the neck following surgery, any administered RAI is preferentially taken up by native thyroid tissue which is more iodine avid than metastatic thyroid cancer, reducing the chance a tumouricidal radiation dose is delivered to malignant cells.

In addition to the thyroid procedure, resection of any evident nodal disease should be performed with a 'compartment-oriented' neck dissection (Box 8.5).[32] For low-risk patients with disease within the thyroid and no evidence of spread beyond the gland, thyroid lobectomy should be sufficient. In such patients, oncological outcomes are excellent, and the morbidity of thyroid lobectomy is significantly lower than that of total thyroidectomy.[18] A more detailed approach to the management of differentiated thyroid cancer is available in British and American Thyroid Association Guideline Documents.[2,3]

The issue of appropriate management of thyroid malignancy in the absence of clinical nodal metastasis (the 'cN0 neck') remains highly controversial. Proponents of both aggressive (total thyroidectomy and prophylactic neck dissection) and conservative (thyroid lobectomy and no regional lymphadenectomy) exist. The reason for the controversy is the excellent and equivalent outcomes enjoyed by low-risk patients with differentiated thyroid cancer. Some studies demonstrate an increased risk of postoperative complications when lymphadenectomy is performed, especially in older patients.[33] As outlined above, if an indication for RAI exists, total thyroidectomy is indicated. If there is evidence of nodal disease at the time of presentation, neck dissection is indicated. For most patients however, disease is limited to the thyroid and 30-year survival in this group is > 95%.

Box 8.3 Thy cytological grading system

THY category	Clinical meaning
THY1	Non-diagnostic sample
THY2	Benign
THY3a	Atypical cells
THY3f	Follicular neoplasm
THY4	Suspicious for malignancy
THY5	Diagnostic for malignancy

Box 8.4 Primary thyroid procedure for malignancy

Total thyroidectomy	Large primary tumour (>4 cm) Evidence of extra thyroid extension Nodal or distant metastatic disease Contralateral nodular disease
Thyroid lobectomy	Small primary tumour Intra-thyroid disease only No evidence of contralateral nodules

Box 8.5 Primary neck procedure for malignancy

Evidence of disease in the central neck (cN1a)	Dissection of levels VI and VII
Evidence of disease in lateral neck (cN1b)	Dissection of levels II–V
No evidence of neck disease (cN0)	Controversial—consider prophylactic surgery if high-risk features (extra thyroidal extension or large primary tumour)

When the American Thyroid Association performed a feasibility analysis of determining the optimal approach to therapy, their power calculation suggested almost 6000 patients would be required for a definitive prospective randomised trial. As such, it is unlikely that a definitive answer will ever be provided.

✔ For patients with thyroid cancer and evidence of nodal metastases, compartment-oriented neck dissection is indicated. For those patients without evidence of nodal metastases, elective nodal dissection should only be considered in those at highest risk of harbouring occult disease.[2,3]

SURGERY FOR PRESSURE SYMPTOMS

As the thyroid enlarges, initial growth is asymptomatic. However, as the gland increases in size, and in particular if it encroaches on the thoracic inlet, pressure on surrounding structures including the oesophagus and trachea may increase. Such patients initially complain of a vague feeling of something in the throat, progressing to dysphagia and even airway compromise in severe cases. Compression of the great vessels may compromise venous return, particularly with the arms raised (Pemberton's sign). Such patients should be considered for surgery.[5] For the vast majority of patients, even those with retrosternal goitre, a cervical approach to surgery is adequate. For those patients with a goitre which exceeds the dimensions of the thoracic inlet and those which involve the posterior mediastinum, sternotomy may be required.[34,35]

Preoperative investigation is similar to that for patients considered at risk of malignancy, with US and FNA as indicated. However, if there is significant retrosternal extension, cross-sectional imaging with CT allows assessment of the relationship of the goitre with mediastinal structures.

When considering such patients, one should remember that although thyroidectomy relieves compression caused by the thyroid gland, entering the pre-tracheal fascia replaces native thyroid tissue with scar. As such, patients with mild throat discomfort and a small thyroid goitre may not notice a significant improvement in symptoms following surgery. Furthermore, if there is injury of the RLN intraoperatively, postoperative symptoms may exceed preoperative symptoms. In such patients, a barium swallow to identify the extent of impingement caused by the gland is useful for counselling the patient in relation to postoperative expectations.

Rates of RLN injury are greater in surgery for large goitres. Not only can the position of the nerve be affected by the unpredictable growth of the gland, but the nerve is in apposition with the gland for a greater distance requiring significant dissection. The RLN will tend to lie deep to the thyroid making visualisation impossible as the gland is mobilised up out of the neck. For this reason, the nerve is at risk throughout the surgery and great care should be taken, particularly in bilateral procedures.

SURGERY FOR HYPERTHYROIDISM

Patients who present with hyperthyroidism require careful investigation to determine the cause and select the most appropriate treatment. The most common cause of hyperthyroidism is Graves' disease, a diffuse toxic goitre. Functioning nodules can also cause hyperthyroidism as an isolated finding or within a multinodular goitre. Investigation of this patient group will include basic thyroid function tests and serum autoantibodies. US is used in conjunction with RAI scanning in order to identify functioning nodules.

Most patients will be considered for non-surgical treatment. Medical therapy with anti-thyroid drugs offers the advantages of avoiding surgery in diffuse toxic goitre, but has a failure rate of up to 50%.[36] RAI can be used to destroy thyroid cells and reduce the function of the gland. This may be suitable for diffuse or nodular toxic disease, but requires quarantine during treatment and pregnancy must be avoided during and for a minimum 6 month period after therapy.

Surgery is considered for patients who have failed non-surgical therapy or for specific subgroups (Box 8.6): for example, large toxic nodular goitres tend to respond poorly to RAI therapy,[37] and patients with significant eye signs from Graves' disease show better response to surgical than non-surgical therapy.[38]

When the decision is made to proceed with surgery, the extent of surgery will depend on the nature of the disease. Patients with diffuse toxic goitre will be candidates for total thyroidectomy and thyroxine replacement therapy. In the setting of a single functioning nodule, lobectomy alone will suffice.[39]

This patient group should be managed by a clinical team including an endocrinologist, not only for non-surgical therapy but also to optimise preoperative preparation and postoperative treatment. Prior to surgery, anti-thyroid drugs should be used to achieve euthyroidism. In patients who cannot be adequately controlled, β-blockers may be used to abolish the systemic features of hyperthyroidism in the perioperative and postoperative period. Oral iodine has also been used to reduce the vascularity of the thyroid prior to surgery.[40,41]

Surgery for Graves' disease (total or near total thyroidectomy)[39] is challenging due to the firm nature of the gland and the inflammatory response that surrounds it. Careful dissection with prompt control of pin-point haemorrhages is required to safely identify the nerves and parathyroid glands during the dissection and minimise the risk of postoperative complications. UK data suggests that patients with Graves' disease who opt for surgery are at a significantly increased risk of complications compared with those operated on for other thyroid conditions.[4]

✔✔ Patients with Graves' disease and associated significant thyroid eye disease have better outcomes following total thyroidectomy than with medical management. However, surgery in these patients is more technically challenging.[4,38]

Box 8.6 Thyroid procedure for hyperthyroidism

Toxic nodule	Thyroid lobectomy
Graves' disease	Total or near total thyroidectomy with thyroxine replacement
Toxic multinodular goitre	Total or near total thyroidectomy with thyroxine replacement

POSTOPERATIVE MANAGEMENT FOLLOWING THYROIDECTOMY

Following surgery, patients require close observation for bleeding and airway compromise. Immediately following extubation, stridor should alert the team to the possibility of a bilateral nerve injury. Ideally in this situation, the larynx is examined with a flexible endoscope. However, if the patient is clinically unstable (tachypnoeic or hypoxic), re-intubation may be required. A decision whether to re-explore the recurrent nerves at this point is best delayed as even if divided nerves are identified and repaired, the acute situation will not resolve immediately. Nerve repair is best undertaken when the patient is stable. The patient is transferred for ventilation and most authors recommend high-dose steroids and a trial of extubation in 24–48 hours. There is evidence to suggest that re-exploration can be beneficial in the long term if injured nerves can be identified and repaired.[42] If there is a certainty about bilateral injury, early tracheostomy will be required. This should be an extremely rare event (~0.1%).[43]

All patients should have regular observation of the wound and be instructed to alert staff if there is swelling or discomfort. It is critical that staff caring for these patients understand the importance of postoperative haematoma and that equipment (stitch cutter or staple remover) is available at the bedside, in order to open the skin and ideally the platysmal layer of sutures to temporarily relieve pressure in the central neck. In addition, those who have had total thyroidectomy require monitoring of serum calcium. Many units have local policies, and measuring levels on the first postoperative day will allow those with hypocalcaemia to be identified. Late hypocalcaemia does occur and patients should be aware of the symptoms so they can seek medical attention if this develops. Some units now prefer to use rapid assessment of parathyroid hormone which can reliably identify those at risk of developing hypocalcaemia. However, this is an expensive resource and unavailable in many centres. The British Association of Endocrine and Thyroid Surgeons website provides further information and a suitable algorithm for managing post-thyroidectomy hypocalcaemia.[44]

After total thyroidectomy, patients should commence replacement therapy (approximately 1.6 μg/kg of thyroxine daily) and this can be fine-tuned in the postoperative period. Following thyroid lobectomy, patients should have assessment of thyroid function 4–6 weeks after surgery to determine the need for thyroxine.

CONGENITAL MASSES

Although many different rare types of congenital mass may arise in the head and neck region, the most commonly occurring are branchial cysts and thyroglossal duct cysts.

As the embryo matures, the branchial arches fuse to obliterate the spaces between. However, if that process is incomplete, a persistent communication between the pharynx and skin may persist, termed a branchial fistula. These are rare, complex and may be associated with structures including the carotid artery and branches of the facial nerve.

More commonly, if mucosal surface connections are lost, a branchial cyst forms. These most commonly present in children and young adults with swelling and pain, often following an infection. The diagnosis can be made clinically, and imaging will demonstrate an isolated cystic structure, medial to the sternomastoid muscle and lateral to the carotid sheath (Fig. 8.2). Classically, this is found at the junction of the upper and middle third of sternomastoid.

Treatment is indicated to prevent further infections and confirm the diagnosis.[45] The main risk of surgery is damage to the marginal mandibular branch of the facial nerve, which lies immediately deep to platysma. In order to prevent permanent damage, a skin crease incision is placed a minimum of two finger-breadths below the mandible. Incision continues through platysma and on to the sternomastoid muscle, raising a plane deep to platysma to maintain the nerve within the skin flap. Although temporary injury can occur from excessive retraction, division of the nerve should be prevented with this approach.

A diagnosis of branchial cyst should raise suspicion in an older patient, or those with risk factors for mucosal head and neck cancer, as there is a risk of malignancy. Previously, 'malignant degeneration of branchial cysts' was thought to be the cause of such cases. However, squamous cell carcinoma from the tonsil or tongue base region of the oropharynx typically presents with cystic masses in the lateral neck and the primary lesion can be small. It is likely that these are the main cause of such cystic metastases rather than a cystic squamous lining undergoing dysplastic change.

As endoscopic and imaging techniques have improved, previously occult head and neck primary tumours can be identified and treated appropriately. As outlined above, diagnosis should avoid open biopsy and therefore all such patients should undergo a full head and neck examination, cross-sectional imaging and FNA biopsy, only considering surgical excision in those with negative results.

As the thyroid gland descends from its initial position at the junction of the anterior two-third and posterior one-third of the tongue (foramen caecum) to its adult position anterior to the second and third tracheal rings, it does so down the thyroglossal duct. If the duct fails to regress, a thyroglossal tract may remain and cells within the tract may present later as a cystic structure. Most lie inferior to the hyoid, but may present anywhere along the route of descent (Fig. 8.3). The classic finding is of a midline mass which moves both on swallowing (adherence to the pre-tracheal fascia) and on tongue protrusion (adherence to the base of the tongue). In contrast, thyroid masses move only on swallowing.

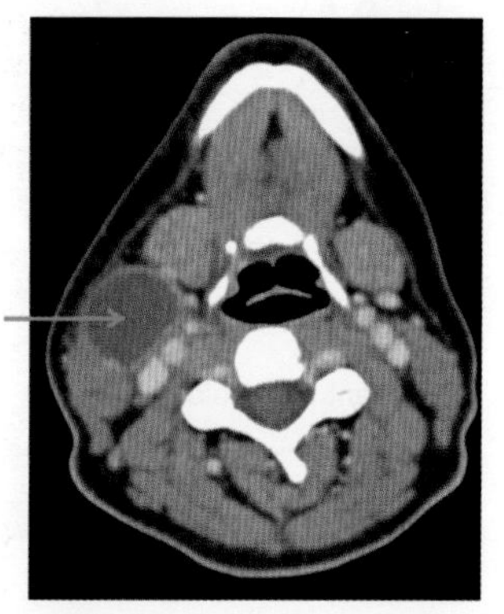

Figure 8.2 Computed tomography scan showing branchial cyst deep to sternomastoid and lateral to the carotid sheath.

Again, US and FNA are the main investigations to guide diagnosis. The majority of patients will be candidates for surgical excision to confirm the diagnosis and prevent recurrent infections. It is said that US and thyroid function tests are mandatory to confirm the presence of a normal thyroid prior to surgery which would otherwise render the patient hypothyroid. However, it is extremely rare to find a patient with no functioning thyroid tissue in the normal position, and if a sole site of ectopic thyroid was identified, most clinicians would consider surgical excision in this unusual setting.

Early attempts at thyroglossal cystectomy resulted in high rates of recurrence. These observations led to the Sistrunk procedure, where the entire tract including the central portion of the hyoid bone and a small cone of tissue towards the base of tongue are excised. This more radical approach has reduced recurrence rates to < 5%. More recently, histological analysis of excised thyroglossal tracts has demonstrated a branching structure.[46] In response, many authors now recommend an en bloc excision of a medial portion of the strap muscles along with the tract to encompass any branches.[47,48]

PARATHYROID DISEASE

The field of parathyroid surgery is complex, demanding multidisciplinary input and an in-depth understanding of the embryological development of the parathyroid glands. The majority of parathyroid surgeons will work within an endocrine team with the support of colleagues in radiology, nuclear medicine, pathology, biochemistry and interventional radiology.

The parathyroids are small, tan coloured glands located in the space around the thyroid gland. The inferior parathyroids develop from the dorsal aspect of the third pharyngeal pouch. They descend, along with the thymus, to lie in the inferior neck. The superior glands arise in the dorsal wing of the fourth pharyngeal pouch and descend along with the thyroid. Due to the longer route of descent, the position of the inferior parathyroid glands is more variable. Over 80% of patients have four parathyroids, 13% have more than four and less than 5% have fewer than four glands.

Primary hyperparathyroidism usually presents with hypercalcaemia detected on routine biochemistry. If severe, it may present with clinical manifestations of hypercalcaemia including fatigue, thirst, dehydration, renal stones, muscle weakness and bone fractures. A raised calcium and raised parathyroid hormone level is diagnostic. Treatment is usually surgical, as medical therapy to reduce calcium levels does not address the pathology directly.

Having made the diagnosis and decided to pursue surgical treatment, the next issue is whether to perform preoperative localisation. Bilateral neck exploration performed by an experienced surgeon cures primary hyperparathyroidism in 95% of cases and localisation studies have historically been inaccurate. However, improvements in imaging in addition to the observation that > 90% of patients will have only one parathyroid adenoma mean that most surgeons now rely on imaging to guide the surgical procedure.

US is cheap, readily available and non-irradiating. However, it is operator dependant and poor at visualising areas in the deep central neck. Therefore, it has significant limitations and is best used in conjunction with other modalities. Cross-sectional imaging with contrast-enhanced CT or MRI is useful for surgical planning, particularly in the re-operative setting. Technetium-99m sestamibi is concentrated in abnormal parathyroid glands and has revolutionised parathyroid surgery (Fig. 8.4). Sestamibi can be combined with CT to produce three-dimensional single-photon emission computed tomography (SPECT) scans to provide further anatomical detail (Fig. 8.5). Furthermore, four-dimensional CT with multiple contrast phases may be used as an adjunct in adenoma localisation. The ability to localise disease to a single gland has made targeted unilateral exploration an alternative to routine bilateral procedures. Interventional radiology can contribute to localisation with targeted angiography (where the parathyroid adenoma is seen as a ‘stain’) or selective venous sampling

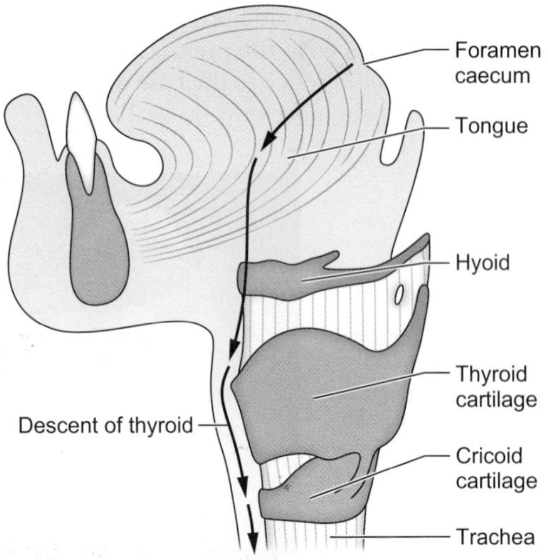

Figure 8.3 Illustration of the route of descent of thyroid and therefore possible locations of a thyroglossal duct cyst.

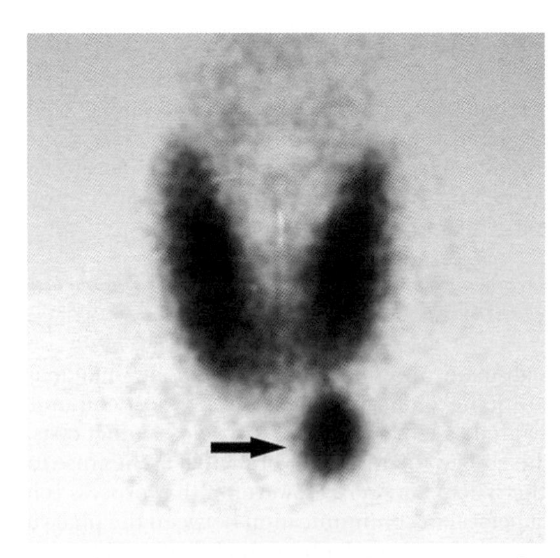

Figure 8.4 Single-isotope dual-phase sestamibi scan. Sestamibi tracer can be seen concentrating in both the thyroid gland and a left lower pole parathyroid adenoma *(arrow)* in this early-phase image. Delayed-phase images would demonstrate washout of tracer from the thyroid gland but not the parathyroid adenoma.

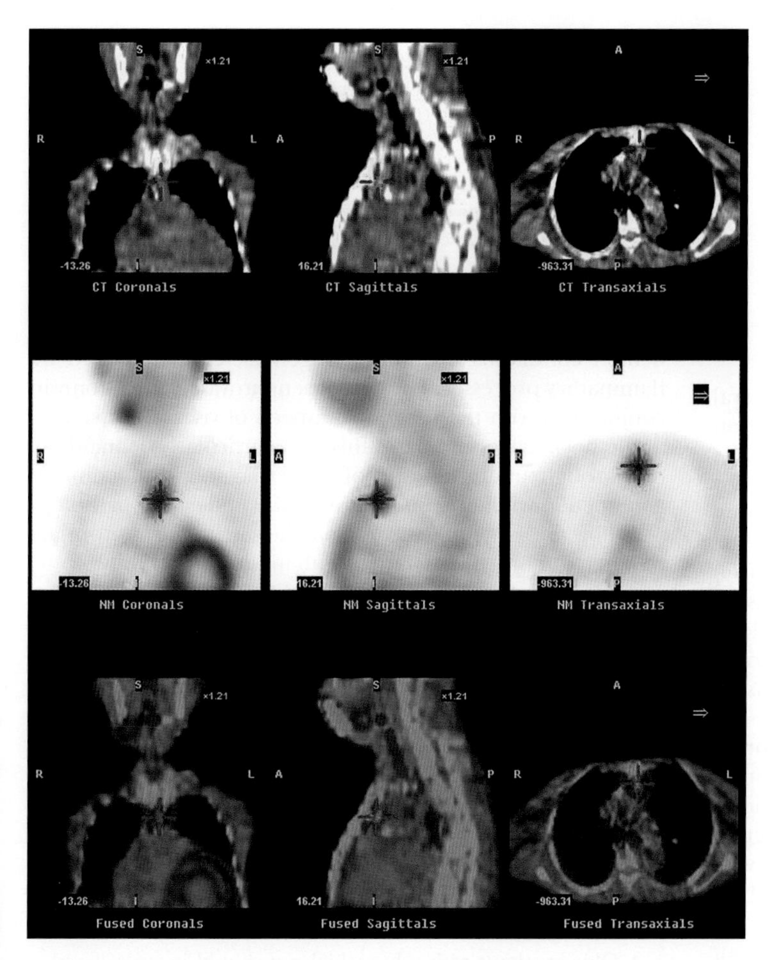

Figure 8.5 Computed tomography (CT)-enhanced single-photon emission computed tomography (SPECT) scan. This image shows a mediastinal parathyroid adenoma identified precisely by SPECT enhancement and CT. The top two rows of images mark the parathyroid adenoma on CT scan (cross-hair). The bottom row of images marks the parathyroid adenoma on SPECT scan.

(Fig. 8.6). Drawbacks of these techniques include the need for nephrotoxic contrast and the risk of embolic events, meaning most centres reserve these for re-operative cases. Although parathyroid adenomas are most frequently identified in the normal position of a parathyroid gland, more rarely they can be found at other anatomical sites including within the thyroid gland, thymus, mediastinum or tracheo-oesophageal groove.

Ninety percent of cases of primary hyperparathyroidism are caused by a single adenoma, 5% by multiple adenomas, 5% by four gland hyperplasia and <1% by carcinoma.[49] The normal gland weighs approximately 40 mg. Diseased glands weigh upwards of 70 mg. Adenomas are either tan or beefy red in colour. Malignancy is difficult to confirm, even on histological analysis. If a parathyroid is palpable, this should alert the clinician to the risk of malignancy, as should extremely high serum calcium. Intraoperative findings may include local invasion, which will confirm the diagnosis clinically, as would regional or distant metastatic disease. If malignancy is suspected, an en bloc resection including the ipsilateral thyroid gland is recommended. If the capsule of the gland is ruptured, recurrent disease presents due to seeding and can be impossible to resect.

Having completed the assessment of a patient with primary hyperparathyroidism, the treating surgeon must decide on the most appropriate operation. For those patients with a single adenoma confirmed on preoperative localisation, unilateral open or minimally invasive surgery may be chosen (Box 8.7). In those with suspicion of multi-gland disease

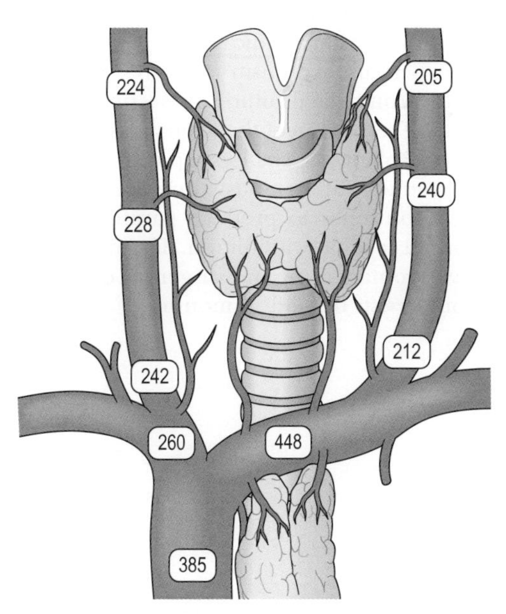

Figure 8.6 Selective venous sampling data. This image of parathyroid hormone values represents an adenoma in the cervical thymus.

(either due to family history or imaging studies), a bilateral exploration will be preferred.[50] This is a controversial subject with conflicting opinions.[51] Improvements in preoperative localisation make a targeted approach attractive. The potential for low morbidity and high success rates have led to an increase in interest in this technique. However,

Box 8.7 Indications for surgical intervention for primary hyperparathyroidism

Symptomatic hypercalcaemia
Nephrolithiasis
Age < 50 years
Serum calcium > 1.0 mg/dL above normal limit
Reduced creatinine clearance
Loss of bone mineral density

some authors report higher recurrence rates with unilateral than standard bilateral exploration, and low complication rates for bilateral procedures in experienced hands. The approach chosen by the clinical team will be influenced by factors including preoperative investigations and local complication rates.[52] Once the suspected parathyroid adenoma is resected, many surgeons advocate immediate fresh frozen section pathology to confirm complete adenoma excision before closing.[53] The more optimal approach, if available, is the use of intraoperative parathyroid hormone monitoring, whereby a significant reduction in levels indicates excision of the adenoma.

Secondary hyperparathyroidism arises when factors other than primary hyperparathyroidism cause overproduction of parathyroid hormone. The most common cause is chronic renal failure which leads to hypocalcaemia and overproduction of parathyroid hormone. Initial medical management is with calcium and vitamin D supplementation and a low-phosphate diet. The definitive therapy is renal transplantation. For refractory cases (5–10%), surgical parathyroidectomy with four gland excision with or without auto transplantation or three and a half gland excision is indicated.[54]

Tertiary hyperparathyroidism is a rare condition where patients with chronic renal failure and secondary hyperparathyroidism have resolution of their renal dysfunction (usually by renal transplant). A small group of these patients will have developed an autonomously functioning parathyroid gland which continues to produce parathyroid hormone without normal feedback inhibition. The majority of these cases resolve spontaneously and surgery is only indicated if the situation persists beyond 12 months.

✔ Preoperative localisation of parathyroid adenomas using imaging techniques such as technetium-99m sestamibi scans or four-dimensional CT imaging is preferable to bilateral neck exploration.

CONCLUSION

A wide spectrum of disease processes present with surgical head and neck manifestations. These comprise malignant and benign conditions including congenital, endocrine and inflammatory processes. The complex neurovascular anatomy in conjunction with the functional aspects of visceral physiology in the neck make surgery in this area particularly demanding. A thorough understanding of embryology and anatomy in conjunction with an appreciation of the underlying pathology will allow the surgeon to investigate the case in the appropriate manner and provide treatment with minimal morbidity.

Key points

- Full head and neck examination is critical in all patients who present with a neck mass.
- When indicated, FNA biopsy is preferred to open biopsy to avoid the risk of seeding.
- Patients with thyroid cancer require US imaging and FNA biopsy.
- In patients at risk of RLN involvement who undergo thyroidectomy, preoperative assessment of laryngeal function is advised.
- During thyroidectomy, identification of the RLN is considered mandatory.
- Older patients with a branchial cyst should be considered at risk of having metastatic squamous cell carcinoma and investigated accordingly prior to excision.
- Thyroglossal duct cysts should be excised with a portion of the hyoid bone to minimise recurrence rates.
- Parathyroid disease is complex and requires multidisciplinary management.
- Surgery for primary hyperparathyroidism can often be targeted with modern preoperative investigations.

References available at http://ebooks.health.elsevier.com/

Human factors and patient safety in surgery

9

Craig McIlhenny | Steven Yule

THE SCALE OF MEDICAL ERROR

As surgeons, we are arguably practitioners of one of the most entitled, rewarded and rewarding occupations in the world. We are empowered to the completely legal action of putting a knife to work in a human body. Unfortunately … our patients are frequently caught in the 'friendly fire' of surgical care – health care providers causing unintentional harm when their only intent was to help.[1]

The practice of healthcare in general, and surgery in particular, is a hazardous business. It was not until the 1990s, however, that the exact nature and scale of that hazard became apparent. In that decade, several high-profile cases of medical error were reported in the USA and in the UK, such as the enquiry into perioperative deaths from paediatric cardiac surgical care in Bristol Royal Infirmary,[2] which threw the adverse effects of medical intervention into stark relief.

This prompted further investigation into the possible scale of harm perpetrated by modern healthcare. The Harvard Medical Practice Study in 1991[3] demonstrated a major adverse incident rate in 3.7% of all patients treated. Studies conducted in Utah and Colorado,[4] Denmark,[5] New Zealand[6] and Canada[7] reported remarkably similar adverse events rates of between 8% and 12% in all patients admitted to acute hospitals, and this range is now generally accepted as being typical of healthcare systems in developed countries. Crucially, throughout these studies about half of all these adverse events are deemed to be preventable.

Not surprisingly, these publications brought about a sharp focus on patient safety, which has now become, quite rightly, a permanent part of healthcare policy. Numerous changes have since been advocated to improve patient safety, including the mandating of minimum nurse-to-patient ratios, reducing working hours of trainee doctors, introduction of 'care bundles', the use of safety checklists and advances in the science of simulation and teamwork training.

ADVERSE EVENTS IN SURGERY

The surgical domain can be seen as more complex and high risk in its delivery of care than other non-interventional specialities. It is therefore not surprising that in the majority of studies of adverse events in healthcare, at least 50% occurred within the surgical domain and the majority of these in the operating theatre. Furthermore, at least half of these adverse events were also deemed preventable.

Just as the multiple studies in the high-income countries have similar figures for adverse events in hospitalised patients across all specialities, there appears to be a similar rate of harm in surgery. A review of 14 studies, incorporating more than 16 000 surgical patients, quoted an adverse event occurring in 14.4% of surgical patients.[8] This was not simply minor harm; a full 3.6% of these adverse events were fatal, 10% severe and 34% moderately harmful.

Gawande, a surgeon, policy and healthcare leader in Boston, made one of the first attempts to clarify the source of these adverse events.[9] This paper pioneered the concept that the majority of adverse events were not due to lack of technical expertise or surgical skill on the part of the surgeon, finding instead that 'systems factors' were the main contributing factor in 86% of adverse events. The most common system factors quoted were related to the people involved and how they were functioning in their environment. Communication breakdown was a factor in 43% of incidents, individual cognitive factors (such as decision-making) were cited in 86%, with excessive workload, fatigue and the design or ergonomics of the environment also contributing. These findings were confirmed in the systematic review of surgical adverse events, where it was found that errors in what were described as 'non-operative management' were implicated in 8.3% of the study population versus only 2.5% contributed to by technical surgical error.[8]

In accordance with other high-risk industries, such as commercial aviation, the majority of these adverse events are therefore not caused by failures of technical skill on the part of the individual surgeon, but rather lie within the wider healthcare team, environment and system. Lapses and errors in communication, teamworking, leadership, situational awareness or decision-making all feature highly in post-hoc analysis of surgical adverse events. This knowledge of error causation has been prominent and acknowledged in most other high-risk industries for many years, but it is only recently that healthcare has appreciated this.

HUMAN FACTORS

Enhancing clinical performance through an understanding of the effects of teamwork, tasks, equipment, workspace, culture and organisation on human behaviour and abilities and application of that knowledge in clinical settings.

Ken Catchpole, https://chfg.org/.

Human factors encompass all the issues to do with humans working in a system—how we see, hear, think, behave and function physically as individuals and teams—which need to be considered to optimise performance and assure safety[10] (Fig. 9.1). The aim is to enhance performance by fitting the task to the human rather than vice versa, and maintaining wellbeing throughout careers. Human factors science extends to the design of tools, machines, systems, tasks and environments to ensure safe and effective human use. So a human factors perspective helps highlight why a piece of clinical equipment that has not taken human strengths and limitations into account in its design, or a work environment and shift pattern that is disruptive and stressful, is more likely to lead to less-than-optimal human performance and result in error and compromised patient safety. In surgery, these human factors issues range from the design of surgical instruments or operating theatres, to services and systems, as well as the working environment and working practices such as rotas, roles, team behaviours and so on.

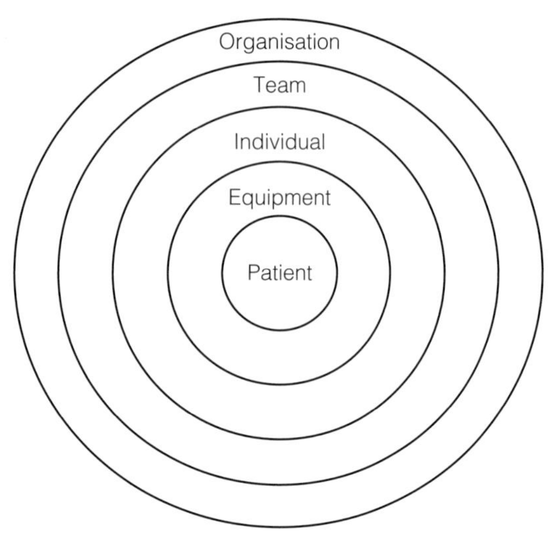

Figure 9.1 Human factors in a healthcare system.

Surgical adverse events are almost invariably preceded by multiple contributing factors, often combining unsafe systems and unsafe behaviours.[11] Unsafe systems (such as poorly managed operating lists) produce unsafe behaviours (such as disruption during swab counts). Equally, unsafe behaviours (such as disrespect towards junior staff) undermine safety processes (such as use of the World Health Organisation Safer Surgery checklist). Examples of poor systems and practices in the National Health Service include: widespread toleration of variation in standard procedures, such as surgical counts; operating lists with multiple changes in list order; failure to adhere to surgical site marking procedures; inadequate staffing; and absent or inadequate training, particularly in team working and human factors; all of which contribute to adverse events.

As evidenced from previous literature, it is apparent that the vast majority of adverse events and errors in surgery occur due to failures in these human factors domains, and can be traced back to poor work design rather than technical ineptitude on the part of the operating surgeon.

The Systems Engineering Initiative for Patient Safety (SEIPS) framework is one of the most widely used systems models for analysing the healthcare system and comprises three components: the work system, the care process and the patient outcome (Fig. 9.2). The 'work system' encompasses five interconnected elements: individual, tasks, tools and technologies, physical environment and organisational conditions. These five interacting elements in turn influence care and other connected processes which in turn have an impact on outcomes. Although we focus a lot on patient outcomes in this chapter, the SEIPS model also focuses on staff outcomes including safety, health, satisfaction, stress and burnout; plus organisational outcomes including rates of turnover, injuries and illnesses, and organisational health.

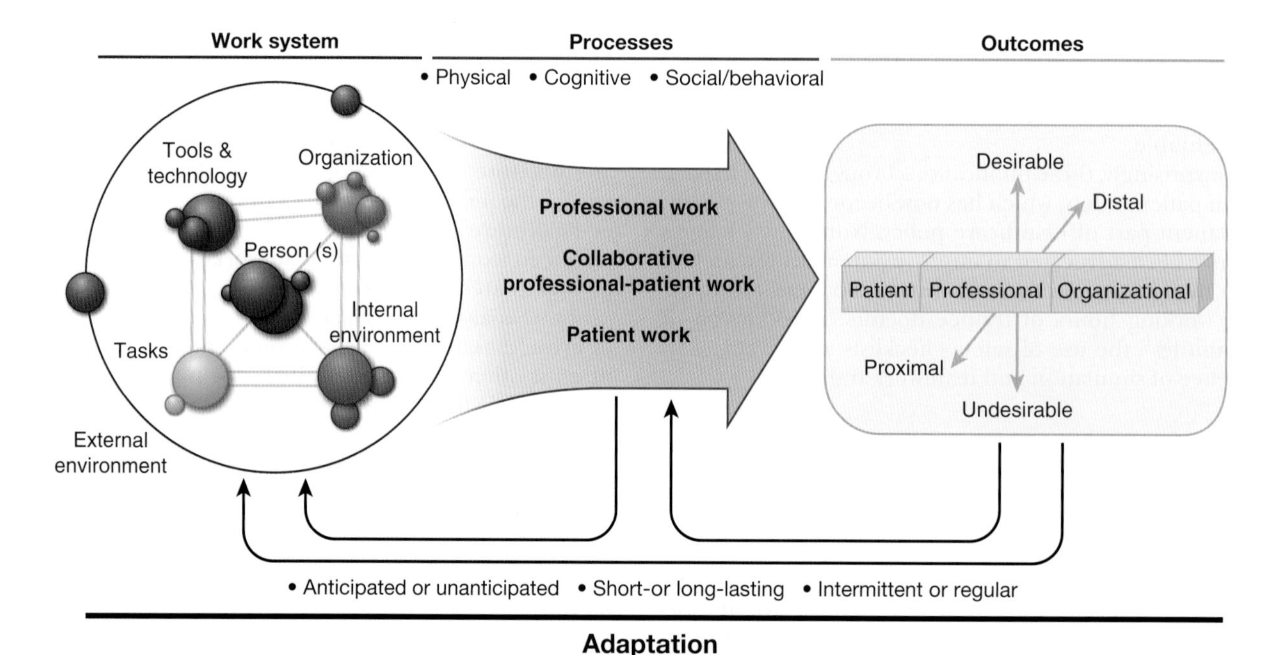

Figure 9.2 Human factors Systems Engineering Initiative for Patient Safety (SEIPS) model.

(i) Individual: The individual at the centre of the work system could be any healthcare provider or team performing patient care related tasks or a patient receiving care or their family and support system. System design must take into account personal characteristics (including age, competence, preferences, ability to manage health information and wellbeing) as well as collective-level characteristics such as team cohesiveness or consistency of knowledge.
(ii) Tools and technologies: These are the items required by the caregiver to do their work. They can range from paper and pencil to computers and include information technology, medical devices as well as physical equipment. These factors can be characteristics such as usability, accessibility, familiarity and automation.
(iii) Tasks: These are those specific actions required by the caregiver to treat the patient e.g. documenting results, talking with patients and team interactions. Task factors can also be attributes of the task such as complexity, variety and ambiguity.
(iv) Organisational factors: Organisation refers to the structures external to a person that organise time, space, resources and activity. Within hospitals, organisation factors can be characteristics of work schedules, management systems, organisational culture, training and resource availability.
(v) Environment: Internal environment refers to the physical environment in which staff work and includes characteristics of lighting, physical layout and protection from hazards.

Many of these human factors can exist in a latent form within our environment, but they affect those of us working in the operating theatre at the 'sharp end', as it is the surgical teams who are the final common pathway for harm to occur to that patient (Fig. 9.3).[12] While in other high-risk industries, considerable work has been done by human factors scientists to engineer out many of these latent threats that lurk in our work systems, in healthcare we are still at a very rudimentary stage in this journey. At present in healthcare, we still need to rely predominantly on humans to act as our final line of defence to prevent harm coming to our patients, and to optimise our surgical outcomes. While technical skills undoubtedly play a part in this, it is equally important that we are able to deploy good non-technical skills to minimise the risk of harm to our patients.

NON-TECHNICAL SKILLS IN SURGERY

Although there is undoubtedly a link between technical surgical skill and patient outcomes,[13] it is clear that the majority of error and unintended harm arises from poor non-technical skills on the part of the surgical team,[14] with loss of situation awareness (SA), poor decision-making, compounded by poor leadership, teamwork and suboptimal communication all implicated. Despite this, until recently there was no way of describing, categorising or rating these non-technical skills, and as a result they were not formally acknowledged, taught or assessed in surgeons.

A collaboration between the University of Aberdeen Industrial Psychology Research Centre and the Royal College of Surgeons of Edinburgh produced the Non-Technical Skills for Surgeons (NOTSS) taxonomy to describe and assess these non-technical skills in the intraoperative environment in the early 2000s.[15] This taxonomy was designed specifically for use in the operating room and is currently the most widely validated tool for rating and classifying surgical non-technical skills.[16]

The NOTSS classification (Table 9.1) describes two cognitive non-technical skill categories—those of situational awareness and decision-making—and two social non-technical skill categories—teamworking and communication, and leadership. Each of the four categories can be subdivided into further three elements that describe each category in detail. This taxonomy can be used to rate and improve the non-technical skills of surgeons in the intraoperative environment—and they will now be considered in turn.

SITUATION AWARENESS

SA can best be simply described as 'knowing what is going on around you'. To delve a little deeper, SA is the awareness of what is going on around you at any one time, the correct

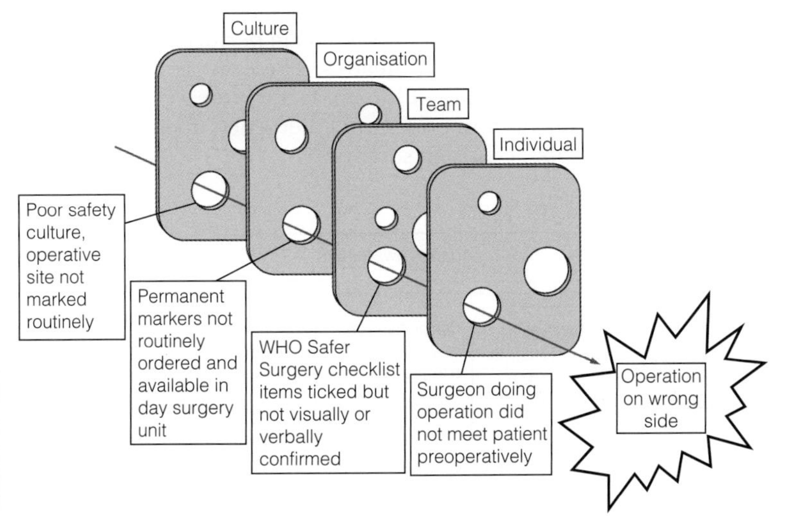

Figure 9.3 The Swiss cheese model applied to a case of wrong site surgery. The slices of cheese are defensive layers within the healthcare system, the holes are transient or permanent gaps in these defences. When the holes align, a significant adverse event occurs.

understanding of what is going on and a projection into the future of what that means is likely to happen next (Fig. 9.4). This three-level model of SA described by Mica Endsley has been well described in aviation and is often referred to as 'What?, So What? and Now What?'.[17]

The concept of knowing what is going on around you in the operating theatre may seem obvious, but as human beings we think that we notice far more of our environment than we actually do. At any one time, there is an overwhelming amount of information available to us, so in order for us to make sense of the world we become very selective in what we consciously attend to, otherwise we would be constantly overwhelmed by masses of competing information. What we focus our attention on depends on the environment (we are easily distracted from a task by loud noises for example), but it also depends on our past experiences—so our knowledge of how the world works will guide us in focusing our attention—for instance, looking out for moving cars when we cross a road.

We have a limited capacity for monitoring our current state, interpreting new incoming information and planning our future actions, and that capacity is easily overwhelmed. This is very powerfully demonstrated in a classic experiment,[18] in which observers were asked to watch a video of a basketball game and count the number of times the ball was passed between team members. In this experiment, 60% of observers were so engrossed in the task of counting the passes that they failed to notice an actor in a gorilla suit walking across their field of vision. This demonstrated eloquently and powerfully how selective our attention can be, and that concentrating on one task can overwhelm our perception of reality and our ability to process and understand information that was clearly available to our senses at the time. (Watch the video at https://www.youtube.com/watch?v=vJG698U2Mvo.)

Maintaining SA is crucial to patient safety and one does not have to look very far to find accidents where loss of SA was implicated. In aviation, loss of SA has been implicated in 88% of aviation accidents in which human performance was implicated.[19] Likewise, in surgery, good SA within the surgical team has been associated with improved operating times and fewer errors during surgery.[20]

Given the importance of SA and the implications of loss of SA and its connection to accidents and adverse outcomes, we should seek to minimise the risks of reduced or absent SA. A simple way to enhance the SA of the whole team is the use of a robust preoperative briefing. This means that everyone starts the day with the same understanding and expectations of the tasks and challenges ahead. A good briefing should ensure that the whole team has a correct mental model of the forthcoming task or operating list. In many other high-risk industries, a pre-task briefing is an accepted safety procedure, such as pilots briefing for an aborted take-off before every flight. In the now famous 'Miracle on the Hudson' US Airways Flight 1549, an Airbus A320 on a flight from New York City's LaGuardia Airport struck a flock of birds shortly after take-off, losing all engine power. Unable to reach any airport for an emergency landing, pilots Chesley Sullenberger and Jeffrey Skiles glided the plane to a ditching in the Hudson River off Manhattan. All 155 people on board were rescued by nearby boats, with few serious injuries and no fatalities. Capt. Sullenberger had studied psychology and human factors, and the pilots had both participated in regular simulation training with emergency checklists as 'cognitive aids' to guide team performance during high-acuity, low-frequency events like the bird strike.

Another method to maintain good SA in your operating theatre is to minimise the incidence of interruptions and distractions. Distractions are common in operating theatres, with pagers and phones going off and multiple conversations occurring between different team members at once. An observational study reported an average of 3.5 procedure-irrelevant conversations occurring per surgical case.[21] They also reported that as the number of interruptions in theatre increased, so did the number of team miscommunications, revealing a direct link between team performance and interruptions occurring in theatres. These surgical flow disruptions are a hallmark of human factors research in operative environments and evident in emergency, open, laparoscopic and robotic-assisted surgery.[22]

Table 9.1 Non-Technical Skills for Surgeons (NOTSS) skills taxonomy v1.2

Category	Elements
Situation awareness	Gathering information
	Projecting information
	Projecting and anticipating future state
Decision-making	Considering options
	Selecting and communicating option
	Implementing and reviewing decisions
Communication and teamwork	Exchanging information
	Establishing a shared understanding
	Coordinating team activities
Leadership	Setting and maintaining standards
	Supporting others
	Coping with pressure

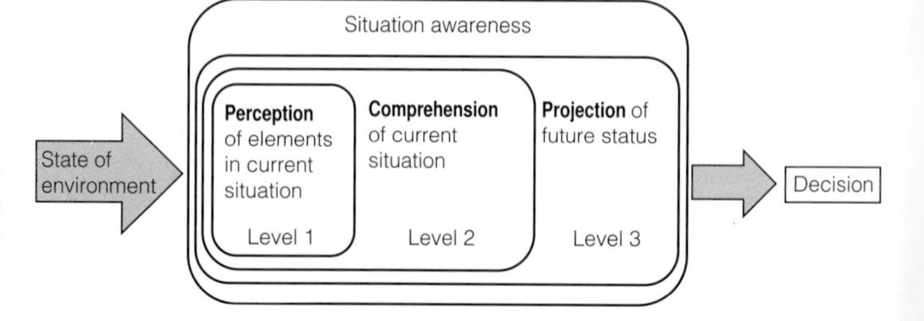

Figure 9.4 Three-level model of situation awareness. (Adapted from Mica R. Endsley (1995) Toward a Theory of Situation Awareness in Dynamic Systems. Human Factors: The Journal of the Human Factors and Ergonomics Society, Volume 37, Issue 1. Available from https://journals.sagepub.com/doi/10.1518/001872095779049543.)

Distractions are just as deadly to SA, and this includes not concentrating on the job at hand. A well-known aviation case involved a DC-9 in the USA. During the approach to the airport, the crew were so busy chatting about matters unrelated to the flight that they failed to notice they were too low, and the aircraft crashed with 74 fatalities. This led to the introduction of the 'sterile cockpit', where the crew are prohibited from performing non-essential duties or conversations during crucial phases of the flight such as take-off and landing. This sterile cockpit rule helps minimise distraction to the flight crew and helps them maintain their SA. There is good evidence from both objective[23] and subjective metrics that surgical team members' cognitive load rises and falls at different rates during the procedure, and there is no uniform high or low of team cognitive load.[24] We therefore need to be mindful of our team members attention capacity and cognitive load as it may differ from ours. In our own institutions, we have implemented a form of sterile cockpit into our operating theatre routine to try to mirror this effect. During these phases, music must be turned off, staff are forbidden to talk about anything not directly related to the current case, staff are not allowed to enter or leave the theatre unless on a task directly related to the case, etc. This sterile cockpit state occurs automatically at certain phases of the surgery such as the surgical pause and the postoperative sign out, and during any instrument counts. In addition, any member of the team can call for sterile cockpit during crucial phases of the case—if the anaesthetist is having airway difficulties for instance, or if the surgeon is approaching a technically challenging part of the case. Of course, as well as sterile cockpit drill, it is important to take simple steps to minimise other interruptions and distractions such as not having bleeps or mobile phones in theatre.

To help maintain both individual surgeon's and the surgical team's SA, it is important to regularly update your mental model and that of the team. Regularly check your current mental model with real-world cues and also with your team's mental model to make sure that they match. And remember that if they do not match, it may not be your mental model that is correct! In this regard it is also important that your team feels empowered to speak up if they see unsafe behaviour, or if their mental model of what is happening does not seem to coincide with either what is going on or what should be going on. Set the tone for this hierarchical challenge culture at your preoperative brief.

Maintaining good time management is also crucial to maintaining good SA. Rushing to get through a procedure, or complete a task, is not conducive to good SA. In a study of aviation accidents, the pilots were found to be behind schedule in 55% of them, and were hurrying to get their flight onto the ground on time. This added time pressure serves as a distraction and also utilises precious cognitive capacity; it is a sure recipe for decreased SA and poor decision-making.

DECISION-MAKING

Decision-making is intrinsically linked to SA—without the correct mental picture of the situation, it is very difficult to make a good decision. As humans, we have two main pathways by which we can make decisions—automatic or analytical.[25] The traditional method of decision-making involves critically assessing the situation, then formulating a series of possible options to take, and then carefully weighing up the pros and cons of each before committing to carrying out one of these options. This analytical method of making decisions has long been taught and studied as the classic method of decision-making, and it involves considerable expenditure of mental effort.

Experienced surgeons, on the other hand, spend most of their time using recognition-primed decision-making, which is an almost unconscious, automatic method of decision-making. This relies on 'fast and frugal' pattern matching to recognise familiar situations and apply actions that have been used successfully in previous similar situations. This system of thinking is, however, entirely dependent on previous experience, so is very accurate in experts but highly prone to error in novices. An example of this would be to think about your drive into work—you made thousands of decisions during this drive, but were probably not aware of any of them as you perform this task now on 'automatic pilot' as you are so familiar with it. If you asked a novice to drive you, the result would be very different and you would see them resort to slow effortful analytical decision-making mode—having to consciously think about every junction and road sign along the way.

In crisis situations, or if we stray into unfamiliar surgical territory, we too will resort to a more analytical mode of decision-making because we may not have a pattern to match to. While this still enables us to make decisions, it takes much more conscious, cognitive 'thinking power' to do this, and it is a much slower method of decision-making, so we will see ourselves slowing down. We must also be conscious in these situations to try to preserve enough space in our working memory to enable us to make these analytical decisions. If this cognitive capacity is exceeded, then there can be a spiralling deterioration in performance. In these situations, stress can act to reduce cognitive capacity, leading to loss of SA, with associated deterioration in decision-making and motor skills that in turn causes more stress. Effective utilisation of leadership and teamwork can help in re-distributing tasks and their associated cognitive load to other team members, thus protecting high performance for successful completion of the surgical task. Effective use of non-technical skills is thus directly related to technical performance of the surgical task.

It is also vital to the rest of the surgical team that they are kept 'up to speed' with the decision-making processes, and the reasoning behind them. Effective teamworking depends on all of the members of the surgical team having the same accurate SA, or mental model. This is especially important when recognition-primed decision-making is being used, as it can look to the team as if you have just plucked a course of action out of nowhere, so it is vital that the course of action, and its reasoning, are verbalised to the rest of the team so that they can update their mental models and make them congruent with your own. Likewise, it is vital for you to review your decision and its consequences—vocalizing 'have we made this situation better or worse?' 'Do we need to implement another course of action?' can be helpful in reviewing decisions and inviting team buy-in and participation.

TEAMWORK AND COMMUNICATION

The practice of surgery is not the premise of an individual, but can only be delivered by an operating theatre team. Teams can only function effectively through good communication—and it is no coincidence that teamwork and communication have been singled out[26] as the 'main contributors to error'.

As surgeons, we tend to think we are better at teamworking than we are—one study found that surgeons thought they are very good at teamworking about 85% of the time, whereas only 48% of the nursing staff agreed.[27] It is now well known that teamworking has a real and demonstrable effect on surgical outcomes, with directly observed poor teamworking behaviours in the operating room having worse outcomes for patients than good teamworking, to the extent that teamworking ability was a more powerful predictor of patient outcome than the American Society of Anesthesiologists status of the patient.[28] In addition, surgical team training has been shown to significantly improve both morbidity and mortality compared with no training.[29] This has been further emphasised in a randomised trial involving over 182 000 operations and 74 hospitals, which demonstrated an 18% reduction in surgical mortality in an intervention group compared with 7% reduction in a control group after initiation of a team training programme.[30]

Teamwork and communication in the NOTSS taxonomy are subdivided into the three practical elements—exchanging information, establishing a shared understanding and coordinating team activities.

The first element emphasises the vital importance of communication within the team. The surgeon should ensure that the entire team feel safe to freely share information. After almost all adverse events, someone will say that they thought that something was going to happen but they either 'could not put their finger' on why things did not feel right, or that they did not feel empowered to speak up. It is therefore essential that the lead surgeon encourages free flow of information amongst team members, best brought about by consciously trying to 'flatten' the hierarchy between team members. The preoperative briefing is a useful opportunity to set this tone and explicitly encourage team members to speak up if they see something concerning. Use of first names, encouraging contribution of team members who may see themselves as lower on the hierarchy, and constant and predictable behaviour are important tools all surgeons can utilise.

Information sharing is a skill, and used to ensure that all team members have a shared understanding of the current situation. SA is key to patient safety, and building shared SA among team members is one of the hallmarks of a high-performing surgical team. Again, the preoperative briefing is the first step to establishing this shared understanding, and continuous progress updates from all team members during the course of the procedure ensure that the team hold a shared mental model at all times.

The lead surgeon should also be instrumental in explicitly coordinating team activities, by assessing team members' abilities and then clearly assigning tasks to team members. In the dynamic situation of an operation it may be necessary to re-assign tasks, and to share workload so that any individual team member does not become cognitively overloaded. This explicit assigned role clarity is often taken as read, but clearly defined roles and monitoring of team members' workload is again a mark of excellence in teamwork. Such re-assignment of tasks can of course be coordinated by any member of the team, such as the floor nurse and anaesthetist, especially in times of stress when the surgeons are deeply occupied.

LEADERSHIP

In the NOTSS taxonomy, the leadership category involves the surgeon leading the operating team and providing a clear direction and goal. It involves demonstrating the highest standards of clinical practice and care, being considerate and supportive of the other members of the operative team, and being able, and seen to be able, to cope with pressure and stressful situations.

Setting and maintaining standards is vital, and being a role model for the rest of the surgical team is crucial. Demonstrating a positive leadership style through modelling positive behaviours has been shown to have a major impact on how patient safety initiatives are viewed and accepted amongst the other members of the medical or surgical team. The surgeon who demonstrates positive attitudes towards protocols and models attention to best surgical practice will be rewarded with a more positive attitude towards safety within the whole team.

The time when modelling good behaviour and being a role model is perhaps most important is during the preoperative briefing. The lead surgeon can set the tone for the entire day with this briefing; simply introducing the briefing with the phrase 'Welcome to today's safety briefing' focuses the entire team onto a safety-oriented footing. Also one can use the introduction to set the tone for the team regarding hierarchy, and encouraging other team members to speak out if they see or think they see unsafe or potentially unsafe events or behaviours.

In addition to setting and maintaining standards within the operating team, it is a vital aspect of leadership that the lead surgeon supports others within the team. Effective leadership means not just focusing on completing the task; truly effective leadership means that the leader must also demonstrate behaviours to improve and enhance team functioning and performance.

The third element in the leadership category is 'coping with pressure'. Demonstration of an outwardly calm demeanour when under increased stress is essential in emphasising to the rest of the team that you have this high-pressure situation under control. This can also mean adopting a forceful manner if such is appropriate in urgent or emergency situations, but without undermining the role of the other team members. This last part is vital as the surgeon who remains completely laid back and laconic even during an emergency situation and who does not convey the urgency or seriousness of the situation is not demonstrating a positive behaviour in this situation.

CONCLUSION

Our next challenge in improving surgical practice is how to make it safer for our patients who are subject to preventable adverse events. The majority of these unintended outcomes are not due to a lack of technical surgical skill, but are down to poor systems, inadequate human factors design and lack of non-technical skills within the surgical team. The SEIPS model allows us to understand the multiple contributory causes of healthcare performance and can be used to examine surgical patient safety from a systems perspective. The NOTSS taxonomy allows us all to classify, rate and improve non-technical skills, both in ourselves and others. An appreciation for the dual benefit of human factors science and non-technical skills can support all surgeons to optimise their performance and make surgery safer for our patients.

Key points

- The incidence of adverse events in surgical patients worldwide is around 10%.
- Human factors play a major role in adverse events.
- Better non-technical skills and team training reduce surgical errors and improve outcomes.

References available at http://ebooks.health.elsevier.com/

SELECTIVE ATTENTION TEST

Recommended video:

- The original awareness test from Daniel Simons and Christopher Chabris – goo.gl/TO804q

KEY REFERENCES

[3] Brennan TA, Leape LL, Laird NM, et al. Incidence of adverse events and negligence in hospitalized patients. Results of the Harvard Medical Practice Study I. N Engl J Med 1991;324(6):370–6. PMID: 1987460

This large review of over 30 000 case records was one of the first studies into iatrogenic harm and reported an adverse event rate of 3.9% in hospitalised patients in the USA. It concluded that many of these adverse events were 'the result of substandard care'.

[4] Gawande AA, Thomas EJ, Zinner MJ, et al. The incidence and nature of surgical adverse events in Colorado and utah in 1992. Surgery 1999;126(1):66–75. PMID: 10418594

This retrospective case review was the first study to specifically look at the incidence of adverse events in surgery. It concluded that of all hospital-related adverse events, 66% occurred within the surgical domain, and crucially, that at least 50% of these were preventable.

[8] Anderson O, Davis R, Hanna GB, et al. Surgical adverse events: a systematic review. AJS 2013;206(2):253–62. PMID: 23642651

This systematic review incorporated over 16 000 surgical patients and found an overall adverse event rate of 14.4%, with preventable adverse events occurring in 5.2%. The review also concluded that errors in 'non-operative management' caused more frequent adverse events than errors in surgical technique.

[9] Gawande AA, Zinner MJ, Studdert DM, et al. Analysis of errors reported by surgeons at three teaching hospitals. Surgery 2003;133(6):614–21. PMID: 12796727

This study was the first to attempt to classify the cause of surgical adverse events by interviewing surgeons about past adverse outcomes. It highlighted that the majority of surgical adverse events occur during the intraoperative phase of care and that most were due to 'system errors' such as poor leadership or communication rather than errors in surgical technique.

[13] Birkmeyer JD, Finks JF, O'Reilly A, et al. Surgical skill and complication rates after bariatric surgery. N Engl J Med 2013;369(15):1434–42. PMID: 24106936

In this study, surgical skill was assessed by blinded review of surgeons' videos of laparoscopic bariatric surgery. Technical skill as measured using OSATS correlated directly with outcomes.

[14] Yule S, Flin R, Paterson-Brown S, et al. Non-technical skills for surgeons in the operating room: a review of the literature. Surgery 2006;139(2):140–9. PMID: 16455321

This paper reviewed the literature on non-technical skills in surgery and was the first to identify 'core categories' of non-technical skills in surgery, namely communication, teamwork, leadership and decision-making.

[15] Yule SS, Flin RR, Paterson-Brown SS, et al. Development of a rating system for surgeons' non-technical skills. Med Educ 2006;40(11):1098–104. PMID: 17054619

This paper analyses the identification of crucial non-technical skills for surgeons through a combination of critical incident analysis, direct observation and interviews. It details how these data were then used to develop the NOTSS skills taxonomy and behavioural ratings system to structure observation and feedback in surgical training.

[28] Mazzocco K, Petitti DB, Fong KT, et al. Surgical team behaviors and patient outcomes. AJS 2009;197(5):678–85. PMID: 18789425

Direct observation of surgical teams was used in this study to ascertain a behaviour marker score that reflected how good surgical teams were at teamworking. Teams with good teamworking had better patient outcomes than those with poor teamworking. The quality of surgical teamworking was a more powerful predictor of patient outcome than the patient's ASA score.

[29] Armour Forse R, Bramble JD, McQuillan R. Team training can improve operating room performance. Surgery 2011;150(4):771–8. PMID: 22000190

This cohort study demonstrated that a surgical team training programme improved the teamworking in surgical teams, and led to a decrease in both morbidity and mortality for surgical patients.

[30] Neily J, Mills PD, Young-Xu Y, et al. Association between implementation of a medical team training program and surgical mortality. JAMA 2010;304(15):1693–700. PMID: 20959579

This randomised trial involving over 182 000 procedures demonstrated an 18% reduction in annual surgical mortality in institutions where a team training programme was implemented for their surgical teams.

10 Principles of organ donation and transplantation

Diana A. Wu | Gabriel C. Oniscu

INTRODUCTION

Organ transplantation has revolutionised the treatment of end-stage organ failure and is arguably one of the greatest medical advances of the last century. Practice in organ donation and transplantation continues to evolve as a result of remarkable innovations in surgical technique, immunosuppression and organ perfusion and preservation. This has led to excellent post-transplantation survival rates (Table 10.1) that have improved year on year.

This chapter summarises the principles of organ donation and abdominal organ transplantation.

PRINCIPLES OF ORGAN DONATION

Organs for transplantation may be donated from deceased donors or living donors. Worldwide, the number of donors falls drastically short of the number of patients in need of a transplant, and this is perhaps the greatest challenge currently faced by the transplant community.

ETHICAL AND LEGAL ASPECTS OF ORGAN DONATION

Consent is the cornerstone of organ donation. The process of consent for organ donation varies according to medical, ethical, societal and legal factors in each country. For deceased organ donation, the legislative framework for consent may be an opt-out system (consent for organ donation is presumed unless the person has specifically registered to opt out) or an opt-in system (explicit consent for organ donation is required). Both systems can be implemented on either a hard basis, where primacy is given to the donor's wishes, or a soft basis, where family members' views are considered (Table 10.2).[1] In recent years, there has been a trend towards conversion to opt-out systems in an effort to improve donation rates. For example, in the UK, soft opt-out systems were introduced in Wales in December 2015,[2] in England in May 2020[3] and in Scotland in March 2021.[4] Under this legislation, all adults who have not opted out, possess the mental capacity to understand the law and have lived in the country for more than 12 months before their death will be deemed to have authorised donation of their organs for transplantation. The legislation is applied softly; thus, if there is objection from family members, organ donation does not proceed. At the time of writing, Northern Ireland still operates under a soft opt-in system but has recently held a consultation on introduction of a soft opt-out system. The benefits of an opt-out approach are hotly debated and evidence is limited. Some studies have shown an association between opt-out systems and higher rates of deceased donation,[1,5,6] while others have shown no significant difference in deceased donation rates between opt-in and opt-out systems[7] but have demonstrated that the latter is in fact associated with lower rates of living organ donation.[8] Introduction of an opt-out system is unlikely to provide the sole solution to increasing deceased organ donation rates as other factors such as intensive care capacity, the infrastructure of the transplantation service, healthcare investment as well as public attitudes and awareness play a role.[9]

Living organ donation generates unique ethical concerns. Subjecting healthy individuals to a major surgical procedure with an inherent risk of harm but no physical benefit challenges the ethical principle of nonmaleficence. However, autonomy and beneficence must also be considered; an individual has the right to make an informed decision about becoming a living donor, they may gain significant psychological benefit from the act and could potentially suffer psychological harm if donation does not take place. Valid consent is the fundamental principle underpinning legislation for living donation. It is crucial to ensure that consent for living donation is given voluntarily, without coercion, without any form of reward and from a person who has full capacity to make informed decisions. In the UK, consent for living donation is an extensive process involving an independent regulator, the Human Tissue Authority (HTA), which assesses each individual living donor and recipient to ensure that valid consent has been given.[10]

The global shortage of organ donors has led to the emergence of unethical practices in transplantation. Organ trafficking, transplant commercialism and transplant tourism (Box 10.1) exploit vulnerable and impoverished people through the illicit removal and sale of their organs. These practices are prohibited by the World Health Organisation (WHO) Guiding Principles on Human Cell, Tissue and Organ Transplantation[11] and the Declaration of Istanbul,[12,13] which provide international ethical standards for organ transplantation.

✔ Organ trafficking, transplant commercialism and transplant tourism are unethical practices that should be prohibited and criminalised, as they exploit vulnerable people, impede equitable access to organ transplantation and prevent countries from achieving self-sufficiency in organ transplantation.[12,13]

Table 10.1 National 1-year and 5-year adult patient survival rates for abdominal organ transplantation in the UK

	1-year patient survival (%)*	5-year patient survival (%)**
Kidney		
Living donor	99	94
Deceased donor	97	88
Pancreas	100	88
Simultaneous Pancreas-Kidney	98	91
Liver		
Elective	95	84
Super-urgent	90	83

Includes transplants performed between 1 April 2017 - 31 March 2021
**Includes transplants performed between 1 April 2013 - 31 March 2017*
Source: NHS Blood and Transplant. Annual Report on Kidney Transplantation 2021/22, Pancreas and Islet Transplantation 2021/22 and Liver Transplantation 2021/22.

Table 10.2 Consent systems for deceased organ donation

	Opt-out	Opt-in
Hard	Consent for deceased organ donation is presumed, unless a person has registered to opt out. If a person has not registered to opt out, organ donation can proceed even if family members object	Consent for deceased organ donation is based on whether a person has registered to opt in. If a person has registered to opt in, organ donation can proceed even if family members object
Soft	Consent for deceased organ donation is presumed, unless a person has registered to opt out. If a person has not registered to opt out, organ donation does not proceed if family members object	Consent for deceased organ donation is based on whether a person has registered to opt in. If a person has registered to opt in, organ donation does not proceed if family members object

Box 10.1 Definitions of unethical practices in organ transplantation as set out by the declaration of Istanbul

Organ trafficking is the recruitment, transport, transfer, harbouring or receipt of living or deceased persons or their organs by means of threat or use of force or other forms of coercion, of abduction, of fraud, of deception, of the abuse of power or of a position of vulnerability, or of the giving to, or the receiving by, a third party of payments or benefits to achieve the transfer of control over the potential donor, for the purpose of exploitation by the removal of organs for transplantation.

Transplant commercialism is a policy or practice in which an organ is treated as a commodity, including by being bought or sold or used for material gain.

Travel for transplantation is the movement of organs, donors, recipients or transplant professionals across jurisdictional borders for transplantation purposes. Travel for transplantation becomes **transplant tourism** if it involves organ trafficking and/or transplant commercialism or if the resources (organs, professionals and transplant centres) devoted to providing transplants to patients from outside a country undermine the country's ability to provide transplant services for its own population.

Source: Reprinted from The Lancet, Vol. 372, Steering Committee of the Istanbul Summit, Organ trafficking and transplant tourism and commercialism: the Declaration of Istanbul, (9632):pages 5-6, Copyright (2008) with permission from Elsevier.

DECEASED ORGAN DONATION

Deceased organ donors may be donors after brain death (DBD) or donors after circulatory death (DCD). Internationally, the majority of organs transplanted from deceased donors are recovered from DBD donors, only a limited number of countries have developed DCD programmes.

DONOR IDENTIFICATION AND REFERRAL

The identification and referral of potential deceased organ donors is a fundamental step in the deceased donation process and should be seen as a routine part of end-of-life care. Failure of this step is one of the main reasons for significant differences in deceased donation rates between countries.[14] All clinicians have a responsibility to recognise if a patient under their care becomes a potential organ donor, and to initiate discussions with specialist nurses in organ donation (SNODs) (previously known as transplant coordinators) as early as possible. The General Medical Council (GMC) has published guidance on the duties of doctors with respect to end-of-life care and organ donation (Box 10.2).[15]

Clinical triggers can aid the identification of potential organ donors. UK National Institute for Health and Care Excellence (NICE) guidelines[16] recommend referral to the SNOD if either of the following criteria are met:

1. A patient with catastrophic brain injury **with**
   - the absence of one or more cranial nerve reflexes **and**
   - a Glasgow Coma Scale (GCS) score of 4 or less that is not explained by sedation **and/or**
   - a decision is made to perform brain stem death tests.

Box 10.2 General Medical Council (GMC) guidance regarding end-of-life care and organ donation

81. If a patient is close to death and their views cannot be determined, you should be prepared to explore with those close to them whether they had expressed any views about organ or tissue donation, if donation is likely to be a possibility.
82. You should follow any national procedures for identifying potential organ donors and, in appropriate cases, for notifying the local transplant coordinator. You must take account of the requirements in relevant legislation and in any supporting codes of practice, in any discussions that you have with the patient or those close to them. You should make clear that any decision about whether the patient would be a suitable candidate for donation would be made by the transplant coordinator or team, and not by you and the team providing treatment.

Source: General Medical Council, Treatment and care towards the end of life: good practice in decision making © 2010 General Medical Council. Available from: http://www.gmc-uk.org/static/documents/content/Treatment_and_care_towards_the_end_of_life_English_1015.pdf.

2. A patient with a life-threatening or life-limiting condition **where**
   - a decision has been made to withdraw life-sustaining treatment **and**
   - this is expected to result in circulatory death.

In order for deceased donation to be successfully realised into a transplant, a sequence of complex steps must be achieved including donor referral, confirmation of brain death (if DBD), assessment of donor suitability, valid consent, tissue typing/screening, coordination of resources for organ retrieval (e.g. operating rooms, anaesthesia, theatre staff etc), allocation of organs and transportation of organs to the accepting centres. It is increasingly recognised that specialised health professionals play an important role in the organ donation and transplantation pathway. In the UK, SNODs facilitate the entire donation process and are trained in communication, family support and end-of-life discussions. When a SNOD is involved in approaching families of eligible donors about deceased donation, the consent rate is significantly higher than when a SNOD is not involved (71% vs 29%, respectively).[17–19] Similar findings have been reported in other countries.[20–22]

✔ When trained specialist organ donation professionals are involved in deceased organ donation discussions, the consent rate is significantly higher.[19,20]

DONATION AFTER BRAIN DEATH

Donation after brain death requires determination of death by neurological criteria. The concept of brain death was first proposed by Harvard Medical School in 1967.[23] Advances in intensive care techniques meant that comatose patients could be maintained on mechanical ventilation, despite loss of brainstem function and therefore loss of the capacity for spontaneous respiration and consciousness. Consequently, it was proposed that such cases of irreversible coma due to permanent damage to the brain could be defined as death. Subsequently, the concept of brain death was gradually accepted more widely. In the UK, a statement by the Conference of Medical Royal Colleges and their Faculties in 1979 concluded for the first time that brain death equated to the death of the whole person.[24,25] The current criteria for the diagnosis of brainstem death in the UK are shown in Table 10.3.[26]

Table 10.3 Criteria for diagnosis of brainstem death in the UK

Preconditions
Patient is deeply comatose, unresponsive and apnoeic with his/her lungs being artificially ventilated
Patient's condition is due to irreversible brain damage of known aetiology
Exclusions
There should be no evidence that this state is due to:
Depressant drugs
Neuromuscular blocking drugs
Hypothermia*
Circulatory, metabolic or endocrine disturbance
Clinical examination
Absence of brainstem reflexes:
Pupils are fixed and do not respond to sharp changes in the intensity of incident light
No corneal reflex
No oculo-vestibular reflex**
No motor responses within the cranial nerve distribution by adequate stimulation of any somatic area
No cough reflex response to bronchial stimulation by a suction catheter placed down the trachea to the carina
No gag reflex to stimulation of the posterior pharynx with a spatula
Apnoea despite an induced moderate hypercarbia and mild acidaemia***

*Core temperature should be > 34°C at the time of testing.
**Caloric test: no eye movements are seen during or following the slow injection of at least 50 mL of ice-cold water over 1 minute into each external auditory meatus in turn. Clear access to the tympanic membrane must be established by direct inspection and the head should be at 30° to the horizontal plane, unless this positioning is contraindicated by the presence of an unstable spinal injury.
***The apnoea test should be the last brainstem reflex to be tested and should not be performed if any of the preceding tests confirm the presence of brainstem reflexes. A controlled rise in arterial $PaCO_2$ (> 6.0 KPa or > 6.5 KPa in the context of chronic CO_2 retention or intravenous bicarbonate) with corresponding acidaemia (pH < 7.40) should be induced whilst maintaining a normal PaO_2 and blood pressure. The patient should be disconnected from the ventilator for 5 minutes to confirm no spontaneous respiratory response. A further confirmatory arterial blood gas sample should be obtained to ensure that the $PaCO_2$ has increased from the starting level by more than 0.5 KPa.
Source: Academy of Medical Royal Colleges. A code of practice for the diagnosis and confirmation of death. 2008. http://aomrc.org.uk/wp-content/uploads/2016/04/Code_Practice_Confirmation_Diagnosis_Death_1008-4.pdf. Reproduced with permission.

The UK code of practice for the diagnosis of death provides clear criteria for confirming brainstem death and circulatory death.[26]

Brainstem death testing must be carried out by two doctors (at least one of which should be a consultant) who have been registered for more than 5 years and are competent in the procedure. Neither doctor should be a member of the transplant team. Testing should be undertaken by the doctors together and on two separate occasions. Death will be confirmed after the second set of tests, but the legal time of death is after completion of the first set of tests. The diagnosis of brainstem death can generally be confirmed by clinical criteria alone, but on rare occasions where there is uncertainty over the completion or interpretation of clinical examination (e.g. extensive facio-maxillary injuries, high cervical cord injury), ancillary tests may be required (e.g. cerebral angiography, electroencephalogram, evoked potentials). There are considerable international differences in the definition of brain death. For instance, in the USA, irreversible loss of all brain function (including the brainstem) must be confirmed, while in the UK confirmation of irreversible cessation of brainstem function is adequate (based upon the fact that the capacity for consciousness and cardiorespiratory function reside in the brainstem).[27] There is also wide variation in the diagnostic criteria for brain death, including whether apnoea testing is required and the way in which it is conducted, the number and seniority of clinicians required for brain death testing and whether ancillary tests are mandatory.[28,29] Furthermore, in some countries brain death is not legally or culturally accepted as the death of an individual under any circumstances.[27]

Brainstem death may result from intracranial causes such as trauma or haemorrhage, or from extracranial causes such as cardiorespiratory arrest leading to impaired cerebral perfusion. Brainstem death triggers complex physiological changes that jeopardise organ function and ultimately lead to cardiac arrest. Effective management of DBD donors involves active care from the time of brainstem death to the point of organ retrieval in order to prevent organ damage and maximise the number of transplantable organs.[30] Around the time of brainstem death there is a rise in intracranial pressure, which limits cerebral perfusion and oxygen delivery. Cushing's reflex describes the compensatory hypertension that ensues as an attempt to restore cerebral perfusion, which stimulates arterial baroreceptors and causes reflex bradycardia. Subsequently, there is a period of intense sympathetic activity (the catecholamine storm), followed by an agonal phase of hypotension with reduced vasomotor tone, impaired cardiac output, neurogenic pulmonary oedema and a systemic inflammatory response.[31] Loss of central regulation results in haemodynamic instability, hypothermia and diabetes insipidus. Without adequate therapy, rapid deterioration and cardiac arrest follow. Optimal donor management is aimed at detecting and correcting the cardiovascular, respiratory and metabolic derangement of brainstem death. Therapy should be based on specific physiological targets (Box 10.3), and typically involves correction of hypovolaemia, vasoconstriction, lung protective ventilation and the administration of hormonal therapy including methylprednisolone, vasopressin and insulin.[32]

Box 10.3 Physiological targets in the management of brainstem death donors

- Pa_{O_2} ≥ 10.0 kPa (Fi_{O_2} < 0.4 as able)
- Pa_{CO_2} 5–6.5 kPa (or higher as long as pH > 7.25)
- MAP 60–80 mmHg
- CVP 4–10 mmHg (secondary goal)
- Cardiac index > 2.1 L/min/m^2
- Sc_{VO_2} > 60 %
- SVRI (secondary goal) 1800–2400 dyn*s/cm^5/m^2
- Temperature 36–37.5°C
- Blood glucose 4.0–10.0 mmol/L
- Urine output 0.5–2.0 mL/kg/h

Source: NHS Blood and Transplant. UK National Organ Donation Commitee. DBD donor optimisation extended care bundle. 2012. https://nhsbtdbe.blob.core.windows.net/umbraco-assets-corp/4522/donor-optimisation-extended-care-bundle.pdf.

Active donor management is continued whilst the donor is transferred to the operating theatre for the multiorgan retrieval procedure and up until the point that the aorta is cannulated and organs are perfused *in situ* with cold preservation fluid.

DONATION AFTER CIRCULATORY DEATH

Donation after circulatory death occurs after the irreversible cessation of cardiorespiratory function. The clinical scenario in which cardiorespiratory arrest occurs can be classified into four different categories known as the Maastricht Classification, which were first described in 1995[33] and subsequently updated in 2013 [34] (Table 10.4). These categories can be described as either 'controlled' or 'uncontrolled', referring to whether cardiac arrest was planned and expected or sudden and unexpected, respectively. In most countries, the majority of DCD donations are 'controlled' Maastricht category III. This is usually in the context of a critically ill patient who does not fulfil the criteria for brainstem death, but where life-sustaining cardiorespiratory support is no longer considered to be in the patient's best interests, and is withdrawn under controlled circumstances. 'Uncontrolled' donation is the predominant type of DCD donation in a limited number of countries (e.g. Spain, France).[35]

The Maastricht classification is the universally accepted method for describing the four categories of donors after circulatory death.[34]

After confirmation of circulatory death, there is a mandatory 'no touch' observation period before organ retrieval can commence. In most countries (including the UK), this period is 5 minutes, but it varies from 2 minutes in Australia to 30 minutes in Russia.[36,37]

Despite a substantial increase in DCD donation in recent years, its practice is not universally accepted. In some countries such as the Netherlands and the UK, DCD donation now accounts for around 40–60% of all deceased donors.[38] However, in most countries DCD donation remains uncommon, and in several countries it is prohibited by the law (e.g. Germany, Greece, Estonia).[36]

Table 10.4 Modified Maastricht classification of donation after circulatory death

Type	Category	Circumstances	Scenario
Uncontrolled	I	Found dead Ia. Out of hospital Ib. In hospital	Sudden unexpected cardiac arrest, with no attempt at resuscitation by a medical team
Uncontrolled	II	Witnessed cardiac arrest IIa. Out of hospital IIb. In hospital	Sudden unexpected cardiac arrest, with unsuccessful attempt at resuscitation by a medical team
Controlled	III	Withdrawal of life-sustaining therapy	Planned expected cardiac arrest, following the withdrawal of life-sustaining therapy
Uncontrolled or Controlled	IV	Cardiac arrest while brain dead	Sudden unexpected or planned expected cardiac arrest after brain death diagnosis, but before organ recovery

Reproduced from Thuong M, Ruiz A, Evrard P, et al. New classification of donation after circulatory death donors definitions and terminology. Transpl Int 2016;29(7):749-59 with permission from John Wiley & Sons, Inc.

A major concern over the use of DCD organs is the exposure to longer periods of warm ischaemia, leading to potentially inferior graft outcomes. Warm ischaemia is of particular concern because at normothermic temperatures full metabolic processes continue, thus inducing more rapid ischaemic damage than under hypothermic conditions when metabolism is slowed. Following withdrawal of life-sustaining treatment in a DCD donor, cardiovascular instability causes organ hypoperfusion. Functional warm ischaemia starts when there is a sustained (at least 2 minutes) fall of systolic blood pressure below 50 mmHg and continues throughout the subsequent period of circulatory arrest until *in situ* cold perfusion is instituted.[39] The definition of functional warm ischemia is not universally agreed and therefore other indicators such as withdrawal time (e.g. time from withdrawal of therapy to circulatory arrest) or true warm ischaemia time (e.g. time from circulatory arrest to *in situ* perfusion) are used in the literature. Once death is verified and the mandatory 'no touch' period is completed, the donor is transferred to the operating theatre and undergoes rapid laparotomy for organ retrieval. It is only when cold perfusion is achieved and the organs are cooled that warm ischaemia is halted and the period of cold ischaemia begins. The same metabolic processes that lead to cell death continue during cold ischaemia but at a much slower rate, and so cells and organs are able to survive for longer periods. Guidelines for maximum functional warm ischaemia times for specific organs are shown in Table 10.5.[40]

DCD organs are associated with a higher risk of post-transplantation complications such as delayed graft function in kidney grafts,[41,42] graft thrombosis in pancreas grafts[43] and biliary complications including ischaemic cholangiopathy in liver grafts.[44–46] Despite this, patient and graft survival rates are comparable between DCD and DBD grafts for kidney,[47] lung[48–50] and pancreas transplantation.[51,52] For liver transplantation, the evidence is less clear, with early reports demonstrating inferior graft and patient survival from DCD compared with DBD livers,[44,45] but more contemporary meta-analysis suggesting this may no longer be the case.[46]

✓✓ DCD liver transplantation is associated with a higher risk of biliary complications including ischaemic cholangiopathy.[45]

Table 10.5 Recommended maximum functional warm ischaemia times for donation after circulatory death

Organ	Stand-down time from the onset of functional warm ischaemia
Liver	30 minutes
Pancreas	30 minutes
Lungs	60 minutes
Kidney	180 minutes

Source: NHS Blood and Transplant. National standards for organ retrieval form deceased donors. MPD1043/8, 2018. Available from: https://nhsbtdbe.blob.core.windows.net/umbraco-assets-corp/12548/mpd1043-nors-standard.pdf.

✓✓ Short- and long-term survival outcomes are similar between DBD and DCD kidney transplantation; however, DCD grafts are associated with a higher risk of delayed graft function.[47]

✓✓ There is no difference in short- and long-term survival outcomes between DBD and DCD pancreas transplantation. DCD grafts are associated with a higher risk of graft thrombosis unless antemortem heparin is administered (antemortem heparin administration is prohibited in some countries including the UK).[52]

There is growing interest in the use of machine perfusion technology to minimise the consequences of ischaemia. These technologies can be applied either *in situ* or *ex situ* and at hypothermic or normothermic temperatures. Normothermic regional perfusion (NRP) is a recent advance in DCD donation. It involves perfusing the abdominal (A-NRP) or thoraco-abdominal organs (TA-NRP) *in situ* with oxygenated blood at body temperature using a modified extracorporeal membrane oxygenator (ECMO) circuit following circulatory arrest and prior to cold perfusion and organ retrieval.[53] Initial results from observational studies suggest that NRP reduces the risk of ischaemic cholangiopathy and improves early graft survival in DCD livers.[54,55] Further evidence from randomised controlled trials and for other organs is awaited. *Ex situ* machine perfusion is also being explored for liver transplantation with encouraging early results.[56–58] These techniques allow for more objective assessment of organ viability and enable organ 'resuscitation' prior to transplantation. *Ex situ* hypothermic machine perfusion is increasingly used in kidneys as an alternative to cold static storage during transport, with good evidence for decreased rates of delayed graft function and better short-term graft survival.[59–61]

DECEASED DONOR ORGAN RETRIEVAL

In abdominal organ retrieval, the primary goal is timely retrieval of organs whilst minimising the risk of damage. In DCD donors and unstable DBD donors, the first priority is rapid cannulation of the aorta in order to start perfusion with ice-cold preservation fluid and organ cooling as soon as possible. In stable DBD donors, a more measured approach can be taken to identify and prepare key vessels and structures during the warm phase whilst the heart is still beating, prior to cold perfusion.

After full midline laparotomy and median sternotomy, the organs are carefully inspected for any aberrant anatomy or unexpected pathology (with urgent biopsy if found). In stable DBD donors, the right colon is mobilised along the white line of Toldt whilst protecting the ureter and gonadal vessels, and this is continued with Cattell-Braasch and Kocher manoeuvres to expose the inferior vena cava (IVC) and aorta. The distal aorta is dissected and two ties are placed around it, ready for cannulation. The origin of the superior mesenteric artery (SMA) is also identified and encircled before attention is turned to the porta hepatis. The common bile duct is divided close to the duodenum and the common hepatic, gastroduodenal and splenic arteries are identified and dissected. It is vital to check for and preserve any aberrant hepatic arteries; the most common variants are a replaced right hepatic artery arising from the SMA, a replaced left hepatic artery (LHA) arising from the left gastric artery (LGA) and an accessory LHA from the LGA.[62,63] Other less common variants can be classified as described by Michels (Fig. 10.1).[63,64] The lesser sac is entered and dissection is continued along the greater curvature of the stomach to expose the pancreas. The supra-coeliac aorta is prepared to allow placement of a clamp under the diaphragm which ensures adequate cold perfusion to the abdominal organs. Following heparinisation and discussions with the cardiothoracic team (if present), the distal aorta is tied above the bifurcation, an arteriotomy is made proximally and a cannula is inserted and secured with the second tie. The supra-coeliac aorta is cross clamped and pressurised cold perfusion is commenced following venous venting. This is most commonly performed in the chest; the IVC is incised just below the right atrium to allow draining of the blood and fluid that is flushed through. Ice-slush is simultaneously packed over the abdominal organs for topical cooling. In DBD donors, heparin is given intravenously prior to cold perfusion, whilst in DCD donors it is mixed with the cold preservation fluid. The next step is cold phase dissection. The liver and pancreas are most often retrieved *en bloc*. The block will include the duodenum which is stapled proximally and distally, a segment of IVC and an aortic patch including the origins of the coeliac trunk and SMA. In contrast,

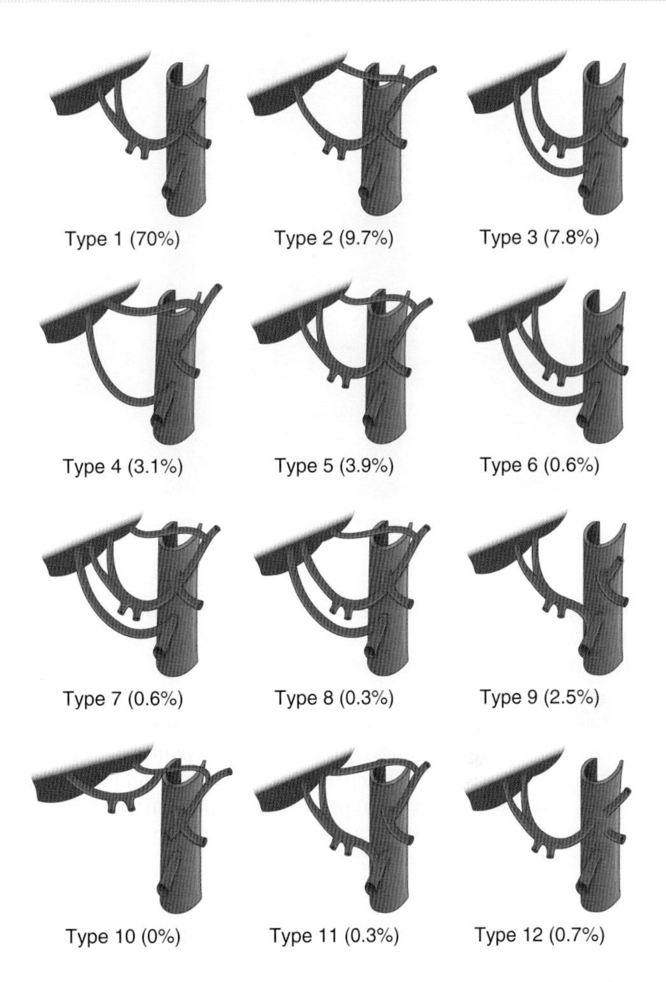

Type 1: CHA arising from coeliac trunk to form gastroduodenal and proper hepatic arteries
Type 2: Replaced LHA from LGA
Type 3: Replaced RHA from SMA
Type 4: Replaced LHA from LGA and replaced RHA from SMA
Type 5: Accessory LHA from LGA
Type 6: Accessory RHA from SMA
Type 7: Accessory LHA from LGA and accessory RHA from SMA
Type 8: Replaced LHA from LGA and accessory RHA from SMA or vice versa
Type 9: CHA from SMA
Type 10: CHA from LGA
Type 11: CHA from SMA and accessory LHA from LGA
Type 12: CHA from aorta

CHA, common hepatic artery; LHA, left hepatic artery; LGA, left gastric artery, RHA, right hepatic artery, SMA, superior mesenteric artery.

Figure 10.1 Hepatic artery variations.

the kidneys are generally retrieved separately. The aorta is split anteriorly and posteriorly in the midline to give an aortic patch with each renal artery. The left renal vein is divided at its confluence with the IVC, leaving the IVC with the right renal vein. The ureters are divided as low as possible and dissected with surrounding tissues to preserve vascularity. A segment of iliac arteries and veins are retrieved for vascular reconstruction during pancreas and liver transplantation. Multiple mesenteric lymph nodes and segments of spleen are also excised and sent with each organ for tissue typing.

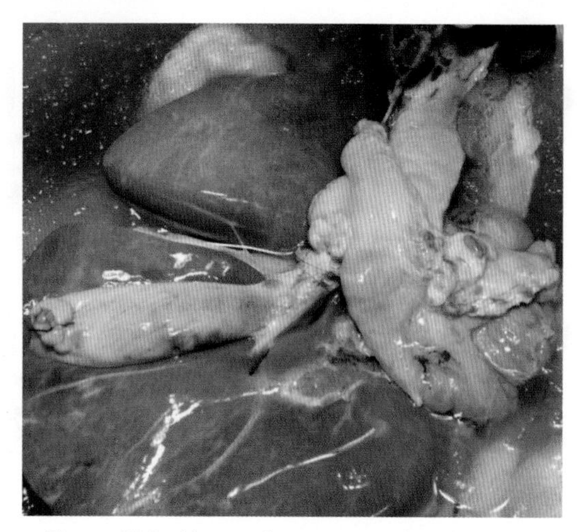

Figure 10.2 Liver and pancreas retrieved *en bloc*.

All organs are inspected on the back table to ensure no damage has occurred, to further flush the organs and separate the organs if retrieved *en bloc* (Fig. 10.2).

✔ During deceased donor organ retrieval, awareness of the most common anatomical variants of the hepatic artery is required: a replaced right hepatic artery arising from the superior mesenteric artery, a replaced left hepatic artery arising from the left gastric artery and an accessory left hepatic artery from the left gastric artery.[62,63]

CONTRAINDICATIONS TO DECEASED DONATION

Absolute contraindications to deceased organ donation are shown in Table 10.6. Any disease with the potential to be transmitted from donor to recipient which could result in morbidity or mortality despite appropriate treatment (e.g. cancer, significant infections) requires a careful risk assessment. It is the responsibility of the recipient transplant team to consider all relevant donor and recipient factors when deciding whether to accept an organ. Organs from all donors will carry some degree of risk, which must be balanced against the benefits of transplantation and the risks of awaiting a further offer of a donor organ.

LIVING ORGAN DONATION

The limited availability of deceased donor organs has led to a significant rise in living donor transplantation. Besides expanding the donor pool, living donor transplantation provides additional advantages. First, living donor organs have not been exposed to the detrimental effects of the dying process or prolonged periods of ischaemia, thus leading to optimal post-transplant organ function. Second, the transplant procedure can be scheduled electively, at a time when both donor and recipient health are optimal, enabling recipients to avoid long waiting times and the associated risk of waiting-list morbidity and mortality. Nevertheless, the benefits of living donor transplantation must be carefully weighed against the small but not insignificant risks to the donor. The safety and welfare of the potential living donor always take precedence over the needs of the potential transplant recipient.[65,66]

Currently, kidney and liver transplantation from living donors is common practice in many countries, while lung and pancreas living donation have been reported in smaller series.[67–69] In the UK, living donation accounts for 30% of all kidney transplants[70] but just 2% of the liver transplants.[71] In contrast, in many Asian and Middle Eastern countries such as Japan, Saudi Arabia and Turkey, the vast majority of transplants are from living donors due to the lack of cultural acceptance of deceased organ donation.[38,72]

Living donation may be 'directed' to a specific identified recipient, or 'non-directed' to an unknown recipient. Altruistic donation, whereby the donor does not have a genetic or pre-existing emotional relationship with the recipient, accounts for an increasing number of transplants. For example, directed altruistic donation may occur when a donor sees a social media campaign for a person in need of a transplant who is not previously known to them, while non-directed donation occurs when a donor decides to donate to any unknown individual and the organ is offered to the most suitable recipient on the waiting list, or through a living donor sharing scheme (see below).

The assessment of all potential living donors is a multistep, multidisciplinary process. A comprehensive medical and psychosocial assessment is required to minimise risk and ensure suitability for donation. Assessment must include functional and anatomical evaluation of the kidneys, general medical fitness of the donor, risk of transmissible disease and psychiatric morbidity.

LIVING KIDNEY DONATION

Compared with deceased donor kidney transplantation, living donor kidney transplantation offers significantly better graft and recipient survival, reduced time on the waiting list and the opportunity for pre-emptive transplantation (transplant prior to starting dialysis) and is therefore the treatment of choice for patients with end-stage renal disease (ESRD).[73] Sharing schemes have been developed to enable blood or human leukocyte antigen (HLA)-incompatible donor-recipient pairs to be matched with other incompatible pairs, in order to achieve compatible transplants. Paired donation includes two pairs, while pooled donation includes at least three pairs (Fig. 10.3). When a non-directed altruistic donor donates their kidney into the paired/pooled scheme, a chain of transplants can ensue, with the organ at the end of the chain offered to the best matched recipient on the national transplant waiting list (Fig. 10.4).

Living donor nephrectomy may be performed using a variety of open, laparoscopic and hand-assisted techniques via a trans- or retroperitoneal approach (Box 10.4). The laparoscopic approaches are now standard in most centres. Several randomised controlled trials have demonstrated shorter hospital stay, less pain, quicker recovery and quicker return to normal activities for laparoscopic versus open techniques, with equivalent complication rates and graft outcomes.[74,75] Compared with the standard laparoscopic procedure, hand-assisted techniques are associated with shorter operative time and warm ischaemic time,[76,77] while retroperitoneoscopic procedures have fewer complications.[77]

Generally, there is a preference for left kidney donation due to the longer left renal vein; however, there is no difference in recipient outcomes using either kidney.[78]

Table 10.6 Contraindications to deceased organ donation (UK guidelines)

General contraindications
Age ≥ 85 years
Primary intracerebral lymphoma
All secondary intracerebral tumours
Any active cancer with evidence of spread outside affected organ within 3 years of donation*
Malignant melanoma
Active (not in remission) haematological malignancy (myeloma, lymphoma, leukaemia)
Definite, probable or possible case of human transmissible spongiform encephalopathy, including CJD and variant CJD, individuals whose blood relatives have had familial CJD, other neurodegenerative diseases associated with infectious agents
Tuberculosis: active and untreated or during first 6 months of treatment
West Nile virus infection
HIV disease (but not HIV infection**)
A history of infection with Ebola virus
Bacillus anthracis (Anthrax)
Dengue virus
Middle East Respiratory Syndrome
Severe Acute Respiratory Syndrome (SARS)
Rabies
Yellow fever
Viral haemorrhagic fevers – including Lassa, Ebola, Marburg and CCHF viruses
Chikungunya virus (Donation can be considered 6 months post recovery)
Progressive Multifocal Leukoencephalopathy
Zika virus (Donation may be considered 6 months post recovery)
Liver specific contraindications
Acute hepatitis of viral, drug or other known aetiology
Serum AST or ALT > 10000 IU/L (if of liver origin)
Cirrhosis
Portal vein thrombosis
Metabolic diseases that would be of harm to the recipient and not treatable (such as haemophilia A and B, inborn errors of metabolism such as oxaluria, tyrosinaemia)
Idiopathic Thrombocytopenia (relative contraindication)
Kidney specific contraindications
Chronic kidney disease (CKD stage 3B or worse, eGFR < 45)
Long-term dialysis (that is, not relating to acute illness)
Renal malignancy: Prior kidney tumours of low grade and previously excised would not necessarily exclude donation
Previous kidney transplant (> 6 months previously)
Pancreas specific contraindications
Insulin-dependent diabetes (excluding ICU-associated insulin requirement)
Non-insulin-dependent diabetes (type 2)
Any history of pancreatic malignancy
Donor BMI > 40 kg/m^2
Donors < 15 kg (except where there is a small paediatric IFALD patient who requires donation of a pancreas with other abdominal organs)
DBD donors ≥ 61 years
DCD donors aged ≥ 56 years

*Active means not in remission; spread outside affected organ includes spread to lymph nodes. Localised prostate, thyroid, in situ cervical cancer and non-melanotic skin cancers are acceptable as possible organ donors.

**HIV infection means people who have infection with HIV but none of the associated complications. Organs from donors with HIV are highly likely to transmit the infection to the recipient and so are used only for those recipients who are already carriers of the virus. Such recipients must be informed and consented about the risks of possible super-infection and transmission of other infective agents that may be present in HIV-infected patients and whose effects may be exacerbated by immunosuppression.

CJD, Creutzfeldt–Jakob disease; HIV, human immunodeficiency virus; CCHF, Crimean-Congo haemorrhagic fever; AST, aspartate transaminase; ALT, alanine transaminase; eGFR, estimated glomerular filtration rate; ICU, intensive care unit; BMI, body mass index; IFALD, intestinal failure-associated liver disease; DBD, donor after brain death; DCD, donor after circulatory death.

Source: NHS Blood and Transplant. Policy POL188/13. Clinical contraindications to approaching families for possible organ donation. 2020. Available from: https://nhsbtdbe.blob.core.windows.net/umbraco-assets-corp/19976/pol188.pdf.

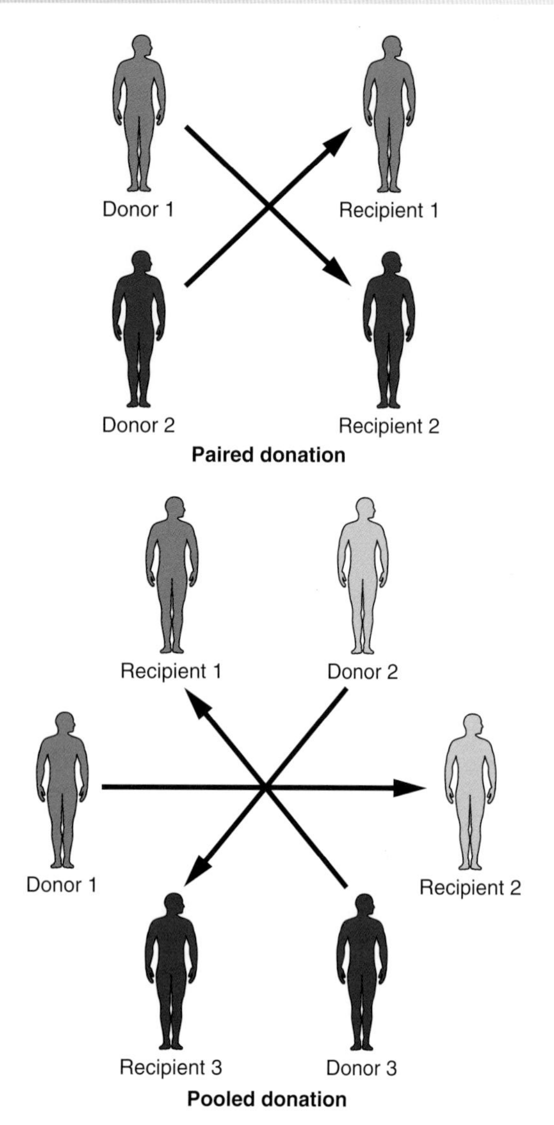

Figure 10.3 Paired and pooled donation.

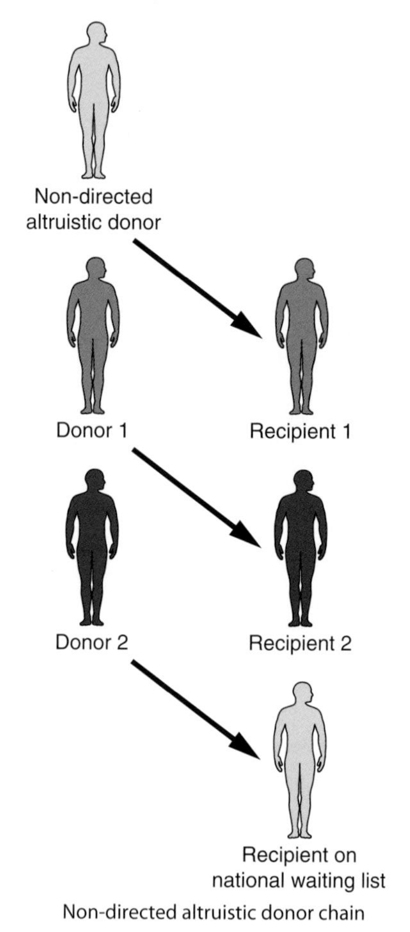

Figure 10.4 Non-directed altruistic donor chains.

Computerised tomography (CT) or magnetic resonance (MR) angiography should be undertaken to assess the renal vasculature and anatomy.[65] Direct measurement of radioisotope (e.g. ^{51}Cr-EDTA, ^{125}Iothalamate) clearance allows accurate evaluation of the glomerular filtration rate (GFR).[65] The recommended GFR thresholds that are considered acceptable for living kidney donation are shown in Table 10.7. Pre-donation GFR thresholds are calculated to ensure that the predicted post-donation GFR remains within the sex- and age-specific normal range throughout the patient's lifetime. This is based on evidence that GFR initially halves post-donation, but then rises to around 75% of pre-donation levels and that GFR declines with age at a faster rate in women than in men.[79,80] Assessment of split renal function is recommended when there is a size disparity of more than 10% between the two kidneys or if there are anatomical abnormalities.[81]

There are few absolute contraindications to living kidney donation. These include active malignancy, chronic infection, nephrolithiasis secondary to a metabolic abnormality, uncontrolled hypertension with end-organ damage, glomerular pathology, inadequate GFR, renal artery disease and sickle cell disease.[81,82] Since age alone is not associated with increased surgical mortality or complications,[83,84] there is no specific age cut-off for kidney donation. Individual risk should be considered within the context of renal function, comorbidities and overall health. Patients with obesity, controlled hypertension and diabetes should undergo careful preoperative evaluation of cardiovascular risk and be counselled about the increased risk of perioperative complications and long-term renal disease.[83]

Box 10.4 Surgical approaches to living donor nephrectomy

- Open
- Mini-incision
- Laparoscopic
  - Transperitoneal
    - Retroperitoneal
    - Anterior
    - Lumbar
- Hand-assisted
  - Transperitoneal
  - Retroperitoneal
- Laparoendoscopic single-site surgery (LESS)
- Robotic-assisted
- Natural orifice transluminal endoscopic surgery (NOTES)

Table 10.7 Recommended GFR thresholds for living kidney donation

Age	Threshold GFR (mL/min/1.73m²)	
	Male	Female
20-29	90	90
30-34	80	80
35	80	80
40	80	80
45	80	80
50	80	80
55	80	75
60	76	70
65	71	64
70	67	59
75	63	54
80	58	49

Source: Fenton A, Montgomery E, Nightingale P, et al. Glomerular filtration rate: new age- and gender- specific reference ranges and thresholds for living kidney donation. BMC Nephrol 2018; 19(1): 336.

Living donor nephrectomy is a low-risk procedure with perioperative mortality consistently reported below 0.03%.[85,86] This is estimated to be six times lower than that of laparoscopic cholecystectomy.[85] In a systematic review of 32 038 minimally invasive living donor nephrectomies, the overall intraoperative complication rate was 2.3% (mainly bleeding), postoperative complication rate 7.3% (mainly infective) and conversion rate 1.1%.[86]

Although the long-term survival of kidney donors is equivalent to that of age- and comorbidity-matched controls,[85,87] there is now sufficient evidence to conclude that donors are at a higher risk of developing ESRD in the long term. A meta-analysis of 118 426 living kidney donors calculated a nine-fold increased risk of ESRD for kidney donors compared with healthy controls.[88] This risk is estimated to be higher for black, hypertensive and male donors.[89] Despite this, the absolute incidence of ESRD amongst kidney donors remains low (<1%) and is lower than that of the general unscreened population.[89,90]

✔✔ Living donor kidney transplantation offers significantly better graft and recipient survival than deceased donor kidney transplantation.[73]

✔✔ Living donor nephrectomy is a low-risk procedure with a perioperative mortality risk of approximately 0.03% and long-term survival equivalent to age- and comorbidity-matched controls.[85,86]

✔✔ Living kidney donors are at a higher risk of developing ESRD compared with non-donors.[88] However, the absolute incidence of ESRD amongst kidney donors is low (<1%).[89,90]

LIVING LIVER DONATION

Living liver donation involves a partial hepatectomy in which a liver lobe or segment is resected. The optimal size of the graft is the smallest possible liver resection to minimise operative risk and ensure an adequate remnant liver volume for the donor, balanced with a graft volume that is sufficient to meet the metabolic demands of the recipient. A graft to recipient body weight ratio (GRWR) of < 0.8% increases the risk of small-for-size syndrome, which is associated with high recipient morbidity and mortality.[91,92] In adult-to-child transplantation, a left lateral segment graft (segments II and III) is most often used. In adult-to-adult transplantation, the full left lobe (segments II, III and IV) may be used, but more commonly the larger volume of a right lobe graft (segments V, VI, VII and VIII) is required. Laparoscopic and hand-assisted techniques have not yet been widely adopted; however, they have been shown to have an equivalent safety profile to the open procedure.[93,94]

CT or magnetic resonance imaging with intravascular contrast are necessary for volumetric analysis, determination of vascular and biliary anatomy, and assessment of hepatic steatosis of the donor liver. It is generally accepted that the donor remnant liver volume should be at minimum 30%.[95,96] Most liver regeneration occurs rapidly within the first week after resection or transplantation.[97] Within 3 months, the donor liver remnant regenerates to around 80% of original liver volume, while the recipient graft reaches 93% of standard liver volume.[98]

Donor hepatic steatosis increases both donor and recipient risk. Although no clear cut-off is defined, usually > 30% steatosis precludes donation.[66] There is insufficient evidence to define an upper age limit for living liver donation, but the increased risk of perioperative complications with older age must be given careful consideration, in conjunction with other risk factors. Obesity increases the risk of surgical complications and is associated with a higher frequency of hepatic steatosis; therefore, a BMI > 35 kg/m² is usually considered a contraindication to donation.[66] Other contraindications include active malignancy and active infection with hepatitis B, hepatitis C and human immunodeficiency virus.[66]

Current data suggest the risk of donor mortality to be 0.2%.[99,100] The overall complication rate is reported to be between 16.1% and 39%; most common complications include biliary complications (e.g. leaks, strictures), infections (e.g. wound, urinary, lung) and incisional hernias.[99,100] Complications are more common and more serious in right lobe donation.[99,101,102] However, most donors return to normal activity within 3–6 months.[99]

✔✔ The overall risk of mortality after living liver donation is 0.2%, and this is higher for right lobe than for left lobe donors.[99]

PRINCIPLES OF ABDOMINAL ORGAN TRANSPLANTATION

TRANSPLANT IMMUNOLOGY

A donor organ that is transplanted into a genetically non-identical recipient is termed an *allograft*, the immune response to the allograft is termed *alloimmune response* and the process of recognising the allograft as foreign is termed *allorecognition*. Understanding the alloimmune response and ways in which to suppress it are key to successful transplantation without allograft rejection. Different organs appear to induce varying levels of alloimmune response, with liver transplant recipients requiring less immunosuppression than kidney transplant recipients.[103]

The alloimmune response is primarily activated through the adaptive immune system which involves recognition of foreign antigens. However, during organ reperfusion in the early stages after transplantation, ischaemic injury of the allograft initially activates the innate immune system which reacts to non-specific damage signals through the complement system, neutrophils, macrophages, natural killer cells and cytokines.[104]

There are three main tissue antigens that can trigger the alloimmune response through the adaptive immune system: ABO blood group antigens, HLA antigens and non-HLA antigens.

ABO blood group antigens are expressed on a wide range of cells including red blood cells and vascular endothelium (Table 10.8). Naturally-occurring anti-A and anti-B antibodies cause antibody-mediated hyperacute rejection and graft loss in ABO-incompatible transplantation.

HLA antigens are cell surface proteins present on most nucleated cells and are a major target for the alloimmune response.[104] These antigens are encoded on major histocompatibility complex (MHC) genes on chromosome 6. Class I HLA antigens includes HLA-A, HLA-B and HLA-C, while class II includes HLA-DP, HLA-DQ and HLA-DR antigens. There are a huge number of different variants of each HLA antigen in the human population. A higher number of HLA mismatches between donor and recipient is associated with increased risk of rejection and graft loss in kidney and pancreas transplantation.[104,105] In contrast, HLA mismatches do not impact on outcomes after liver transplantation.[106] Sensitisation to HLA antigens can occur through blood transfusions, pregnancy and previous transplantation resulting in antibodies to specific HLA antigens. The level of sensitisation can be measured as the calculated reaction frequency (cRF); the percentage of donors to which the patient has pre-formed HLA antibodies. The higher the cRF, the more difficult it is to find a compatible donor.

Table 10.8 ABO blood group antigens

Blood group	Antigen	ABO antibodies	Compatible donor blood groups
A	A	Anti-B	A and O
B	B	Anti-A	B and O
AB	A and B	None	A, B, AB, O
O	None	Anti-A and anti-B	O

Non-HLA antigens, also known as minor histocompatibility (miH) antigens may play a minor role in allograft rejection, however their clinical significance is currently unknown.[103]

Allorecognition leads to T-cell activation, cytokine production, cellular cytotoxicity, the humoral response, a delayed-type hypersensitivity reaction and ultimately immune-mediated destruction of the allograft i.e. rejection (Table 10.9).[103] Numerous immunosuppressive medications have been developed to target different parts of the alloimmune response, however rejection remains one of the major barriers to successful transplantation.

Following a transplant, the most widely used immunosuppressive regimen is triple therapy with:

1. A calcineurin inhibitor (e.g. tacrolimus or ciclosporin)
2. An antiproliferative agent (e.g. azathioprine or mycophenolate mofetil)
3. A corticosteroid (e.g. prednisolone)

Other options include polyclonal antibodies (e.g. antithymocyte immunoglobulin [ATG]) and monoclonal antibodies (e.g. interleukin-2 T-cell receptor antibody – basiliximab) for induction and mammalian target of rapamycin (mTOR) inhibitors (e.g. sirolimus or everolimus) for maintenance therapy.[107] Calcineurin inhibitors must be kept within a narrow therapeutic range and thus require regular monitoring. Since

Table 10.9 Types of rejection

Rejection type and usual time of onset	Underlying mechanism(s)	Treatment
Hyperacute rejection (minutes to hours)	• Presence of pre-formed antibodies (either anti-ABO or anti-HLA) in high volumes directed against the graft • Rapid deposition of antibodies on the graft activates the complement cascade, leading to cell destruction, graft thrombosis and necrosis	• If it occurs it is irreversible • Can be prevented by transplanting ABO-compatible organs into recipients without significant volumes of anti-donor HLA antibodies
Acute rejection (weeks to months)	• Cell-mediated: macrophages, CD8 T cells and neutrophils within the graft causing organ damage • Antibody-mediated: anti-donor antibodies produced by B cells causing complement deposition etc.	• Cell-mediated: mild-moderate episodes can be treated with high-dose iv methylprednisolone; severe episodes require additional anti-thymocyte globulin (ATG) to deplete T cells • Antibody-mediated: iv methylprednisolone + plasmapheresis + IVIG (consider splenectomy, eculizumab, ATG also)
Chronic rejection (months to years)	• Chronic, indolent alloimmune responses (cell- or antibody-mediated)	• Optimize immunosuppressive therapy • Control other long-term risk factors for graft dysfunction (BP, lipids, smoking)

BP, blood pressure; IVIG, intravenous immunoglobulin

Source: Phillips BL, Callaghan C. The immunology of organ transplantation. *Surgery (Oxford)* 2020; 38(7): 353-60 with permission from Elsevier.

Table 10.10 Common immunosuppressive drugs used in transplant recipients and their main side-effects

Immunosuppressive drug	Side-effects
Tacrolimus	Nephrotoxicity Diabetes Hypertension Neurotoxicity
Ciclosporin	Nephrotoxicity Hypertension Gingival hypertrophy Hirsutism
Azathioprine	Pancytopenia Pancreatitis
Mycophenolate mofetil	Pancytopenia Diarrhoea
Prednisolone	Diabetes Pancreatitis Peptic ulcer disease Impaired wound healing
Sirolimus/everolimus	Hypertension Pancytopenia Impaired wound healing Hypertriglyceridaemia

sirolimus is associated with poor wound healing, it is generally avoided in the immediate postoperative period.[103,108]

✔✔ Since sirolimus is associated with poor wound healing, it should generally be avoided in the immediate postoperative period.[108]

Lifelong immunosuppression is associated with significant side effects (Table 10.10) as well as an increased risk of opportunistic infections and a two-fold higher risk of malignancy compared with the general population.[109]

ABO- and HLA-incompatible transplantation is a novel approach that has been investigated in living donor kidney transplantation whereby antibodies are removed from the recipient via plasma exchange or immunoabsorption in the weeks leading up to transplant. However, graft outcomes are inferior to antibody compatible transplants and further work is required to improve these new technologies.[110]

KIDNEY TRANSPLANTATION

For patients with ESRD, kidney transplantation offers better life expectancy, quality of life and cost-effectiveness compared with dialysis.[111–113] Living donor transplants and in particular, pre-emptive living donor transplants provide the best outcomes[73,114]; however, access to such optimal grafts is inequitable, with patients from socioeconomically deprived and minority ethnic backgrounds significantly less likely to receive them.[115]

✔ Pre-emptive kidney transplantation provides better graft survival than transplantation after the start of dialysis.[114]

Patients must be fit enough to undergo major surgery and chronic immunosuppression. Comorbidities are common in patients with ESRD and must be carefully assessed. Peripheral vascular disease, obesity, heart failure, cerebrovascular disease, chronic liver disease and diabetes are associated with poorer survival outcomes.[116]

The kidney transplant procedure is most commonly undertaken through a curvilinear incision in the right or left iliac fossa in an extraperitoneal plane. The renal artery is most commonly anastomosed to the external iliac artery with an end-to-side anastomosis; however, an end-to-end anastomosis to the internal iliac artery can also be utilised and provides equivalent outcomes.[117] The renal vein is anastomosed to the external iliac vein. A ureteroneocystostomy is created to anastomose the ureter to the bladder. The Lich-Gregoir technique is associated with a lower rate of urinary leakage than the Politano-Leadbetter and U-stitch techniques.[118] Meta-analyses have demonstrated that routine ureteric stenting significantly lowers the risk of urological complications such as urine leak and stenosis, however prophylactic antibiotics should be given to reduce the risk of urinary tract infection associated with stenting.[119,120]

✔✔ Routine ureteric stents with prophylactic antibiotics are recommended in kidney transplantation to reduce the risk of urological complications such as urine leak and stenosis.[119,120]

PANCREAS TRANSPLANTATION

Pancreas transplantation offers improved survival and quality of life for patients with insulin-dependent diabetes, with the potential for freedom from insulin and halting of progressive diabetic complications. Pancreas transplantation may be undertaken as simultaneous pancreas-kidney (SPK), pancreas-after-kidney (PAK), pancreas alone or islet transplantation, depending on whether the primary indication is end-stage diabetic nephropathy or brittle diabetes with severe hypoglycaemic events and lack of awareness of hypoglycaemia.

The pancreas transplantation procedure is ordinarily performed through a midline laparotomy. The pancreas is usually implanted on the right-sided iliac vessels whilst venous drainage can be into the systemic system (anastomosis between the donor portal vein and the distal IVC) or portal venous system (anastomosis between donor portal vein and recipient SMV). The arterial anastomosis requires an extension Y graft fashioned using the donor iliac artery bifurcation which is anastomosed to the donor SMA and splenic arteries. The arterial Y graft is then anastomosed to the recipient common iliac artery. Exocrine drainage can be achieved usually through a duodenojejunal (enteric) anastomosis although a duodeno-vesical (bladder) anastomosis can be considered in pancreas-alone transplantation.

LIVER TRANSPLANTATION

This is covered in the Hepatobiliary Companion Series volume.

GENERAL SURGERY IN THE TRANSPLANT PATIENT

The management of transplant recipients requiring elective or emergency general surgery is complex and raises several key issues. First, transplant recipients may have risk factors relating to their primary disease which need to be taken into account when estimating perioperative risk, e.g. renal transplant recipients have a three- to five-fold increased risk of premature cardiovascular disease compared with the general population.[121] Second, all transplant recipients require potent life-long immunosuppression, which complicates both the presentation and management of general surgical diseases. Finally, the transplanted organ must be given due consideration in the planning of any general surgical procedure, as it may present technical issues and is at particular risk of ischaemic injury. A multidisciplinary team approach is essential and the transplant team should be involved as early as possible in the course of management.

Immunosuppression presents particular issues in the context of general surgery given their side effects (Table 10.10). These side effects may be responsible for general surgical presentations (e.g. pancreatitis, peptic ulcer disease), increased perioperative risk (e.g. hypertension, diabetes) or complicated post-surgical recovery (e.g. impaired wound healing, pancytopenia, increased infection risk). Most commonly used immunosuppressive drugs require close monitoring to keep them within their narrow therapeutic range and therefore they must be continued throughout the perioperative period. Therefore, the transplant team should be involved in assessing whether changes to the immunosuppressive regimen are indicated.

PRINCIPLES OF PERIOPERATIVE MANAGEMENT

- The function of the transplanted graft must be closely monitored throughout the perioperative period.
- Anaesthetic drugs, analgesia and antibiotic choices and doses should be guided by organ function and potential interactions with immunosuppressive medication.
- Non-steroidal anti-inflammatory drugs should be avoided due to their nephrotoxic effects.
- Avoidance of haemodynamic instability is key to maintaining adequate perfusion to the graft.
- Gentle handling of tissues is particularly important due to the effects of immunosuppression on tissue integrity.

Key points

- There is considerable international variation in the legislative framework for organ donation and all surgeons have a responsibility to be familiar with the current legislation in their country.
- Donation after brain death (DBD) requires confirmation of brain death by neurological criteria, while donation after circulatory death (DCD) occurs after irreversible cessation of cardiorespiratory function.
- The perioperative mortality risk for living kidney donation and living liver donation is low. Living kidney donation is associated with a small increased long-term risk of ESRD.
- Rejection remains one of the major barriers to successful transplantation and can be hyperacute, acute or chronic.
- Transplant patients require lifelong immunosuppression which is associated with significant side-effects and increased risk of malignancy.

References available at http://ebooks.health.elsevier.com/

KEY REFERENCES

[45] O'Neill S, Roebuck A, Khoo E, Wigmore SJ, Harrison EM. A meta-analysis and meta-regression of outcomes including biliary complications in donation after cardiac death liver transplantation. Transpl Int 2014;27(11):1159–74.

This systematic review and meta-analysis included 62 184 liver transplant recipients from 25 retrospective cohort studies. DCD transplants were associated with a 2.4-fold increased risk of biliary complications and a 10.5-fold increased risk of ischaemic cholangiopathy compared with DBD transplants.

[47] Gavrilidis P, Inston NG. Recipient and allograft survival following donation after circulatory death versus donation after brain death for renal transplantation: a systematic review and meta-analysis. Transplant Rev 2020;34(4):100563.

This systematic review and meta-analysis included 19 137 patients from 12 observational studies, and found no significant difference in graft and patient survival between DCD and DBD kidney transplants, despite a higher rate of delayed graft function among DCD transplants.

[52] Shahrestani S, Webster AC, Lam VW, et al. Outcomes from pancreatic transplantation in donation after cardiac death: a systematic review and meta-analysis. Transplantation 2017;101(1):122–30.

This systematic review and meta-analysis included 643 patients from 18 observational studies and demonstrated no significant difference in graft and patient survival between DCD and DBD pancreas transplantation. There was a higher rate of graft thrombosis in the DCD group, but this was not the case if antemortem heparin was administered.

[73] Terasaki PI, Cecka JM, Gjertson DW, et al. High survival rates of kidney transplants from spousal and living unrelated donors. N Engl J Med 1995;333(6):333–6.

This landmark registry study demonstrated that despite a higher degree of HLA mismatching, the graft survival of living unrelated donor kidneys was superior to that of deceased donor kidneys.

[85] Segev DL, Muzaale AD, Caffo BS, et al. Perioperative mortality and long-term survival following live kidney donation. JAMA 2010;303(10):959–66.

This US case-control study of 80 347 live kidney donors found that long-term risk of death was no higher for kidney donors than for age- and comorbidity-matched controls (n = 9364) from the NHANES III survey. Overall 90-day surgical mortality was 3.1 per 10 000 donors. Both short- and long-term mortality was higher in male, Black and hypertensive donors.

[88] O'Keeffe LM, Ramond A, Oliver-Williams C, et al. Mid- and long-term health risks in living kidney donors: a systematic review and meta-analysis. Ann Intern Med 2018;168(4):276–84.

This systematic review and meta-analysis of 118 426 living kidney donors and 117 656 non-donors demonstrated a nine-fold increased long-term risk of ESRD among donors.

[99] Middleton PF, Duffield M, Lynch SV, et al. Living donor liver transplantation. Adult donor outcomes: a systematic review. Liver Transpl 2006;12(1):24–30.

This systematic review of living liver donor outcomes (214 studies) found overall donor mortality to be 0.2% (13/6000 procedures, 117 studies), with mortality for right lobe donors (0.23–0.5%) higher than for left lobe donors (0.05–0.21%). The rate of donor morbidity was 16.1% (131 studies); most commonly biliary leaks and strictures (6.2%, 97 studies) and infections such as wound infections, urinary tract infections and pneumonia (5.8%, 50 studies). Median hospital stay was 9 days (58 studies) with return to normal activities within 3–6 months (18 studies).

[108] Dean PG, Lund WJ, Larson TS, et al. Wound-healing complications after kidney transplantation: a prospective, randomized comparison of sirolimus and tacrolimus. Transplantation 2004;77(10):1555–61.

This randomised trial found a higher incidence of wound-healing complications in sirolimus-based versus tacrolimus-based immunosuppressive regimens.

[120] Wilson CH, Bhatti AA, Rix DA, Manas DM. Routine intraoperative ureteric stenting for kidney transplant recipients. Cochrane Database Syst Rev 2005;(4):Cd004925.

This Cochrane systematic review of 7 RCTs (1154 patients) showed that prophylactic ureteric stenting of the vesico-ureteric anastomosis in kidney transplantation significantly reduces the risk of urine leaks and ureteric stenosis, however it is associated with a higher rate of UTIs unless patients are prescribed antibiotics.

Early assessment of the acute abdomen

11

Hugh M.Paterson

The acute abdomen may be defined as 'abdominal pain of non-traumatic origin with a maximum duration of 5 days'.[1] There is a long list of causes ranging from the entirely benign, requiring no particular management other than reassurance, to the rapidly fatal where swift diagnosis and appropriate surgical treatment is life-saving. Abdominal symptoms may be manifested by conditions that are entirely extra-abdominal, and intra-abdominal conditions may present with extra-abdominal symptoms. Thus there are many pitfalls for the unwary, and many abdominal surgeons will readily attest that the emergency 'take' is the most challenging part of their activities.

Acute abdominal pain (for the purposes of this chapter, the terms 'acute abdominal pain' and 'acute abdomen' are used interchangeably) remains a common cause for seeking medical attention. In the USA, between 5% and 10% of all emergency department (ED) consultations are for abdominal pain.[2] In the UK, there has been a substantial increase in emergency surgical admissions to hospitals in the last 20 years, reflecting the increase in all emergency admissions to secondary care.[3] The acute abdomen has long been the bread-and-butter of the general surgeon, with clinical experience in surgical decision-making honed in an era without recourse to extensive diagnostic investigations. Although there has been no major change to the incidence of most of the common diagnoses (with the exception of a substantial reduction in prevalence of peptic ulcer disease[4]), new challenges have arisen. As the population in developed countries becomes more elderly, frailty and multi-morbidity complicate surgical assessment and treatment. The hospital environment continues to evolve due to centralisation of services, reduced hospital inpatient capacity and/or resource limitation. And with the development of subspecialist training, surgeons themselves no longer have the breadth of surgical experience that characterised the previous generation.

CONDITIONS ASSOCIATED WITH ABDOMINAL PAIN

The list of potential causes of the acute abdomen is extensive. An exhaustive account is not the purpose of this chapter, and readers will find the latest guidance on diagnosis and management of common conditions elsewhere in this book or the Companion to Specialist Practice series. It is now over 30 years since Irvin et al.[5] documented the diagnoses presenting with acute abdominal pain to a UK general surgery department. At that time, the most common diagnosis (over a third of the cohort) was non-specific abdominal pain (NSAP), twice as frequent as the next most common condition (acute appendicitis, 17%).

NSAP may be defined as 'pain for which no immediate cause can be found following examination and baseline investigations and specifically does not require surgical intervention'. A variety of causes have been proposed (Box 11.1). Historically, clinicians worried that a label of NSAP might mask serious undiagnosed pathology. However, data from children with abdominal pain suggests NSAP is a safe diagnosis: a large retrospective study of > 3000 admissions with NSAP in children over 20 years found a 'missed' appendicitis rate of only 0.2%.[6] A record linkage study of a cohort of > 250 000 children with NSAP 1999–2011 from English national data found that only 5.8% were subsequently hospitalised for bowel disorders, the most likely conditions being appendicitis, IBD and IBS.[7] In adults, increased use of diagnostic imaging in the past 10–20 years (see below) suggests that a diagnosis of NSAP is likely to be much more secure than when de Dombal et al.[8] observed that 10% of patients over 50 years old labelled as NSAP presented subsequently with an intra-abdominal malignancy (most commonly colorectal cancer).

Irvin's audit has been updated in a 2009 multicentre study of 1021 adult patients presenting with acute abdominal pain to EDs in the Netherlands (Table 11.1). Although the frequency of individual diagnoses remained broadly similar over time, it is notable that the frequency of NSAP was substantially less in the Dutch study and no doubt reflects the more advanced imaging strategies employed. However, that depends on referral pathways: the proportion of non-surgical causes of acute abdominal pain admitted to a New Zealand surgical unit increased during the same 10-year period despite greater use of diagnostic imaging.[9]

A small number of medical conditions can present with acute abdominal pain, and although uncommon are mentioned here for the benefit of surgeons in training. Inferior myocardial infarction, lower lobar pneumonia and some metabolic disorders can all be excluded by examination and/or basic investigations (ECG, chest radiograph and serum glucose); failure to recognise them is associated with significantly increased morbidity and mortality.

INITIAL ASSESSMENT: HISTORY, EXAMINATION AND SIMPLE TESTS

A careful medical history and clinical examination remains the keystone of initial assessment and should lead to formulation of a differential diagnosis from the conditions listed

Box 11.1 Causes of non-specific abdominal pain[9]

Viral infections
Bacterial gastroenteritis
Worm infestation
Irritable bowel syndrome
Gynaecological conditions
Psychosomatic pain
Coeliac disease[10]
Abdominal wall pain[11]

- Peripheral nerve injuries
- Hernias
- Myofascial pain syndromes
- Rib tip syndrome
- Nerve root pain

Table 11.1 Final diagnoses in 1021 patients with acute abdominal pain

Final diagnoses in 1021 patients	*n* (%)
Urgent	
Acute appendicitis	284 (28)
Acute diverticulitis	118 (12)
Bowel obstruction	68 (7)
Acute cholecystitis	52 (5)
Acute pancreatitis	28 (3)
Gynaecological diseases	27 (3)
Urological diseases	22 (2)
Abscess	14 (1)
Perforated viscus	13 (1)
Bowel ischaemia	12 (1)
Pneumonia	11 (1)
Retroperitoneal or abdominal wall bleeding	9 (1)
Acute peritonitis	3 (0.3)
Total urgent diagnoses	661 (65)
Non-urgent	
Non-specific abdominal pain	183 (18)
Gastrointestinal diseases	56 (5)
Hepatic, pancreatic and biliary diseases	43 (4)
Inflammatory bowel disease	30 (3)
Urological diseases	20 (2)
Gynaecological diseases	9 (1)
Malignancy	5 (0.5)
Hemia	2 (0.2)
Other	12 (1)
Total non-urgent diagnoses	360 (35)

Reproduced from Lameris W, van Randen A, van Es HW, et al. Imaging strategies for detection of urgent conditions in patients with acute abdominal pain: diagnostic accuracy study. BMJ 2009;338: b2431. With permission from BMJ Publishing Group Ltd.

in Table 11.1. In a review of abdominal pain assessment errors in the ED, failure of history taking was one of the biggest contributors.[10] Age is an important determinant of likely diagnoses; the differential of, for example, right iliac fossa pain in teenagers is quite different in octogenarians.

It is now well established that adequate (usually opiate) analgesia for patients presenting with an acute abdomen does not mask abdominal signs and is not detrimental to surgical assessment or decision-making.[11]

✔✔ Analgesia does not mask clinical signs in assessment of the acute abdomen and should not be withheld.[11]

However, as previous generations of general surgeons knew well, in managing the acute abdomen there is an important distinction between assessing *urgency* and making an accurate *diagnosis*. Although some conditions are recognised reliably by clinical assessment (particularly acute diverticulitis[12] and small bowel obstruction[13]), in general the accuracy of clinical diagnosis in the acute abdomen is only moderate. The Acute Abdominal Pain Study Group found that diagnostic accuracy was less than 50% with substantial interobserver variation, particularly in eliciting physical signs, but distinguishing urgent from non-urgent conditions was more reliable.[14] In the previous era, the main decision for the general surgeon was when to operate immediately, when to observe and when not to operate at all. A precise diagnosis was less of a priority, partly because the diagnostic armamentarium was limited. Consequently, the prevailing negative laparotomy rate at the time was considerable ('better to look and see than wait and see'). In the patient with peritonitis and septic shock, it may still be argued that a precise diagnosis is less important than rapid intervention to resuscitate and achieve source control (and the diagnosis) by laparotomy. However, for patients in whom the need for operation is less obvious, in modern practice a precise preoperative diagnosis has important implications:

- Subspecialisation in general surgery is now the norm in many countries, hence diagnosis is important for onward referral to the appropriate subspecialty (which may be in a different hospital). The emergence of the emergency general surgeon in UK practice has embedded this process in many hospitals.
- To avoid unnecessary admission to hospital in an increasingly resource-limited service. Although time is a key determinant in the evaluation of the acute abdomen, and active observation is a well-established and safe practice, hospital bed occupancy is costly.
- For selection of the appropriate treatment option depending on severity (operative vs non-operative; laparoscopic vs open surgery).

A number of studies have sought to improve the accuracy of clinical diagnosis by systematic documentation of clinical variables to develop risk prediction scoring systems, applied most frequently to acute appendicitis (e.g. Alvarado score,[15] Appendicitis Inflammatory Response score[16]). A comprehensive comparison of appendicitis risk prediction models in a large UK 'snap-shot' audit of > 5000 patients has recently been published (overall, the Adult Appendicitis Score performed best, with a failure rate of 3.7%).[17] In current practice, these scoring systems probably have greatest application in allowing less experienced or non-surgical clinicians to triage patients that may safely avoid hospital admission, to select patients for diagnostic imaging and to provide a framework for clinical reassessment.[18,19]

INITIAL INVESTIGATIONS

BLOOD TESTS

'Routine' blood tests are useful for assessing severity of illness (indeed the physiology component of the P-POSSUM risk stratification score relies heavily on these) but have limited diagnostic utility. Serum amylase and/or lipase assays are requested routinely in assessment of (upper) abdominal pain in most centres and are reasonably reliable.[20,21] It is important to note that both enzymes may be significantly elevated in non-pancreatic aetiologies of the acute abdomen, and a normal value does not always exclude acute pancreatitis.

Diabetic ketoacidosis (DKA) as a first presentation of diabetes mellitus can mimic an acute abdomen quite convincingly; serum glucose measurement is a cheap and reliable way of excluding serious diabetic complications such as DKA or hyperosmolar hyperglycaemic state (HHS). Bear in mind, though, that occasionally DKA is associated with a primary abdominal pathology such as acute pancreatitis,[22] while HHS may be provoked by intra-abdominal sepsis.[23]

White cell count (WCC) and C-reactive protein (CRP) have limited discriminatory value in diagnosis of acute abdominal pain, although trends over time may be of value in assessing response to treatment in some cases. Gans et al.[24] summarised three large prospective studies examining the utility of WCC and CRP in acute abdominal pain: even at thresholds of WCC > 15 × 10/L and CRP > 50 mg/L, over 80% of urgent diagnoses were missed.

Some novel biomarkers have been evaluated in assessment of the acute abdomen. Plasma procalcitonin use has not progressed beyond experimental interest.[25] Biomarker panels may be of value in discriminating low-risk patients in some healthcare settings, particularly where over-reliance on radiological imaging is prevalent.[26] Perhaps surprisingly, given the prognostic value of elevated serum lactate in the assessment of sepsis, there is relatively little data examining its use as a triage test in the acute abdomen. It has very limited discriminatory power in the diagnosis of acute mesenteric ischaemia.[27]

DIAGNOSTIC IMAGING

Contemporary surgical practice in the developed world is aided considerably by availability of sophisticated radiological investigations that would have been the envy of our predecessors. The use of plain and contrast radiographs is diminishing as computed tomography (CT) becomes the dominant investigation of choice, but remains relevant to practice in developing countries and will be discussed here.

PLAIN RADIOGRAPHS

Plain radiographs of the erect chest and supine abdomen have been embedded in assessment of the acute abdomen for decades. They are viewed as cheap and easy to obtain, but in fact consume time and resource, result in unnecessary radiation exposure and can be uncomfortable for patients. Their role in contemporary practice in developed countries is gradually diminishing. The erect chest X-ray has limited ability to identify a perforated intra-abdominal viscus by

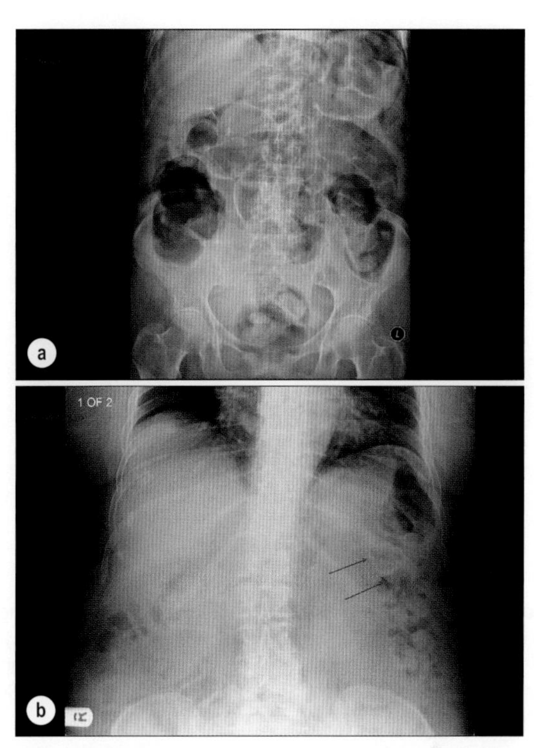

Figure 11.1 Plain supine abdominal radiographs demonstrating free intraperitoneal air **(a)** in a patient with a perforated duodenal ulcer and retroperitoneal air **(b)** in a patient with perforated diverticular disease.

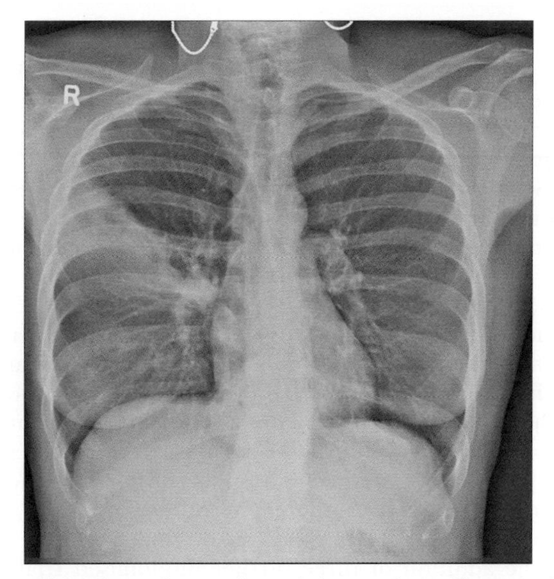

Figure 11.2 Erect chest radiograph in a patient with acute right-sided pneumonia.

demonstrating free intraperitoneal air (Fig. 11.1).[28] It is indicated if lower lobar pneumonia is being considered (Fig. 11.2). Abdominal radiographs have very low yield if requested as part of the routine assessment of acute abdominal pain, although by most radiological guidelines this is inappropriate anyway. Their main indication is in the diagnosis of bowel obstruction (Fig. 11.3).[29] Since symptoms and signs of bowel obstruction can be readily identified from the clinical assessment, its primary function is to distinguish small

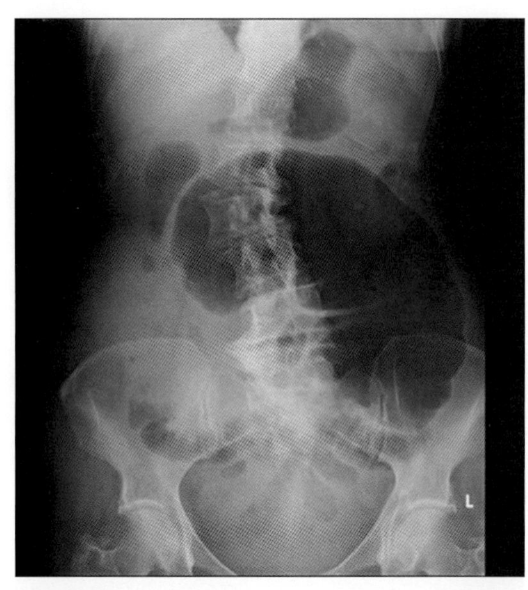

Figure 11.3 Plain abdominal radiograph in a patient presenting with acute vomiting 1 week after closure of a defunctioning ileostomy. This is the characteristic appearance of caecal volvulus. (With thanks to Dr Tom Blankenstein, Specialty Trainee in Radiology, Western General Hospital, Edinburgh.)

from large bowel obstruction to guide early management, but even here CT is markedly superior.[30]

CONTRAST RADIOGRAPHS

Only water-soluble contrast is discussed, as barium-based studies are relatively contraindicated in the emergency setting due to the presence or high possibility of developing intestinal perforation. The main indications are in the management of adhesive small bowel obstruction, and in demonstrating the presence (or absence) of ongoing leakage from intestinal perforation. CT scan has superseded water-soluble contrast enemas in the diagnosis of colonic obstruction in most institutions.

There is strong evidence from meta-analysis of a number of studies that water-soluble contrast followed by an abdominal radiograph will reliably predict the likelihood of resolution of adhesive small bowel obstruction. If contrast reaches the colon within 24 hours, obstruction will resolve in 99% of patients, reducing hospital stay for those not requiring surgery compared to conventional 'drip and suck' management (Fig. 11.4). Since the original Cochrane analysis, the addition of three further randomised trials has shown that this practice also reduces the need for surgery. These studies form the basis for the Bologna guidelines for diagnosis and management of adhesive small bowel obstruction.[31–33]

The role of contrast radiography in suspected gastroduodenal perforation has largely been replaced by oral contrast-enhanced CT. However, in resource-limited settings, patients diagnosed by erect chest X-ray to have a perforation may be selected for non-operative management using contrast to demonstrate whether the leak has sealed or there is ongoing leakage.[34] This topic is discussed in further detail in Chapter 12.

✔✔ Early use of water-soluble contrast in adhesive small bowel obstruction reduces the need for surgery, accurately selects patients for operative/non-operative management and reduces length of stay.[33]

ULTRASONOGRAPHY

Ultrasound is cost-effective, harmless, readily available and in experienced hands has high diagnostic accuracy in specific acute abdominal conditions. Its disadvantage is that accuracy is user-dependent and images lack the spatial resolution useful to surgical planning afforded by CT. In direct comparison with CT, ultrasound was less sensitive in diagnosis of appendicitis and diverticulitis (76% vs 94% and 61% vs 81%, respectively), though positive predictive values were similar.[35] It should not be used as an unguided initial investigation of the acute abdomen and is best targeted to confirm or refute specific diagnoses. It is the investigation of choice for acute biliary disease, with sensitivity of 90–95% in detecting gall bladder inflammation, gallstones and biliary dilation, and is recommended as the first-line investigation in the Tokyo Guidelines for acute cholecystitis.[36] CT may be required in equivocal cases (Fig. 11.5).[37]

In the assessment of right iliac fossa/lower abdominal pain, ultrasound is effective in evaluating the pelvic organs in women to triage acute ovarian/pelvic organ pathology requiring direct referral to gynaecology. The data available for its use in the diagnosis of appendicitis are inconsistent, reflecting user-dependency and constraints of patient habitus. Specific diagnostic features (non-compressible appendix > 7 mm, periappendiceal inflammation or abscess; Fig. 11.6) are associated with high sensitivity (74%) and specificity (97%), but both normal and perforated appendixes can be difficult to visualise ultrasonically. A multicentre observational trial in 870 patients concluded that there was no clinical benefit of ultrasound of the appendix in routine clinical diagnosis.[38]

Ultrasound can also be useful in detecting abdominal wall problems such as hernias and rectus sheath haematoma (Fig. 11.7). It may have a role in some settings for assessing the aorta and renal tract, but increasingly CT is the investigation of choice in these areas. In resource-poor healthcare settings, ultrasound can be used by surgeons themselves with satisfactory results.[39,40]

COMPUTED TOMOGRAPHY

Over the past 20 years, there has been a substantial increase in the use of CT scans for assessment of the acute abdomen in patients of all ages, particularly in North America.[41] In the UK, use of CT has increased as the test has become more available, but there has always been reluctance to subject younger patients, particularly children, to the ionising radiation (IR) exposure of CT. In the USA, IR exposure concerns may be less of a priority given the high risk of litigation associated with misdiagnosis. However, awareness of the risks associated with radiation exposure is growing. It has been estimated that a 10-mSV CT in a 25-year-old patient is associated with a risk of induced cancer of 1 in 900 individuals and a risk of fatal cancer in 1 in 1800 individuals.[42] Contrast-induced nephropathy and contrast allergies are other recognised complications of CT scan.

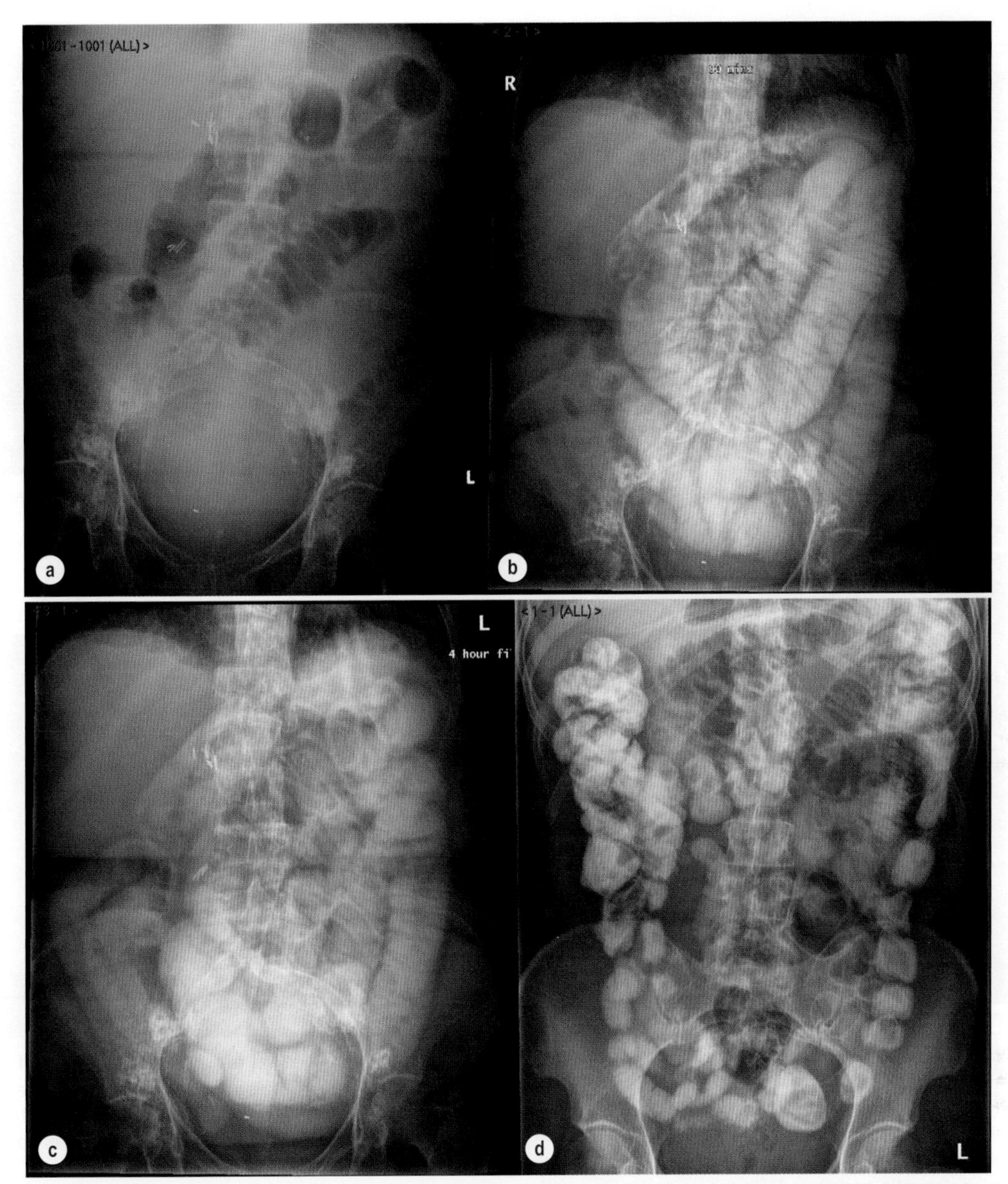

Figure 11.4 Supine abdominal radiograph in a patient with adhesive small bowel obstruction **(a)**, 90 minutes **(b)** and 4 hours **(c)** after oral administration of 50 mL of water-soluble contrast material. Note failure of contrast to reach the caecum and the obvious small bowel obstruction. Laparotomy confirmed small bowel obstruction due to adhesions. **(d)** A post-contrast 4-hour film in a patient with suspected small bowel obstruction from the plain abdominal radiograph but on this occasion contrast has reached the colon by 4 hours and no surgery was required.

However, there is good evidence that CT is accurate across a range of diagnoses. It is sufficiently reliable to allow appropriate triage of acute abdomen patients in the ED (particularly by non-surgeons),[43] improves the accuracy of clinical diagnosis[44,45] and has a demonstrable impact on patient management plans in a substantial proportion of cases, both by avoiding admission but also by prompting immediate surgery in equivocal cases (Figs. 11.8–11.10).[46,47]

CT is highly accurate in diagnosing acute appendicitis. In one randomised trial, mandatory CT was associated with a negative appendicectomy rate (NAR) of 3% compared with 14% where CT was used selectively.[48] A recent meta-analysis comprising 26 cohort studies and two randomised trials concluded that CT was associated with a reduced NAR compared with clinical assessment alone (8.7% vs 16.7%); this benefit was particularly apparent in women.[49] On the other hand, a USA single institution review over 10 years found that increased use of CT from 18% (1998) to 93% (2007) of cases was associated with reduced NAR only in women under 45 years of age.[50] Although CT is accurate in acute appendicitis, in view of the concerns regarding radiation in a predominantly young patient group, selective use in cases where the clinical picture is unclear is a sensible policy.

The impact of widespread use of CT on other clinical outcomes is less clear. In a comparison of CT diagnosis before and after emergency laparotomy in 361 adult patients, the CT report was judged inaccurate in 43 (12%) cases, which included five negative laparotomies.[51] Thus although CT was not infallible, the contemporary negative laparotomy rate was 10-fold lower than in series from 30 years ago. This observation seems to be supported by other studies, in

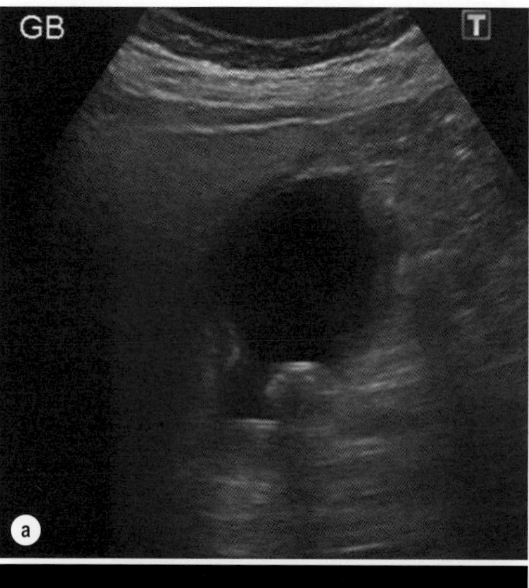

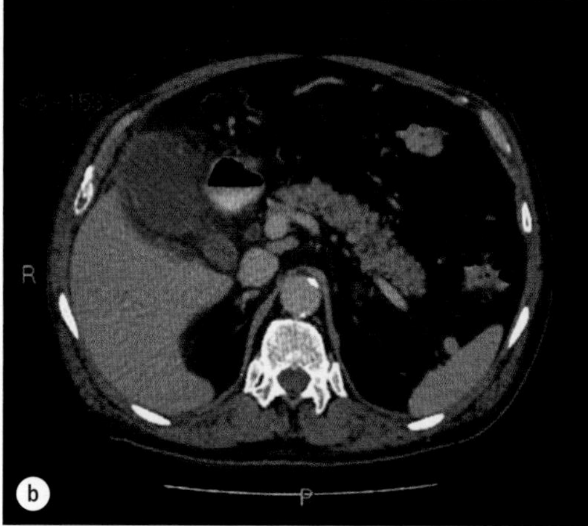

Figure 11.5 **(a)** Ultrasound image of acute cholecystitis due to gallstones. Note the characteristic acoustic shadowing from the impacted gallstone, with associated features of gallbladder distension and wall thickening. There may also be evidence of pericholecystic fluid. **(b)** CT scan of patient with acute cholecystitis following equivocal ultrasound scan. This image demonstrates gallbladder distension, wall thickening and pericholecystic oedema. (With thanks to Dr Domenyk Brown, Consultant Radiologist, Western General Hospital, Edinburgh.)

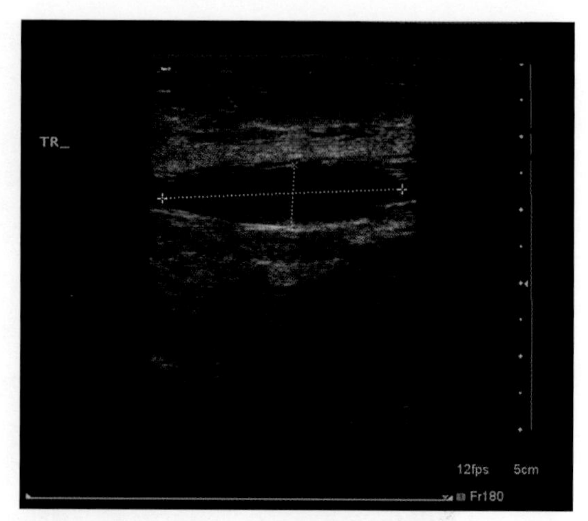

Figure 11.7 Ultrasound of the abdominal wall demonstrating a rectus sheath haematoma.

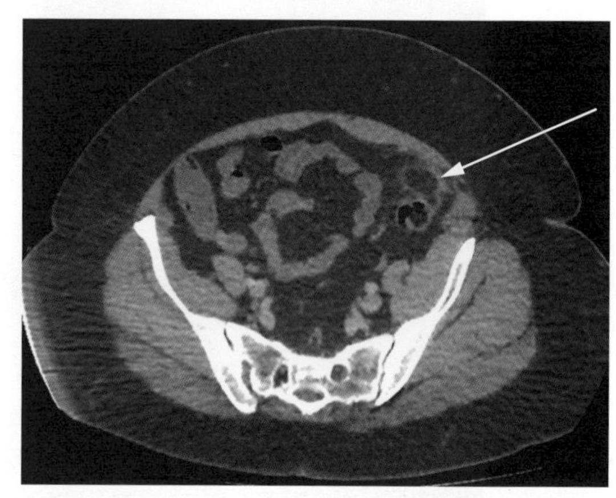

Figure 11.8 This patient presented with left iliac fossa pain and localised tenderness to palpation suggestive of acute sigmoid diverticulitis. CT shows epiploic appendagitis (*arrowed;* note the colon immediately below the arrowed area of inflammation is normal), which does not require hospital admission and is treated with simple analgesia. (With thanks to Dr Tom Blankenstein, Specialty Trainee in Radiology, Western General Hospital, Edinburgh.)

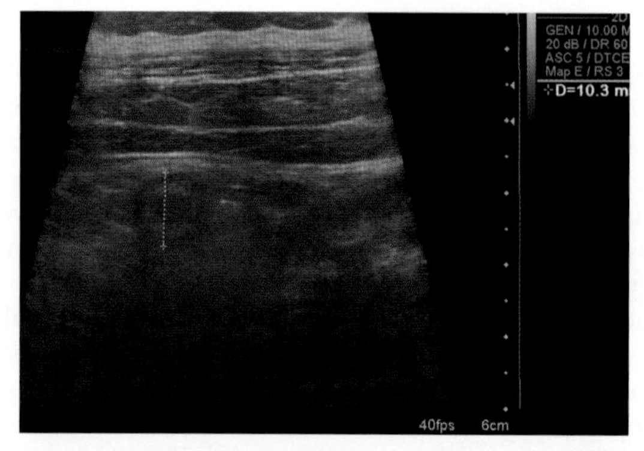

Figure 11.6 Ultrasound examination on a patient with acute appendicitis. Note the non-compressible thick-walled hollow organ (appendix) beneath the probe.

which much of the benefit of CT was to reduce the number of patients deemed to require urgent surgery compared with clinical assessment alone.[47]

Sala et al.[52] conducted a randomised controlled trial of routine CT versus standard clinical assessment in 205 patients with acute abdominal pain. Although the diagnostic accuracy was higher in the CT group, there was no difference in length of hospital stay or mortality. Ng et al.[53] also showed no significant difference in length of stay in a similar randomised trial of 120 patients, but there were fewer missed serious diagnoses in the routine imaging group. A randomised trial in 300 patients with acute abdominal pain compared selective investigation with routine CT: length of stay and treatment costs were significantly higher in the CT group.[54] However, the same group found in a subsequent

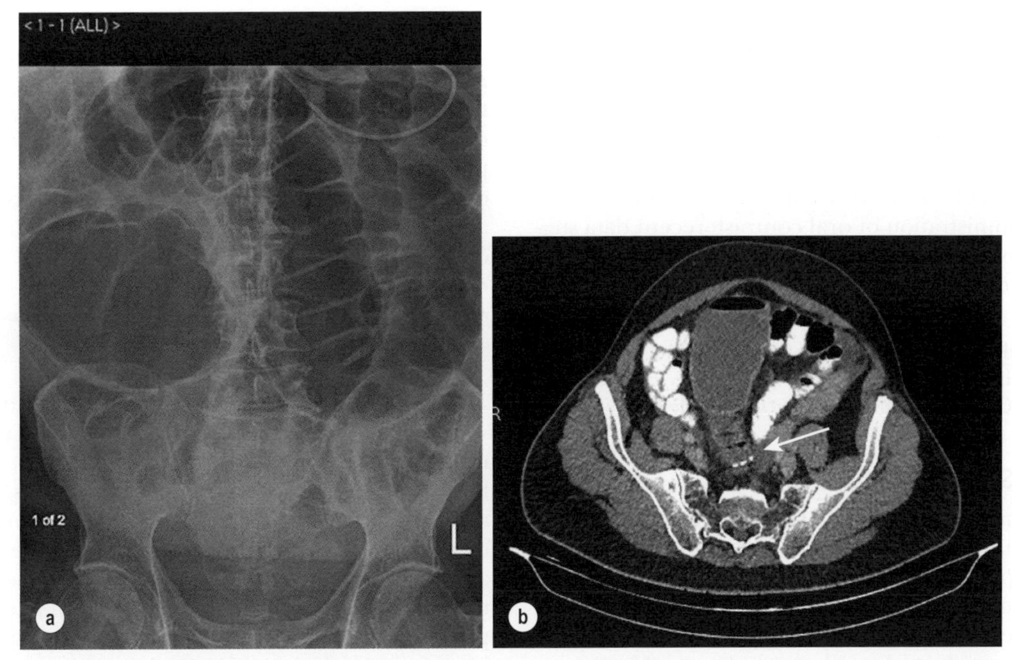

Figure 11.9 CT not diagnostic in this case of acute large bowel obstruction 18 months after laparoscopic anterior resection for sigmoid adenocarcinoma **(a)**. CT showed obstruction at the anastomosis suggesting anastomotic stricture (*arrow*) **(b)**. Laparotomy revealed a volvulus of the transverse colon under the descending colon, creating a 360-degree twist at the anastomosis and rendering it ischaemic.

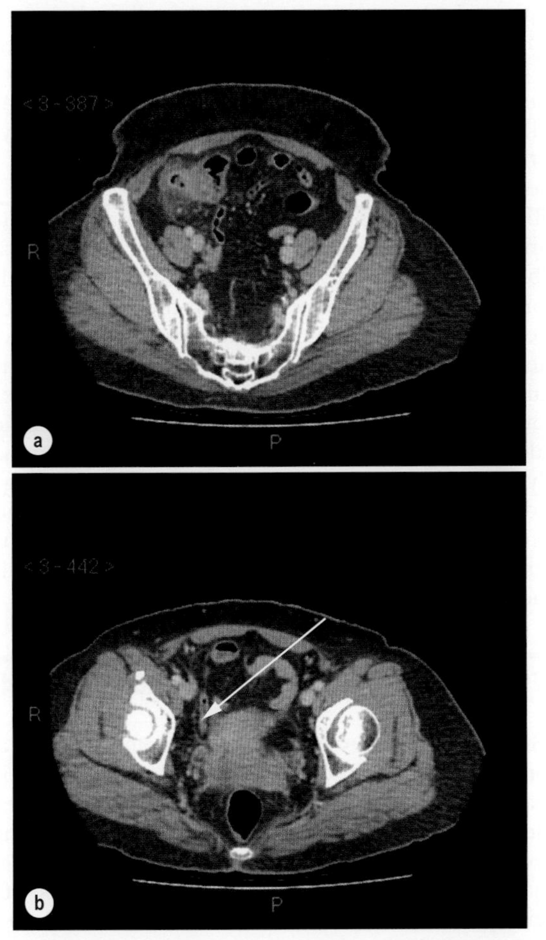

Figure 11.10 CT images of caecal acute diverticulitis **(a)** in a 56-year-old woman presenting with right iliac fossa pain; note clear views of the normal appendix (*arrow*) in **(b)**.

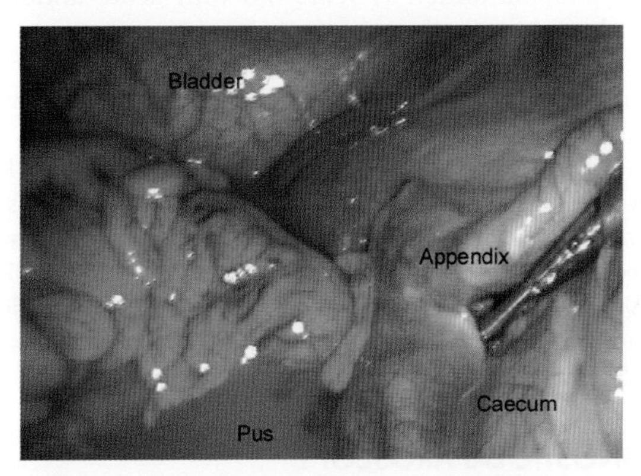

Figure 11.11 Laparoscopy showing an acutely inflamed appendix with pelvic peritonitis.

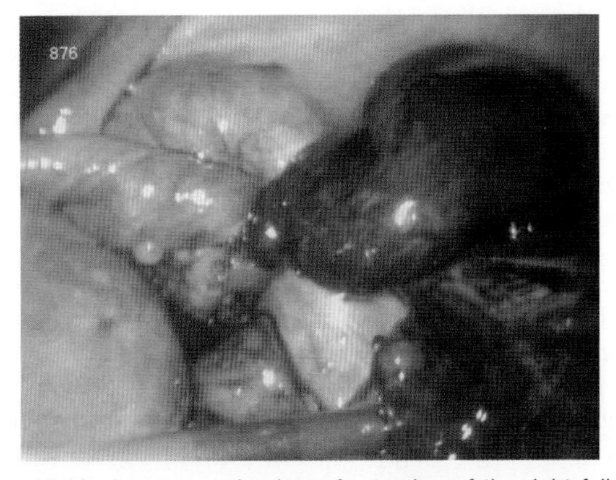

Figure 11.12 Laparoscopic view of a torsion of the right fallopian tube with ischaemia of the distal tube and ovary.

study that as well as increasing diagnostic accuracy, routine CT increased the confidence to treat operatively compared with the selective imaging group.[55]

As technological innovation continues, both IR dose and time delays in obtaining urgent CT are being reduced. Low-dose CT can give comparable results to standard CT protocols,[56] while some of the CT-associated delay can be reduced by avoiding administration of oral contrast; recent data suggests omitting oral contrast does not reduce diagnostic power in acute abdomen assessment.[57]

✓✓ Routine CT scan in acute abdominal pain does not reduce mortality, complications or length of stay compared with selective CT imaging and is not recommended.[52]

MAGNETIC RESONANCE IMAGING

Magnetic resonance imaging (MRI) is a highly sensitive and specific examination in acute abdominal pain.[58] It avoids IR but is more expensive, takes longer and is less readily available than CT in most settings. Patients with claustrophobia struggle to tolerate the examination, and it is contraindicated in patients with implanted metal/devices. Most experience has been obtained in children and younger adults, including pregnancy, where it is effective in diagnosis of a range of conditions including appendicitis.[59] In a UK series of 468 patients under 60 years old with acute abdominal pain selected for further imaging after surgical review, overall diagnostic accuracy of MRI was 99%.[60] As yet, there are no randomised data on its use or cost-effectiveness in assessment of the acute abdomen.

Magnetic resonance cholangiopancreatography (MRCP) has a key role in evaluating the biliary tree in patients presenting with symptomatic gallstones, being effective in demonstrating common bile duct stones with a sensitivity of > 90%. It has the obvious advantage over endoscopic retrograde cholangiopancreatography of being non-invasive. MRCP is discussed in more detail in Chapter 14.

DIAGNOSTIC LAPAROSCOPY

The role of diagnostic laparoscopy has become less clear as accurate diagnostic imaging becomes more widely available and minimally invasive techniques replace open surgery for appendicectomy. It has been used most frequently in the management of women of child-bearing age presenting with lower abdominal or right lower quadrant pain, where NSAP and acute gynaecological conditions widen the differential diagnosis compared with males of equivalent age. A meta-analysis of four randomised trials (811 patients) comparing laparoscopy with active observation found that laparoscopy was associated with a reduced number of patients leaving hospital without a diagnosis but did not affect complications, readmission rates or length of stay.[61] Its role depends on availability of imaging locally, but in general it should only be used where imaging is inconclusive and high suspicion of an urgent cause remains (Figs. 11.11 and 11.12). This patient group remains a challenge for the emergency general surgeon: routine CT scan would be costly, is less accurate in diagnosing pelvic organ pathology and IR dose remains a concern; diagnostic laparoscopy is invasive, costly and carries a (albeit low) risk of operative complications; active observation is time-consuming for the clinician and resource-heavy. An interesting observation comes from national data from England comparing readmission rates after diagnostic laparoscopy alone versus laparoscopic normal appendicectomy: readmission within 1 year occurred in 33% of the cohort (19 000 patients), but laparoscopic normal appendicectomy was associated with substantially reduced odds of readmission.[62]

SPECIAL POPULATIONS

Two groups are worth highlighting for consideration.

The acute abdomen in pregnancy is a relatively common presentation. Delay in diagnosis and treatment can have poor outcomes for mother and foetus. Assessment is complicated by the physiological and anatomical changes of pregnancy: uterine enlargement displaces other organs and may alter clinical signs; the abdominal wall is lax; pregnancy often induces a mild physiological leucocytosis; both patient and clinicians may be reluctant to use radiological investigations due to concern about the foetal impact of IR. Ultrasound is the imaging modality of choice, but has limitations as noted above. MRI avoids IR and appears to be very accurate; its limitation is availability.[63] CT should be avoided if possible but if there is sufficient clinical concern, particularly given the factors above prejudicing clinical assessment, diagnostic imaging should not be withheld. The American College of Obstetricians and Gynecologists' Committee on Obstetric Practice has issued summary recommendations for diagnostic imaging procedures during pregnancy and lactation.[64]

Elderly patients may also be difficult to assess.[65] They exhibit atypical presentations due to impaired ability to mount normal physiological responses such as tachycardia or abdominal guarding as a consequence of physical limitations, underlying comorbidity or the treatment thereof (e.g. beta-adrenoceptor antagonists, corticosteroids). Acute surgical illness may exacerbate pre-existing cognitive impairment or induce acute delirium. In view of the limitations of clinical assessment in these patients, clinicians should have a low threshold for diagnostic imaging, particularly as the range of potential diagnoses in this age group is wide. CT scan is usually the investigation of choice in the elderly patient with acute abdominal pain. In patients with severe renal impairment, non-contrast CT should be considered.[66]

PATHWAYS/GUIDELINES FOR ASSESSMENT

A USA institutional review of ED management of the acute abdomen over 35 years concluded that while diagnostic imaging had increased sixfold between 1993 and 2007 (increasing ED delays and patient charges), there had been no change in rates of hospital admission or missed surgical illness.[67]

Imaging costs continue to rise and the risks of CT-associated morbidity have been noted above. Therefore, there is a need to optimise imaging strategies in patients with acute abdominal pain in order to achieve timely identification of urgent conditions, without using imaging unnecessarily.

A systematic review of diagnostic pathways for patients presenting with acute abdominal pain found that routine imaging increased diagnostic accuracy, but was not associated with a reduction in length of stay, complication rate or mortality.[68] Similar conclusions were reached in a meta-analysis of four randomised controlled trials comparing routine CT and selective CT: there was no difference in correct diagnoses, mortality or length of hospital stay.[69]

An important prospective multicentre study examined imaging strategies in acute abdominal pain in 1101 adults. All patients underwent routine clinical assessment, plain radiography, US and CT scan. Sensitivity and specificity for detecting urgent conditions were recorded for 11 diagnostic strategies, comprising single test strategies (e.g. CT alone), conditional strategies (e.g. CT if ultrasound inconclusive), strategies defined by patient characteristics (age, BMI) and strategies driven by location of pain. CT detected more urgent diagnoses than ultrasound. The highest sensitivity was obtained by a conditional strategy of CT after negative or inconclusive ultrasonography, missing only 6% of urgent cases and reducing use of CT to 49% of cases (though to date this strategy has not been evaluated prospectively). Alternative strategies guided by BMI, age, or location of pain resulted in a loss of sensitivity.[70]

Clinical reassessment remains an important part of management of the acute abdomen, and we should not discard results from a previous era that still stand up to comparison with modern imaging.[71] The increase in patients presenting for assessment to secondary care in the UK has seen the creation of 'hot clinics' to reduce hospital admissions, with good evidence that selected patients can be managed safely in an outpatient fashion, reducing costs, with high patient satisfaction.[72,73]

In the UK, recognition that there was considerable inter-hospital variation in outcomes from emergency laparotomy led to the establishment of the National Emergency Laparotomy Audit (www.nela.org).[74] Early decision-making and use of investigations in the acute abdomen by experienced clinicians is key to improvement.[75,76] Reducing variation is also aided by following guidelines for effective practice: the Royal College of Surgeons of England and the Association of Surgeons of the Netherlands have published recommendations for management of acute abdominal pain.[1,77] The American College of Radiologists publishes regularly updated guidance developed by consensus methodology on imaging strategies in a variety of clinical presentations.[78,79] A number of guidelines for management of acute general surgical conditions are provided by the World Society of Emergency Surgeons (www.wses.org.uk). In 2010 a national guideline for management of acute appendicitis was introduced in the Netherlands, mandating preoperative imaging in all suspected cases. A snapshot audit of national practice in 2015 found that over 99% of cases underwent preoperative diagnostic imaging, with NAR of 2.2%.[80] When compared with a UK audit in which preoperative imaging took place in only one third of patients and NAR ranged up to 36%,[81] it is difficult to avoid the conclusion that the combination of practice guideline based on confirmatory imaging has been effective. Future research should help to inform effective and appropriate imaging strategies, evaluating criteria based on patient subgroups, anatomical pain location and clinical scoring systems.

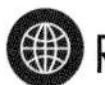 Clinical assessment has limitations even in experienced hands, therefore imaging is an essential part of the diagnostic pathway.[14,70]

Key points

- The foundations for good management of the acute abdomen are accurate history and careful examination allied to an appreciation of the wide range of surgical and non-surgical conditions that may present with abdominal pain.
- Analgesia does not mask clinical signs in assessment of the acute abdomen and should not be withheld
- Early use of water-soluble contrast in adhesive small bowel obstruction reduces the need for surgery, accurately selects patients for operative/ non-operative management and reduces length of stay
- Although clinicians are able to distinguish urgent from non-urgent conditions on clinical grounds alone, they are less good at making an accurate diagnosis
- Modern radiological imaging is highly accurate in identifying the correct diagnosis and informing choice of management by the clinician. The challenge in the acute setting is to use the available modalities effectively.

References available at http://ebooks.health.elsevier.com/

KEY REFERENCES

[11] Manterola C, Vial M, Moraga J, Astudillo P. Analgesia in patients with acute abdominal pain. Cochrane Database Syst Rev 2011;(1):CD005660

Convincing meta-analysis confirming that early use of opioid analgesia for acute abdominal pain does not adversely affect patient evaluation..

[14] Acute Abdominal Pain Study Group. Diagnostic accuracy of surgeons and trainees in assessment of patients with acute abdominal pain. Br J Surg 2016;103(10):1343–9

Diagnostic accuracy by senior clinicians was no better than by trainees and was less than 50% overall, illustrating the challenge of making a clinical diagnosis. Both groups were better at distinguishing urgent from non-urgent conditions.

[17] Bhangu A, RIFT study group. Evaluation of appendicitis risk prediction models in adults with suspected appendicitis. Br J Surg 2020;107(1):73–86

Comprehensive prospective comparison of appendicitis risk prediction models in patients presenting with acute right iliac fossa pain.

[33] Di Saverio S, Coccolini F, Galati M, Smerieri N, Biffl WL, Ansaloni L, et al. Bologna guidelines for diagnosis and management of adhesive small bowel obstruction (ASBO): 2013 update of the evidence-based guidelines from the world society of emergency surgery ASBO working group. World J Emerg Surg 2013;8(1):42

Early use of water-soluble contrast in adhesive small bowel obstruction reduces the need for surgery, accurately selects patients for operative/non-operative management and reduces length of stay.

[68] de Burlet KJ, Ing AJ, Larsen PD, Dennett ER. Systematic review of diagnostic pathways for patients presenting with acute abdominal pain. Int J Qual Health Care 2018;30(9):678–83

Early abdominal CT in patients with acute abdominal pain improves diagnostic certainty, but not length of hospital stay or 6-month mortality.

[70] Lameris W, van Randen A, van Es HW, van Heesewijk JP, van Ramshorst B, Bouma WH, et al. Imaging strategies for detection of urgent conditions in patients with acute abdominal pain: diagnostic accuracy study. BMJ 2009;338:b2431

Carefully designed study seeking to evaluate a variety of imaging strategies in acute abdominal pain.

[80] van Rossem CC, Bolmers MD, Schreinemacher MH, van Geloven AA, Bemelman WA, Snapshot Appendicitis Collaborative Study Group. Prospective nationwide outcome audit of surgery for suspected acute appendicitis. Br J Surg 2016;103(1):144–51.

Mandatory preoperative imaging in suspected acute appendicitis was associated with low negative appendicectomy rate.

[81] National Surgical Research Collaborative. Multicentre observational study of performance variation in provision and outcome of emergency appendicectomy. Br J Surg 2013;100(9):1240–52

Some contrasting results from two national audits of management of appendicitis.

Perforations of the upper gastrointestinal tract

12

Adam Frankel | Chris Deans

OVERVIEW

Perforation of the upper gastrointestinal (UGI) tract is a relatively common surgical emergency. Most cases are due to peptic ulceration, but other causes, although uncommon, may be challenging to diagnose and manage (e.g. oesophageal perforation). Perforation secondary to endoscopic procedures is also increasingly seen in recent times due to technological advancement and more widespread integration of these techniques into mainstream practice.

Perforation can be free or contained. Free perforation into a body cavity (peritoneal or pleural cavities or the mediastinum) results in gross contamination and the clinical features often correlate with the site, degree and nature of contamination. For example, free intra-abdominal perforation causes generalised abdominal pain and generalised peritonitis. The nature of the leaking contents is determined by the location of the perforation. In the UGI tract, the contamination will be microbial and chemical (e.g. acidic rich fluid from the stomach and bile-rich fluid from the duodenum). Further, the rapidity of symptom development can also correlate with the nature of the contents being leaked (chemical peritonitis results in sudden and severe pain, while the development of infection can take time).[1] Less commonly, the contamination can be contained, such as rapid 'walling-off' of an intraperitoneal perforation by the omentum, or a retroperitoneal perforation. This scenario often gives more localised clinical features and frequently results in abscess formation.

A high index of suspicion with appropriate and timely investigation will lead to early diagnosis, which has been shown to reduce length of stay, reduce the need for reintervention and a reduction in mortality.[2,3] All general surgeons should be capable of caring for patients with gastroduodenal perforations, but better outcomes are seen with more complex cases, such as oesophageal perforation, when they are cared for in an experienced centre.[4]

This chapter will outline the main principles of management of perforations of the UGI tract, including diagnosis, initial management and surgical techniques, follow-up care, and complications. Areas of controversy will be highlighted and novel techniques will be considered. The specific management of anastomotic leak is covered elsewhere in this book series.

EPIDEMIOLOGY AND PATHOGENESIS

Perforations of the UGI tract affect the oesophagus, stomach or duodenum. The aetiology varies according to site. The causes of UGI tract perforation may be considered according to the relationship with the gastrointestinal tract: intra-luminal, mural or extra-luminal or classified according to underlying pathology (Table 12.1). Perforations may be due to disease (peptic ulcer disease [PUD] or malignancy), iatrogenic (following endoscopy or gastric band erosion), following foreign body ingestion (batteries or caustic liquids), medication-related (non-steroidal anti-inflammatory drugs [NSAIDs]) or spontaneous (Boerhaave's syndrome). Peptic ulcer perforations occurring in the duodenum and stomach are by far the most common.

PEPTIC ULCER DISEASE

PUD is by far the commonest cause of UGI perforation with an annual incidence of 4–14 per 100 000 individuals.[5] However, the incidence is reducing, presumably related to a better understanding and treatment of *Helicobacter pylori* and reduced rates of smoking.[6–8] Approximately 98% of peptic ulcers are located in or around the pylorus with 80% occurring in the first part of the duodenum. Ulcers located elsewhere, especially in the proximal stomach, raise the possibility of malignant aetiology and multiple ulcers may suggest less common conditions such as Zollinger-Ellison syndrome. Peptic ulceration occurs due to an imbalance between the gastroduodenal mucosal protective defences and potentially damaging forces. *H. pylori* has been identified in 80–90% of patients with duodenal ulceration. *H. pylori* increases damaging forces by increasing local gastric acid secretion contributing to the pathogenesis of ulcer formation. Drugs, particularly NSAIDs, are associated with 20–30% of peptic ulcers. Smoking and alcohol are also implicated due to the adverse effect on protective mucosal defences.

CLINICAL FEATURES

In general, patients will present with an acute illness. Epigastric pain usually predominates which is often sudden onset. There may be a history of dull epigastric pain in the

Table 12.1 Causes of perforation of the upper gastrointestinal tract

Oesophageal	Iatrogenic: endoscopic (especially therapeutic endoscopy) Trans-oesophageal ECHO catheter placement Barotrauma (Boerhaave's syndrome) Malignant Secondary to foreign body ingestion/caustic ingestion (e.g. batteries or bleach) Trauma (mainly penetrating injuries)
Gastric	Peptic ulcer disease Malignant (adenocarcinoma, lymphoma, GIST, NET) Iatrogenic (e.g. endoscopic mucosal resection, gastric band erosion)
Duodenal	Peptic ulcer disease Iatrogenic (e.g. ERCP) Foreign body Drugs (e.g. biologicals)

ERCP, endoscopic retrograde cholangiopancreatography; *GIST*, gastrointestinal stromal tumour; *NET*, neuroendocrine tumour.

preceding days or weeks. Diaphragmatic irritation causes pain to radiate to the shoulders. Generalised abdominal pain implies free perforation and generalised peritonitis. Some patients, especially the elderly or immunocompromised, may have surprisingly little pain and few signs. Other features may include nausea, vomiting, history of dyspepsia, or small volume haematemesis. History taking should include a detailed drug history and documentation of comorbidity and a pre-morbid functional assessment. Many patients will appear unwell and exhibit systemic signs and symptoms of sepsis or shock, including fever, sweating, hypotension and clamminess. Abdominal examination will usually reveal generalised guarding due to peritonitis. Vital signs should be assessed and initial supportive measures commenced in a timely and systematic manner.

Differential diagnoses include many conditions that present with an acute abdomen, such as acute pancreatitis, perforated appendicitis and intestinal ischaemia. A plain chest X-ray may demonstrate subphrenic free gas, but this sign is only evident in around 70% of cases (Fig. 12.1a).[9] Computed tomography (CT) is the gold standard for the investigation of suspected UGI perforation[10] (Fig. 12.1b). The presence of pneumoperitoneum and free fluid is diagnostic and may even help locate the site of perforation. Patterns of pneumoperitoneum may help predict upper versus lower gastrointestinal perforation (e.g. periportal free air is suggestive of UGI perforation) and the location of inflammatory changes and/or wall discontinuity may also be visible on the images.[11–13] Oral contrast is not routinely used in the initial imaging of the acute abdomen but may be useful in selected cases where the diagnosis remains in doubt or an attempt at non-operative management is appropriate and it is necessary to demonstrate that there is no evidence of ongoing leakage.

MANAGEMENT

Initial management should focus on resuscitation in a systematic process. In some instances, it may be necessary to initiate resuscitative measures at the same time as making the initial clinical assessment. Consideration should be given to involve critical care teams early. Critical care support is indicated in the presence of organ dysfunction, where there is evidence of abnormal physiology (e.g. elevated serum lactate), and where the patient is predicted high risk on relevant scoring systems (e.g. NELA or P-POSSUM risk predictors). Oxygen therapy should be administered, intravenous access achieved and adequate doses of parenteral analgesia should be provided. Intravenous fluids should be prescribed and broad-spectrum antibiotics should be commenced as soon as possible in accordance with the principles of the 'Sepsis 6' care bundle.[14] Surgery is the mainstay treatment for most patients with perforated PUD. Patients should proceed to theatre as soon as is practical and following appropriate resuscitation. Delay to surgery is a clear prognostic factor and mortality increases by approximately 2.5% per hour after admission.[15]

✔✔ Delay to definitive treatment is an important determinant of poor outcome for patients with UGI tract perforation. Delay to surgery is an established adverse prognostic factor with mortality rates increasing for every hour of delay. These findings are equally valid for the management of both peptic perforation and oesophageal perforation. Every effort should be taken to ensure patients are diagnosed, resuscitated and receive definitive treatment in a timely fashion.

Omental patch repair and thorough peritoneal lavage are the principles of surgical management and are sufficient for most patients. The patch is usually a well vascularised omental pedicle but in instances where there is paucity of omentum or it is absent, the falciform ligament may be used.[16] It is the author's opinion that no attempt should be made to primarily close the ulcer but simply to cover with a viable omental patch (Fig. 12.2). A thorough and extensive peritoneal washout is vital. The value of placing an abdominal drain remains controversial, although there is some evidence that drainage provides no benefit and may indeed be harmful.[17] A drain should therefore be used selectively.

There are several studies including a meta-analysis of randomised controlled trials as well as a large propensity score-matched series favouring minimally invasive surgery over conventional open surgery for selected patients.[18,19] These reviews confirm a significant reduction in postoperative morbidity (particularly surgical site infection rates), reduced length of hospital stay and a possible mortality benefit. Indeed, there is now sufficient evidence that laparoscopic repair is the standard of care in centres with appropriate equipment and expertise. However, appropriate patient selection is vital to ensure good outcomes. Limitations of minimally invasive surgery are the requirement for a pneumoperitoneum, difficulty removing large food debris and possibly longer operating times. Therefore, patients who are clinically unstable, the elderly patient and in situations where there is gross peritoneal contamination may be better managed with open surgery.[15] Whatever approach is used, the priority should always be the provision of safe and effective surgery.

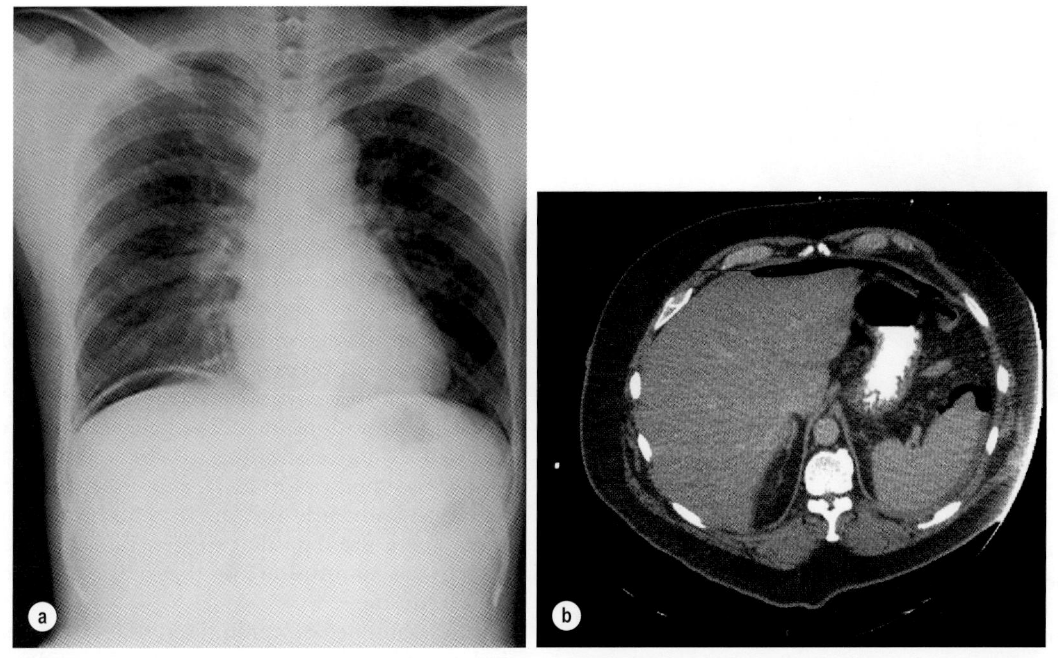

Figure 12.1 (a) Chest X-ray demonstrating right subphrenic free gas secondary to a perforated peptic ulcer. (b) Transverse section of an abdominal computed tomography scan demonstrating free intraperitoneal gas (*arrow*) in a patient presenting with a perforated peptic ulcer with normal erect chest X-ray appearances.

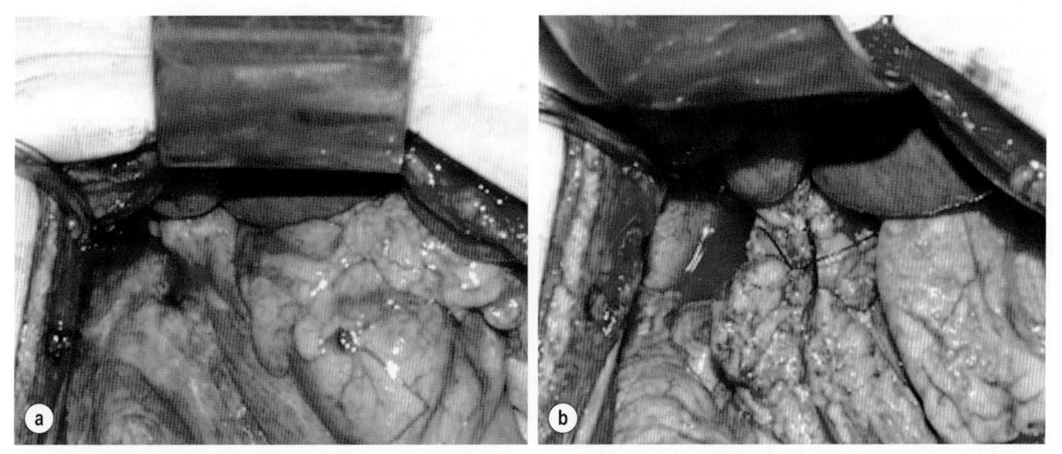

Figure 12.2 (a) A small perforation at the juxtapyloric area. (b) Pedicle omental patch repair on the perforation site secured with absorbable sutures.

✔✔ There is some evidence that minimally invasive surgery has advantages over open surgery in the management of perforated PUD. Laparoscopic surgery is associated with a reduction in wound complications and length of hospital stay without any difference in leak rate, abscess formation or mortality. However, it is important to emphasise that not all patients are suited to a minimally invasive approach and appropriate patient selection is vital to ensure a good outcome.

Gastric ulcers should always be biopsied as they carry a small risk of malignancy. In some circumstances ulcer excision may be a better option where there is sufficient redundant stomach to allow limited resection of the ulcer to ensure healthy tissue for closure and to maximise the amount of tissue for histological assessment. This remains the preferred approach even in circumstances where there is a high index of suspicion that the gastric perforation is malignant. Retrospective analyses demonstrate increased morbidity and mortality when a gastrectomy is performed rather than a simple repair and urgent rather than elective gastrectomy results in an increased positive surgical margin rate, increased inpatient mortality and decreased overall survival.[20,21] Major oncological resections are best done electively after normal physiology is restored, appropriate work-up including staging is completed, and the full range of treatment options has been discussed at a multidisciplinary team meeting (such as considering a role for preoperative chemotherapy). Similar oncological outcomes including overall survival can be achieved for selected patients by adopting this approach when comparing perforated and non-perforated gastric cancers treated with a curative resection, suggesting there is no reason to rush.[20,22]

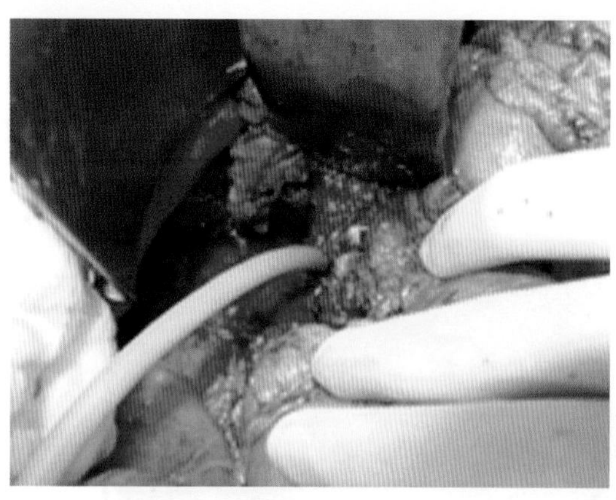

Figure 12.3 A catheter duodenostomy for managing a difficult duodenal stump.

✔ For perforated gastric ulcers, a simple repair (omental patch or local ulcer excision) is the best management option even when malignancy is suspected. There is no role for attempted cancer resection in this setting.

However, there are circumstances where a simple omental patch or limited ulcer excision is not possible or is considered likely to fail. This may occur with large duodenal perforations where the defect may be several centimetres and the surrounding tissue may be extremely friable. There are several procedures described to manage this scenario. The simplest procedure is to create a controlled fistula by placing a tube drain or T-tube into the duodenal defect and approximating the surrounding tissue (Fig. 12.3). This creates a definite leak and therefore should probably be reserved for instances where the patient is very unwell and abnormal physiology dictates a simpler and faster approach. It may be a better option to attempt to repair the duodenum, possibly with a double layer repair or an overlying omental patch, and placing adjacent drains. If the repair leaks, then the drains will create a controlled fistula. In some circumstances, it might be appropriate to consider a resection of the ulcer tissue. This would normally involve an antrectomy with Roux-en-Y reconstruction. This procedure carries the advantage of removing the ulcerated tissue and allowing earlier introduction of enteral nutrition. However, managing the duodenal stump remains challenging and this procedure should only be considered in patients with normal physiology. There are many other techniques described to manage this challenging scenario including a Finney pyloroplasty and creating a duodenojejunostomy. Many of these procedures are now considered historical. Selecting the best approach for an individual patient is the key to maximising chances of a favourable outcome.

NON-OPERATIVE MANAGEMENT

Non-operative management of peptic ulcer perforation may be appropriate for selected patients.[23] Patients who are clinically well, with normal physiology and vital signs and without evidence of peritonitis, may be considered suitable for a trial of non-operative management. Cross-sectional imaging with oral contrast is also useful to support a conservative treatment approach. Minimal peritoneal contamination and no leak of oral contrast would favour a successful outcome.[15] Patients should be maintained nil by mouth, have nasogastric drainage, intravenous fluids, intravenous proton pump inhibitors (PPI) and antibiotics. Frequent review by an experienced clinician is mandatory and any deterioration in the condition of the patient should be interpreted as a failure of non-operative management. Up to 70% of patients may avoid surgery by adopting this strategy and with appropriate patient selection, although it is important to note that non-operative management in patients over 70 years old is associated with a poorer outcome.[6,23] There is no role for endoscopic management, such as application of clips, in the management of these patients.[15]

Although there are relatively few trials of PPI in relation to UGI perforations including PUD, there is a considerable body of evidence showing a large reduction in bleeding and re-bleeding risk in PUD, and it seems logical that there would be both early and late benefits in relation to perforation. There are data that suggest intermittent dosing is as effective as an infusion and that oral is as effective as intravenous dosing.[24,25]

In the absence of randomised trials, experienced clinical judgement and local practice should guide antimicrobial choice.[26] Antibiotics are generally continued for 7 days and should be administered by the intravenous route until oral intake is established. In most centres, antifungal agents are reserved for high-risk patients (such as immunosuppressed patients) or those with a positive culture and clinically severe infection.[15]

COMPLICATIONS AND FOLLOW-UP CARE

A leak from the omental patch repair suggests technical failure and subsequent management will be determined by the condition of the patient and whether the leak is controlled through drainage. Optimisation of non-operative management and the use of additional radiologically placed drains may be sufficient. In other instances, a return to the operating theatre will be mandatory. Special consideration should be given to addressing nutritional support during this time. Intra-peritoneal abscess formation usually presents with deterioration in the clinical condition of the patient. Collections most commonly occur in the subphrenic space or pelvis. These manifest with features of sepsis (fever, tachycardia) and signs and symptoms relating to the site of the abscess, e.g. diarrhoea secondary to a pelvic collection or shoulder pain and respiratory compromise due to a subphrenic collection. Small abscesses can be treated medically, whilst larger ones are better suited to percutaneous drainage.

We favour empirical treatment for *H. pylori* for every patient who presents with peptic ulcer perforation. All patients should receive a course of oral eradication therapy with PPI treatment. Efficacy of eradication should be confirmed at 6–8 weeks with a urea breath test or faecal antigen test. Endoscopy is indicated for all gastric ulcers 6–8 weeks post-discharge to check for healing, and repeat biopsies should be taken irrespective of the results of the initial biopsies taken at the time of surgery. Most patients will likely require long-term PPI treatment and other possible risk factors should be addressed prior to discharge, such as smoking cessation and stopping NSAID use.

OTHER CAUSES OF GASTRIC AND DUODENAL PERFORATION

PUD is by far the commonest cause of perforation of the stomach and duodenum. Less common causes are listed in Table 12.1. Perforated malignancy is more common with ulcerated tumours and is seen in adenocarcinoma, lymphoma, gastrointestinal stromal tumour (GIST) and neuroendocrine tumour (NET) in order of incidence. Perforation by an endoscope can be due to the instrument itself, barotrauma, or more commonly, a therapeutic procedure such as endoscopic retrograde cholangiopancreatography (ERCP), polypectomy, endoscopic mucosal resection (EMR) or endoscopic submucosal dissection (ESD), thermal treatment (e.g. argon plasma coagulation), or foreign body removal. Iatrogenic injuries are conceptually different to other causes. The perforation is often recognised immediately or soon after and as the patient is fasted, the degree of contamination is reduced. Perforation following ERCP may be more challenging as the site of perforation is often retroperitoneal. Therefore, a high index of suspicion is required for patients who are not quite right following an ERCP and timely cross-sectional imaging should be undertaken, usually with oral contrast. More detailed management of ERCP-related perforation is described elsewhere in this book series, but the same principles described above for the management of perforated PUD should be followed irrespective of the aetiology of the perforation.

OESOPHAGEAL PERFORATION

Oesophageal perforation can be very challenging but is comparatively rare. The Finnish National Registry reports an incidence of 1/100 000 person years.[4] The majority are iatrogenic and usually occur secondary to endoscopic interventions. Even then the risk of perforation remains very low; a single centre over a 10-year period involving nearly 150 000 endoscopic procedures reported a perforation rate of 0.02%.[27] However, risk varies with procedure type and expertise.[28–30]

Less common causes of oesophageal perforation are spontaneous secondary to barotrauma (Boerhaave's syndrome), perforated malignancy or foreign body ingestion (including caustic liquid ingestion) (Table 12.2).[3] Traumatic injury to the oesophagus is extremely rare. Early diagnosis and treatment is crucial to improve outcomes following oesophageal perforation; mortality is 10–25% if treatment is commenced within 24 hours, rising to 40–60% if commenced beyond 48 hours.[31] Outcomes are further improved when cases are treated in high-volume centres involving teams that are more familiar in the management of these complex cases.[4]

CLINICAL FEATURES

Pain is the predominant feature and may correlate with the site of perforation; for example, cervical oesophageal perforation may produce neck pain and intra-thoracic oesophageal perforation often results in retrosternal/interscapular pain with pleuritic pain. Dysphagia and odynophagia are often present and prior history of other gastrointestinal symptoms should be sought as they may indicate an underlying pathology. Sepsis may be the presenting feature in patients with delayed presentation and some patients may be acutely unwell with features of septic shock. Other patients may present several days following a perforation and appear relatively well and only exhibit respiratory symptoms such as pleuritic chest pain and dyspnoea. Examination may reveal the presence of subcutaneous emphysema, pneumothorax or pleural effusion. Vital signs should be assessed and initial supportive measures commenced in a timely and systematic manner.

Table 12.2 Causes of oesophageal perforation

Endoscopic (per oral endoscopic myotomy [POEM], dilatation, stent, endoscopic mucosal resection [EMR] or submucosal dissection [ESD], thermal treatment [argon plasma coagulation, photodynamic therapy, Nd:YAG laser], sclerotherapy, tube insertion, foreign body removal, diverticulum)
Boerhaave's syndrome (barotrauma secondary to forceful retching against a closed glottis)
Malignancy (carcinoma, GIST, NET, lymphoma; can be spontaneous or after treatment (chemotherapy, radiotherapy, stent)
Trauma (intraluminal foreign body, external blunt or penetrating, caustic ingestion)

GIST, gastrointestinal stromal tumour; *NET*, neuroendocrine tumour.

A high index of clinical suspicion is vital to ensure timely diagnosis and management. The oesophageal perforation may be immediately apparent, for example at the time of endoscopic dilatation, but for other patients further investigation is required to confirm the diagnosis. The key step is to consider the diagnosis at the outset, particularly for patients who do not appear quite as they should after an endoscopic procedure. A plain chest X-ray may show a hydropneumothorax which is pathognomonic of the condition (Fig. 12.4). In other situations, there may only be a subtle sign of mediastinal free gas that is easily missed without specifically looking for it. CT with oral contrast has a low sensitivity for perforation (19–42%), but if extravasation is present, it is highly specific and can be very helpful to localise the defect[32,33] (Fig. 12.5). CT also provides details on surrounding anatomy, degree of contamination and does not require the patient to be able to sit up and comply with instructions. Fluoroscopy is a more sensitive modality for demonstrating a perforation and provides good anatomical localisation of the defect, but the patient must be able to swallow on demand and protect their airway. Endoscopy is very sensitive and therefore is also a useful modality to exclude oesophageal perforation. When perforation is present, it can precisely define the site of the defect and identify whether there is an associated stricture present[3] (Fig. 12.6). Gas insufflation at the time of endoscopy may result in a tension pneumothorax and therefore it is often prudent to place a chest drain in patients with evidence of a pneumothorax prior to performing the endoscopy.

MANAGEMENT

Initial management should follow the processes already described for peptic ulcers. Prompt recognition of the

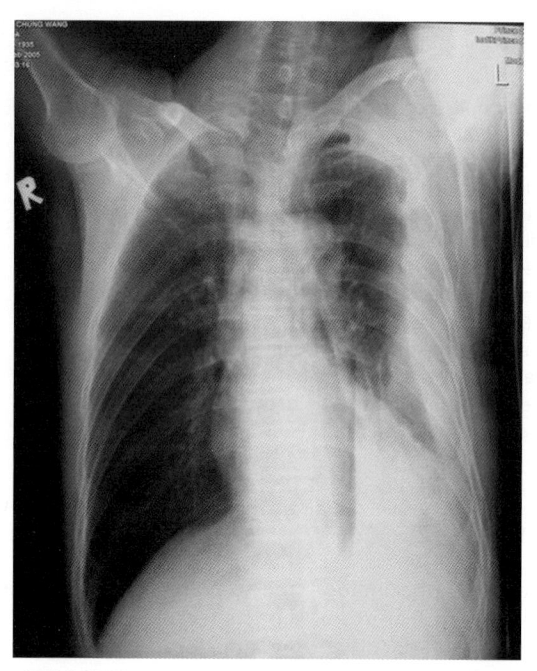

Figure 12.4 Plain radiograph of a patient with surgical emphysema in the neck due to a mid-oesophageal perforation following endoscopic ultrasound examination and transmural biopsy.

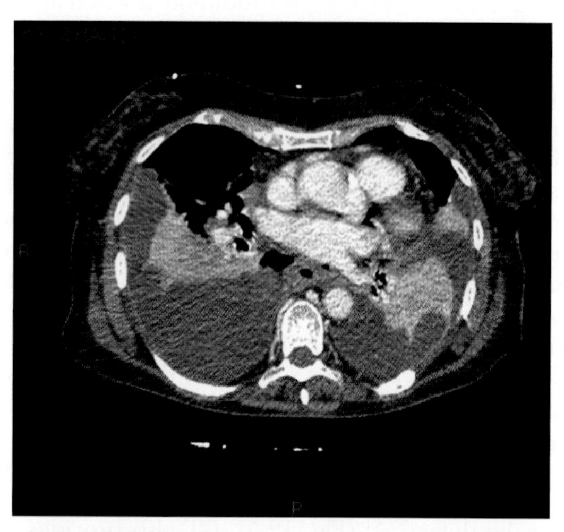

Figure 12.5 Bilateral hydropneumothoraces and mediastinal free gas secondary to Boerhaave's syndrome.

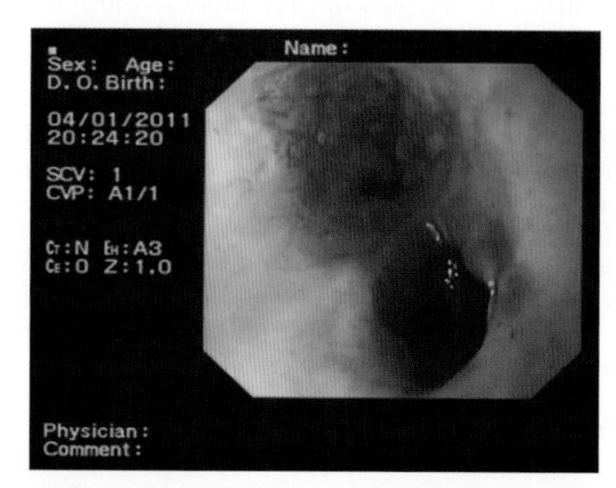

Figure 12.6 Endoscopic view of the distal oesophagus showing a perforation in a patient with Boerhaave's syndrome.

unwell patient should result in a focus on resuscitation with consideration given to early involvement of critical care teams. Patients should be kept nil by mouth, broad-spectrum antibiotics and antifungal agents administered and intravenous PPI treatment commenced. A chest drain should be placed into patients with a hydropneumothorax—the presence of enteric contents into the drain bottle confirms the diagnosis of oesophageal perforation. Subsequent management is heavily guided by patient factors, aetiology of the perforation and the time delay to diagnosis. Patient comorbidity and pre-morbid functional status should be considered in deciding management strategy. As with all aspects of surgical care, good practice dictates that decisions to limit treatment should be ideally taken in conjunction with the patients and their family. Many of these patients are old, frail and comorbid, and not all treatment approaches will be appropriate.

The second consideration in management decision-making relates to the underlying aetiology. Spontaneous oesophageal perforation with significant pleural contamination usually mandates surgery. In contrast, an endoscopic perforation following dilatation of a malignant stricture is better managed with a stent. These specific scenarios will be discussed in more detail later in this chapter.

The final consideration is the time delay from perforation to diagnosis. There is clear evidence that a longer delay to definitive treatment is associated with worse outcome.[34] In some instances, the patient is responsible for the delay in diagnosis due to delayed presentation. Patients often fit into two categories within this group; one group of patients are extremely unwell with sepsis and shock and account for the poor outcome for these patients. The second group are relatively well and often have a contained collection and have proven themselves to be likely survivors. In other circumstances, the delay in diagnosis and hence delay to definitive treatment is usually due to a lack of clinical appreciation. Once again a high index of clinical suspicion is vital to ensure timely diagnosis and management to ensure a good outcome for these patients.

Some authors have proposed a severity scoring system to aid management decision-making for patients with oesophageal perforation. The Pittsburgh Severity Score is a clinical scoring system that aims to stratify patients into low-, medium- and high-risk groups and the authors go on to propose a treatment algorithm according to the severity score.[35] As is the case with many scoring systems, there are variable reports of usefulness within the clinical setting and the true value may lie in facilitating comparison of outcomes between different centres.

Between 1996 and 2007, Finnish registry data reported 90-day mortality following oesophageal perforation was 22% with 5-year mortality of 46%.[4] Early mortality was similar with benign and malignant causes, while unsurprisingly, malignancy had a worse prognosis at later time points. 'Invasive treatment' was necessary for 41% of oesophageal perforations (31% endoscopic stenting and 69% underwent surgery). The proportion of patients receiving stents as definitive management increased with time. The evidence for non-surgical management remains relatively sparse and appropriate patient selection remains the most important determinant for a successful outcome.

OPERATIVE MANAGEMENT

The general principles of surgery, whatever the underlying aetiology, are debridement, washout, drainage and nutrition. Following appropriate resuscitation and chest drain insertion, a lateral thoracotomy is usually required with single lung ventilation. The site of perforation is often readily identified. All devitalised tissue should be debrided and a thorough washout of the pleural cavity and mediastinum should be undertaken. Several techniques are described to manage the perforation and include primary closure of the defect, patching the defect with a vascularised pedicle of tissue (such as an intercostal muscle flap), oesophageal diversion with an oesophagostomy, and even performing an oesophagectomy.[34] It is the author's preference to close the defect around a drain, such as a large-calibre T-tube, to create a controlled fistula. Additional drains are then placed around the site of repair. A nasogastric tube can be advanced into the stomach at the time of surgery to ensure effective gastric drainage. A feeding jejunostomy is then sited through a mini-laparotomy to establish good access for enteral nutrition postoperatively. Generally, these procedures are performed as open procedures but in experienced centres, minimally invasive techniques have been described.[36]

NON-OPERATIVE MANAGEMENT

The success of non-operative management depends very much on appropriate patient selection. Candidates for conservative treatment may declare themselves due to frailty, comorbidity or critical illness as being unsuitable for surgery. For other patients, an attempt at non-operative management may be considered in patients with no features of sepsis and imaging suggests that there is minimal pleural or mediastinal contamination. Alternatively, some patients may present several days after the perforation and remain generally well but have a contained collection. These patients will require radiological drainage (often multiple), endoscopic procedures (often multiple) and nutritional support. Non-operative management of oesophageal perforation requires high levels of expertise and constitutes a significant workload.[37] It should not be viewed as an easier option when compared with surgery.

ENDOSCOPIC PERFORATION

Two recently published guidelines recommend endoscopic treatment as first-line management for endoscopic oesophageal perforations.[34,38] The European Society of Gastroenterology (ESGE) guidelines recommend perforations in the cervical region will usually respond to conservative care, while more distal injuries should generally be treated with endoscopic options, such as application of clips or covered stents.[38] However, it should be acknowledged that there are no randomised studies in this field. Endoscopic management appears to bring similar success rates to surgery, but with reduced morbidity, possibly due to delivering more timely endoscopic treatment when compared with delay to proceeding with surgery.[28,39] Surgery to address an endoscopic injury is generally reserved for circumstances where expert endoscopic treatment is not available, for injuries that are not technically possible to fix endoscopically, or if endoscopic treatment has failed.[40] The main limitation of endoscopic management is the inability to address source control, but contamination should be minimised due to the fact that the patient is usually fasted and the perforation is usually identified early. Regardless of treatment modality, iatrogenic perforation carries a good prognosis overall when compared with outcomes following oesophageal perforation from other causes, but overall health-related quality of life is reduced even beyond 5 years.[41]

✔✔ The European Society of Gastroenterology (ESGE) and World Society of Emergency Surgery (WSES) have recently produced guidelines recommending endoscopic treatment as first-line management for endoscopic perforations of the oesophagus. Endoscopic techniques may include clip application and/or stent deployment among others. The choice of technique will likely vary according to local expertise. The evidence for endoscopic management of oesophageal perforation secondary to other causes remains unclear due to a lack of good quality evidence.

BOERHAAVE'S SYNDROME

Due to the pathogenesis of Boerhaave's syndrome, the condition is often associated with significant contamination of the mediastinum or pleura. Therefore, for appropriate patients, surgery is generally the management of choice and should be performed urgently due to the well-documented correlation of delay with mortality.[34] The site of perforation usually occurs just above the level of the gastro-oesophageal junction and is more common towards the left side. Preoperative imaging and/or endoscopy should confirm the exact position of the defect and which side is involved (Fig. 12.6). It is well described that the mucosal defect is often greater than the muscular defect, necessitating myotomy above and below the muscular defect to fully expose the extent of injury and allow appropriate debridement. The principles of operative repair are described above.

The data for non-operative management is generally retrospective with modest numbers of patients. For example, in 117 patients with benign intrathoracic perforation from a single centre, a 95% success rate was achieved with a stent and drainage. The stent was removed at a mean of 19 days (range 7–51) once certain criteria were met (return of gut function, normal observations, satisfactory volume and character of chest tube drainage, normal inflammatory markers, no effusion on chest X-ray, and no leak on contrast swallow). The authors concluded that as soon as these criteria are met, the stent should be removed, which should ideally be within 4 weeks.[42] Predictors of treatment failure using a stent include a very proximal or distal perforation, a long injury (>6 cm), or the presence of a second perforation distally.[40] The same group advocate waiting at least 48 hours to get a contrast swallow; 6% had contrast leaking around the stent at initial imaging at 24 hours, but they remained clinically stable and were kept fasted for 48 hours and then re-imaged, at which time extravasation had resolved in all of them. Presumably, this relates to the stent needing time to fully deploy.

A recent systematic review of oesophageal stent usage for benign perforation (including anastomotic leak) demonstrated that a covered metal stent has superior technical success rate to a plastic stent, although clinical success rates were similar (87%).[42] However, the authors acknowledge that the quality of evidence was generally poor.

By the nature of the condition, there are no randomised controlled trials in this clinical area. Patient numbers are small, publications report heterogeneous patient groups and case selection often remains obscure making meaningful and accurate conclusions on clinical management challenging.

FOLLOW-UP

Most patients will require a prolonged inpatient stay and many patients develop long-term health issues following discharge from hospital. Dysphagia is common following oesophageal perforation due to stricturing and the patient may require several episodes of endoscopic dilatation. Nutritional support may be required for some period following discharge and nutritional supplementation may be necessary, and this is best done with input from a dietitian. Routine medical advice should be provided, including counselling on alcohol abuse if relevant.

NEW AND FUTURE DEVELOPMENTS

Developments in technology along with increasing expertise has led to a rapid expansion of novel endoscopic techniques in the management of UGI tract perforations. At the present time, however, there remains a paucity of good quality evidence to support their routine use. It is important to note that much of the literature relates to the management of operative complications such as anastomotic leak. Some of the novel endoscopic techniques that have been described include the application of endoscopic clips (either through-the-scope clips [TTSC] or over-the-scope clips [OTSC]), applying fibrin sealant, endoscopic suturing, endoloop closure, deployment of a self-expanding covered stent, and endoscopic vacuum therapy (EVT).[43–46] For example, in a cohort of 69 patients with an anastomotic leak, 80% of patients responded to endoscopic therapy (OTSC) despite a median age of defect being 9 days.[47] It is plausible that this approach could be extended to non-operative perforations. Much of the published 'evidence' for these techniques is limited to case reports.

EVT has been introduced as a novel technique in the armoury for endoscopic management of oesophageal perforation and may show more promise.[48] This technique is based on a continuous negative pressure applied to the site of perforation through a sponge which is placed into the defect endoscopically (Fig. 12.7). The rationale is the same as that for a surgical wound vacuum device. Most data comes from the management of anastomotic leakage; however, a recent systematic review and meta-analysis reported 92% clinical success rate for 76 cases of iatrogenic oesophageal perforation treated with EVT.[49] In a review of 24 patients, there was a 90% clinical success rate with EVT.[49] Early experience with a novel combination metal stent and vacuum device has been recently described in a small number of patients with oesophageal perforation with a reported success rate of 70%.[50] The efficacy of EVT in the management of oesophageal perforation should be clarified on the completion of a trial which is currently recruiting with results expected to be available in early 2023. A limitation of EVT is the requirement for the vacuum sponge to be changed every 2–4 days making this technique labour intensive and highly dependent on local expertise.

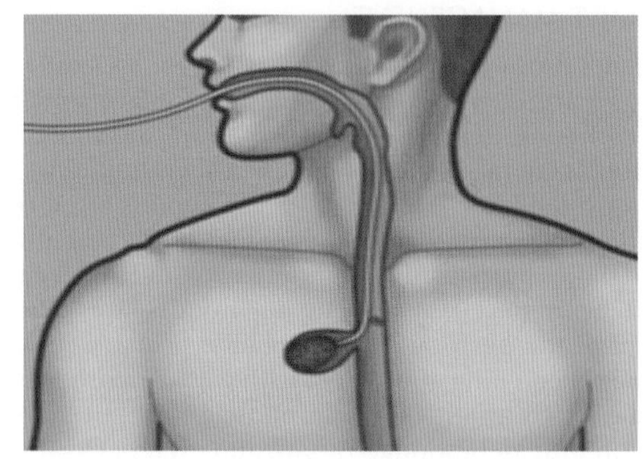

Figure 12.7 A diagram demonstrating the use of a vacuum therapy sponge for the treatment of an oesophageal perforation. The sponge is endoscopically placed into the defect cavity and attached to a low pressure suction device (EsoSponge[R], B. Braun Medical Ltd. Sheffield, Chapeltown.).

Endoscopic management will continue to evolve rapidly and the indications outlined above are likely to expand as experience is gained.[28] Many of the techniques described currently remain in the domain of the enthusiast requiring skills and experience not yet widely adopted into practice and without a strong evidence base.

✔ Endoscopic vacuum therapy has been introduced as a novel technique in the endoscopic management of oesophageal perforation. A recent small systematic review involving only 100 patients reported a clinical success rate of 94% with the remaining patients requiring conversion to surgical treatment. Further trials on this technique are ongoing and the results are awaited.

Key points

- Peptic ulceration occurring in the duodenum and stomach is by far the most common cause of UGI tract perforations encountered in clinical practice.
- Delay to definitive treatment is a clear prognostic factor for peptic ulcer perforations. Every effort should be taken to ensure patients are diagnosed, resuscitated and receive definitive treatment in a timely fashion.
- Surgery is the mainstay management for perforated peptic ulcer disease, and an omental patch repair and thorough peritoneal lavage are the principles of surgical management and are sufficient for most patients.
- For perforated gastric ulcers, a simple repair (omental patch or local ulcer excision) remains the best management option even when malignancy is suspected. Major cancer resections are best undertaken in patients with normal physiology, ideally following MDT discussion and by specialist cancer surgeons.
- There is some evidence that minimally invasive surgery has advantages over open surgery in the management of perforated peptic ulcer disease, but not all patients are suited to a minimally invasive approach and appropriate patient selection is vital to ensure a good outcome. Whatever approach is used, the priority should always be the provision of safe and effective surgery.
- Non-operative management of peptic ulcer perforation may be appropriate for selected patients. Up to 70% of patients can avoid surgery by adopting this strategy and with appropriate patient selection.
- All patients should receive a course of oral *Helicobacter pylori* eradication therapy with PPI treatment. Efficacy of eradication should be confirmed at 6–8 weeks with an appropriate test.
- Endoscopy is indicated for all gastric ulcers 6–8 weeks post-discharge to check for healing and repeat biopsies should be taken.
- The majority of causes of oesophageal perforation are iatrogenic and usually occur secondary to endoscopic interventions.
- Early diagnosis and treatment is crucial to improve outcomes following oesophageal perforation; mortality doubles if treatment is delayed by 24 hours. Outcomes are further improved when cases are treated in high-volume centres involving teams that are more familiar in the management of these complex cases.
- Two recently published guidelines recommend endoscopic treatment as first-line management for endoscopic oesophageal perforations. Endoscopic techniques may include clip application and/or stent deployment among others with the choice of technique likely to vary according to local expertise.
- The evidence for endoscopic management of oesophageal perforation secondary to other causes remains unclear due to a lack of good quality evidence.
- The general principles of surgery for the management of oesophageal perforation, whatever the underlying aetiology, are debridement, washout, drainage and nutrition.
- Developments in technology along with increasing expertise has led to a rapid expansion of novel endoscopic techniques in the management of UGI tract perforations. At the present time, however, there remains a paucity of good quality evidence to support their routine use.

References available at http://ebooks.health.elsevier.com/

KEY REFERENCES

[15] Tarasconi A, Coccolini F, Biffl WL, et al. Perforated and bleeding peptic ulcer: WSES guidelines. World J Emerg Surg 2020;15(1):3. https://doi.org/10.1186/s13017-019-0283-9.

Recently produced international guidelines addressing several aspects in the management of peptic ulcer complications.

[18] Quah GS, Eslick GD, Cox MR. Laparoscopic repair for perforated peptic ulcer disease has better outcomes than open repair. J Gastrointest Surg 2019;23(3):618–25.

Data from a meta-analysis of seven RCTs showed reduced wound infections with laparoscopic surgery compared with open surgery (2.2% vs 6.3%), shorter length of stay (6.6 days vs 8.2 days) and reduced overall morbidity (8.9% vs 17%). There were no significant differences in leak rate, abscess formation or mortality.

[19] Vakayil V, Bauman B, Joppru K, et al. Surgical repair of perforated peptic ulcers: laparoscopic versus open approach. Surg Endosc 2019;33(1):281–92.

This retrospective review of over 6000 patients compared open and laparoscopic surgery for the management of perforated peptic ulcers. Propensity score matching was used to mitigate selection bias. The authors found lower rates of wound complications (infection and dehiscence) and reduced mortality. However, it is worth noting that only 10% of patients in the study cohort had minimally invasive surgery.

[20] Melloni M, Bernardi D, Asti E, Bonavina L. Perforated gastric cancer: a systematic review. J Laparoendosc Adv Surg Tech 2020;30(2):156–62.

This systematic review included 964 patients with perforated gastric ulcers. Malignant perforation was rare but mortality was significantly reduced when simple closure was performed rather than resection (1.9% vs 11.4% mortality). Staged gastrectomy outcomes were similar to non-perforated cancers for selected patients.

[21] Fisher BW, Fluck M, Young K, Shabahang M, Blansfield J, Arora TK. Urgent surgery for gastric adenocarcinoma: a study of the National Cancer Database. J Surg Res 2020;245:619–28.

This retrospective review compared outcomes between gastric cancer patients who had urgent surgery versus elective surgery. Urgent surgery was associated with lower lymph node counts, higher rates of positive resection margins, higher inpatient mortality and reduced overall survival.

[22] Wang S-Y, Hsu C-H, Liao C-H, et al. Surgical outcome evaluation of perforated gastric cancer: from the aspects of both acute care surgery and surgical oncology. Scand J Gastroenterol 2017;52(12):1371–6.

This review from a single institution found that malignant gastric perforation is rare, but comparable survival outcomes may be achieved with appropriate surgical management.

[31] Kaman L, Iqbal J, Kundil B, Kochhar R. Management of esophageal perforation in adults. Gastroenterology Res 2010;3(6):235–44.

This study reports an increased mortality from oesophageal perforation with delay in diagnosis and treatment: 10–25% mortality when treatment is initiated within 24 hours compared with 40–60% mortality when treatment is delayed beyond 48 hours.

[34] Chirica M, Kelly MD, Siboni S, et al. Esophageal emergencies: WSES guidelines. World J Emerg Surg 2019;14(1):26.

Recently produced international guidelines addressing several aspects in the management of oesophageal emergencies.

[38] Paspatis GA, Arvanitakis M, Dumonceau J-M, et al. Diagnosis and management of iatrogenic endoscopic perforations: european Society of gastrointestinal endoscopy (ESGE) position Statement–Update 2020. Endoscopy 2020;52(09):792–810.

Recently produced international guidelines addressing several aspects in the management of endoscopic oesophageal perforations.

[49] Fahmawi Y, Hammad F, Abdel-Aziz Y, et al. Endoscopic vacuum therapy for esophageal perforation - are we there? a systematic review and meta-analysis. Official Journal of the American College of Gastroenterology 2020;115:S213.

A small systematic review involving only 100 patients reporting a clinical success rate of 94% with EVT for patients with oesophageal perforation. The remaining patients required conversion to surgical treatment.

13 Acute non-variceal upper gastrointestinal bleeding

Shannon Melissa Chan | James Lau

INTRODUCTION

A major audit of upper gastrointestinal (UGI) bleeding in the UK carried out over 20 years ago reported an incidence of 103 patients per 100 000 adults per year.[1] There is a twofold increase in likelihood of requiring hospitalisation among those residents from more deprived socioeconomic areas.[2] Overall mortality from an episode of UGI bleeding was 14% in the UK study and a marked increase in mortality (33%) was observed if bleeding occurred following hospitalisation with another complaint.[1] A more recent audit of patients admitted to UK hospitals during 2007 demonstrated a marked reduction in the proportion of patients requiring surgery, as well as a reduction in overall mortality (10% vs 14%), and a reduction in mortality rate for inpatients (26% vs 33%).[3] This study also identified an increase in the proportion of patients admitted with variceal bleeding.[3] Mortality rate in patients admitted with peptic ulcer bleeding decreased from 8.8% to 5.8%.

The typical patient with severe peptic ulcer bleeding is now elderly, often with medical comorbidities and taking antiplatelet therapy and/or on anticoagulants. Such patients are at greater risk of death despite skilled intervention and are less able to withstand surgery should this be necessary. Although the need for surgical intervention is now much reduced with the widespread availability of skilled endoscopic haemostasis, mortality following surgery remains high. As a result, alternatives to surgical intervention are increasingly being employed and will be discussed in this chapter.

AETIOLOGY

In the earlier study reported in 1995 by Rockall,[1] only 4% of patients had UGI bleeding due to varices, with the majority (35%) being attributed to peptic ulcer disease (PUD). Of some concern was the 25% of patients in this study where no cause for bleeding was identified, particularly as this group had a mortality of 20%. Similar figures were reported in the later study[3] where, in patients with a diagnosis made, approximately 25% were due to duodenal ulcer and 25% to peptic ulceration in the stomach, oesophagus or a combination of sites. The other causes were due to a number of other conditions, including oesophagitis, gastritis and duodenitis, malignancy or Mallory–Weiss syndrome. In this later audit, the proportion of patients with variceal bleeding had increased to 11%, whereas the overall proportion with peptic ulcer remained unchanged.

INITIAL ASSESSMENT AND TRIAGE

Patients with acute UGI bleeding present with haematemesis, melaena or a combination of the two. Haematemesis is indicative of significant bleeding from a site proximal to the ligament of Treitz. Melaena usually indicates a bleeding site in the UGI tract, although bleeding from the small bowel or even the right colon may present in a similar way, depending on speed of passage. Presentation with haematemesis is associated with an increased risk of mortality compared with melaena.[4] Coffee-ground vomiting is no longer considered a serious stigma of UGI bleeding. Patients with UGI blood loss may occasionally present with frank rectal bleeding (haematochezia), but this is indicative of major blood loss and, not surprisingly, is associated with an increased need for transfusion, surgery and mortality.[5] A good example of this would be a patient who has previously undergone aortic aneurysm surgery who subsequently develops an aortoduodenal fistula related to the aortic graft.

SCORING SYSTEMS

Risk stratification in patients with UGI haemorrhage is important as it assists decision-making in the need for emergency intervention and feasibility of safe outpatient management. Published guidelines suggest routine use of validated stratification tools in these patients.[6] Multiple scoring tools have been previously reported, with the Rockall score and the Glasgow Blatchford score (GBS) being most extensively validated. Using data from the first National UK Audit, Rockall et al.[5] derived a scoring system based on five significant risk factors for mortality. The Rockall system consists of an initial score from clinical parameters and a complete composite score after endoscopic assessment. Patients with an initial score of 0 (i.e. age < 60, no tachycardia, no hypotension and no comorbidity) had a very low mortality.

The composite Rockall system, incorporating endoscopic information including cause of bleeding and stigmata of haemorrhage, has been validated in prospective studies,[7–9] but is more accurate in predicting mortality than the risk of re-bleeding.[7,8]

The GBS aimed to allow early assessment of the need for intervention rather than risk of death (Table 13.1).[10] Based entirely on clinical risk markers before endoscopy, the GBS performed significantly better than the Rockall score at predicting the need for intervention and has now been validated in prospective studies from the UK[11] and Hong Kong[10]. In a prospective multicentre international validation study of 3012 patients, GBS was better in predicting the need for endoscopic treatment (AUROC = 0.75) when compared with the Rockall score and several other scores. A GBS of 7 or more is the optimal threshold (sensitivity of 80% and specificity of 57%).[12] The small proportion of patients with a GBS of 0 or 1 have minimal chance of requiring intervention as well as risk of re-bleeding and death, thus outpatient management of these patients is considered safe and cost-effective.[13] Given the superiority of GBS over Rockall score at predicting the need for intervention, GBS is now the stratification system of choice in many centres.

Despite recommendations from guidelines, published nationwide registries consistently report a low adherence to the use of risk stratification tools in real-life practice. In the 2007 UK audit, only 19% (1250/6750) of patients had either Rockall score or GBS recorded in the medical notes.[14] Risk stratification systems should be adopted into clinical management protocol for all patients presenting with UGI haemorrhage, as routine use of such a system would assist in detecting patients at high risk of re-bleeding or death, as well as increase cost-effectiveness by reducing unnecessary admission of low-risk patients.

Table 13.1 Glasgow Blatchford score for predicting risk of re-bleeding or death in non-variceal upper gastrointestinal haemorrhage

Admission risk marker	Score component value
Blood urea (mmol/L)	
≥ 6.5 < 8.0	2
≥ 8.0 < 10.0	3
≥ 10.0 < 25.0	4
≥ 25	6
Haemoglobin (g/L) for men	
≥ 120 < 130	1
≥ 100 < 120	3
< 100	6
Haemoglobin (g/L) for women	
≥ 100 < 120	1
< 100	6
Systolic blood pressure (mmHg)	
100–109	1
90–99	2
< 90	3
Other markers	
Pulse ≥ 100 (per min)	1
Presentation with melaena	1
Presentation with syncope	2
Hepatic disease	2
Cardiac failure	2

Modified from Blatchford O, Murray WR, Blatchford M. A risk score to predict need for treatment for upper-gastrointestinal haemorrhage. Lancet 2000;356(9238):1318–21.

✔ The most recently published comprehensive guidelines on the management of UGI bleeding include data from published meta-analyses as well as expert opinion.[6,15,16]

INITIAL MANAGEMENT

While it may be appropriate to consider discharge for young patients with no haemodynamic compromise and a GBS of 0, particularly where there has been no witnessed frank haematemesis, most patients with a history of UGI bleeding will be admitted for observation and endoscopy. This will entail insertion of a large-bore intravenous cannula, administration of pre-warmed fluid to expand the intravascular volume and immediate blood samples taken for crossmatch, biochemistry, full blood count, coagulation screen and arterial blood gases. There is also some evidence that admission to a dedicated UGI bleeding unit is associated with a reduction in mortality.[17] Such a unit requires a 24-hour on-call service for immediate endoscopy if required and early (within 24 hours) consultant-led endoscopy for all patients. Indications for urgent (out-of-hours) endoscopy vary, but the main factor determining the degree of urgency is the necessity for endostasis. Therefore, patients with evidence of ongoing haemorrhage, declared either by fresh haematemesis or haemodynamic instability despite initial fluid resuscitation, require emergency endoscopy. Most stable patients will undergo UGI endoscopy within 24 hours (usually on the morning after admission). In such patients, the purpose of endoscopy is twofold: first, patients with minor bleeds undergo full diagnostic assessment and if considered at low risk of re-bleeding can be discharged home; second, to identify the group of patients who have significant lesions and who require endoscopic therapy to reduce the risk of re-bleeding.

MASSIVE HAEMORRHAGE

In those patients who have evidence of haemodynamic compromise, initial resuscitation should follow the appropriate guidelines and the local major haemorrhage protocol should be activated.[17] Early intensive haemodynamic resuscitation is recommended for such patients. In an observational study of patients suffering from UGI haemorrhage with haemodynamic instability, intensive haemodynamic resuscitation was associated with a lower risk of myocardial infarction and mortality than the control 'observation' group.[18] The type of intravenous fluid used for resuscitation remains contentious. A Cochrane review of 55 trials found no evidence to favour the use of colloid rather than crystalloid solutions during resuscitation in critically ill patients.[19] As colloid solutions are more expensive, initial resuscitation with appropriate crystalloids is recommended.

USE OF BLOOD AND BLOOD PRODUCTS

Red cell replacement is likely to be required when 30% or more of the blood volume is lost. This can be difficult to assess, particularly in young patients, and clinical assessment of blood loss, coupled with the response to initial volume replacement, must guide the decision on the necessity of transfusion. While blood transfusion may achieve intravascular volume replenishment and enhance tissue oxygen delivery, a liberal transfusion strategy could be associated with worse clinical outcomes. In a randomised trial, 921 patients with acute UGI haemorrhage were randomised to restrictive transfusion strategy (target haemoglobin: 7–9 g/dL) and liberal transfusion strategy (target haemoglobin: 9–11 g/dL) groups.[20] The restrictive RBC transfusion group had a significantly improved 6-week survival (95% vs 91%; hazard ratio [HR] 0.55, 95% confidence interval [CI] 0.33–0.92) and reduced re-bleeding (10% vs 16%; HR 0.68, 95% CI 0.47–0.98). Of note, patients with massive exsanguinating haemorrhage as well as significant medical comorbidities were excluded from the trial. A cluster randomised controlled trial (RCT) was subsequently conducted in the UK. Six university hospitals were randomised to either a restrictive or a liberal transfusion strategy (transfusion threshold of 8 g/dL vs 10 g/dL). The RCT enrolled 936 patients. Fewer patients in the restrictive transfusion group received red cell transfusion (33% vs 46%). Mean red cell transfused was 0.7 U compared with 1.2 U. No difference in clinical outcomes was observed between groups.[21] However, in patients with significant cardiopulmonary disease, a higher target haemoglobin level should be considered in order to increase oxygen-carrying capacity.

Administration of platelets should aim to maintain a platelet count of more than 50×10^9/L, while coagulation factors are likely to be required when more than one blood volume has been lost. These are most commonly given in the form of fresh frozen plasma (FFP). The use of platelets, FFP and other agents, such as recombinant factor VIIa, should be guided by local protocols and early involvement of a haematologist.

MANAGEMENT OF PATIENTS ON ANTIPLATELET AGENTS AND ANTICOAGULANTS

Antiplatelet agents and anticoagulants are in common practice, and UGI haemorrhage is a serious complication for patients taking these drugs. Patients taking vitamin K antagonists (VKA) should be admitted with the drug withheld. In patients suffering from major bleeding with haemodynamic compromise, urgent reversal of VKA should be undertaken. This could be achieved by administration of prothrombin complex concentrates (PCC) or FFP. PCC contain clotting factors prepared from pooled and concentrated human plasma. The major advantages of PCC are faster onset of action and a smaller transfusion volume, thus a lower risk of fluid overload. PCC was associated with a quicker correction of international normalised ratio in a recent small-scale non-randomised study.[22]

In recent years, use of non-VKA oral anticoagulants (NOACs) is increasingly popular in patients with non-valvular atrial fibrillation and venous thromboembolism. The risk of UGI haemorrhage is at least similar to that of VKA. These agents have a short and predictable anticoagulation effect, but rapid reversal in the setting of life-threatening haemorrhage is difficult. Vitamin K and FFP have not been found useful. The only reversal agent of dabigatran, idarucizumab, has been recently approved by the FDA. Administration of PCC or use of haemofiltration should be considered when urgent reversal of NOACs is necessary.

In patients with UGI haemorrhage who are taking antiplatelet agents, further management would depend on the severity of the bleeding, indication and the type of antiplatelet agents used. In general, patients on low-dose aspirin for secondary cardiovascular prophylaxis should have the drug resumed as soon as satisfactory haemostasis is confirmed after endoscopy. In a randomised study, patients who received continuous aspirin had a significantly lower all-cause short-term mortality compared with placebo, with the difference being attributable to cardiovascular, cerebrovascular or GI complications.[23] Patients who are taking dual antiplatelet agents should at least continue with low-dose aspirin to avoid cardiovascular events. Patients on other antiplatelet agents such as clopidogrel, prasugrel or ticagrelor should consider switching back to low-dose aspirin or an early cardiology consultation if high-risk endoscopic stigmata was identified during endoscopy.

EARLY PHARMACOLOGICAL TREATMENT

UGI endoscopy is the mainstay of investigation and management of UGI bleeding, but there may also be a role for early treatment with acid suppression therapy. *In vitro* studies have shown that, at pH < 6, platelet aggregation and plasma coagulation are markedly reduced,[24] a situation exacerbated by the presence of pepsin. It is therefore reasonable to expect acid suppression therapy to promote clot formation and stabilisation. A Cochrane review summarised six RCTs comparing proton pump inhibitors (PPIs) to either placebo or an histamine-2 receptor antagonist initiated prior to endoscopy.[25] No significant impact of PPI therapy was demonstrated on mortality, surgery or re-bleeding rates. There was, however, a reduction in the proportion of patients with stigmata of recent haemorrhage at the time of endoscopy, and a reduction in the requirement for endoscopic therapy at the index endoscopy. A post-hoc cost-effective analysis was reported using data from a large randomised study in Asia.[26] The study concluded that the strategy of pre-emptive use of PPI infusion was cost-saving because of reduced endoscopic therapy and hospitalisation, offsetting the cost of PPI therapy.[27] It therefore seems reasonable to propose pre-endoscopic

PPI therapy in patients admitted with UGI bleeding, but this should not delay or act as a substitute for early endoscopic intervention. There is no evidence to support the use of other agents such as somatostatin, octreotide or vasopressin in the pre-endoscopy setting, except where variceal bleeding is suspected.

✔✔ Pre-endoscopy treatment with a PPI is recommended as it reduces the number of actively bleeding ulcers and increases the number of clean-based ulcers seen at the time of endoscopy.[28] Early use of PPI reduces the need for endoscopic intervention and hospitalisation.

The use of pre-endoscopy prokinetic agents has also been advocated to improve endoscopic visualisation by reducing blood clots within the gastrointestinal tract lumen. Earlier meta-analysis showed that prokinetic agents reduced the need for repeat endoscopy.[29] In another recent meta-analysis, pre-endoscopy erythromycin infusion significantly improved gastric mucosal visualisation, decreased the need for second-look endoscopy, red cell transfusion and duration of hospital stay.[30]

Tranexamic acid, an antifibrinolytic agent, may also aid in haemorrhage control by reducing clot breakdown and its use in acute trauma has been proven in a recent large randomised study.[31] In a recently conducted Cochrane review, the use of tranexamic acid in UGI haemorrhage appeared to be associated with a reduction in overall mortality.[32] Unfortunately most of the included trials in the review were performed before the routine use of PPI and there was also a high dropout rate in some of the trials. In a large-scale placebo-controlled multicentre trial that enrolled 12 009 patients, the use of high-dose tranexamic acid infusion (intravenous tranexamic acid 1 g loading followed by 3 g infusion over 24 hours) did not reduce death from acute UGI bleeding (4% in the tranexamic acid and placebo group, respectively). The rate of venous thrombotic events (deep vein thrombosis and pulmonary embolism) was increased by twofold in those who received tranexamic acid (0.8% vs 0.4%). The use of tranexamic acid is not routinely recommended.[33]

ENDOSCOPY

UGI endoscopy is required for any patient with significant UGI bleeding. Patients with haemodynamic instability or evidence of continuing haemorrhage require emergency endoscopy, whereas the majority of patients will undergo endoscopy within 24 hours of admission. A systematic review of the literature supports a policy of early endoscopy, as this allows the safe discharge of patients with low-risk haemorrhage and improves outcome for patients with high-risk lesions.[34] A recent randomised controlled trial that included 516 high-risk patients compared endoscopy within 6 hours of consultation to endoscopy the next morning.[35] These patients belonged to a high-risk group (i.e. with an admission GBS of 12 or more) but were haemodynamically stable at randomisation. The primary outcome was 30-day mortality from all causes, which was 8.9% in the endoscopy within 6-hours group and 6.6% in the endoscopy within 24-hours group. (HR 1.35; 95% CI 0.72–2.54; $P = 0.34$).[35] There was a higher rate of ulcers with active bleeding or visible vessels found at endoscopy within 6-hours group (66.4% vs 47.8%) and therefore a higher rate of endoscopic treatment. Most stable patients can safely receive endoscopy the next morning, although they should be monitored carefully for signs of further bleeding.

✔✔ Early endoscopy is recommended for all patients with UGI haemorrhage.[34]

✔✔ In patients who are haemodynamically stable, urgent endoscopy within 6 hours does not improve mortality when compared with endoscopy within 24 hours (although patients require close haemodynamic monitoring).

ENDOSCOPIC TECHNIQUE

Endoscopy for UGI bleeding requires the support of a dedicated endoscopic unit with trained staff, availability of additional endoscopes and equipment, ready access to anaesthesia and operating theatre, and, increasingly, access to interventional radiology services. These procedures should be performed or supervised by experienced senior members of staff.

For the majority of stable patients, procedures can be safely carried out using standard diagnostic endoscopes. In the unstable patient or where continuing haemorrhage is suspected, the twin-channel or large (3.7 mm) single-channel endoscope is preferable and allows better aspiration of gastric contents as well as more flexibility with regard to the use of heater probes and other instruments. In unstable or obtunded patients, anaesthetic support is mandatory as an endotracheal tube should be passed before endoscopy to guard against aspiration. The use of a tilting trolley allows repositioning of the patient, which can facilitate visualisation of the proximal stomach when obscured by blood and clot. Initially, placing the patient in a head-up position may suffice, and if necessary rolling the patient into a right lateral and head-up position may be needed for complete visualisation of the gastric fundus. In general, lavage is more successful in achieving visualisation than endoscopic aspiration, as endoscope working channels rapidly block with clot. Lavage can be achieved using repeated flushes of saline down the endoscope working channel or with the use of the powered endoscopic lavage catheters such as that provided with the heater probe. With experience, it should rarely be necessary to proceed to surgery or angiography because of inability to visualise the bleeding site due to blood and clot in the stomach or duodenum.

Bleeding gastric ulcers are most likely within the antrum or at the incisura (77%), or less commonly higher on the lesser curve (15%), with ulcers at other sites within the stomach being uncommon. Ulcers at the incisura and proximal lesser curvature can be readily overlooked unless the endoscope is retroflexed within the stomach. The most common site for a bleeding duodenal ulcer is the posterior wall, sometimes with involvement of the inferior and superior walls of the first part of the duodenum. Anterior duodenal wall ulcers can ooze, but usually these ulcers perforate. Ulcers elsewhere in the duodenum are seen in less than 10% of patients.[36] The presence of active bleeding at the time of endoscopy and the size of the ulcer, rather than its anatomical site, are the main endoscopic determinants of the risk of therapeutic failure.

MANAGEMENT OF BLEEDING DUE TO CAUSES OTHER THAN PEPTIC ULCERATION

GASTRITIS/DUODENITIS

Bleeding due to gastritis or duodenitis may be associated with non-steroidal anti-inflammatory drug (NSAID) therapy or ingestion of alcohol. It may also be due to *Helicobacter pylori* and can be severe enough to cause superficial erosions. Such bleeding, however, is almost always self-limiting in the absence of bleeding disorders, and therapeutic intervention is not required at the time of endoscopy. Treatment with appropriate acid suppression therapy and early discharge is usually appropriate in the absence of other comorbid illness.

MALLORY–WEISS SYNDROME

Mallory–Weiss syndrome was first described in 1929 and refers to haematemesis following repeated or violent vomiting or retching. It is caused by a linear tear of the mucosa close to the oesophagogastric junction. It accounts for approximately 5% of patients with UGI haemorrhage and most will settle without the need for therapeutic intervention. However, if bleeding is seen at the time of endoscopy, several approaches have been described. The simplest and most readily available technique is the injection of 1:10 000 adrenaline, as for bleeding peptic ulcers, which is sufficient in the great majority of patients.[37] Mechanical methods of endostasis such as endoscopic band ligation or clip application have not been shown to be superior to adrenaline injection alone but are appropriate alternatives, particularly when major bleeding or shock has occurred or where adrenaline injection fails to achieve endostasis.[37,38]

OESOPHAGITIS

Gastro-oesophageal reflux disease is responsible for approximately 10% of cases of UGI haemorrhage and is rarely severe. Following diagnosis, treatment is with oral PPI therapy.

NEOPLASTIC DISEASE

Major bleeding is occasionally associated with oesophageal, gastric or duodenal tumours. Gastrointestinal stromal tumours (GISTs) may present with bleeding, which can be severe in some patients. Malignancies of the UGI tract commonly cause occult, chronic bleeding but major bleeding can occur and may be difficult to control endoscopically. Management will be dependent on the specific circumstances and may include endoscopic techniques such as argon plasma coagulation, angiographic embolisation or, as a last resort, surgical resection. Where possible, however, if a malignancy is suspected, non-operative methods of achieving haemostasis should be employed, allowing full staging investigations to be organised to guide appropriate management. Some patients with ongoing but slow blood loss from non-curable gastric malignancy can be helped by a single treatment of radiotherapy.

DIEULAFOY'S LESION

This rare cause of UGI bleeding is due to spontaneous rupture of a submucosal artery, usually in the stomach and often within 6 cm of the cardia. The characteristic endoscopic appearance is of a protruding vessel with no evidence of surrounding ulceration. They are commonly missed due to their small size and relatively inaccessible position. Endoscopic clip application or band ligation offers durable and definitive treatment when the lesion is identified. In a small randomised trial,[39] haemoclip application was associated with a lower rate of re-bleeding than adrenaline injection, although both achieved similar rates of initial haemostasis.

ENDOSCOPIC MANAGEMENT OF BLEEDING PEPTIC ULCERS

Endoscopy has a central role in the management of non-variceal UGI bleeding. It enables an early diagnosis and allows for risk stratification. Endoscopic signs or stigmata of bleeding are of prognostic value and, in patients with actively bleeding ulcers or stigmata associated with a high risk of recurrent bleeding, endoscopic therapy stops ongoing bleeding and reduces re-bleeding. When compared with placebo in pooled analyses, endoscopic therapy has been shown to reduce not only recurrent bleeding but also the need for surgery and mortality.[40,41]

ENDOSCOPIC STIGMATA OF BLEEDING

Forrest et al.[42] categorised endoscopic findings of bleeding peptic ulcers into those with active bleeding, stigmata of bleeding and a clean base, and a modified nomenclature has been in common use in the endoscopy literature since then. Laine and Peterson[43] summarised published endoscopic series of ulcer appearances in which endoscopic therapy was not used and provided crude figures for both the prevalence and rate of recurrent bleeding associated with these stigmata of bleeding. In ulcers that are actively bleeding (Fig. 13.1) or exhibit a non-bleeding visible vessel (NBVV; Fig. 13.2), endoscopic treatment should be offered. There has, however, been observer variation in the interpretation of endoscopic signs[44] and the National Institutes of Health Consensus Conference[45] defined an NBVV as 'protuberant discoloration' (Fig. 13.2). The endoscopist should search the ulcer base diligently in patients judged to have bled significantly or when there is circumstantial evidence of ongoing or recent bleeding, e.g. presence of fresh blood or altered blood or blood clot in the gastroduodenal tract. There has been until recently a controversy whether to wash away adherent clot overlying an ulcer (Fig. 13.3).

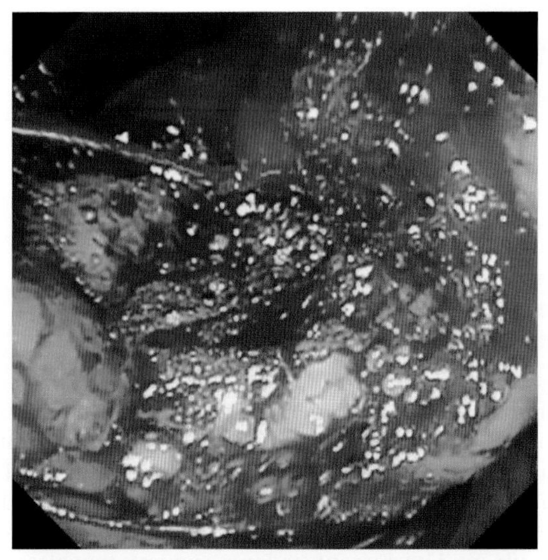

Figure 13.1 Bleeding vessel in base of ulcer.

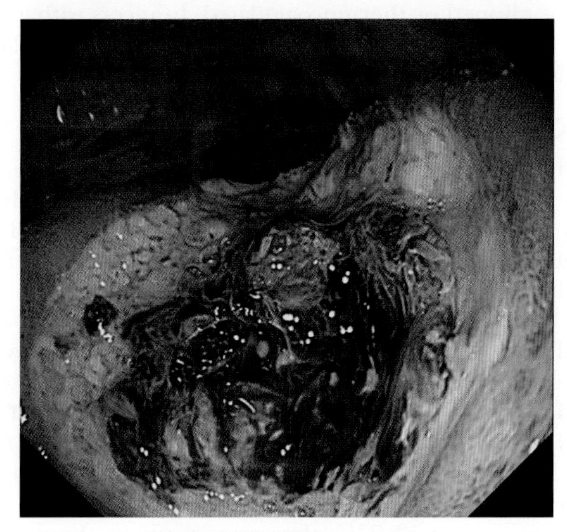

Figure 13.2 Visible vessel.

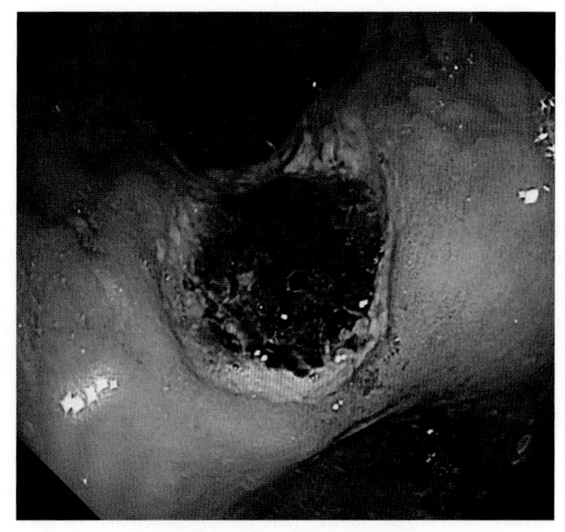

Figure 13.3 Adherent clot.

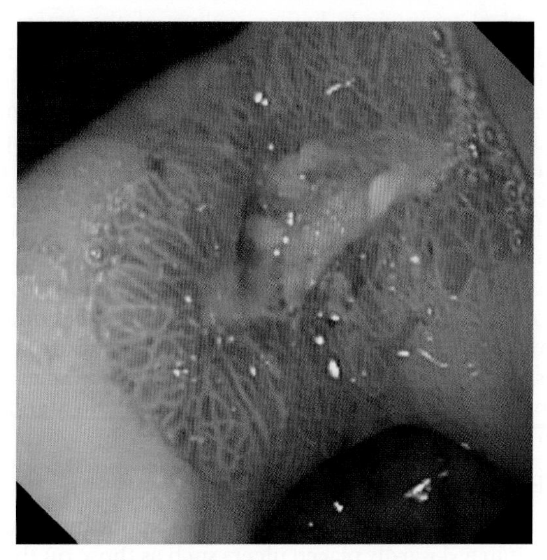

Figure 13.4 Ulcer with clean base.

Endoscopists vary in their vigour in clot irrigation before declaring a clot adherent. There have been several randomised studies and a pooled analysis has demonstrated that recurrent bleeding is reduced following clot elevation and treatment to the underlying vessel when compared with medical therapy alone.[46] Techniques for clot elevation include target irrigation using a heat probe and cheese-wiring using a snare with or without pre-injection with diluted adrenaline. One should, however, be cautious in elevation of clots overlying large deep bulbar and lesser curve ulcers as some of these may have eroded into large arteries. A recourse to angiographic embolisation without clot elevation and possible provocation of bleeding may be a better option in such patients. Ulcers with flat pigmentation and a clean base (Fig. 13.4) are associated with minimal risk of recurrent bleeding. Stable patients with such ulcers can be discharged home early on medical treatment (Table 13.2).

✔✔ Endoscopic therapy should be applied where there is active bleeding or a non-bleeding visible vessel in the ulcer base. Adherent clot should be removed and endoscopic therapy applied to the underlying vessel.[46]

ENDOSCOPIC TREATMENT

Modalities of endoscopic treatment can be broadly categorised into: injection, contact thermocoagulation, clipping and, recently, the use of topical haemostatic powder and over-the-scope-clips (OTSCs).

INJECTION

Injection therapy has been widely used because of its simplicity. Injection therapy works principally by volume tamponade. Aliquots (0.5–1 mL) are injected near the bleeding point at four quadrants using a 21- or 23-gauge injection needle. Adrenaline 1:10 000 has an added local vasoconstrictive effect. There is no role for the use of a sclerosant as there have been fatal case reports of gastric necrosis following its injection, and the added injection of a sclerosant such as polidocanol or sodium tetradecylsulphate after pre-injection of diluted adrenaline does not confer any advantage over injection of diluted adrenaline alone. Injection of fibrin or thrombin has been shown to be effective in some studies, but repeated injections are required. These products are costly.[47,48]

Table 13.2 Prevalence and outcomes of ulcers based on endoscopic appearance

Endoscopic signs	Prevalence (%)	Further bleeding (%)	Surgery (%)	Death (%)
Clean base	42	5	0.5	2
Flat spot	20	10	6	3
Adherent clot	17	22	10	7
Non-bleeding visible vessel	17	43	34	11
Active bleeding	18	55	35	11

Data from Laine L, Peterson WL. Bleeding peptic ulcer. N Engl J Med 1994;331(11):717–27.

THERMAL METHODS

In a canine mesenteric artery model, contact thermocoagulation is superior to injection therapy and non-contact coagulation such as laser photocoagulation in securing haemostasis. Contact thermocoagulation using a 3.2-mm probe consistently seals arteries up to 2 mm in diameter in *ex vivo* models. Johnston et al. emphasised the need for firm mechanical tamponade before sealing of the artery with thermal energy, introducing the term 'coaptive thermocoagulation'. Mechanical compression alone stops bleeding, reduces heat-sink effect and dissipation of thermal energy. The footprint after treatment provides a clear endpoint to therapy. Non-contact thermocoagulation in the form of laser photocoagulation is no longer used as a laser unit is bulky and difficult to be transported. At least in animal experiments, non-contact coagulation in the form of laser photocoagulation is not as effective as contact thermocoagulation.[49] There has also been interest in the use of argon plasma thermocoagulation, with a meta-analysis that summarised clinical trials comparing this to injection sclerotherapy or heat-probe treatment, respectively.[50] No significant difference in outcome was demonstrated.

MECHANICAL METHODS

Haemoclips are commonly used. Their application may be difficult in awkwardly placed ulcers such as those on the lesser curvature of the stomach and the posterior bulbar duodenum. In a meta-analysis of 15 studies with 390 patients[51] that compared haemoclipping versus injection and thermocoagulation, successful application of haemoclips (81.5%) was superior to injection alone (75.4%) but comparable to thermocoagulation (81.2%) in producing definitive haemostasis. In this pooled analysis, haemoclipping also led to a reduced need for surgery when compared with injection alone.

SINGLE VERSUS COMBINED METHODS

Soehendra introduced the concept of combination treatment that involved pre-injection with adrenaline allowing a clear view of the vessel, which then permitted targeted therapy using a second modality to induce thrombosis. In a meta-analysis of 16 studies and 1673 patients,[52] adding a second modality after adrenaline injection further reduces bleeding from 18.4% to 10.6% (odds ratio [OR] 0.53, 95% CI 0.4–0.69), emergency surgery from 11.3% to 7.6% (OR 0.64, 95% CI 0.46–0.90) and mortality from 5.1% to 2.6% (OR 0.51, 95% CI 0.31–0.84). In an independent meta-analysis of 22 studies (2472 patients),[53] dual therapy was shown to be superior to injection alone. However, treatment outcomes following combination treatments were not better than either mechanical or thermal therapy alone. Based on the above pooled analyses, adrenaline alone should no longer be considered an adequate treatment for bleeding peptic ulcers. The current evidence suggests that after initial adrenaline injection to stop bleeding, the vessel should either be clipped or thermocoagulated. In ulcers with a clear view to the vessel, direct clipping or thermocoagulation should yield similar results.

HEMOSPRAY®

Recently the endoscopic use of a haemostatic powder has been FDA approved for endoscopic use in the USA. Hemospray consists of bentonite powder with aluminium phyllosilicate as the main ingredient. During endoscopy, the tip of a catheter is placed 1–2 cm from the ulcer. With the push of a button, the powder is then power-sprayed onto the bleeding point using a canister pressurised with carbon dioxide (Fig. 13.5). In a small series of 20 patients with actively bleeding peptic ulcers,[54] it was successful in the control of bleeding in 19 of the 20 patients. In two European registries, Hemospray was applied in a variety of actively bleeding non-variceal lesions including GI cancers and post-surgical bleeding, and in 53–73% of cases, as a rescue therapy with high rates of success between 93% and 96.5% of cases in the control of bleeding. Rate of recurrent bleeding after initial control was high (27–33%). Currently the use of Hemospray should be considered only as a temporary measure to stop bleeding.[55,56] From another multicentre European registry, 314 patients with non-variceal UGI haemorrhage received endoscopic haemostasis with Hemospray.[57] Immediate haemostasis was achieved in 89.5% patients, rebleeding rate was 10.3%, 7-day and 30-day all-cause mortality was 11.5% and 20.1%, respectively. Similar haemostasis rates were achieved with Hemospray monotherapy, combination therapy and rescue therapy. The above findings were confirmed by a recent meta-analyses, concluding that Hemospray is a reasonable alternative to conventional haemostatic methods.[58] Comparative studies, however, are required to determine the efficacy of this haemostatic powder, but the simplicity of its application certainly appeals to endoscopists.

PUD was the most common pathology (167/314 = 53%) and Forrest Ib the most common bleed type in PUD (100/167 = 60%). A total of 281 patients (89.5%) achieved immediate haemostasis after successful endoscopic therapy with Hemospray. Re-bleeding occurred in 29 (10.3%) of the 281 patients who achieved immediate haemostasis.

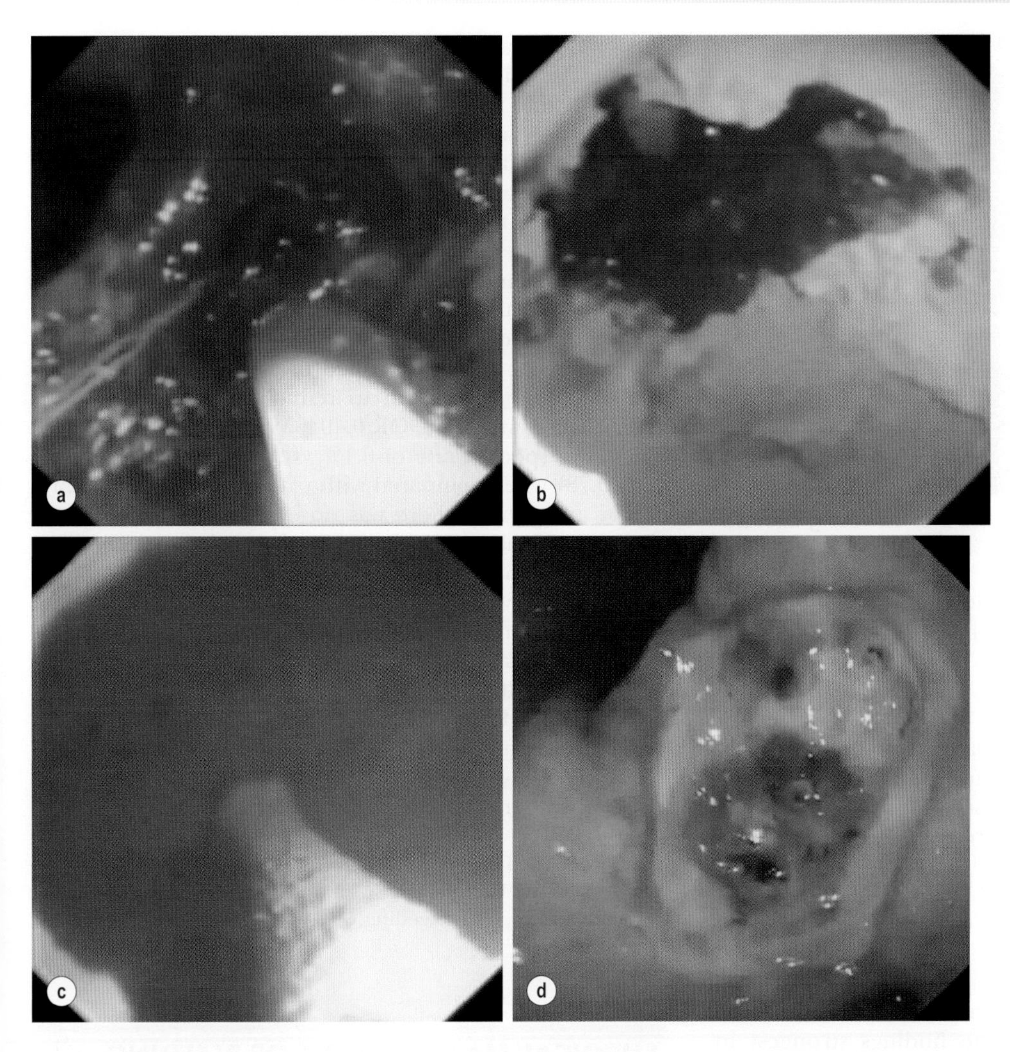

Figure 13.5 The use of Hemospray in an active bleeding ulcer. (a) Active spurter over incisura ulcer with difficult haemostasis. (b) Hemospray being applied. (c) Immediately after Hemospray applied. (d) Second-look endoscopy the next day showing visible vessels

Furthermore, 7-day and 30-day all-cause mortality were 11.5% (36/314) and 20.1% (63/314), respectively (lower than the predicted rates as per the Rockall score). Similar haemostasis rates were noted in the Hemospray monotherapy (92.4%), combination therapy (88.7%) and rescue therapy (85.5%) groups.

'OVER-THE-SCOPE CLIP'

The over-the-scope clip (OTSC) is a cap-mounted nitinol clip that has the ability to grasp the full thickness of the wall of the gastrointestinal tract. A transparent cap with the clip is mounted onto the tip of the endoscope. Before deployment of the OTSC, gentle suction is applied to allow approximation of the target lesion and the application cap (Fig. 13.6). An anchoring device is also available to target the bleeding vessel and to pull tissue into the cap before OTSC deployment (Fig. 13.6). A multicentre German randomised trial (STING study) showed that OTSC was more effective than standard therapy for recurrent bleeding of peptic ulcers.[59] Recently, Jensen et al.[60] randomised 53 patients with bleeding peptic ulcers and Dieulafoy's lesions to receive either OTSC or standard treatment. Recurrent bleeding occurred in only 1 of 25 patients treated by OTSC compared with 8 of 28 in the standard treatment group ($P = 0.017$). The Mayo Clinic reported its experience with the use of OTSC. The indications for use were vessels greater than 2 mm in size, deep, penetrating or excavating fibrotic ulcers and those who fail other endoscopic treatment.[61] The clinical success rate was 81.3% and patients with coronary artery disease have an increased risk of rebleeding even after OTSC, suggesting need for escalating therapies.

✔✔ Endoscopic therapy for bleeding peptic ulcers should use dual therapy or mechanical therapy rather than adrenaline injection alone in order to reduce the risk of rebleeding.[53,62]

LIMIT OF ENDOSCOPIC THERAPY

As mentioned previously, the size of the bleeding artery is a critical determinant in the success of endoscopic treatment. In an *ex vivo* model, a vessel size of 2 mm could be consistently sealed by a 3.2-mm contact thermal device.[50] In clinical studies that examined factors that might predict failure of endoscopic treatment, ulcer size greater than 2 cm, ulcers on the lesser curvature of the stomach and ulcers on the superior or posterior wall of the bulbar duodenum were consistently identified as major risk factors for recurrent bleeding. These ulcers erode into large artery complexes such as the left gastric artery and the gastroduodenal artery, which are usually sizeable. Consideration should therefore be given to prophylactic measures against recurrent

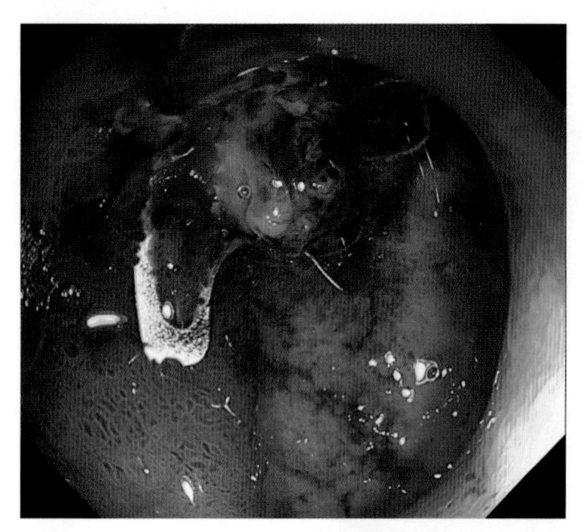

Figure 13.6 Over-the-scope clip applied over a bleeding duodenal ulcer.

bleeding in these ulcers judged endoscopically to be at significant risk of re-bleeding. This will be discussed later.

SECOND-LOOK ENDOSCOPY

Many endoscopists re-scope their patients 24–48 hours later and re-treat ulcers that have residual stigmata of bleeding. In a pooled analysis on the role of second-look endoscopy,[63] the authors found a modest 6.2% reduction in the absolute risk of re-bleeding. The number needed to treat [NNT]) to reduce one episode of recurrent bleeding was 58, and the NNT to reduce the requirement for surgical intervention was 97. A subsequent meta-analysis and a third meta-analysis carried out for an international consensus conference confirmed that routine second-look endoscopy did reduce the incidence of re-bleeding, with the findings strongest in studies that included a high proportion of high-risk ulcers. However, in many of these trials, adrenaline injection alone was used and the role of second-look endoscopy following dual therapy or mechanical therapy remains unclear. In addition, adjuvant treatment with PPI therapy following endoscopic haemostasis can be expected to reduce the benefit of second-look endoscopy even further. In the latest meta-analysis including nine RCTs, the authors confirmed that single endoscopy with adequate haemostasis is not inferior to second-look endoscopy at reducing re-bleed rates, mortality and need for surgery.

✓✓ Second-look endoscopy is not indicated as a routine if primary optimum endoscopic haemostasis has been performed.[6]

PHARMACOLOGICAL MANAGEMENT OF BLEEDING PEPTIC ULCERS

ACID SUPPRESSION

It has been shown in an *in vitro* study that platelet aggregation is dependent on plasma pH. It is thought that a pH of 6 is critical for clot stability and an intragastric pH above 4 inactivates stomach pepsin, preventing the digestion of clots.[24] To raise intragastric pH consistently above 6, a high-dose PPI given intravenously is required. The antisecretory effect of histamine receptor antagonists, due to tolerance, is less reliable than PPIs. In a study from the Hong Kong group,[64] a 3-day course of high-dose omeprazole infusion given after endoscopic therapy to bleeding ulcers reduced the rate of recurrent bleeding from 22.5% to 6.7% at day 30. The majority of recurrent bleeding occurred within the first 3 days of endoscopic treatment. This trial demonstrated the importance of early endoscopic triage, selecting only the high-risk ulcers for aggressive endoscopic treatment followed by profound acid suppression. In a Cochrane systematic review of 24 controlled trials and 4373 patients,[65] PPI treatment was shown to reduce re-bleeding (pooled rate of 10.6% vs 17.3%, OR 0.49, 95% CI 0.37–0.65) as well as surgery (pooled rate of 6.1% vs 9.3%, OR 0.61, 95% CI 0.48–0.78) when compared with placebo or histamine-2 receptor antagonist. There was no evidence of an effect on all-cause mortality, although when the analysis was confined to patients with high-risk stigmata (active bleeding or visible vessels), there was an associated reduction in mortality with PPI therapy. A multicentre randomised study of 767 patients from 91 hospitals in 16 countries compared intravenous esomeprazole with placebo following successful endoscopic haemostasis.[66] Esomeprazole was associated with significant reductions in re-bleeding and endoscopic re-intervention rates and non-significant reductions in mortality and the need for surgery.

✓✓ High-dose intravenous PPI therapy (80 mg omeprazole followed by 8 mg/h for 72 hours) is recommended for patients with active bleeding or visible vessels at the time of endoscopy.[66]

SURGICAL MANAGEMENT OF BLEEDING PEPTIC ULCERS

The first UK audit revealed a mortality of 24% in those patients (251 of 2071, 12%) who required surgery for bleeding peptic ulcers.[1] However, in 78% of these patients no previous attempt at endoscopic haemostasis had been made. In the most recent UK audit,[3] surgery was required in only 1.9% of patients, but mortality remained high in this group (30%). The high mortality is probably related to a combination of an aged population with high incidence of comorbidity, as well as surgery being utilised as a salvage therapy after failed endoscopic haemostasis. Bleeding ulcers that fail endostasis are typically 'difficult' ulcers—larger chronic ulcers that erode into major arterial complexes. The decline in elective ulcer surgery also means the atrophy of surgical expertise in dealing with these ulcers. Ideally, a specialist team with an experienced UGI surgeon should be involved in managing these patients.

Although emergency ulcer surgery has diminished significantly, it has an important gatekeeping role in the management algorithm. The clear indication for surgery is loosely defined as 'failure of endoscopic treatment'. In a patient with massive bleeding that cannot be controlled by endoscopy, immediate surgery should obviously follow. However, the difficulty lies in deciding the exact role of surgery in ulcers judged to have a high risk of recurrent bleeding (e.g. > 2 cm and at difficult locations), in which endoscopic haemostasis has been initially successful. Increasingly, angiographic embolisation is replacing emergency surgery in these circumstances.

CHOICE OF SURGICAL PROCEDURE FOR BLEEDING PEPTIC ULCERS

The choice of surgical procedure for bleeding peptic ulcers, when required, has not been adequately examined in the era following routine eradication of *H. pylori* and high-dose PPI therapy. Many surgeons maintain that under-running of ulcers alone combined with acid suppression using high-dose PPI therapy is safer than definitive surgery by either gastric resection or vagotomy. In the era of PPI therapy, the role of vagotomy has now completely disappeared. A proper ligation of the gastroduodenal artery complex including the right gastroepiploic and the transverse pancreatic branches is the key to avoid recurrent bleeding.

In a survey of UK surgeons reported in 2003, more than 80% of respondents rarely or never perform vagotomy for bleeding peptic ulcer.[67] Despite the absence of recent randomised evidence, surgeons have clearly adopted a more conservative approach based on the efficiency of PPI treatment and *H. pylori* eradication in the healing of peptic ulceration. With improvements in endoscopic therapy and the increasing age and comorbidity of patients, the risks of definitive ulcer surgery may outweigh any potential benefit from reduction in re-bleeding. For duodenal ulcer haemorrhage, longitudinal duodenotomy is carried out and control of bleeding achieved by digital pressure or by grasping the posterior duodenal wall in tissue forceps. If possible, preservation of the pylorus is preferred, but extension of the duodenotomy to include the pylorus may be required if access is difficult. Control of bleeding may be aided by mobilisation of the duodenum (Kocher's manoeuvre), allowing pressure to be applied posteriorly. In the majority of patients, simple under-running of the bleeding vessel can be achieved using 0 or 1/0 absorbable sutures above and below the bleeding point, ensuring deep enough tissue penetration to completely occlude the vessel. Due to the variation in anatomy of the gastroduodenal artery (Fig. 13.7), four or five sutures should be placed to ensure enduring haemostasis. The duodenotomy can then be closed longitudinally or converted into a formal pyloroplasty if the pylorus has been divided.

In cases of a massive duodenal ulcer, it may be necessary to exclude the ulcer, perform a distal gastrectomy and close the duodenum distal to the ulcer. This can be a challenging procedure in an elderly, unstable patient, particularly where duodenal thickening and scarring prevent safe stump closure. In this situation, it is reasonable to attempt duodenal closure as best as possible, leaving large drains to the area, which will permit a leak to be managed non-operatively. Some surgeons advocate forming a controlled duodenal fistula by closing the duodenal stump around a Foley catheter or drain rather than attempting more complex closures.

In the case of surgery for a bleeding gastric ulcer, the common scenario is for the ulcer to be located high on the lesser curve of stomach. Anterior gastrotomy, identification of the bleeding site and simple under-running of the ulcer

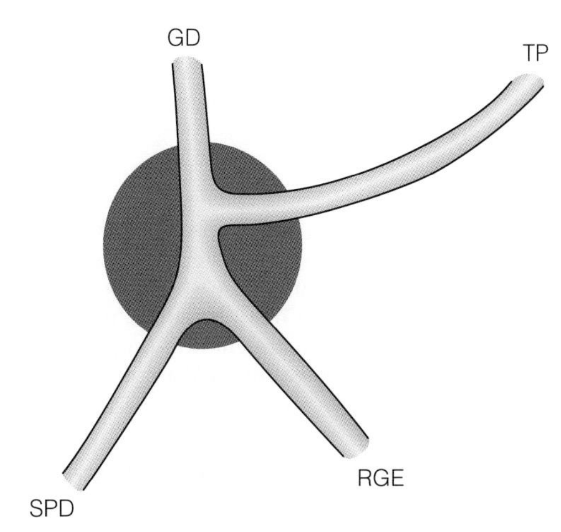

Figure 13.7 The anatomy of the gastroduodenal (GD) artery complex with confluence of several branches into the artery itself. *RGE,* right gastroepiploic; *SPD,* superior pancreatico-duodenal; *TP,* transverse pancreatic. (Reproduced from Berne CJ, Rosoff L. Peptic ulcer perforation of the gastroduodenal artery complex: clinical features and operative control. Ann Surg 1969; 169: 141–4. With permission from Lippincott, Williams & Wilkins.)

(with biopsy of the ulcer edge) is the procedure of choice, and is also suitable for rare cases of Mallory–Weiss tear or a Dieulafoy lesion that does not respond to endoscopic management. In the rare case of a distal gastric ulcer that does not respond to endoscopic therapy, there may occasionally be a case for ulcer excision or even distal gastrectomy, but it is difficult to justify such a course of action in the hands of a non-specialist surgeon, and simple under-running should be the aim in the majority of patients.

✔ The choice of operation in patients with bleeding peptic ulcers who have failed endoscopic treatment should involve, where possible, simple under-running of the bleeding ulcer, without either vagotomy or gastric resection. Biopsies should be taken from the edge of a gastric ulcer.

MANAGEMENT OF RECURRENT BLEEDING

The decision on management of patients who re-bleed after initial endoscopic control can be difficult. In a randomised study that compared endoscopic re-treatment to surgery in such patients,[68] endoscopic re-treatment secured bleeding again in 75% of patients. With intention-to-treat analysis, complications following endoscopic re-treatment were significantly less in patients when compared with those who underwent surgery. The gastrectomy rate in the surgery group was 50%. In a subgroup analysis, those re-bleeding with hypotensive shock from ulcers greater than 2 cm were less likely to respond to a repeat endoscopic treatment. It is therefore suggested that a selective approach can be used in re-bleeding patients. Patients with smaller ulcers and subtle signs of re-bleeding should undergo repeated endoscopic therapy, with surgery reserved for those who fail haemostasis. Patients with large chronic ulcers who are unstable should go straight to surgery without recourse to endoscopic re-treatment. Some of these patients identified as 'high risk of re-bleeding' may, however, benefit from early pre-emptive angiographic embolisation (see below). 'Elective/pre-emptive' surgery for high-risk ulcers for re-bleeding is becoming less common.

✔ Management of re-bleeding following successful endostasis will depend on the specific circumstances. Further endoscopic haemostasis may be appropriate for many patients,[68] but high-risk ulcers, particularly those where good endostasis was difficult to achieve at the first procedure, may be better considered for pre-emptive treatment with prophylactic transarterial angiographic embolisation (TAE).

THE ROLE OF ANGIOGRAPHIC EMBOLISATION

TAE is an alternative rescue procedure for bleeding gastroduodenal ulcers and the technique has been in use for over three decades. In the 1980s, there were reports of visceral infarcts[69,70] following angiographic embolisation, and its use was restricted to a small group of patients with refractory bleeding considered unfit for surgical intervention. With advances in embolisation techniques and specifically the use of coils and other agents (Fig. 13.8) and improvements in expertise, the success rate in the control of bleeding has been reported to be between 64% and 91%, and mortality between 5% and 25%. In patients where endoscopic haemostasis failed, a population-based cohort study from Sweden showed that although TAE had higher risk of re-bleeding than surgery (HR 2.48, 95% CI 0.37–1.35), there was no difference in 30-day mortality (HR 0.70, 95% CI 0.37–1.35) with a shorter median hospital stay (8 vs 16 days; 95% CI 0.45–0.77) and lower risk of complications (8.3% vs 32.2%; $P < 0.0001$).[71] The results of another meta-analysis including 13 studies with a total of 1077 patients echoed

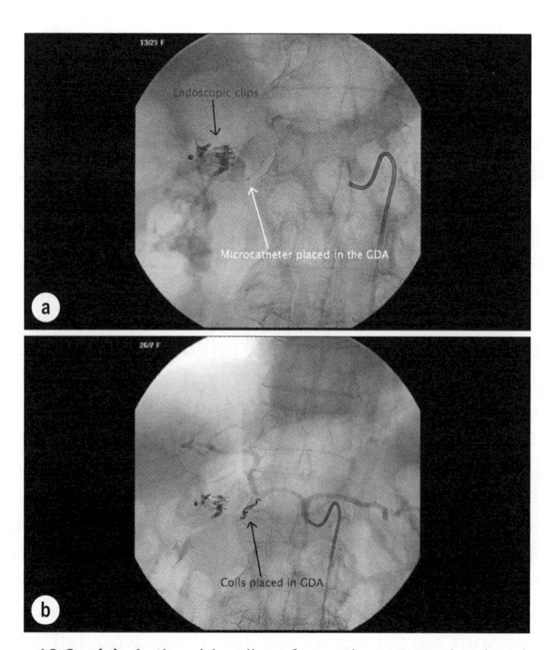

Figure 13.8 (a) Active bleeding from the gastroduodenal artery complex during transfemoral angiography. **(b)** Coils were used to embolise the artery leading to cessation of bleeding.

with this study.[72] These findings suggest that angiographic embolisation may be at least as good an option as surgery in the management of refractory ulcer bleeding, especially in those patients at advanced age with high risk of surgical morbidities.

The potential role of angiographic embolisation as a prophylactic measure following successful endostasis for patients considered at high risk of re-bleeding or death is also a subject worth investigating. Results of a randomised study of 222 patients with high-risk peptic ulcers, of whom 109 were randomised to receive prophylactic angiographic embolisation were recently reported.[73] On per-protocol analysis, there was a trend of reduced re-bleeding after angiographic embolisation (4.4% vs 10.9%, $P = 0.08$). Subgroup analysis of those with ulcer size ≥ 1.5 cm demonstrated a significant risk reduction in re-bleeding after prophylactic angiographic embolisation (5.0% vs 23.2%, OR 0.173, 95% CI 0.036–0.850, $P = 0.027$). These large ulcers are likely to erode into larger subserosal arteries; therefore, embolisation of such feeding arteries would be particularly effective at securing adequate haemostasis.

✔ Angiographic embolisation should be considered in patients who re-bleed following surgery for bleeding peptic ulcers and as an alternative to surgery when endoscopic haemostasis has failed, provided appropriate facilities and expertise are available. This may be particularly useful in elderly patients with medical comorbidity. It should also be considered as a possible pre-emptive treatment option for patients who are at high risk of re-bleeding after endostasis.

HELICOBACTER PYLORI ERADICATION

A Cochrane review[74] concluded that *H. pylori* eradication was associated with a significant reduction in the risk of re-bleeding compared with no *H. pylori* eradication, from 20% to 2.9%. If antisecretory therapy was continued, the risk was 5.6%, still significantly higher than that achieved with *H. pylori* eradication. The overall risk of re-bleeding following *H. pylori* eradication was less than 1% per year. While it was indeed a concern that in a UK review of consultant surgical behaviour reported in 2003, fewer than 60% routinely tested patients for *H. pylori* following treatment for complicated peptic ulcers[67] the same is very unlikely to still be the case now.

✔✔ Following treatment for bleeding duodenal ulcer, all patients should be tested for *H. pylori* and receive eradication therapy where appropriate. Patients should have further testing to ensure successful eradication.[75]

USE OF NON-STEROIDAL ANTI-INFLAMMATORY DRUGS

In patients who continue to require NSAIDs, co-therapy with PPI reduces recurrence in peptic ulcers and bleeding. In these patients, *H. pylori* should first be tested and

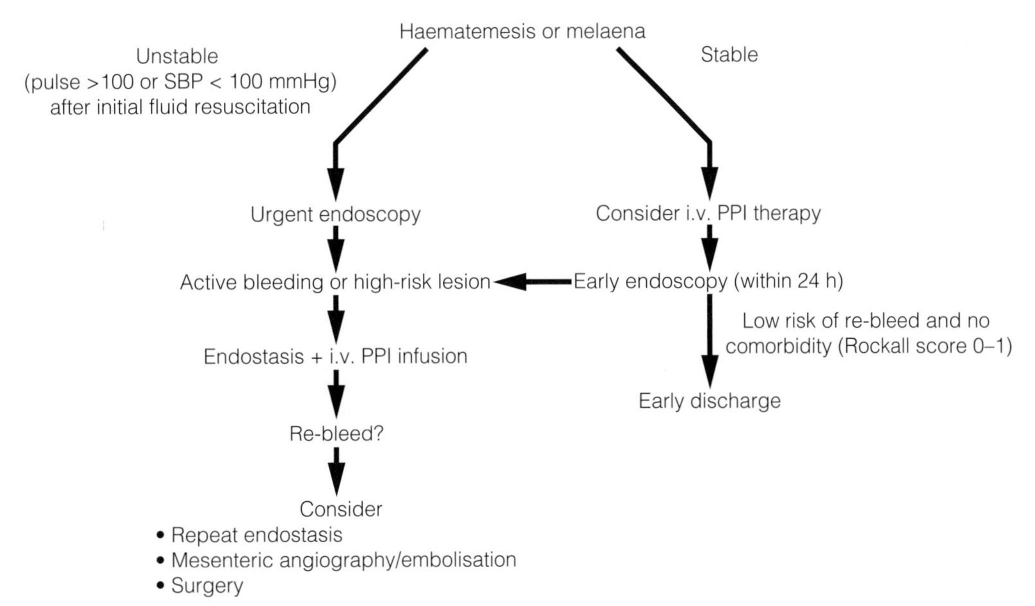

Figure 13.9 Management algorithm. PPI, proton pump inhibitor; *SBP*, systolic blood pressure.

treated if confirmed. An RCT compared the use of a traditional NSAID plus a PPI to COX-2 inhibitors and found that the rate of further ulcer complications is around 5% at 6 months.[76] A subsequent randomised trial combined the use of COX-2 inhibitor to PPI and compared them with the use of a COX-2 inhibitor alone.[77] At 1 year, the use of COX-2 inhibitor alone was associated with a rate of 9% in recurrent bleeding. The risk of recurrent bleeding was completely abolished in those who received the combined treatment. COX-2 inhibitor plus PPI appears to offer the best protection to these high-risk patients.

SUMMARY

The challenge posed by peptic ulcer bleeding has altered with the increasing age of the population at risk and the increasing availability of skilled therapeutic endoscopy. Endoscopy is the mainstay of management for these patients. Failure of endoscopic haemostasis is increasingly uncommon, but the surgical challenge presented by the elderly patient with refractory bleeding from a large ulcer is considerable. Successful management of UGI bleeding will involve the close cooperation of a multidisciplinary team, which will increasingly include interventional radiologists, aided by local protocols based on evidence-based best practice (Fig. 13.9).

Key points

- A risk stratification system should be utilised for all patients with UGI bleeding.
- Pre-endoscopy treatment with PPIs is recommended as it reduces the risk of active bleeding at the time of endoscopy and may reduce the need for endoscopic intervention.
- Early endoscopy should be performed on all patients with UGI bleeding.
- Endoscopic therapy should be applied where there is active bleeding or a non-bleeding visible vessel in the ulcer base. Adherent clot should be removed and endoscopic therapy applied to the underlying vessel.
- Endoscopic therapy for bleeding peptic ulcers should involve use of dual therapy or mechanical therapy rather than adrenaline injection alone in order to reduce the risk of re-bleeding.
- High-dose intravenous PPI therapy (80 mg omeprazole followed by 8 mg/h for 72 hours) is recommended for patients with active bleeding or visible vessels at the time of endoscopy.
- The choice of operation in patients with bleeding peptic ulcers who have failed endoscopic treatment should involve, where possible, simple under-running of the bleeding ulcer, without gastric resection unless it is not possible to close the duodenotomy. There is no longer any place for vagotomy.
- Management of re-bleeding following successful endoscopic haemostasis will depend on the specific circumstances. Further endoscopic haemostasis may be appropriate for many patients but those with high-risk ulcers, particularly where good endostasis was difficult to achieve at the first procedure, may be better considered for surgery or transarterial angiographic embolisation.
- Following treatment for a bleeding duodenal ulcer, patients should receive *H. pylori* eradication therapy and patients should be tested to ensure successful eradication.

References available at http://ebooks.health.elsevier.com/

RECOMMENDED VIDEOS

- Hemoclip application for bleeding gastric ulcer – https://youtu.be/DwF_yyWWTvQ
- OTSC application for bleeding duodenal ulcer – https://youtu.be/VJTFxyFf654

KEY REFERENCES

[6] Gralnek IM, Dumonceau JM, Kuipers EJ, et al. Diagnosis and management of nonvariceal upper gastrointestinal hemorrhage: european Society of Gastrointestinal Endoscopy (ESGE) Guideline. Endoscopy 2015;47(10):a1–46. PMID: 26417980.

These are the most recently published comprehensive guidelines on the management of UGI bleeding based on studies published to date and include data from published and new meta-analyses as well as expert opinion.

[28] Sreedharan A, Martin J, Leontiadis GI, et al. Proton pump inhibitor treatment initiated prior to endoscopic diagnosis in upper gastrointestinal bleeding. Cochrane Database Syst Rev 2010;7:CD005415. PMID: 20614440.

This systematic review of randomised trials found no effect of pre-endoscopy PPI therapy on mortality, but there was a significant reduction in active bleeding and the need for intervention at the time of endoscopy.

[34] Spiegel BM, Vakil NB, Ofman JJ. Endoscopy for acute nonvariceal upper gastrointestinal tract hemorrhage: is sooner better? A systematic review. Arch Intern Med 2001;161(11):1393–404. PMID: 11386888.

This systematic review of 23 studies concluded that early endoscopy improved outcome in patients with UGI bleeding in all risk categories.

[46] Kahi CJ, Jensen DM, Sung JJ, et al. Endoscopic therapy versus medical therapy for bleeding peptic ulcer with adherent clot: a meta-analysis. Gastroenterol 2005;129(3):855–62. PMID: 16143125.

A pooled analysis of several randomised studies demonstrated that recurrent bleeding is reduced following clot elevation and treatment to the underlying vessel when compared with medical therapy alone.

[53] Marmo R, Rotondano G, Piscopo R, et al. Dual therapy versus monotherapy in the endoscopic treatment of high-risk bleeding ulcers: a meta-analysis of controlled trials. Am J Gastroenterol 2007;102(2):279–89. quiz 469. PMID: 17311650.

These two meta-analyses provide compelling evidence that addition of a second endoscopic therapy is better than adrenaline alone.

[62] Calvet X, Vergara M, Brullet E, et al. Addition of a second endoscopic treatment following epinephrine injection improves outcome in high-risk bleeding ulcers. Gastroenterol 2004;126(2):441–50. PMID: 14762781.

This meta-analysis of randomized trial showed that additional endoscopic treatment after epinephrine injection reduces further bleeding, need for surgery, and mortality in patients with bleeding peptic ulcer.

[65] Leontiadis GI, Sharma VK, Howden CW. Proton pump inhibitor treatment for acute peptic ulcer bleeding. Cochrane Database Syst Rev 2006;1:CD002094. PMID: 16437441.

This Cochrane review of randomised trials found that high-dose PPI therapy reduced re-bleeding, surgery and mortality rates following endotherapy for high-risk ulcers.

[74] Gisbert JP, Khorrami S, Carballo F, et al. Meta-analysis: *helicobacter pylori* eradication therapy vs. antisecretory non-eradication therapy for the prevention of recurrent bleeding from peptic ulcer. Aliment Pharmacol Ther 2004;19(6):617–29. PMID: 15023164.

This Cochrane review included seven studies and a reduction in re-bleeding rates following H. pylori eradication compared with antisecretory therapy and no eradication.

Pancreatico-biliary emergencies

14

Saxon Connor | Matthew Leeman

INTRODUCTION

As a general surgeon it is important to be competent in the management of the common emergency presentations associated with calculous biliary disease as these patients comprise a significant component of the acute workload.[1] In addition, recognising the patient who will benefit from specialised hepato-biliary-pancreatic (HPB) surgical care and transferring the patient after appropriate initial management is a key component of this process. The aim of this chapter is to provide an evidence-based approach to the management of acute calculous biliary disease and acute pancreatitis (AP) appreciating that the management of severe or complicated acute and chronic pancreatitis, pancreatic tumours and pancreatico-biliary trauma are dealt with in the HPB volume of the companion series.

GALLSTONES

The cumulative incidence of gallstones in the Western world has been reported as 0.60% per year with an overall prevalence of 9% in females and 10% in males.[2,3] Risk factors identified included increasing age, female sex, obesity, elevated non-high-density lipoprotein cholesterol and gallbladder polyps.[2] The underlying contributing aetiologies and risk factors are shown in Fig. 14.1. It is important to understand the differences in stone composition by geographical area or ethnicity. In parts of Asia, pigment stones predominate, while in Western countries mixed-type or cholesterol-based stones predominate. Although most gallstones remain asymptomatic, acute presentation can be divided into complications from local obstruction of the gallbladder due to cholecystolithiasis or migration of stones into the bile duct (choledocholithiasis) via the cystic duct.

CHOLECYSTOLITHIASIS AND ASSOCIATED COMPLICATIONS

CLINICAL PRESENTATION AND DIAGNOSIS

The underlying aetiology and pathogenesis of biliary colic and its sequelae are shown in Figs. 14.2 and 14.3, respectively. The commonest presentation is right upper quadrant (RUQ) pain with nausea or vomiting.[4] Clinical examination reveals tenderness in the RUQ and the arrest of inspiration during palpation is known as Murphy's sign and is associated with acute cholecystitis (AC).[3] Biliary colic usually has a short history without signs of clinical or biochemical inflammation. As the disease progresses, RUQ peritoneal inflammation develops and systemic inflammation can be present either clinically or biochemically. Following development of a mucocele or empyema, an RUQ mass may be palpable although this is rare.[4] The Tokyo guidelines are a series of international multi-society, multispecialty guidelines regarding the management of AC and cholangitis (also available as a mobile application). The 2013 Tokyo guidelines (TG-13) have defined a definitive diagnosis of AC as requiring a combination of clinical and imaging findings and were most recently updated in 2018 (TG-18) (Table 14.1).[4] The sensitivity and specificity of the TG-13 criteria for AC are 91% and 97%, respectively although the World Society of Emergency Surgery (WSES) guidelines have questioned the generalisability of these figures given the limitations of the supporting study.[3,4] Ultrasound (US) is the investigation of choice given its ubiquitous availability; however, the sensitivity and specificity in diagnosing AC are only moderate, reported as 81% (95% CI: 75–87%) and 83% (95% CI: 74–89%), respectively.[4] In contrast, the sensitivity and specificity of US for detecting cholecystolithiasis is 84% and 99%, respectively.[3] The key ultrasonographic findings of AC are thickened gallbladder wall (>3 mm), peri-cholecystic fluid and tenderness on gallbladder compression (radiological Murphy's sign). Although nuclear medicine imaging has been shown to have higher sensitivity and specificity than ultrasonography, it is not widely used given its limited availability and practicality.[3] More common alternatives include cross-sectional imaging such as computed tomography (CT) or magnetic resonance cholangiopancreatography (MRCP). CT findings indicating AC include gallbladder distension, wall thickening, subserosal oedema, mucosal enhancement or peri-cholecystic fat stranding.[4] Other findings include transient focal enhancement of the liver adjacent to the gallbladder.[4] This is due to increased blood flow and subsequent venous drainage through the draining cholecystic veins.[4] Occasionally, gas will be seen within the gallbladder or within a peri-cholecystic abscess in event of contained perforation.[4] Loss of gallbladder wall enhancement suggests gangrenous cholecystitis.[5] Similarly, magnetic resonance imaging (MRI) is thought to be at least comparable with abdominal US in terms of accuracy; however, these conclusions are based on relatively poor underlying patient

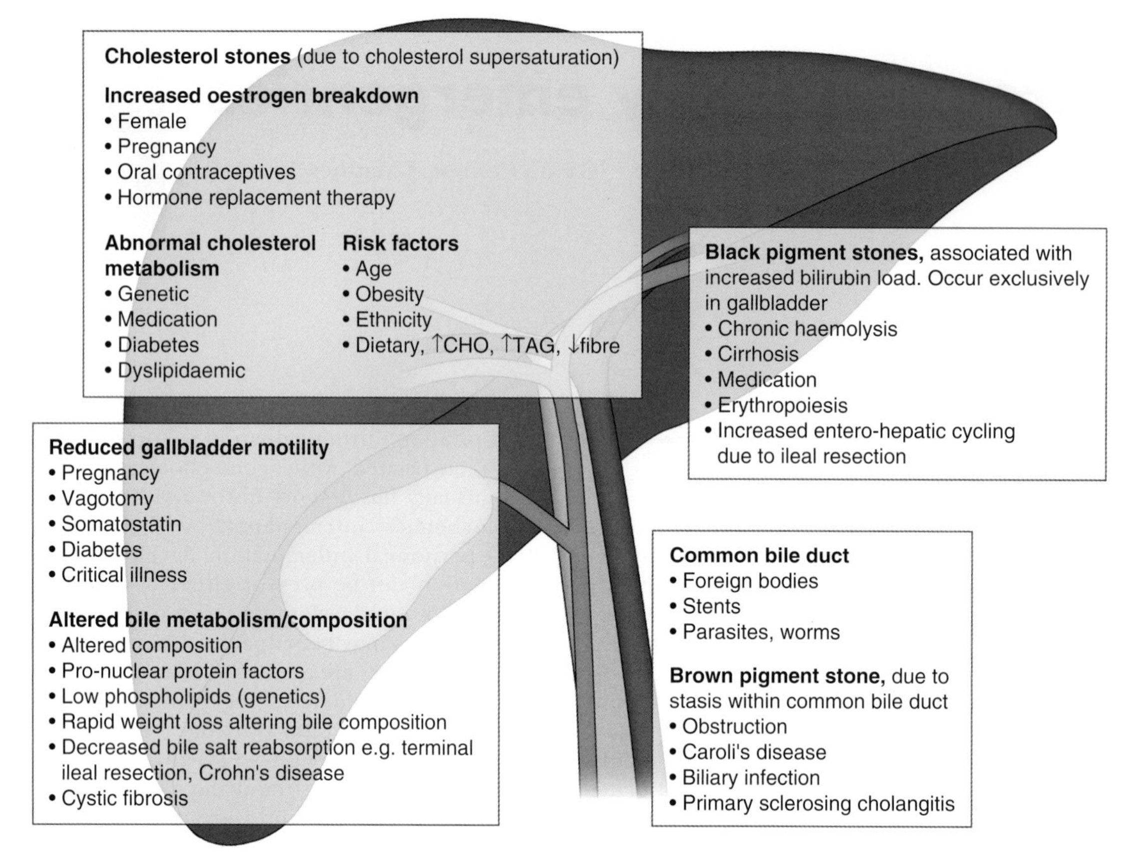

Figure 14.1 Aetiology and risk factors for cholelithiasis and choledocholithiasis.

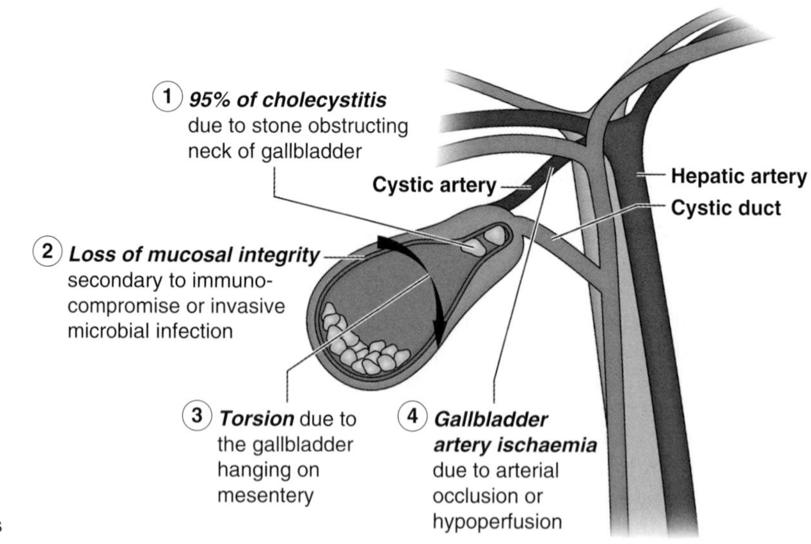

Figure 14.2 Aetiology of acute cholecystitis and its complications.

datasets.[3] The TG-13 guidelines classified the severity of AC into three grades in an aid to guide management.[4] Mild AC is defined as a healthy patient with no organ dysfunction or local complications.[4] Moderate AC is defined as AC with local complications secondary to marked inflammation but without organ dysfunction.[4] Local inflammatory complications include gangrenous or emphysematous cholecystitis, peri-cholecystic or hepatic abscess or biliary peritonitis. Severe AC is defined as AC with associated organ dysfunction.[4]

Markers of moderate AC include grossly elevated white count (>18000/mm^3), palpable mass or symptoms > 72 hours.[4] An elevated C-reactive protein (CRP) has also been associated with severe inflammation. In large retrospective study (n =1843), a CRP of > 67 mg/L predicted moderate and severe histological changes of AC with a 96% sensitivity and 100% specificity with an AUC of 100%.[5] CRP also correlates well with gangrenous cholecystitis (CRP > 200 mg/dL has 50% PPV and 100% NPV, 100% sensitivity and 87.9% specificity)[6] and gallbladder perforation.[7]

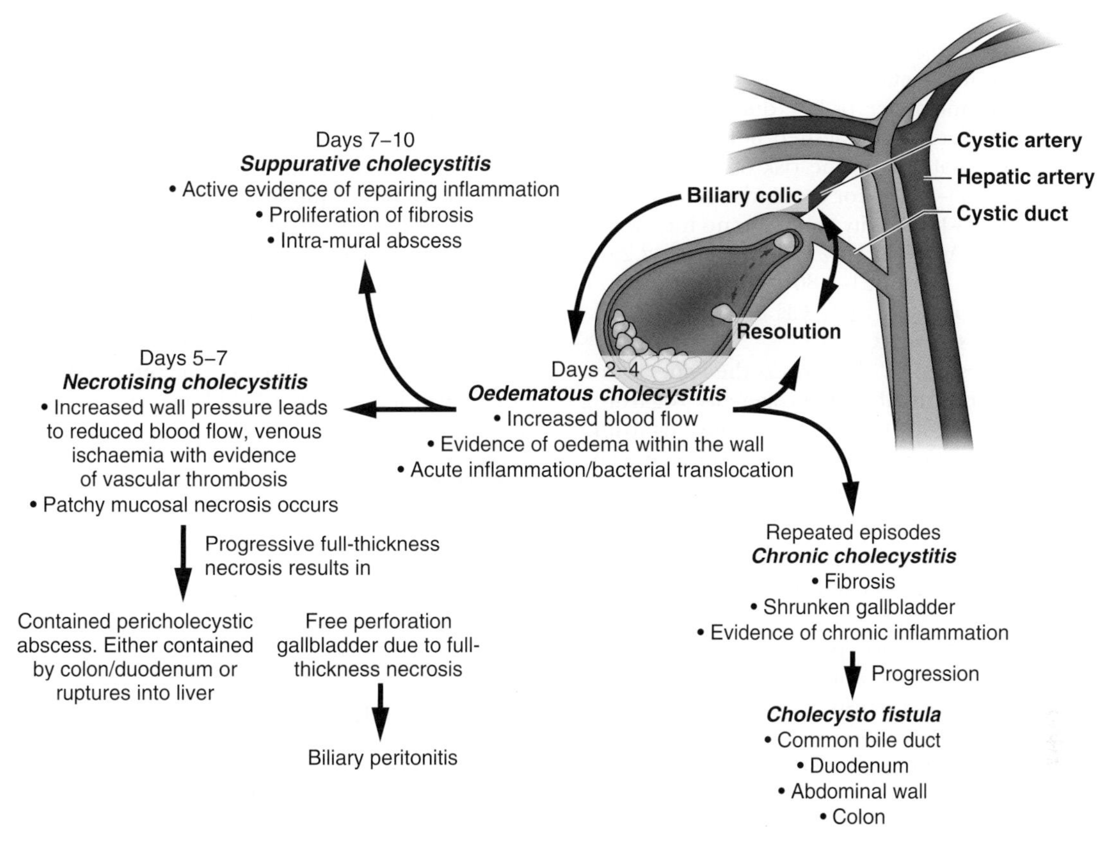

Figure 14.3 Pathogenesis of acute cholecystitis and its complications.

Table 14.1 Tokyo guidelines 2018 criteria for diagnosis of acute cholecystitis[4]

Local signs of inflammation	Murphy's sign, RUQ tenderness, pain or mass
Systemic signs of inflammation	Fever, raised C-reactive protein or white blood count
Imaging findings	Characteristics of acute cholecystitis

Suspected diagnosis = One item each from local and systemic signs of inflammation.
Definitive diagnosis = One item from each category.

✔ Elevated white count or CRP, symptoms > 72 hours or a palpable mass are predictors of complicated cholecystitis.

MANAGEMENT OF ACUTE CHOLECYSTITIS

AC should be managed according to the TG-18 severity classification.[8] In an updated evidence-based review of the literature, the authors of TG-18 recommend patients with mild AC undergo acute cholecystectomy if the patient does not have significant underlying comorbidity as defined by American Society Anesthesiologists (ASA) score or Charleston comorbidity index (CCI).[8] Both TG-18 and WSES guidelines strongly recommend a laparoscopic approach for those with mild AC based on several randomised controlled trials (RCTs) and a meta-analysis showing better short-term outcomes with laparoscopic cholecystectomy (LC) as compared with open cholecystectomy.[8] The WSES guidelines[3] do, however, acknowledge the low level of evidence to support cholecystectomy *per se* as the standard of care and made the following statements with regard to other options in management of AC:

- Antibiotics should be suggested as supportive care; they are effective in treating the first episode of AC, but a high rate of relapse can be expected. Surgery is more effective than antibiotics alone in the treatment of AC.
- Surgery is superior to observation of AC in the clinical outcome and shows some cost-effectiveness advantages due to the gallstone-related complications and to the high rate of re-admission and surgery in the observation group.
- Since there are no reports on surgical gallstone removal (cholelithotomy) in the setting of AC, surgery in the form of cholecystectomy remains the main option.
- There is no role for gallstones dissolution, drugs or extracorporeal shock wave lithotripsy or a combination in the setting of AC.

For patients with moderate AC, LC remains the treatment of choice in experienced centres in patients deemed fit enough to withstand surgery (ASA ≤ 2, CCI ≤ 6).[8] The authors of TG-18[8] rightly highlight some of the limitations of the data that were used to come to the above conclusion. Many of the trials had strict exclusion criteria based on patient comorbidity or complicated biliary disease and availability of surgeons skilled in LC. Surgeons should also be aware that although clinical and financial short-term outcomes are improved from an early approach to cholecystectomy, the trials and meta-analyses are underpowered to detect whether the incidence of bile duct injury (BDI) remains equivalent. A recently published population study from Sweden showed that overall the risk of BDI doubled (OR [95% CI] 1.97 [1.05–3.72]) for those with AC.[9] However, when stratified by TG-13 severity, there was no increase in BDI for those with mild AC (OR [95% CI] 0.96 [0.41–2.25]), a twofold (OR [95% CI] 2.41 [1.21–4.80]) increase for moderate AC and an eightfold (OR [95% CI] 8.43 [0.97–72.9]) increase for those with severe AC.[9]

The WSES guidelines and TG-18 address the issue of timing of LC. There is considerable heterogeneity regarding the definition of early versus late LC, especially regarding duration of symptoms versus time from admission. The WSES guidelines[3] make the following statements:

- Early LC is preferable to delayed LC in patients with AC as long as it is completed within 10 days of onset of symptoms. Earlier surgery is associated with shorter hospital stay and fewer complications.
- LC should not be offered for patients beyond 10 days from the onset of symptoms unless symptoms suggestive of worsening peritonitis or sepsis warrant an emergency surgical intervention. In patients with more than 10 days of symptoms, delaying cholecystectomy for 45 days is better than immediate surgery.

✔✔ Laparoscopic cholecystectomy remains the treatment of choice for patients with acute cholecystitis. Early surgery is associated with reduced length of stay, reduced gallstone-related complications and a reduction in re-admissions due to ongoing symptoms.

Population studies have shown benefits of early LC (defined as within 72 hours of emergency presentation) in terms of reduced complications, BDI, shorter length of stay and fewer re-admissions.[10] Nonetheless, in TG-18 the authors removed the previous limitation of 72 hours on LC for moderate AC, instead suggest progressing with surgery irrespective of time if surgical expertise and patient comorbidity permit.[8] For those patients deemed unfit for surgery, then conservative management with antibiotics for those with mild AC is appropriate, but the consideration of early and urgent percutaneous drainage (PTGD) should be considered for those with moderate AC.[8]

For patients with severe local inflammation or severe AC, urgent gallbladder drainage should be carried out.[8] However, it is important to be aware in the presence of biliary peritonitis, gallbladder torsion, emphysematous, gangrenous, or purulent cholecystitis, urgent surgery is required[8] (Fig. 14.4). TG-18 also makes adjustment to the recommendation for surgery in a select group of patients with severe AC. If a patient appropriately responds to resuscitative measures (no ongoing neurological or respiratory dysfunction), has appropriate ASA score (≤2) or CCI (≤3) and total bilirubin < 2 mg/dL and there is appropriate surgical expertise, then surgery can be considered.[8]

In TG-18, the authors stress the new concept of de-escalation of antimicrobial therapy such that the antibiotic spectrum is narrowed as soon as sensitives of the underlying organism are known.[11] Common organisms associated with biliary infections include *Escherichia coli*, *Klebsiella* spp., *Pseudomonas* spp. and *Enterococcus* spp.[11] For mild AC, ampicillin with aminoglycoside, cephalosporin, carbapenem or fluroquinolone based therapies are all potential options.[11] Blood cultures are not required and antimicrobial therapy can be stopped once source control is achieved for mild AC.[3,11] For more severe infections, culture of bile, blood and, where possible, tissue are recommended.[11] Piperacillin may be used instead of ampicillin.[11] Duration should be extended for 4–7 days.[11] A recent systematic review of the true role of antibiotics in AC also failed to come to definitive conclusions given low quality of evidence despite 12 randomised trials.[12]

✔✔ The routine use of antibiotics in the management of acute cholecystitis remains unclear due to poor quality evidence. Antimicrobial therapy may be stopped once source control is achieved in mild and moderate AC. Systemic antimicrobial treatment should be continued for 4–7 days for more severe infections.

PERCUTANEOUS GALLBLADDER DRAINAGE

When considering the role of PTGD, it is important to have considered the results of the CHOCOLATE trial.[13] This was a multicentre RCT performed across 11 Dutch hospitals. The aim of this study was to compare PTGD with LC in 'high-risk' patients with AC. Although the authors used the TG-13 diagnosis of acute calculous cholecystitis, the definition of high-risk patients was defined as patients with an APACHE score between 7 and 14, excluding those patients with APACHE score > 14, with underlying cirrhosis or requiring ICU admission at the time of diagnosis of AC, or with symptoms > 7 days duration. All LC were performed by experienced surgeons. The primary outcomes were death within 1 year and occurrence of major complications within 1 month, or the need for re-intervention or recurrent biliary disease within 1 year. After recruitment met 50% of the trial target (n = 138 patients), interim independent data analysis recommended cessation of the trial due to superior outcomes for those undergoing LC (major complications 8/66 vs 44/68 patients, RR [95% CI] 0.19 [0.10–0.37], $P < 0.001$). In addition, there was a significant increase in healthcare costs and resource utilisation. The question arising from this study is whether early elective cholecystectomy in those treated with PTGD could have improved outcomes. A recent population study showed a higher risk of overall complications and longer hospital stay in 1211 patients who underwent surgery within 8 weeks of PTGD compared with 1787 patients who underwent surgery after 8 weeks.[14] BDI rate was high but not influenced by timing of surgery.

In patients who undergo PTGD, it is important to realise the effect of increased delay to drainage on short- and long-term outcomes. Yeo et al.[15] have shown that increasing time to drainage increases both inpatient and 30-day mortality. While Yamada et al.[16] demonstrated an increase in operative

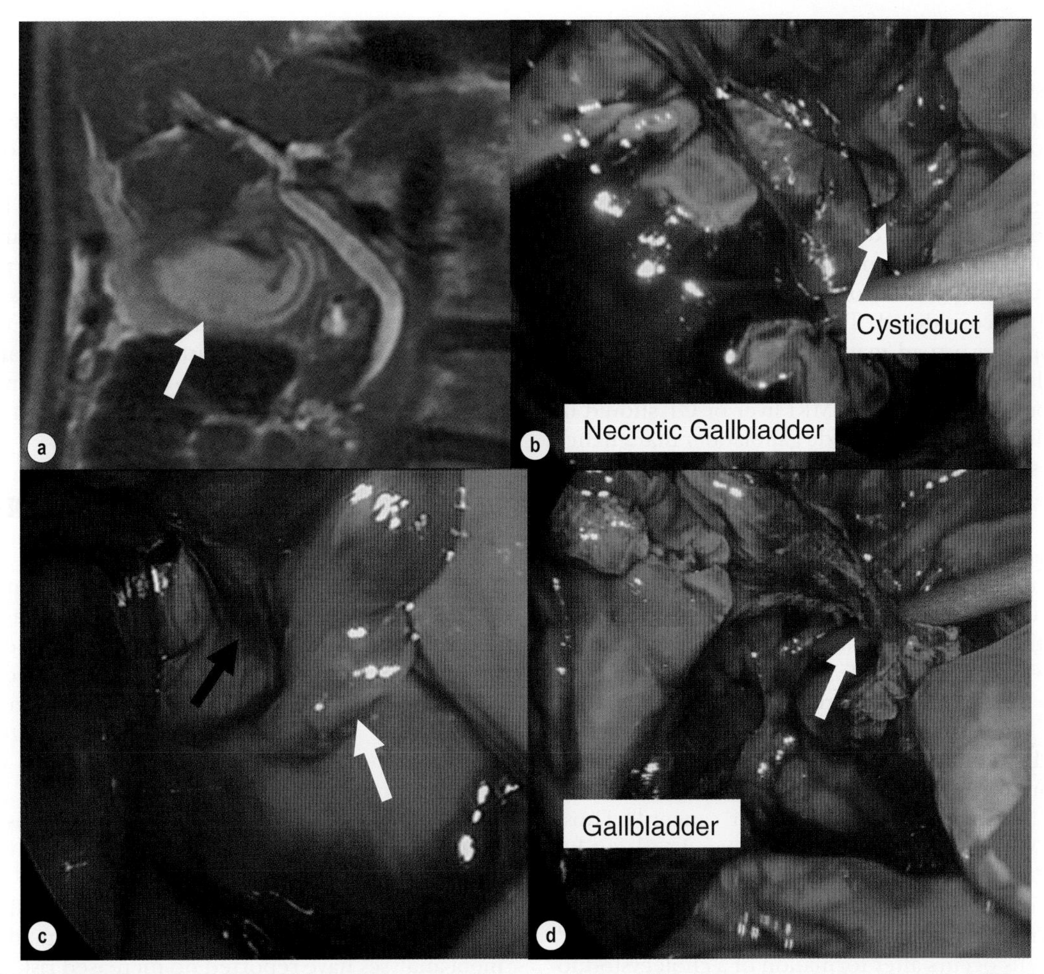

Figure 14.4 An 86-year-old man presents with predicted moderate acute cholecystitis. Magnetic resonance imaging (MRI) shows features of cholecystitis. Note transverse orientation of gallbladder on MRI (a, *white arrow*). At surgery, a necrotic gallbladder secondary to acute torsion is observed **(b)**. The cystic duct is twisted (**c**, *white arrow*) and a narrow mesentery can be seen (**c**, *black arrow*) and the gallbladder lies free of the hepatic surface. With the gallbladder detorted and small mesentery divided the gallbladder can be seen attached by cystic duct alone (**d**, *white arrow*). Caution is required given lack of classical landmarks to guide safe cholecystectomy.

difficulty and conversion in those patients in whom drainage was delayed > 74 hours from onset of symptoms. Therefore, early decision-making regarding surgery or PTGD is required.

In a study of 103 patients[15] with a median age of 80 years in whom PTGD was used, short- and long-term outcomes were described. The inpatient mortality was 13%, indicating the severity of disease and comorbidity in this group of patients. Eventually only 41% underwent cholecystectomy with a 15% rate of conversion. Wang et al.[17] describe 279 (24%) patients who presented with AC undergoing PTGD. Of these patients, 3% died during initial illness and 31% underwent delayed cholecystectomy. Thus, 184 (66%) patients were deemed symptom-free (drainage into cystic duct and no symptoms after clamping) at follow-up and underwent PTGD removal. At 1 year, 60 (33%) patients had undergone LC, 5 (3%) patients had died and 17 (9%) patients developed recurrent AC. Factors associated with recurrent AC were complicated cholecystitis, antibiotic duration < 10 days and PTGD > 32 days.

✔ Acute cholecystectomy is the standard of care of 'high-risk' patients with acute cholecystitis.[13] If percutaneous drainage is employed, the decision should be made early and subsequent elective cholecystectomy should be delayed longer than 8 weeks to reduce complication rates.[14]

COMPLICATED CHOLECYSTITIS

Although specific complications, such as emphysematous cholecystitis, mucocele, empyema, peri-cholecystic abscesses and cholecystoenteric (most commonly to duodenum or colon) fistula, can develop as a sequelae of AC, acute LC remains the standard of care.[8] The exceptions are Mirizzi syndrome and gallstone ileus both of which deserve further consideration as the management differs.

Mirizzi syndrome is due to a large gallstone compressing or eroding into the common bile duct (CBD). It usually presents with symptoms and biochemical signs of AC or cholangitis. Mirizzi syndrome has been classified into four types[18] based on absence (type 1) or presence of a fistula (type 2–4).

Types 2–4 are split by degree of erosion of circumference of the bile duct, <1/3, <2/3 or complete destruction, respectively.[18] The key concept is that there is a high probability that the hepatobiliary triangle has been obliterated due to fibrosis and so the surgeon must be aware that pursing the critical view of safety (CVS) and complete cholecystectomy may be dangerous and lead to BDI. If suspected on US (by the presence of intrahepatic duct dilatation with normal distal CBD and a large stone impacted in Hartmann's pouch), then further imaging in the form of MRCP and MRI liver or CT should be considered. The MRCP should provide a detailed preoperative road map of the biliary and vascular anatomy so that a planned approach to the hepatobiliary triangle can be formulated. The MRI liver or CT should be added as the differential will include gallbladder malignancy.

In type 1, subtotal cholecystectomy can be performed, while types 2–4 likely require a hepaticojejunostomy. Thus, referral to a hepatobiliary surgeon is recommended for more advanced disease, especially if malignancy cannot be excluded. In a recent study of 169 patients with Mirizzi syndrome, the incidence was 2.1% of all cholecystectomies.[19] Median duration of symptoms was 8 months. Presentation by types 1–4 was 20%, 57%, 17% and 6%, respectively.[19] Of concern, only 32% of patients were diagnosed preoperatively. Important co-existent findings were 41% incidence of CBD stones, 14% incidence of coexisting fistula into adjacent hollow organs, 33% incidence of xanthalomatous cholecystitis and 5% incidence of gallbladder cancer.[19] Those patients with Mirizzi type 2–3 who were treated without hepaticojejunostomy had higher rates of bile leak and a non-significant doubling of morbidity.[19] The authors therefore concluded in favour of hepaticojejunostomy for type 2–3.[19]

Gallstone ileus occurs after formation of a cholecystoduodenal fistula and migration of a large stone (>2 cm) into the small bowel lumen.[20] The incidence is 0.3–0.5% of patients with cholelithiasis and is more common in female elderly patients.[20] The distal ileum is the narrowest part of the GI tract and is the usual site of obstruction although proximal obstruction at the duodenal bulb can occur (Bouveret syndrome). Radiological signs include pneumobilia and a luminal calcified mass at the point of obstruction. Management of the bowel obstruction is not controversial with enterotomy and stone extraction the standard approach. However, it is worth noting that if possible the stone should be milked proximally to perform an enterotomy as the obstruction point is likely to be oedematous and potentially ischaemic secondary to pressure from the offending stone. A thorough search for upstream stones should be conducted. The dilemma is the management of the gallbladder and the cholecystoduodenal fistula. Historically, although a selective two-stage approach was recommended, a more contemporary approach is a single definitive procedure given high reported rates of recurrence and cholangitis.[20] Most recommendations are however based on small patient series.[20] A tailored approach is needed. In the frail, elderly or unstable patient at high risk of perioperative mortality, a simple enterolithotomy can be performed.

✔ In gallstone ileus, definitive simultaneous or metachronous management of the gallbladder may be determined by symptoms and presence or absence of cholecystolithiasis or choledocholithiasis.

In those with a clear CBD and empty gallbladder, spontaneous closure of the fistula may occur. Endoscopic management of choledocholithiasis by stone extraction with or without temporary covered stenting of a patent cystic duct may be appropriate for those with choledocholithiasis only. In those patients with persistent cholecystolithiasis, the gallbladder is likely to be shrunken and therefore formal dissection of the hepatobiliary triangle may be hazardous. Simply opening the fundus, extracting the stones, performing a cholangiogram (to ensure a clear CBD), closing the cystic duct if patent from within and then closing the duodenal fistula either primarily or with an omental patch would be the standard of care. Failure to assess the common duct may result in cholangitis once the fistula is closed if distal CBD obstruction remains.

PATIENT-SPECIFIC FACTORS FOR CONSIDERATION IN ACUTE CHOLECYSTITIS

There is an increased incidence of gallstones in patients with cirrhosis and such patients are at risk of increased morbidity and mortality from liver failure in the postoperative period which is proportional to the severity of the liver disease.[3] In addition, in patients with portal hypertension, cholecystectomy carries a significant risk of haemorrhage. Therefore, consideration should be given to referring patients with cirrhosis and AC to HPB units familiar with perioperative management of liver failure and techniques associated with minimising bleeding during cholecystectomy including laparoscopic subtotal cholecystectomy.

During pregnancy, up to 0.8% of patients will present with symptomatic gallstone disease.[21] Two systematic reviews and meta-analyses have reported no increased risk of preterm labour (3.8%) or foetal mortality (1.5%) associated with cholecystectomy and improved maternal and foetal outcomes with LC as compared with open cholecystectomy.[21,22] The data were unable to be analysed by presentation type, comorbidity or by gestational age. Recommendations were that in a well patient with non-complex disease, LC in first and second trimester would appear to be treatment of choice. A further American study using the National Inpatient Sample database identified 23 939 pregnant women with administrative coded cholecystitis.[23] Of these patients, 36%, 60% and 4% underwent non-operative treatment, LC or open cholecystectomy, respectively. Significant improvements in outcomes were observed in those undergoing early LC. Importantly, each day delay to LC resulted in an increased daily risk of 1.173x for pre-term delivery, labour or abortion, 1.073x risk of antepartum haemorrhage, and 1.121x increased risk of amniotic infection. Unfortunately, no data was available regarding the gestational age, and those undergoing LC were clearly patients with improved access to healthcare. Although not specific to AC, Fong et al.[24] did analyse outcomes for women presenting in third trimester with symptomatic biliary disease and compared those who underwent LC antepartum with those in early postpartum period. Both maternal and foetal outcomes were worse for those undergoing LC in third trimester and where possible the authors recommended delaying intervention until the postpartum period. Clearly involvement and support of obstetric, neonatal teams and ensuring the patient is well informed of the risks of all treatment options is a must.

✔ Laparoscopic cholecystectomy is the treatment of choice for uncomplicated symptomatic gallstone disease in the first and second trimester. Outcomes are worse in the third trimester and therefore intervention should be delayed until the postpartum period if possible.

In terms of age alone, Fuks et al.[25] retrospectively analysed 414 patients who had been enrolled in a non-related randomised trial and underwent LC for mild or moderate AC of < 5 days duration. Patients were divided by those older than (n = 78) or younger than (n = 336) 75 years of age. There was no difference in postoperative outcomes by age group, even in those greater than 85 years of age (n = 20) or by performance status. The authors concluded that acute LC is safe in elderly patients with early mild or moderate AC.[25] The WSES guidelines simply acknowledge age > 80 years as a risk factor for greater severity of disease, morbidity and mortality.[3]

ACALCULOUS ACUTE CHOLECYSTITIS

This is defined as AC without the presence of gallstones and is said to contribute 14% of all patients presenting with AC.[26] The aetiology is not well understood but thought to be due to a combination of change in bile salt composition, loss of mucosal integrity and microcirculatory disturbances.[26] Patients tend to be older with associated complications of atherosclerosis.[28] Although traditionally associated with critically ill patients, up to 88% of patients will present from the community.[26] Importantly there are higher rates of gangrenous cholecystitis (31%) than gallstone-induced AC (6%).[27] For those who are fit for surgery, LC is the treatment of choice; otherwise PTGD is recommended.[27] Importantly, the recurrence rates following conservative treatment are less than 2%, so delayed cholecystectomy is not usually indicated.[27]

CHOLEDOCHOLITHIASIS AND ASSOCIATED COMPLICATIONS

Gallstones can migrate into the bile duct via the cystic duct or form within the CBD primarily (primary duct stones). Primary duct stones may form in response to foreign bodies (including parasitic infection), stasis or abnormal bile metabolism. In Western populations, part of the traditional definition for a primary duct stone was for the gallbladder to be absent for > 2 years although this is not relevant when associated with foreign bodies or Asiatic cholangiohepatitis. Complications of CBD stones usually result from biliary obstruction leading to acute bacterial cholangitis (ABC) or AP which occasionally may coexist.

Many CBD stones are found incidentally, while others cause transient obstruction resulting in disordered liver function tests (LFTs) or clinical jaundice. Although RUQ or back pain may be present, it is not always a symptom.[28] The level of bilirubin may fluctuate as the obstruction can be transient and tends not to be as high (<180 µmol/L) or unrelenting as that seen with malignancy.[28] The alkaline phosphatase (ALP) and aspartate aminotransferase (AST) tend to rise proportionally (2x upper limit normal) with stone disease, while ALP is more markedly raised (4x upper limit of normal) in those with malignant obstruction.[28] The AST rise in stone disease is associated with biliary pain and can rise and fall very quickly at a rate much greater than that seen with ALP.[28] Normal LFTs have a high negative predictive value (>95%) for CBD stones,[3,29] but while elevated LFTs may increase the clinical suspicion of underlying choledocholithiasis they lack clinically useful levels of sensitivity or specificity to proceed directly to therapeutic intervention (endoscopic retrograde cholangiopancreatography [ERCP] or surgery) without further diagnostic confirmation.

Abdominal US does not accurately assess for the presence or absence of CBD stones. At a median pre-test probability of 41% for a CBD stone, the post-test probability (95% CI) associated with a positive US was 0.85 (0.75–0.91) and a negative US was 0.17 (0.08–33).[29] Appreciating how these figures will change with the pre-test probability based on a selected group of patients is an important consideration regarding utility and cost-effectiveness of further investigation. Further radiological investigation of the CBD can be performed either metachronously or synchronously regarding cholecystectomy depending on the clinical situation. In the metachronous scenario (pre- or post-cholecystectomy), MRCP or endoscopic ultrasound (EUS) have replaced ERCP as the investigation of choice given the risks associated with diagnostic ERCP. Both MRCP and EUS are highly accurate in the assessment of the presence or absence of CBD stones. At a median pre-test probability of 41%, the post-test probabilities associated with positive or negative results have been reported to be 0.94–0.96 and 0.03–0.05, respectively.[30] Therefore, either can be used depending on availability and individual patient preference or co-existing contraindications. However, resource utilisation is often an important consideration for such specialised tests since intraoperative cholangiography is generally cheaper and more readily available. At a median pre-test probability of 35% for a CBD stone, the post-test probability of a positive and negative intraoperative cholangiogram (IOC) has been shown to be 0.98 and 0.01, respectively.[31]

✔ Preoperative and intraoperative investigations can be considered equivalent tests, and their place in the management of patients with suspected CBD stones will be dependent on the planned management strategy.

Although cost analysis supports laparoscopic ultrasonographic assessment of the CBD, its use has generally been restricted to those surgeons with a strong HPB interest.[32] Fluorescent intraoperative cholangiography is an emerging method of reducing bile duct injuries by demonstrating the anatomy in real time; however, there are currently no data regarding its effectiveness in detecting CBD stones.

MANAGEMENT OF CHOLEDOCHOLITHIASIS

To optimise the management of any condition it is important to understand the natural history. For patients with 'silent' or incidental stones, the seminal and definitive paper is by Collins et al.[33] A total of 962 patients with cholelithiasis and no current suspicion of CBD stone (defined normal CBD on

US, absence of jaundice) underwent LC and successful IOC. Acute patients and those with altered LFTs or a history of AP were included. At the completion of the cholangiogram, the catheter was left *in situ* with no attempt to manage the CBD stones. A follow-up cholangiogram at 48 hours and 6 weeks was performed. Of the 962 patients, 46 (4.7%) were found to have filling defects. At 48 hours, 12 patients had normal cholangiogram (these patients were interpreted as having false-positive IOC). At 6 weeks, 12 of the 34 patients with abnormal cholangiogram at 48 hours had a normal cholangiogram. None of these 12 patients had complications from passage of stones and only 2 described an episode of pain. Of the remaining 22 patients, 20 underwent successful ERCP while 2 did not and neither developed any symptoms after 5-years of follow-up. This study highlighted several important points. Although increasing age and raised ALP predicted presence of CBD stones, no factors (including bile duct size or number of stones) predicted those CBD stones that were more likely to pass spontaneously. The data also showed that in a group of patients without complications of CBD stones, the potential long-term morbidity is low and likely less than 2.5%. This needs to be considered against the morbidity of intervention.

✔ Expectant management has been recommended if the pre-test probability of a CBD stone is < 3% or if intraoperative imaging is suboptimal.[32]

For those patients with CBD stones that warrant intervention, the options are surgical or endoscopic. Either may be performed synchronously or metachronously with cholecystectomy. There has been considerable literature dedicated to whether an endoscopic or laparoscopic approach is superior. A recent meta-analysis including 13 studies with 1757 patients compared the two most commonly utilised and published approaches of LC and bile duct exploration (LCBDE) with preoperative ERCP and LC. LCBDE was superior to preoperative ERCP and LC both in terms of improved stone clearance rates (94.1% vs 90.1%, OR 1.56) and lower perioperative complications (7.6% vs 12.0%, OR 0.67), conversion to other procedure, retained stones (1.2% vs 7.9%, OR 0.34), recurrent stones, operative time, length of stay (4.94 vs 6.62 days) and costs.[34]

The treatment algorithm employed should be tailored to the individual patient (fitness/frailty assessment, organ dysfunction), their anatomical and technical features (duct size, stone size or position, difficulties of endoscopic or laparoscopic access, gallbladder *in situ*, body habitus, previous surgery) and available resources and expertise (proficiency with LCBDE, availability of appropriate equipment, access/availability to ERCP) (Fig. 14.5). Long-term outcomes after LCBDE have shown recurrence rates to be low (2%) and importantly even in a series where a transverse choledochotomy and T-tube were used routinely, no biliary strictures were reported (46 patients, median follow-up of 17 years).[35] Long-term outcomes following ERCP and sphincterotomy have raised the possibility of association with cholangiocarcinoma, but the level of evidence is poor.[28] However, because of this potential association, some authors have recommended caution in using this approach in very young patients.[36]

ACUTE BACTERIAL CHOLANGITIS

Similar to AC, the definition, investigation and management of ABC has been subjected to expert systematic review.[11,37–40] ABC has been defined as acute inflammation and infection of the bile duct. It requires combination of biliary obstruction and the presence of bacteria. The obstruction generates increased intraductal pressure, allowing translocation of bacteria and toxins into the venous or lymphatic systems. The incidence of ABC in those with asymptomatic gallstones is 0.3–1.6% at 5–10 years.[37] The diagnostic criteria for ABC from TG-13 have been further validated and adopted unchanged in TG-18 (Table 14.2). The authors acknowledged the high specificity associated with the traditional diagnosis of Charcot's triad, but its low sensitivity (21–26%) prohibited it as a useful definition.[38,41] Validation studies have shown a 92% sensitivity and 78% specificity with the described diagnostic criteria.[38,41] The importance of the inflammatory component is that it is rarely seen in acute hepatitis, but if there is concern virology and serology should be performed.[37] This does mean that patients with mild ABC may not be captured by the TG-18 definitions.[42]

US will confirm biliary dilatation (or differential diagnoses such as hepatic abscess or AC) providing evidence to support the diagnosis and facilitating early intervention, particularly in those patients with moderate or severe ABC, although it may be inaccurate in detecting the underlying aetiology. Both MRI and CT will show evidence of periportal inflammation and altered perfusion within hepatic parenchyma due to reduced portal venous flow and increased hepatic arterial flow. MRI is more useful for determining aetiology.[38] ABC can be graded as: severe (any associated organ dysfunction including haematological (INR > 1.5, platelets < 100000/mm^3), moderate (any two of the following: white cell count < 4 or > 12 × 10^3/mm^3, temperature > 39°C, age > 74 years, bilirubin > 85 μmol/L, albumin < 0.7x lower limit of normal) or mild without any of the above.[38]

Patient series have shown urgent biliary drainage results in significantly lower 30-day mortality in moderate ABC[41] and reduced length of stay in mild ABC.[42] It has been suggested that severe ABC may benefit from even more urgent biliary decompression, and this is the subject of ongoing research. Importantly, re-assessment of severity should be performed regularly as patients can deteriorate rapidly. There is no correlation between severity grade and 30-day mortality in patients with malignant biliary obstruction.[41]

✔✔ The recommended treatment for acute cholangitis is antibiotics with additional urgent biliary drainage in those classified with moderate or severe disease.[38,39]

Case series have shown a correlation between elevated procalcitonin and severity of ABC, so this may be useful in identifying patients who would benefit from emergency biliary drainage.[43–45] If this correlation is confirmed in further studies and the test made more readily available in clinical practice, it may become a useful adjunct in the management of ABC.

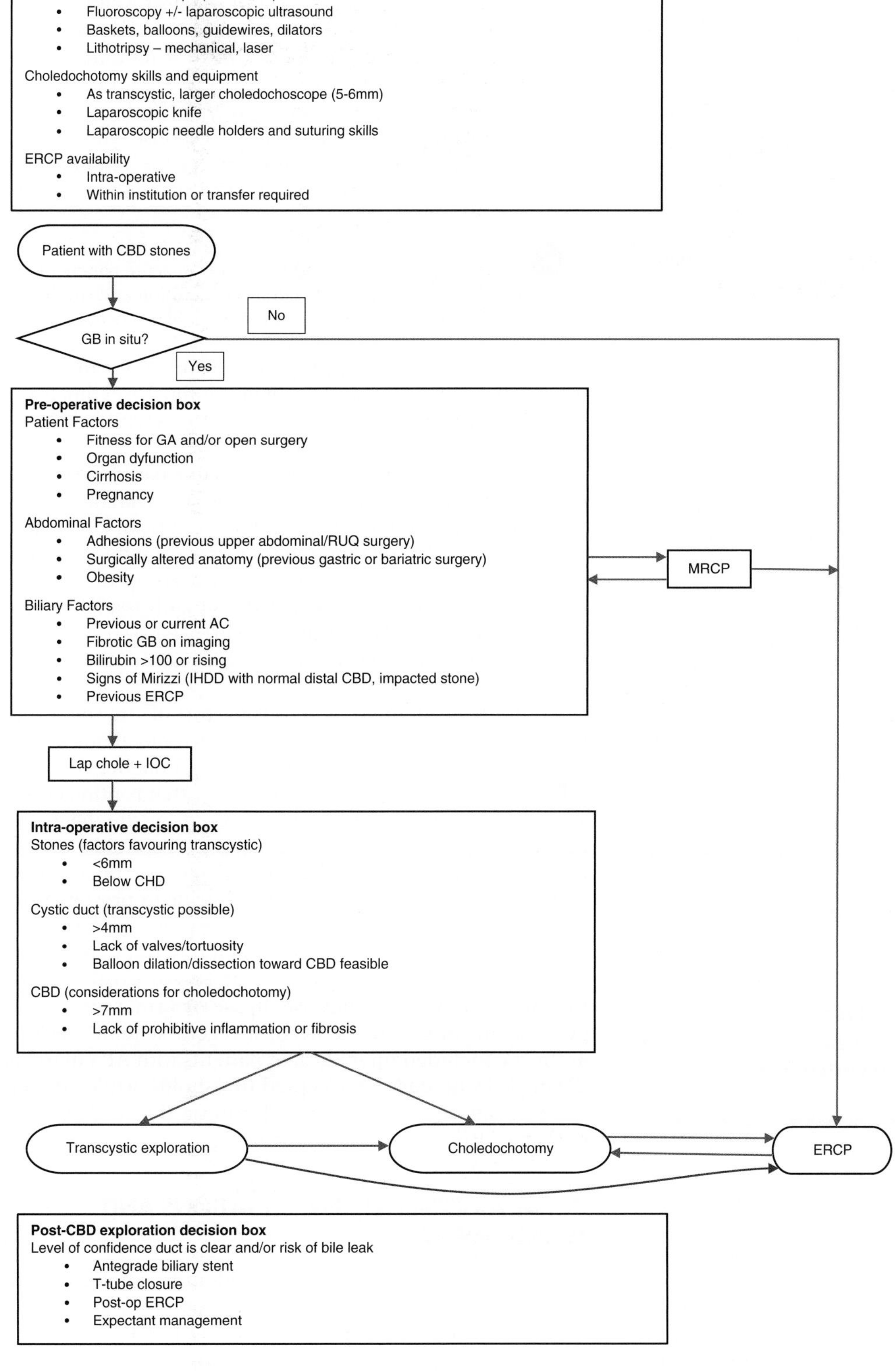

Figure 14.5 Considerations for the management of CBD stones. *CBD,* common bile duct; *CHD,* common hepatic duct; *ERCP,* endoscopic retrograde cholangiopancreatography; *GA,* general anaesthetic; *GB,* gallbladder; *IHDD,* intrahepatic duct dilatation; *IOC,* intraoperative cholangiogram; *RUQ,* right upper quadrant.

In those with severe disease, the principles and interventions associated with managing severe sepsis should be included in the treatment algorithm.[39] Antibiotics of choice are similar to those discussed for management of AC (see preceding section) and are dependent on local patterns of resistance.[11] Once source control is achieved, then a short course of 4–7 days is indicated.

BILIARY DRAINAGE

In terms of biliary drainage, endoscopic drainage has been recommended; however, in a proportion of patients, percutaneous transhepatic biliary drainage (PTBD) will be required when drainage via the papilla cannot be obtained.[40] Surgical drainage has been associated with higher mortality and should be reserved when all other options have been

Table 14.2 TG-18/TG-13 criteria for diagnosis of acute cholangitis[41]

Systemic signs of inflammation	T > 38°C and/or shaking/ chills Abnormal white count (<4, or > 10/mL) or raised C-reactive protein (>10 mg/L)
Biochemical evidence of cholestasis	Bilirubin >34 μmol/L or Raised (>1.5x upper limit normal) liver function tests
Imaging findings	Biliary dilatation or evidence of aetiology (e.g. stones, stricture, stent)

Suspected diagnosis = One item systemic signs of inflammation and one from either biochemistry or imaging.
Definitive diagnosis = One item from each category.

explored. In performing an endoscopic approach, the overriding aim is to achieve transpapillary drainage with the use of an endoscopic stent or nasobiliary drain.[40]

Endoscopic sphincterotomy and stone removal can be attempted at the index procedure in patients with mild–moderate acute cholangitis and stones small enough to not require more invasive techniques such as endoscopic papillary balloon dilatation. This approach is preferable as it reduces hospital stay and costs. Patients with larger stones, those who are coagulopathic and possibly those on antithrombotic agents are best served by a decompressing stent at the index procedure and a second, elective procedure for stone extraction.

In the event of failed endoscopic transpapillary drainage, TG-18 guidelines include endoscopic ultrasound-guided biliary drainage (EUS-BD) as an alternative to PTBD,[40] although the results from community practice may not be equivalent to those in the high-volume centres where the evidence is generated. Hence, if available EUS-BD can be considered, otherwise PTBD should be performed.

Mortality associated with cholangitis has steadily decreased and is now < 3% in most reported series.[38]

ACUTE PANCREATITIS

AP is a common reason for patients to present to acute general surgical services with an underlying incidence of 13–45/100 000 population.[46] It ranges from a mild self-limiting illness to a fulminant and rapidly fatal disease that affects all age groups. Its aetiology is multifactorial, with alcohol and gallstones being the commonest causes although hypertriglyceridemia is now reported to account for 9% of AP.[47] The pathophysiology of AP is complex and there is a lack of a unifying theory possibly due to the multifactorial aetiology.[48] It is thought that the aetiological stimulus results in intracellular activation of pancreatic enzymes such as trypsin.[48] This then triggers a local inflammatory response resulting in release of both pro- and anti-inflammatory mediators and chemokines.[48] This further results in microcirculatory disturbance including increased capillary permeability and microcirculatory intravascular coagulation and ischaemia.[49] If the inflammatory response is confined to a local response, the outcome is mild pancreatitis and usually resolves within a week without systemic or local complications.[48] However, if a systemic inflammatory response (SIRS) is mounted, then moderate or severe pancreatitis ensues. If sustained, multi-organ dysfunction will develop.[48] After 7–10 days, there is transition through to a compensatory response syndrome.[48] In this phase, there is downregulation of the immune system, thus explaining why pancreatic infection peaks in weeks 2–5 after onset.[48]

✔ Understanding this cascade of events in acute pancreatitis is important so that early accurate recognition and stratification into those with mild and severe disease can occur.

This serves to ensure appropriate treatment for those patients with mild disease and facilitates optimal and timely intervention which may include transfer to a specialised HPB unit for those patients with severe disease.

Although there is an extensive guideline-based literature, many are of variable quality. In 2013, the International Association of Pancreatology (IAP) and the American Pancreatic Association (APA) collaborated to produce a systematic and evidence-based guideline compiled by a group of international multidisciplinary experts.[46] This highly readable document provides the best available evidence-based summary of the literature and forms the basis for many of the recommendations in this section.

AP has been defined as requiring two of the following criteria: clinical (upper abdominal pain), biochemical (3x upper limit of normal lipase or amylase), imaging (US, CT, MRI).[46] It is important to note, however, that routine cross-sectional imaging is not usually required for the diagnosis particularly in those with mild disease. It should only be used in the initial phase if there is diagnostic uncertainty or there has been prolonged period prior to presentation in which case the enzyme rise may have passed.[46] Although other biochemical markers have been described, their use has been limited by availability.[48] It is also worth noting the fallibility of serum amylase, lipase or urinary trypsinogen-2 as diagnostic markers. In a recent systemic review, authors concluded up to 25% of patients with AP fail to be diagnosed with current accepted thresholds, while 10% of those diagnosed by biochemical criteria do not have underlying AP.[50]

INITIAL ASSESSMENT, INVESTIGATIONS AND MANAGEMENT

Initial investigations are targeted to identify aetiologies and predict severity or complications that require urgent intervention. In those with a SIRS response and obstructive LFTs with or without jaundice, or a dilated bile duct with evidence of gallstones on abdominal US, co-existing cholangitis (Table 14.2) can be diagnosed. For patients with suspected co-existing cholangitis, antibiotics should be commenced and urgent ERCP should be performed.[11,46] ERCP is not indicated for those with non-biliary pancreatitis or mild biliary pancreatitis without cholangitis.[46] In patients with predicted severe biliary pancreatitis with or without cholestasis but without cholangitis, a multicentre RCT has shown that early

ERCP (within 72 hours) is not associated with a reduction in the incidence of major complications or mortality (45/117 [38%] vs 50/113 [44%], $P = 0.37$) and therefore is not recommended.[51]

✔✔ Urgent ERCP and antibiotics are indicated for patients with co-existing acute biliary pancreatitis with cholangitis. Urgent ERCP is not indicated for patients with acute pancreatitis without cholangitis.

Serum triglycerides (TAG) should be measured especially in those with lipaemic specimens. Although mildly elevated TAG are commonly associated with AP, grossly elevated levels (>1000 mg/dL) indicate hypertriglyceridemia as an aetiology.[47] However, it should be acknowledged there is no uniformly accepted cut-off to act as a definition.[47] Early diagnosis of hypertriglyceride-induced pancreatitis is important as rapid reduction in serum TAG levels can be achieved by with a combination of insulin infusion, anti-hyperlipidaemic medication, dietary manipulation and plasmapheresis.[47] Plasmapheresis has been shown to reduce abdominal pain and APACHE II scores but not morbidity or mortality, although the possibility of a type II error exists.[47] These patients are complex in terms of physiology, nutritional requirements and management and so a multidisciplinary approach with lipid and transfusion specialists, interventional radiologists and dietitians are required. Randomised data is however lacking about the true effect of any of these interventions.

Although abdominal US is the mainstay for the diagnosis of a biliary aetiology, an ALT > 150 U/L within 48 hours has been shown to have a positive predictive value of a biliary aetiology of > 85%.[46] Taking a history for alcohol intake, recent ERCP, trauma, family history of pancreatitis are also important but do not necessarily change immediate management other than management of alcohol withdrawal and vitamin supplementation.

There have been multiple proposed predictors of severity; however, the IAP/APA guidelines have taken a pragmatic approach in using SIRS criteria (Table 14.3) given its ease of use, early applicability and widespread uptake.[46] A recent systematic review of potential biomarkers has identified IL-6 > 50 pg/mL as the best predictor of moderate severe or severe AP with an 87% (69–95) and 88% (80–93) sensitivity (95% CI) and specificity (95% CI), respectively.[52] The widespread real-time availability of IL-6 may however limit its practical usefulness.

For those with predicted severe disease, early CT does not alter the management or improve prediction of outcome and may in fact be harmful due to contrast toxicity to both the pancreas and kidneys.[46] Exceptions to this include those patients in whom bowel ischaemia or hollow viscera perforation is suspected. It has been estimated that it takes 72 hours for pancreatic necrosis to become radiologically evident, although in the future CT perfusion scans may allow earlier detection. In stable patients with a persistent inflammatory state, imaging can be delayed much longer as it is unlikely to change management in the first 4 weeks.

✔ Contrast-enhanced (arterial and portal venous phase) CT should be delayed at least for 96 hours after onset of symptoms.[46]

EARLY MANAGEMENT OF SEVERE DISEASE

Appropriate resuscitation has come into focus in recent times as the enhanced recovery literature has increased understanding of the iatrogenic harm caused by over resuscitation. It is important to keep in mind the reason for fluid resuscitation in AP. The aim is to restore and maintain the macrocirculation but also restore the microcirculation in terms of stabilising the capillary permeability, reducing the inflammatory reaction and sustaining the intestinal barrier function.[49] The purpose is to restore homeostasis with the hope of minimising the development of pancreatic necrosis. However, it should be realised that many of the microcirculatory changes are time dependant and irreversible changes may have occurred by the time the patient presents.[49] The effect of time to presentation on the outcome of fluid resuscitation has not been well studied within the literature.

Currently, it is recommended that an isotonic semi-balanced crystalloid solution (Ringer's lactate or Hartmann's solutions) rather than normal saline or colloid be used for the initial resuscitation.[46] This is based on evidence that balanced crystalloid solutions reduce the incidence of SIRS as compared with normal saline, while colloid solutions have been associated with increased mortality in patients with severe sepsis.[46] Yet, there is some evidence that AP differs from sepsis and that colloids may help protect and stabilise the microcirculation by preventing inflammatory mediators reaching the acinus.[49] Some authors would suggest limiting the use of colloids to those patients with AP

Table 14.3 Definitions that predict severity in acute pancreatitis based on variables contributing to systemic inflammatory response syndrome (SIRS)[49]

Variable	Criteria	
Temperature	<36°C or >38°C	
Heart rate	>90/min	
Respiratory rate	>20/min	
White blood cell count	<4 × 10^9/L or > 12 × 10^9/L or 10% bands	
Terminology	Criteria	Outcome
SIRS	2 or more of above criteria	
Transient SIRS	SIRS < 48 hours	25% mortality
Persistent SIRS	SIRS > 48 hours	8% mortality

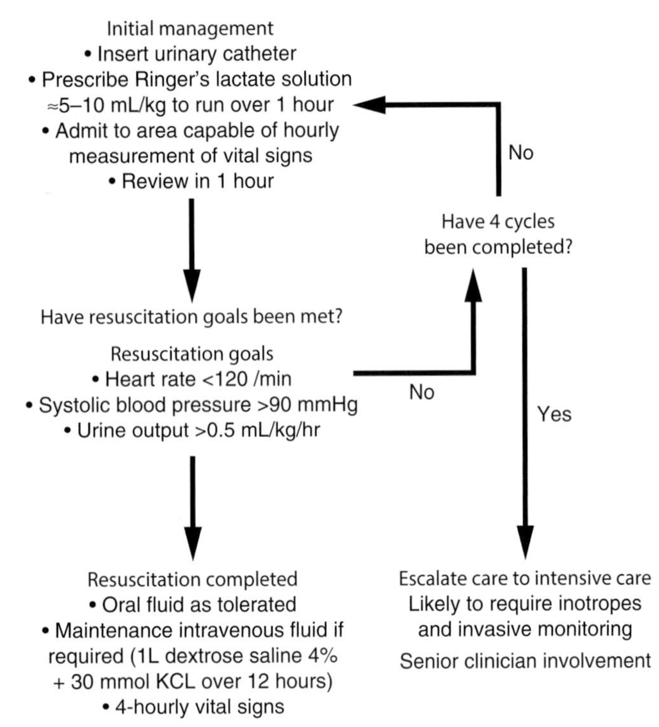

Figure 14.6 Goal-directed resuscitation for patients with systemic inflammatory response syndrome (SIRS) and acute pancreatitis (predicted severe).

and low haematocrit (<25% or albumin < 20 g/L).[49] There is now some evidence to support the use of hypertonic saline.[49] Clearly this area is fraught with confounding factors, and further evidence will be required.

The infusion rate is also important with goal-directed therapy of 5–10 mL/kg/hr to be used until resuscitation goals are met. This has been shown to reduce the incidence of SIRS, need for mechanical ventilation, sepsis and mortality as compared to higher (10–15 mL/kg/hr) rates of resuscitation.[46,49] The evidence for proposed goals as the ideal physiological endpoints to resuscitation remains poor. It has been recommended that non-invasive goals be defined as heart rate < 120/min, mean arterial pressure 65–85 mmHg, urine output 0.5–1 mL/kg/hr and maintain haematocrit between 35% and 44%, while invasive measures include stroke volume variation.[46] This concept may not be easy to implement in a ward setting as traditional intravenous fluid prescribing is based on time not by response. Therefore, new prescribing algorithms are required (Fig. 14.6). It is also important to note that these same principles may not apply to those with mild AP. An RCT looking at aggressive intravenous hydration (20 mL/kg bolus followed by 3 mL/kg/hr, repeated 12 hourly until biochemical and clinical improvement) with lactated Ringer's in patients with mild AP improved the rate of clinical improvement compared with a standard rate of hydration (10 mL/kg bolus followed by 1.5 mL/kg/hr).[53]

✔✔ Infusion of an isotonic semi-balanced crystalloid solution at 5–10 mL/kg/hr should be used until resuscitation goals are achieved.

EARLY THERAPIES AIMED AT MODIFYING SEVERITY OF DISEASE

There has been a long history of unsuccessful pharmacological therapies aimed at mitigating the clinical course of predicted severe AP.[54] Huang et al.[55] have now reported on the use of cyclooxygenase-2 (COX-2) inhibitors in patients with predicted severe AP. The authors performed a single-centre, non-blinded, non-placebo RCT in which patients were randomised to standard of care as recommended by the Chinese society of gastroenterology (it is worth noting this included somatostatin infusion at 50 μg/hr for 3 days) versus standard of care + parecoxib 40 mg daily injection for 3 days, followed by celecoxib 200 mg po bd for 7 days. Inclusion criteria included patients aged 18–70 years, symptoms to admission < 48 hours, APACHE score ≥ 8. The primary endpoint was occurrence of severe AP as defined by persistent (>48 hours duration) organ failure. Secondary outcomes included measures of inflammation, early and late clinical outcomes, and financial costs. In total, 188 patients were analysed. There was a significant reduction in the occurrence of severe AP in the COX-2 group (21% vs 40%, $P = 0.005$); in addition, markers of severity of inflammation at day 4 and 8 including APACHE scores, CRP, IL-6 and TNF were all significantly lower in the treatment group. Clinical outcomes were also improved with reduction in pain and late local complications. Patients in the treatment group had shorter hospital stay and lower overall cost.[55] As with all good research, this trial raises questions especially about the potential adverse effect on renal function and low mortality in those with persistent organ failure; however, it should stimulate further studies. Epidural analgesia may also have an important role to play in helping improve pancreatic perfusion,[56] but further trials are needed.[57]

A recent development is an RCT in patients with severe AP and intra-abdominal hypertension showing more rapid resolution of intra-abdominal pressure with regular intramuscular neostigmine.[58]

The need for nutritional support is widely adopted as the standard of care for those with established severe AP and will be covered within the HPB volume of the companion series. However, the aim of this section is to discuss the role of early feeding in both mild and severe pancreatitis. Historically non-randomised data had suggested that early (<48 hours from admission) nasoenteric feeding could reduce infectious complications and mortality.[59] Subsequently, several meta-analyses and systematic reviews have attempted to clarify the effect of the timing of enteral nutrition (EN). However, many of these reviews have included trials with control arms that have used parenteral nutrition. Doing so may skew the conclusions if parental nutrition has an adverse effect. Therefore, it is better to examine two randomised controls trials which aim to compare either EN with nil by mouth (NBM) or early versus delayed EN.[59,60] Stimac et al.[60] enrolled 214 patients within 24 hours of admission with APACHE II score ≥ 6 and AP. Patients were randomised to NBM or EN with the primary endpoint being a reduction in incidence of persistent (>48 hours) SIRS. The incidence of persistent SIRS at 48 hours was 45% in the EN group versus 48% in the NBM group, $P = 0.681$. None of the secondary outcome measures of severity of inflammation, local pancreatic specific complications, organ failure or mortality showed a reduction in the treatment arm, although the possibility of type II error existed. It is worth noting that prophylactic antibiotics were used in this trial and the patients in the NBM group received higher volumes of IV fluid resuscitation. No measure of time from onset of symptoms was provided. The second RCT by the Dutch pancreatitis study group[59] enrolled 208 patients to either early nasoenteric feeding (within 24 hours of admission) versus NBM for 72 hours (unless patients requested food) and then oral diet with nasoenteric supplementation if required. The primary endpoint was a composite of major infection or death within 6 months. Inclusion criteria was limited to those with APACHE II score > 7 or CRP > 150 mg/L. Patients were stratified by APACHE II score < or ≥ 13. There was no difference in the primary endpoint (30% in early enteral feeding vs 27% in oral diet group, P = 0.76) or secondary outcomes such as incidence necrosis or amelioration of the inflammatory response. No benefit was seen in the subgroup analysis based on the APACHE II score. Thus at this time, there is no evidence to support the statement that early EN will reduce SIRS or mortality in severe AP.[59] Future work in such patients will need to address the issue of feed type as early use of polymeric formulas have been associated with chylous ascites.[61] The data surrounding nutrition is difficult to interpret given the heterogeneity in inclusion criteria, variation in the control groups and the therapies administered. In addition, variable endpoints further confound the data. A large multicentre randomised double-blind clinical trial looking at high versus low energy administration in early phase of AP (GOULASH trial) has been registered[62] including patients with mild AP and aims to recruit almost 1000 patients.

For those with mild disease, the relevant clinical question relates to NBM versus allowing early institution of normal diet. There are three RCTs[63–65] that have tested clear liquid diets against solid diets, all showing reduced length of stay (2 days) in those who were allowed to eat normally. In addition, a further RCT in patients with mild to moderate AP showed reduced pain scores and need for opiates in those fed early.[66]

✔✔ There is strong evidence that allowing patients with mild or moderate acute pancreatitis to eat early and on demand is beneficial.

PREVENTING SECONDARY INFECTIOUS COMPLICATIONS

Prophylactic antibiotics have been extensively studied in a systematic review by Wittau et al.,[67] in which 14 trials consisting of 841 patients were included. There was no reduction in infectious complications, surgical intervention or mortality associated with prophylactic antibiotic use and so they cannot be recommended.[67]

MANAGEMENT OF MILD BILIARY PANCREATITIS

The PONCHO trial[68] randomised 266 patients to same admission cholecystectomy or interval (25–30 days) cholecystectomy. Inclusion criteria were CRP < 100 mg/L, pain-free and eating and ASA < 4 or if > 75 years, ASA < 3. The composite primary endpoint was re-admission for gallstone-related complications or mortality within 6 months. The primary endpoint was reduced from 17% to 5%, P = 0.002. There was no difference in operative safety endpoints between the groups. In those patients who underwent interval cholecystectomy, 51% reported gallstone pain during the interval that did not bring them to hospital.

✔✔ Patients with mild biliary pancreatitis should undergo laparoscopic cholecystectomy on the same admission.

It is clear that early LC is highly desirable for patient-centred care, but it is important to be aware of those patients who may harbour acute peri-pancreatic fluid collections or an acute necrotic collection. In patients with raised inflammatory markers or blood urea nitrogen > 20 mg/dL or packed cell volume > 44%, cross-sectional imaging should be considered to identify those with acute fluid or necrotic collections.[69] Such patients should be excluded from early LC as early LC has been associated with increased infectious pancreatic complications and need for intervention.[70] The natural history of acute peri-pancreatic fluid collections is resolution, while acute necrotic collections may become infected early (5/80), resolve (33/80) or develop walled off necrosis (30/80) which may become infected (8/39), remain sterile (7/39) or resolve (23/39).[69] Therefore, such patients should be left for 6–10 weeks prior to cholecystectomy.

In patients who are not fit enough for LC, definitive endoscopic sphincterotomy should be considered.[71,72] Population data from the UK has shown a reduced rate of gallstone pancreatitis re-admission in patients who underwent ERCP (5.3%) compared with those who had no definitive treatment (13.2%) with 1-year follow-up.[71] A similar study from the USA showed reduced 2-year readmissions in ERCP patients (31.1%) compared with patients receiving no definitive treatment (48.5%) and the re-admissions were less likely to be for gallstone pancreatitis.[72] ERCP does not reduce the risk of other gallstone-related complications.[73]

WHEN SHOULD A PATIENT WITH SEVERE ACUTE PANCREATITIS BE TRANSFERRED?

This will be dependent on the local services (interventional and endoscopic) and the critical care and surgical skill sets at the local hospital. The IAP/APA guidelines have defined which patients should be admitted to an intensive care unit and what determines a tertiary centre for management of AP.[46] The authors of IAP/APA guidelines recommend patients with severe AP be managed in a specialist centre based on population data suggesting improved outcomes from high-volume centres.[46] However, many health systems face physical and resource constraints with regard to the ability to transfer all patients into regional intensive care units especially with the increasing centralisation of HPB cancer services. To get around this, some services have developed the concept of a regional 'hub and spoke' model with remote advice and management given by the tertiary centres; however, no data exists on the outcomes of this approach as compared to early physical transfer. If such an approach is to be taken, close links between the referring and receiving centre will be required with ability for efficient and timely transfer as required.

FOLLOW-UP FOR NON-BILIARY, NON-ALCOHOL-INDUCED PANCREATITIS

Although a rare cause of AP, hypercalcemia should be screened for as further attacks can be prevented by early diagnosis. Other aetiologies include medications which can be difficult to prove given the latency of exposure and presentation with AP. Sphincter of Oddi dysfunction should be considered in those with disordered LFTs. An interval MRI pancreas should be considered looking for structural abnormalities such as pancreas divisum or neoplasm including pancreatic intraductal papillary mucinous neoplasms. EUS is also useful to detect occult gallstones or structural changes of chronic pancreatitis. In patients with family history or recurrent attacks at an early age, genetic screening should be considered in conjunction with a genetic service.

Recent literature also raises an important issue regarding long-term outcomes for all patients irrespective of severity of the AP. In a systematic review[74] of 24 prospective clinical studies involving 1102 patients who presented with their first attack of AP, the prevalence of prediabetes, diabetes and treatment with insulin was 16%, 23% and 15%. By 5 years, there was a 2.7-fold increase in the diagnosis of new-onset diabetes.

✔ Patients and primary practitioners should be informed of the risk of diabetes to ensure appropriate long-term follow-up and awareness of symptoms.

TECHNICAL CONSIDERATIONS FOR PROCEDURES USED IN ACUTE BILIARY DISEASE

Emergency LC has been associated with an increased risk of BDI in those with moderate or severe AC.[9] It is therefore important that surgeons undertaking LC have a construct on how to mitigate the risk of such injuries as has been outlined in the recently published multi-society practice guideline.[75] Although achieving the CVS has been widely promoted as the key to avoiding BDI, randomised data is lacking mainly due to the large numbers of patients that would need to be enrolled given the low rate of transectional BDI.[76] Using error analysis methodology, key steps have been proposed that will allow the identification of stopping points when it is unsafe to proceed with obtaining the CVS.[77] Instead, when faced with difficult pathology and unclear anatomy, it is recommended that consideration be given to calling for help, abandoning the operation or considering subtotal cholecystectomy.[77] Fundus-first cholecystectomy is not recommended as it has been associated with severe vasculobiliary injuries.[78]

Intraoperative cholangiography as a 'preventer' of BDI is a polarising topic with many surgeons lacking individual equipoise, but considerable equipoise exists across the profession. Again, quality randomised data is lacking due to large numbers of patients that would be required to adequately power such a trial.[79] Population data suggests that intraoperative cholangiography may be associated with a reduction in the incidence of BDI, but causality cannot be inferred from such data.[79] A population-based case control study[9] demonstrated that an intention to perform intraoperative cholangiography was associated with 52% reduced risk of BDI. Liberal use of IOC to mitigate the risk of BDI is recommended in the multi-society practice guideline.[75] (Safe Cholecystectomy Summary Box 14.1)

Following LC, postoperative drainage would not appear to be beneficial. In an RCT which included patients with mild or moderate AC, routine use of a drain to the subhepatic fossa post-LC did not reduce risk of postoperative complications (9.6% vs 9.1%, $P = 1.00$).[80]

SUBTOTAL CHOLECYSTECTOMY

A subtotal cholecystectomy should be considered when it is deemed not safe to pursue the CVS. Advanced laparoscopic techniques such as subtotal cholecystectomy are associated with a reduction in BDI compared with historical figures. In fact, a contemporary population-wide study in the USA found that conversion to open surgery associated with an increased relative risk of BDI of 65.44 (12 BDI in 83 patients),[81] raising the question as to whether conversion remains the safest bail out option in the modern era.

The terminology surrounding subtotal cholecystectomy has recently been rationalised and classified into fenestrating and reconstituting subtypes.[82] Subtotal fenestrating cholecystectomy involves removal of the free, peritonealised portion of the gallbladder, except for a lip at the lower end. All stones are extracted and the mucosa may be ablated. The cystic duct can be closed from the inside with a purse-string suture. Care must be taken with the depth of bites in this technique and any attempts to ligate the cystic duct outside the gallbladder run the risk of BDI. A fenestrating cholecystectomy by definition does not result in a remnant gallbladder lumen and therefore has a lower risk of recurrent stone formation but at the expense of an increased risk of bile leakage in the postoperative period, particularly if it is not possible to suture the cystic duct orifice from within the gallbladder lumen, as is often the case.

Subtotal reconstituting cholecystectomy involves removing the free peritonealised portion of the gallbladder and all stones are removed. The lowest safely accessible portion of the gallbladder is then closed with sutures or staples. This typically results in a more reliable seal to the biliary system and therefore carries a lower risk of bile leak. However, a small portion of gallbladder lumen is reconstituted in which more stones may form. In either technique, the hepatic surface of the gallbladder ('back wall') can be left *in situ*. Most series describe the routine use of a postoperative abdominal drain.

A recent meta-analysis of 39 studies including 1784 patients found that fenestrating cholecystectomy had a higher incidence of open conversion, retained stones, intra-abdominal

Box 14.1 Safe laparoscopic cholecystectomy summary box

In mild AC, perform LC within 72 hours of symptom onset
In AC or a history of AC – low threshold for IOC or LUS
Multi-port laparoscopic technique
Use CVS for anatomic identification of CD and artery
Pause to confirm the CVS before clipping or transecting
When CVS cannot be achieved consider STC
Low threshold for calling for help from another surgeon

AC, acute cholecystitis; *CD*, cystic duct; *CVS*, critical view of safety; *IOC*, intraoperative cholangiogram; *LC*, laparoscopic cholecystectomy; *LUS*, laparoscopic ultrasound; *STC*, subtotal cholecystectomy.

Table 14.4 Randomised trials showing benefit of aggressive hydration with lactated Ringer's in preventing endoscopic retrograde cholangiopancreatography pancreatitis.

Variable	Choi et al. 2016[85]		Shaygan-Nejad et al. 2015[87]		Buxbaum et al. 2014[86]	
N	510		150		62	
Aggressive hydration	10 mL/kg before procedure 3 mL/kg/hr during procedure and continue for 8 hours Bolus 10 mL/kg post procedure		3 mL/kg/hr during and for 8 hours post procedure 20 mL/kg bolus post procedure			
Standard hydration	1.5 mL/kg/hr during and for 8 hours post procedure					
Rectal NSAID	No		Not stated		No	
Outcomes (%)	Aggressive	Standard	Aggressive	Standard	Aggressive	Standard
Hyper-amylasemia	7	16	23	44*	23	39
Pain			5	37*	8	22
Pancreatitis	4	10*	5	23*	0	17*

*$P < 0.05$.

collections, surgical site infections, postoperative ERCP and need for re-operation.[83] Given the breadth of complications and the fact that not all would seem directly attributable to the differences in technique, these results are at significant risk of publication bias between the two techniques. Nonetheless, some of the increased risk of complications may be related to the difficulty in suturing the cystic duct orifice laparoscopically in the setting of advanced cholecystitis and fibrosis.

ERCP

Although ERCP is often performed by gastroenterologists, surgeons should be aware of peri-procedural factors that can mitigate the risk of post-ERCP pancreatitis. There is strong evidence for the use of rectal non-steroidal anti-inflammatory drugs[84] which have been associated with 7.7% absolute risk reduction (number needed to treat = 13)[84] in post-ERCP pancreatitis. Currently the recommended dose is 100 mg rectal indomethacin either before or after the procedure.[84] Importantly, IV or PO formulations have not been shown to be beneficial.[84] There are now three RCTs[85–87] that have shown a reduction in post-ERCP pancreatitis with the use of aggressive hydration with lactated Ringer's in peri-procedure period (Table 14.4). In the largest trial by Choi et al., aggressive fluid hydration was also shown to reduce the severity of the pancreatitis ($P = 0.04$) and the effect of reduction was greatest in those at highest risk of post-ERCP pancreatitis (25% vs 9%, $P = 0.04$).[85] The number needed to treat was 18. Important exclusion criteria (other than those deemed at low risk of pancreatitis) in all three trials[85–87] were elderly patients (>70–75 years) and those with significant cardiac, renal or respiratory co-morbidity.

PERCUTANEOUS GALLBLADDER DRAINAGE

For those patients meeting the criteria for PTGD, TG-18 recommends percutaneous transhepatic gallbladder puncture as the standard of care but acknowledge that direct gallbladder puncture and endoscopic approaches have also been described.[88] High-level evidence to strongly support one technique over another is lacking, but one should be aware of the differing complication profiles. Direct gallbladder puncture is associated with increased risk of dislodgement[15] and subsequent bile leak, while transhepatic gallbladder puncture has increased risk of hepatic haemorrhage. Early outcomes of endoscopic gallbladder drainage techniques such as EUS-guided placement of lumen apposing stents seem excellent in highly specialised units.[88]

EUS-GUIDED BILIARY DRAINAGE

The approaches being developed are intrahepatic bile duct drainage by transgastric/transjejunal approach, extrahepatic bile duct drainage by transduodenal/transgastric approach or EUS-guided antegrade stenting. Early peritonitis rates of 10–30%[40] were reported, although this should be reduced with increased experience, improvements in technology and ongoing device innovations such as dedicated lumen-apposing stents for choledochoduodenostomy.

Key points

- Acute cholecystitis can be graded by severity based on degree of systemic inflammation and organ dysfunction.
- For patients without organ failure, early laparoscopic cholecystectomy is the treatment of choice while for those patients who are critically ill, antibiotics and urgent percutaneous gallbladder drainage is the standard of care.
- Acute cholangitis can be graded by degree of systemic inflammation and requires a combination of antibiotics and urgent biliary decompression.
- The natural history of common bile duct stones is that many will pass spontaneously without symptoms and therefore in a population with a low prevalence (<3%), systematic screening for them may not be cost-effective.
- The management of common bile duct stones is dependent on several factors including anatomical, presence or absence of the gallbladder, local services and skill sets. Recent meta-analysis recommends laparoscopic duct exploration as the preferred treatment.
- Acute pancreatitis requires complex timely decision-making depending on severity and aetiology. Therefore, surgical services are encouraged to implement an evidence-based approach and consider optimising clinical work flows to ensure maximal compliance with evidence-based guidelines.

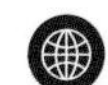
References available at http://ebooks.health.elsevier.com/

VIDEO RECOMMENDATION

- Avoiding bile duct injury. https://www.youtube.com/watch?v=UGhkI6ltAfw
- Difficult cholecystectomy. https://www.youtube.com/watch?v=HeYgOu8C3y4&feature=youtu.be
- Subtotal fenestrating cholecystectomy. https://doi.org/10.1111/ans.16435
- Laparoscopic transcystic CBD exploration. https://www.youtube.com/watch?v=hMYfsqqlKX4
- Choledochotomy and stent insertion. https://www.youtube.com/watch?v=w2vD75t_keA

KEY REFERENCES

[3] Ansaloni L, Pisano M, Coccolin F, Peitzmann AB, Fingerhut A, Catena F, et al. 2016 WSES guidelines on acute calculous cholecystitis. World J Emerg Surg 2016;11:25.

[8] Okamoto K, Suzuki K, Takada T, Strasberg SM, Asbun HJ, Endo I, et al. TG-18 flow chart for the management acute cholecystitis. J Hepatobiliary Pancreat Sci 2018;25:55–72.

[11] Gomi H, Solomkin JS, Schlossberg D, Okamoto K, Takada T, Strasberg SM, et al. TG18: antimicrobial therapy for acute cholangitis and cholecystitis. J Hepatobiliary Pancreat Sci 2018;25:3–16.

[13] Loozen CS, van Santvoort HC, van Duijvendijk P, Besselink MG, Gouma DJ, Nieuwenhuijzen GA, et al. Laparoscopic cholecystectomy versus percutaneous catheter drainage for acute cholecystitis in high risk patients (CHOCOLATE): multicentre randomised clinical trial. BMJ 2018;8(363):k3965.

Dutch Multicentre RCT comparing PTGD with LC in 'high-risk' patients with AC. Exclusions were APACHE score > 14, underlying cirrhosis or requiring ICU admission at the time of diagnosis of AC, or symptoms > 7 days duration. The primary outcomes were death within 1 year and occurrence of major complications within 1 month, or the need for re-intervention or recurrent biliary disease within 1 year. Interim independent data analysis recommended cessation of the trial due to superior outcomes for those undergoing LC.

[14] Altieri MS, Yang J, Yin D, Brunt LM, Talamini MA. Pryor AD Early cholecystectomy (≤ 8 weeks) following percutaneous cholecystostomy tube placement is associated with higher morbidity. Surg Endosc 2020;34(7):3057–63.

Population study showed a higher risk of overall complications and longer hospital stay in 1211 patients who underwent surgery within 8 weeks of PTGD compared with 1787 patients who underwent surgery after 8 weeks.14 BDI rate was high but not influenced by timing of surgery.

[30] Giljaca V, Gurusamy KS, Takwoingi Y, Higgie D, Poropat G, Stimac D, et al. Endoscopic ultrasound vs. magnetic resonance cholangiopancreatography for CBD stones. Cochrane Database Syst Rev 2015;(2): Art No.:CD011549.

[33] Collins C, Maguire D, Ireland A, Fitzgerald E, O'Sullivan G. A prospective study of CBD calculi in patients undergoing laparoscopic cholecystectomy. Ann Surg 2004;239:28–33.

Prospective observational study of patients with CBD stones on cholangiogram. At the completion of the cholangiogram, the catheter was left in situ with no attempt to manage the CBD stones. Follow-up cholangiogram at 48 hours and 6 weeks was performed. 46 (4.7%) were found to have filling defects, 12 false positives. At 6 weeks, 12 of the 34 patients with abnormal cholangiogram at 48 hours had a normal cholangiogram.

[34] Pan L, Chen M, Ji L, Zheng L, Yan P, Fang J, Zhang B, Cai X. The safety and efficacy of laparoscopic common bile duct exploration combined with cholecystectomy for the management of cholecysto-choledocholithiasis. Ann Surg 2018;268:247–53.

[39] Miura F, Takada T, Strasberg SM, Solomkin JS, Pitt HA, Gouma DJ, et al. TG13 flowchart for management of acute cholangitis and cholecystitis. J Hepatobiliary Pancreat Sci 2013;20:47–54.

[46] Working group IAP/APA acute pancreatitis guidelines. IAP/APA evidence based guidelines for the management of acute pancreatitis. Pancreatology 2013;13:e1–15.

[49] Aggarwal A, Manrai M, Kochhar R. Fluid resuscitation in acute pancreatitis. W J Gastroenterol 2014;20:18092–103.

[51] Schepers NJ, Hallensleben NDL, Besselink MG, Anten MPGF, Bollen T, et al. Urgent ERCP with sphincterotomy vs conservative treatment in predicted severe acute pancreatitis (APEC). Lancet 2020;396:167–76

This trial randomised 232 patients with predicted severe acute biliary pancreatitis without cholangitis to urgent ERCP or conservative treatment. The primary endpoint (composite of mortality or major complications such as new-onset persistent organ failure, cholangitis, bacteraemia, pneumonia, pancreatic necrosis or pancreatic insufficiency) occurred in 45/117 (38%) in the urgent ERCP group versus 50/113 (40%) of those in conservative group. Although there was a higher rate of subsequent cholangitis in the conservative group, it did not affect outcomes. Ultimately only one third of patients in the conservative group went onto delayed ERCP.

[55] Huang Z, Ma X, Jia X, Wang R, Liu L, Zhang M, Wan X, Tang C, Huang L. Prevention of severe acute pancreatitis with cyclooxygenase-2 inhibitors: a randomized controlled clinical trial. Am J Gastroenterol 2020;115(3):473–80

This trial showed convincing evidence that early use of COX-2 inhibitors in patients with predicted severe AP reduces the incidence of persistent organ failure and improves clinical outcomes. It limited inclusion to adults < 70 years of age and excluded patients with renal or cardiac impairment. All patients also received somatostatin infusion for 3 days.

[59] Dutch pancreatitis study group. Early vs on demand nasoenteric tube feeding in acute pancreatitis. N Eng J Med 2014;371:1983–93.

[63] Sathiarai E, Murthy S, Mansard MJ, Rao GV, Mahukar S, Reddy DN. Clinical trial:oral feeding with soft diet compared with liquid diet as initial meal in mild Acute pancreatitis. Aliment Pharmacol Ther 2008;28:777–81.

[64] Moraes JM, Felga GE, Chebi LA, Franco MB, Gomes CA, Gaburri PD, et al. A full solid diet as the initial meal in mild acute pancreatitis is safe and results in shorter length of hospitalisation: results of prospective randomised controlled double blind clinical trial. Pancreas 2013;42:88–91.

[65] Rajkumar N, Karthikeyan VS, Ali SM, Sistla SC, Kate V. Clear liquid diet vs. soft diet as the initial meal in patients with mild acute pancreatitis: a randomised interventional trial. Nutr Clin Pract 2013;28:365–70.

[66] Petrov MS, McIlroy K, Grayson L, Phillips AR, Windosr JA. Early nasogastric tube feeding vs. NBM in mild to moderate pancreatitis: a randomised controlled trial. Clin Nutr 2013;32:697–703.

[68] Dutch pancreatitis study group. Same admission vs. interval cholecystectomy for mild gallstone pancreatitis: a multicentre randomised trial. Lancet 2015;386:1261–8.

Dutch randomised controlled trial of 266 patients of same admission cholecystectomy versus interval (25–30 days) cholecystectomy. Inclusion criteria were CRP < 100 mg/L, pain-free and eating and ASA < 4 or if > 75 years, ASA < 3. The composite primary endpoint was re-admission for gallstone-related complications or mortality within 6 months. The primary endpoint was reduced from 17% to 5%, P = 0.002. There was no difference in operative safety endpoints between the groups.

[80] Kim EY, Lee SH, Lee JS, Yoon YC, Park SK, Choi HJ. IS routine drain insertion after laparoscopic cholecystectomy for acute cholecystitis beneficial: a multicentre prospective randomised controlled trial. J Hepatoobilairy Pancreat Sci 2015;22:551–7.

[81] Mangieri CW, Hendren BP, Strode MA, Bandera BC, Faler BJ. Bile duct injuries (BDI) in the advanced laparoscopic cholecystectomy era Surgical. Endoscopy 2019;33:724–30.

[85] Choi JH, Kim HJ, Lee BU, Kim TH, Song IH. Vigorous periprocedural hydration with lactated Ringer's solution reduces the risk of pancreatitis after retrograde cholangiopancreatography in hospitalized patients. Clin Gastroenterol Hepatol 2016:1542–3565.

[86] Buxbaum J, Yan A, Yeh K, Lane C, Nguyen N, Laine L. Aggressive hydration with lactated Ringer's solution reduces pancreatitis after endoscopic retrograde cholangiopancreatography. Clin Gastroenterol Hepatol 2014;12(2):303–7.

[87] Shaygan-Nejad A, Masjedizadeh AR, Ghavidel A, Ghojazadeh M, Khoshbaten M. Aggressive hydration with Lactated Ringer's solution as the prophylactic intervention for post endoscopic retrograde cholangiopancreatography pancreatitis: a randomized controlled double-blind clinical trial. J Res Med Sci 2015;20(9):838–43.

Acute conditions of the small bowel and appendix

15

Timothy Forgan | Robert Baigrie

INTRODUCTION

Acute disease of the small bowel, from which appendicitis is considered separately, contributes substantially to both the urgent and emergency workload of the abdominal surgeon. The pattern of acute small-bowel disease varies with the age of the patient, some being more common in young people, others in older patients. It primarily manifests itself in one of three ways: obstruction, inflammation (peritonitis) and haemorrhage. These are not mutually exclusive and may co-exist in each clinical episode. Treatment may be operative or non-operative, and the timing of surgical intervention is often critical, particularly when bowel ischaemia/infarction is concerned.

SMALL-BOWEL OBSTRUCTION

Although there are many causes of small-bowel obstruction (Box 15.1), the commonest in the developed world is adhesions secondary to previous surgery (approximately 60% of episodes) and malignancy. By comparison, in the developing world, the most common cause is hernia. A large retrospective study using Scottish National Health Service data estimated that 5.7% of all hospital admissions following abdominal and pelvic surgery over a 10-year period were directly related to adhesions.[1] While an attempt should be made to diagnose the cause of the obstruction preoperatively (see Chapter 11) to eliminate conditions that might require special treatment, in practice, the cause of the obstruction is often made only at operation. A meta-analysis published in 2013 showed that the incidence of adhesive small-bowel obstruction (ASBO) requiring surgery was 2.5%. Adhesive obstruction requiring surgery has been found to be highest after paediatric surgery and surgery to the lower gastrointestinal (GI) tract. This review also showed significantly lower incidence of adhesions after laparoscopic (1%) versus open surgery (4%).[2]

MECHANISM

The small bowel responds to obstruction by the onset of vigorous peristalsis. As the obstruction develops, the proximal intestine dilates and fills with fluid, producing systemic hypovolaemia. Further fluid is lost through vomiting, which occurs early if the obstruction is proximal. If the process continues and the blood supply is compromised, infarction and perforation will occur. If the blood supply remains intact and the bowel is decompressed by vomiting and nasogastric drainage, peristalsis will stop, leaving dilated, non-functioning bowel.

PRESENTATION

The typical clinical presentation of small-bowel obstruction is central abdominal colicky pain, vomiting (usually bile-stained), abdominal distension and a reduction or absence of flatus. If the blockage is in the distal ileum, early vomiting may be less of a feature and abdominal distension more obvious. The vomiting often becomes 'faeculent' as the stagnant small-bowel contents become degraded by bacterial colonisation. Bowel sounds increase and may be audible to the patient. Localised peritonitic pain and tenderness suggests ischaemia and incipient strangulation. In some patients there may be an obvious cause, such as an irreducible hernia or scars from previous surgery.

Although small-bowel obstruction can occur without the development of abdominal pain, the absence of this symptom should be viewed with caution. This is particularly the case in postoperative patients, where small-bowel obstruction and intestinal ileus can be difficult to differentiate.

The history and examination of the patient should be sufficiently thorough to identify small-bowel obstruction and its possible causes, as well as any suspicion of ischaemia or perforation aroused by tenderness and peritoneal irritation. Evaluation of the patient's general state, particularly dehydration and its consequences, will ensure adequate resuscitation prior to any planned surgical treatment.

INITIAL MANAGEMENT

The aim of management is adequate resuscitation, confirmation of the diagnosis and the appropriate timing for surgery (when indicated).

Fluid resuscitation usually requires several litres of crystalloid fluid (ideally Hartmann's solution/Ringer's lactate) in the first few hours after admission. With proximal bowel obstruction, ongoing emesis leads to additional loss of fluid containing Na, K, H and Cl and metabolic alkalosis may occur. Continuous assessment of resuscitation using urinary output and lactate is essential. Monitoring of central venous pressure may be required in the elderly or patients with co-existing morbidity. Adequate fluid and electrolyte replacement should be given before any surgical intervention is planned.

Although mild adhesive obstruction may resolve without a nasogastric tube (NGT), its use in established small-bowel

Box 15.1 Causes of small-bowel obstruction

Within the lumen

- Gallstone
- Food bolus
- Bezoars
- Parasites (e.g., *Ascaris*)
- Enterolith
- Foreign body

Within the wall

Tumour

- Primary
  - Small-bowel tumour
  - Carcinoma
  - Lymphoma
  - Sarcoma
  - Carcinoma of caecum
- Secondary

Inflammation

- Crohn's disease
- Radiation enteritis
- Postoperative stricture
- Potassium chloride stricture
- Vascultides (e.g., scleroderma)

Outside the wall

Adhesions

- Congenital
- Bands
- Acquired
- Postoperative
- Inflammatory
- Neoplastic
- Chemical (e.g., starch, talc)
- Pharmacological (e.g., practolol)
- Intussusception

Hernia

- Primary
  - Congenital (e.g., diaphragmatic)
  - Acquired (e.g., inguinal, femoral, etc.)
- Secondary
  - Incisional hernia
  - Internal postoperative hernia (e.g., lateral space, mesenteric defect)

obstruction will reduce vomiting, decompress the bowel and reduce the risk of aspiration. Nasogastric losses should be replaced with additional electrolyte-rich intravenous crystalloid fluids and potassium supplementation if necessary. Adequate analgesia should be given early and will not mask signs of peritonitis, so there is no justification for withholding adequate analgesia while awaiting further clinical assessment.[3] The analgesia requirement should be reviewed regularly, especially in the early stages, as a persistent requirement for increasing amounts may indicate developing strangulation. Anti-thromboembolic prophylaxis should be commenced early and continued until at least discharge from hospital.

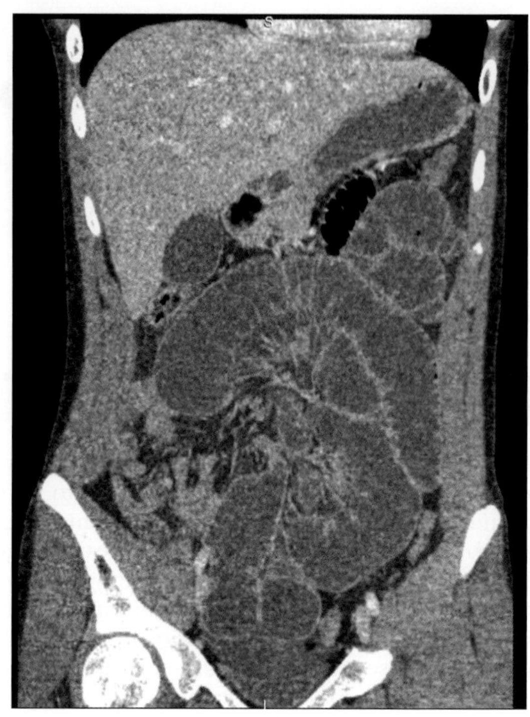

Figure 15.1 Multislice computed tomography with intravenous contrast demonstrating small-bowel obstruction.

INVESTIGATIONS

These are aimed at:

1. Assessing the general state of the patient
2. Confirming the diagnosis of small-bowel obstruction and possible cause
3. Identifying those patients who need early surgery (those with a high risk of strangulation) and those in whom a non-operative approach is appropriate

Contrast-enhanced computed tomography (CT) (Fig. 15.1) is increasingly used in the early assessment of patients with small-bowel obstruction, both to identify the underlying cause (particularly malignancy) and to identify features of possible strangulation. CT features of intraperitoneal free fluid, mesenteric oedema and lack of the 'small-bowel faeces sign', in combination with a history of vomiting, have been reported to be highly predictive of requiring operative intervention.[4] A subtle sign on contrast-enhanced CT scanning is hyperaemia of a segment of bowel, which indicates ischaemia. Identifying patients with possible strangulation remains difficult, and where concern persists, early surgery (laparoscopic or open) is advised. The small-bowel faeces sign refers to the presence of particulate faeculent material mingled with gas bubbles in the lumen of the small intestine (as seen in the colon on CT). It is believed to be the result of delayed intestinal transit and to be caused by incompletely digested food, bacterial overgrowth or increased water absorption of the distal small-bowel contents due to obstruction.

NON-OPERATIVE MANAGEMENT

Adhesive obstruction may initially be treated non-operatively, with a 'drip and suck' regimen, i.e. intravenous fluids and NGT aspiration. Spontaneous resolution can be expected in the majority of adhesive obstructions managed in this way. This treatment plan should be abandoned at the first suggestion of underlying strangulation. These patients are good candidates for a water-soluble contrast medium (WSCM), which has both diagnostic and therapeutic properties. The radiological appearance of contrast in the colon within 24 hours from administration predicts resolution in 99% of patients.[5,6] Although non-operative management (NOM) can be continued for several days in the absence of any suggestion of strangulation, surgical exploration is generally indicated if the obstruction fails to resolve after 48–72 hours, or the WSCM test fails. It might be worth waiting longer in some patients with known extensive adhesions from multiple previous explorations where surgery is likely to be complex, prolonged and high risk. In this setting, attention should be paid to intravenous nutritional support.

✔✔ Adhesive bowel obstruction with the absence of clinical or CT signs of strangulation (free fluid, mesenteric oedema, small-bowel faeces sign, devascularised bowel or hyperaemia), or for patients with partial obstruction, initial non-operative management is appropriate. These patients are good candidates for a trial of orally administered water-soluble contrast medium with both diagnostic and therapeutic purposes. The appearance of water-soluble contrast in the colon on X-ray within 24 hours from administration predicts resolution. The use of contrast is safe and reduces the need for surgery, time to resolution and hospital stay.[5] In the absence of signs of strangulation or peritonitis, non-operative treatment can be prolonged up to 72 hours (Bologna Guidelines for Diagnosis and Management of Adhesive Small Bowel Obstruction).[6]

Box 15.2 Small-bowel obstruction: indications for surgery

Absolute indication (surgery as soon as patient resuscitated)

- Generalised peritonitis
- Visceral perforation
- Irreducible hernia
- Localised peritonitis

Relative indication (surgery within 24 hours)

- Palpable mass lesion
- 'Virgin' abdomen
- Failure to improve (continuing pain, high nasogastric aspirates)

Trial of initial conservative treatment (with further investigations)

- Incomplete obstruction
- Previous surgery
- Advanced malignancy
- Diagnostic doubt (possible ileus)

Self-evaluation questions:

1. Adhesive small bowel obstruction is mainly caused by which two types of surgery?
2. If doing an anastomosis after resection of a small bowel radiation stricture, what is critical to know about the two ends of bowel being joined together?
3. What is the potential 5-year recurrence rate of appendicitis after successful antibiotic management?
4. Are interval appendicectomies indicated after successful conservative management of complicated appendicitis?
5. What is the best management of a low-grade mucinous neoplasm of the appendix?

SURGICAL MANAGEMENT

The particular circumstances of any given patient determine the need for surgical intervention, but some of the commonest features in decision-making are listed in Box 15.2.

OPERATIVE PRINCIPLES

Once a decision to operate has been made, patients should be resuscitated, their co-morbidity optimised, and the stomach emptied with an NGT. The wide range of possible surgical procedures should be explained to the patient, including the possibility of a stoma. Antibiotic and antithromboembolic prophylaxis should be administered.

A midline incision has the most utility when the diagnosis is unknown. Where there is a previous midline incision, this should be utilised and extended cranially or caudally so that the peritoneal cavity can be entered through a 'virgin' area. Loops of small bowel may be densely adherent to the back of the old scar and care taken to avoid an inadvertent enterotomy of the attenuated, dilated bowel.

In open surgery, having entered the abdominal cavity, the first step is to identify the point between dilated and collapsed bowel. It is important to demonstrate this transition as it confirms the diagnosis of mechanical obstruction and identifies the obstructing point. The presence of uniformly dilated small bowel, or no definite point of change in diameter of the bowel, suggests that the clinical diagnosis of mechanical obstruction may be incorrect.

The fluid within the bowel makes it heavy and if it is removed from the abdominal cavity, it should be handled and supported carefully, utilising surgical assistants to ensure the mesentery is not damaged or twisted. The large surface area of dilated loops results in considerable insensible fluid loss, and if it is anticipated that the viscera will lie outside the abdominal cavity for a significant length of time, it should be placed in a transparent 'bowel' bag or wrapped in moist swabs.

Having identified the point of obstruction, it should be released (Fig. 15.2). Although it is not necessary or helpful to divide every adhesion within the abdomen (as these will inevitably re-form), enough should be divided to confirm that there remains no possible site of obstruction between the duodenojejunal flexure and the caecum. It is essential to recognise the patient in whom the clinical diagnosis of mechanical small-bowel obstruction is incorrect, as the presence of adhesions does not in itself confirm the diagnosis.

The small bowel should be resected if it is irreversibly ischaemic, or there is disease or fibrotic narrowing in the bowel at the point of obstruction and anastomosed if both ends of the bowel are healthy and the patient has no other contraindication from associated co-morbidity. If the viability of a

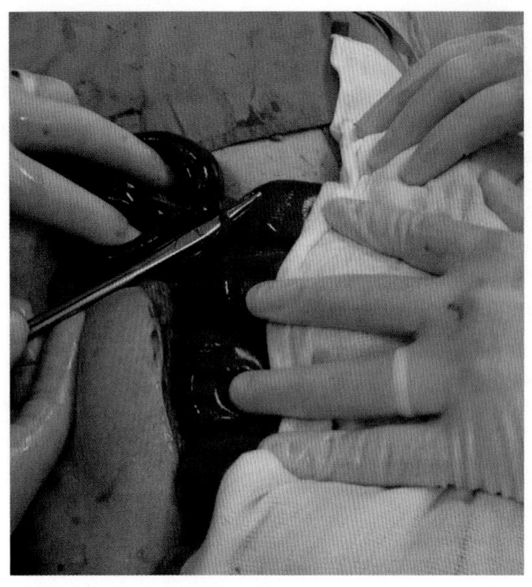

Figure 15.2 Loop of small bowel obstructed by an adhesive band. (With thanks to Dr Bernie Maree, Consultant Surgeon, Cape Town.)

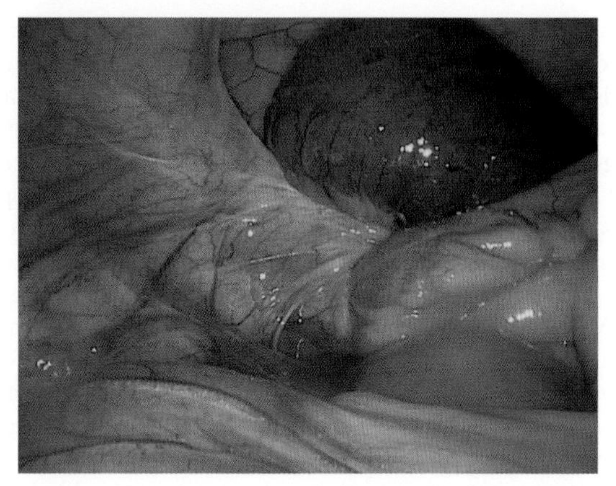

Figure 15.3 Laparoscopic view of a dilated loop of small bowel proximal to an adhesive band from a gynaecological procedure. (With thanks to Dr Bernie Maree, Consultant Surgeon, Cape Town.)

segment of bowel is unclear, it should be wrapped in warm moist swabs for several minutes (approximately 15 minutes while you continue with other parts of the operation) and re-examined. If available, vascular status of the bowel may be assessed using near-infrared imaging with indocyanine green (ICG). Where viability remains in doubt, the segment should be resected, or a planned re-look laparotomy arranged 24–48 hours later. Even after removing the obstruction, exteriorisation of the bowel may be indicated if there is generalised disease of the bowel and when there is a high risk of anastomotic dehiscence. In patients who are septic and unwell, stapling off the ends of resected bowel with a planned re-look in 24–48 hours (such as is carried out in the trauma setting) is useful, with subsequent anastomosis performed in more favourable conditions. An ileostomy may be indicated in patients with Crohn's disease as part of their long-term management, and this possibility should be considered and discussed with the patient beforehand.

LAPAROSCOPY

In suitable patients, laparoscopy can be attempted as an alternative to laparotomy using an open access technique. Laparoscopic adhesiolysis, with a low threshold for conversion, may be suitable during the first episode of small-bowel obstruction, particularly when there has been limited previous surgery and a single band is anticipated, for example in a patient with a virgin abdomen or who has had an appendicectomy, oophorectomy or hysterectomy (Fig. 15.3).[6,7] If laparoscopic adhesiolysis is to be attempted, the obstructed bowel must be manipulated with great care to prevent perforation as it is usually thin-walled and distended.

REDUCING ADHESION FORMATION

There has been considerable research aimed at reducing the development of further adhesions after surgery. Anti-adhesion barriers are compounds that do not actively interfere with inflammation and wound healing. Rather, they act as a spacer that separates injured surfaces of the peritoneum, allowing these surfaces to heal without forming fibrinous attachments, which eventually lead to adhesions. To accomplish this task, such barriers should ideally be inert to the human immune system and be slowly degradable. Anti-adhesion barriers have been demonstrated to reduce adhesion formation and the incidence of subsequent complications.[8] There is moderate evidence that a hyaluronate carboxymethylcellulose adhesion barrier can reduce the incidence of reoperations for ASBO in colorectal surgery. In three trials involving 1132 patients undergoing colorectal surgery, hyaluronate carboxymethylcellulose reduced the incidence of reoperations for ASBO (RR 0.49, 95% CI 0.28–0.88). In surgery for adhesive bowel obstruction,[6] there is evidence that the intraperitoneal administration of icodextrin 4% solution at the end of surgery reduces intra-abdominal adhesion formation and the risk of re-obstruction.[6]

DIFFICULT CLOSURE

There are some patients in whom, after relief of obstruction, the oedematous bowel makes closure impossible. These patients may have had repeated procedures, and in this setting the use of a low-pressure vacuum-assisted closure dressing may allow delayed closure.

SPECIAL CONDITIONS

RADIATION ENTERITIS

Patients can present with an acute abdomen during radiotherapy due to radiation enteritis or with acute-on-chronic attacks many years later. Patients in the former scenario can present considerable diagnostic difficulties, as they are often neutropenic or suffering other side-effects of their treatment. The possibility of a primary pathology, such as acute appendicitis (AA), arising during the course of radiotherapy must also be borne in mind but, where possible, surgical exploration is best avoided. Laparoscopy may be useful here for both diagnosis and management.

A more common acute presentation is with adhesions due to previous radiotherapy, and these patients normally have obstructive symptoms (Fig. 15.4). Again, a prolonged period of NOM, even with intravenous nutritional support, may be preferable to surgery. These adhesions are often dense and, if the small bowel is injured, there is a significant risk that it might not heal whether it is repaired or anastomosed. If an anastomosis is necessary, it is important to adhere to the

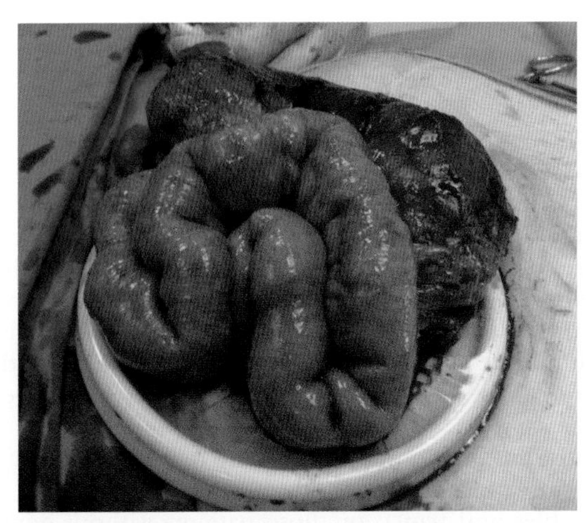

Figure 15.4 Obstructing loop of irradiated small bowel (closest loop) identified at laparoscopic exploration. Note the pale colour, minimal vascular markings and thickened bowel wall of the irradiated bowel.

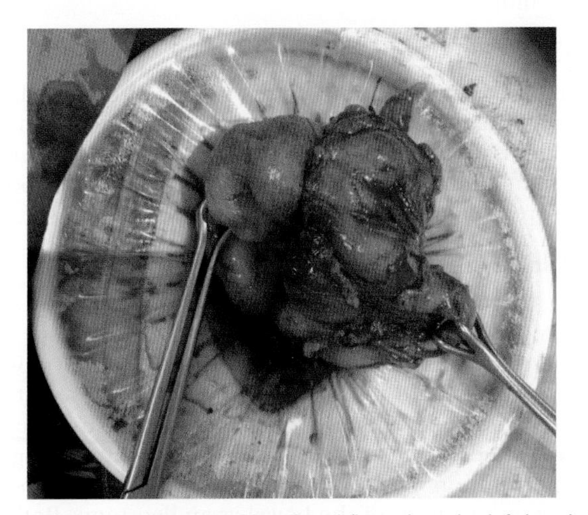

Figure 15.5 Anastomosis of irradiated (bowel on the left-hand side of the image) to unirradiated small bowel.

principle that irradiated bowel should only be anastomosed to non-irradiated bowel[9] (Fig. 15.5).

MALIGNANT OBSTRUCTION

Primary tumours of the small bowel are rare but may cause acute small-bowel obstruction. The surgical approach will depend on the nature and location of the disease. A more common problem is the patient with advanced intra-abdominal malignancy, with or without a past history of surgical treatment for malignancy, who presents with bowel obstruction (Fig. 15.6). Imaging with CT is important in identifying a single area of obstruction, which might be amenable to surgery, as compared to extensive intra-abdominal disease without a single point of obstruction, where surgery has little role to play.

In the presence of advanced and disseminated malignancy, laparotomy should be avoided. However, if the obstruction fails to resolve and the patient is in reasonable condition, surgical bypass may provide relief in some patients, allowing them temporary palliation and to leave hospital. The benefits of surgical bypass in this setting are generally short-lived, and this has stimulated increasing expertise among palliative care physicians in the medical management of intestinal obstruction.[10]

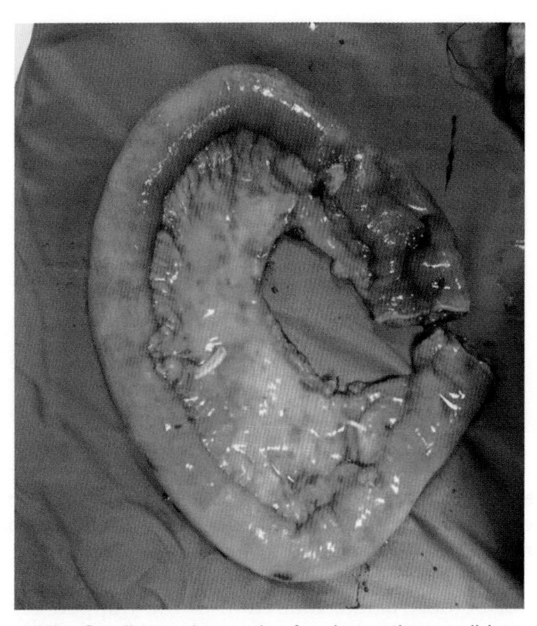

Figure 15.6 Small-bowel resection for obstructing small-bowel metastases from a previously resected oesophageal adenocarcinoma. Note the stricturing, scirrhous nature of the metastasis. Two other smaller metastases are adjacent to the white clips.

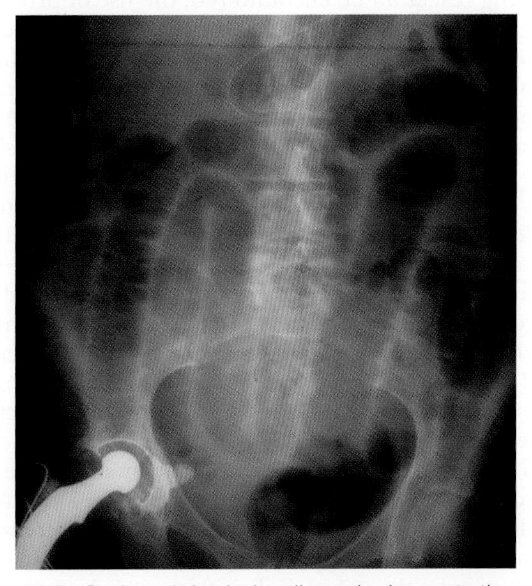

Figure 15.7 Supine abdominal radiograph demonstrating small-bowel obstruction in a patient with an irreducible femoral hernia.

Not all patients have obstruction due to their malignant process and have uncomplicated adhesional obstruction. One study of patients who presented with obstruction following previous treatment of intra-abdominal malignancy reported that in one-third of such patients the obstruction was due to a cause other than secondary malignancy.[10] This may be a particularly appropriate setting for diagnostic laparoscopy, depending on the extent of the previous surgery.

ABDOMINAL WALL HERNIA

Any hernia can present with intestinal obstruction (Figs. 15.7 and 15.8), with delayed presentation and gangrene necessitating bowel resection. A Richter's hernia traps only part of the circumference of the bowel wall and the lumen

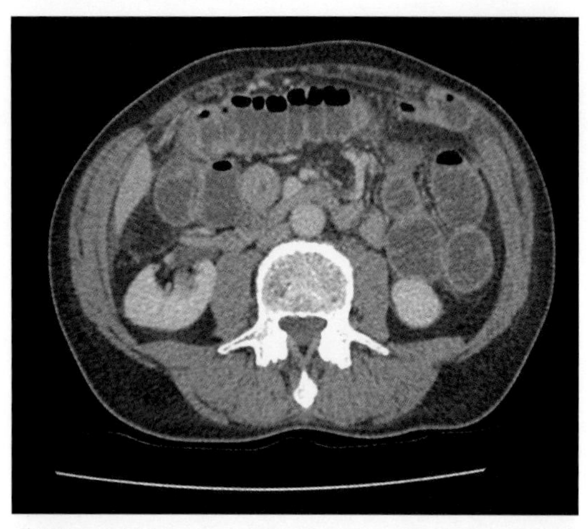

Figure 15.8 Multislice computed tomography image with intravenous contrast demonstrating small-bowel obstruction secondary to a left-sided Spigelian hernia.

may not be obstructed. Infarction of the trapped segment can still occur, with marked localised tenderness over the hernia site.

Any patient with an acute irreducible hernia should undergo urgent surgery. Should necrotic bowel or bowel requiring resection be encountered, the use of prosthetic mesh versus suture repair of the hernia is controversial. Randomised studies on this topic have been conducted and a recent meta-analysis has found that mesh repair for incarcerated or strangulated hernias is feasible with a great benefit of lower recurrence rates without significant increase in the incidence of infection rates (even when bowel resections were needed).[11] Mesh should be avoided when there has been gross contamination due to perforation.

The incarcerated hernia may reduce spontaneously under general anaesthesia and in this instance, it is unlikely that there was strangulation and infarction. However, the bowel loops should be inspected from within the hernia sac to ensure that a gangrenous loop of bowel or a strictured segment has not dropped back into the abdominal cavity. If it is not possible to inspect the viability of the entire bowel through the hernia sac, laparoscopy may be indicated. A useful approach is to place the laparoscope though the hernia and create a sealed pneumoperitoneum by placing tissue graspers on the defect. Failing this, a standard open laparoscopy through a sub-umbilical incision cut down should be used.

A final consideration is the patient with a long history of an uncomplicated hernia who develops acute intestinal obstruction, whereupon the hernia becomes irreducible. The intestinal obstruction raises intra-abdominal pressure, which produces the irreducible hernia, which may be difficult to reduce resulting in it becoming tender. In this setting, a plain abdominal radiograph may demonstrate a dilated colon or the absence of dilated small-bowel loops, suggesting the possibility that the apparently 'incarcerated' hernia is a secondary effect of some other intra-abdominal pathology. In such circumstances, a CT is indicated. If the surgeon proceeds and finds the apparently incarcerated hernia easy to release, the wound should be extended to allow further exploration, or closed and a laparotomy carried out.

ENTEROLITH OBSTRUCTION

Enterolith obstruction is rare, the commonest types being gallstones and bezoars.

Gallstone ileus typically occurs in elderly females and follows development of a cholecystoduodenal fistula after cholecystitis with ongoing inflammation. A visible gallstone (if radio-opaque) and gas in the biliary tree are the classic features of a plain radiograph. At surgery, the stone should be removed via a proximal enterotomy and the proximal intestine palpated to exclude a second stone. The gallbladder should be left alone, as cholecystectomy and duodenal closure can be difficult and dangerous and are generally unnecessary.

Obstructing bezoars may accumulate in psychiatric patients (hair), or after over-indulging in particular types of food (vegetables and fruit), or those patients without dentures who have swallowed inadequately chewed food. Rarely described, an obstructing bezoar can accumulate in a jejunal diverticulum.

INTUSSUSCEPTION

In children, acute presentation is usually to the paediatric department and the main differential diagnosis is GI infection. This is discussed in more detail in Chapter 18. Intussusception in adults is usually caused by tumours of the bowel, which are usually resectable at laparotomy.

CONNECTIVE TISSUE DISORDERS

There are several systemic connective tissue disorders that can affect the GI tract and result in a loss of peristaltic power. These patients generally present with chronic symptoms and are usually hard to characterise. NOM of these patients should be pursued whenever possible, and a gastroenterologist consulted. In the rare event that this condition progresses to perforation of the bowel, consideration should be given to exteriorisation of the bowel as an ileostomy. Both the ischaemic and healthy bowel should be submitted for histology to attempt to identify the connective tissue disorder. Prolonged postoperative ileus is common, and the differentiation of a further episode of mechanical obstruction or continuing ileus presents a diagnostic challenge. The temptation to re-look after several days without progress should be resisted. A WSCM should be tried first, and parenteral nutrition and prolonged NGT drainage may be needed. For the surgeon, this is a particularly uneasy and challenging postoperative scenario.

CHRONIC INTESTINAL PSEUDO-OBSTRUCTION

Chronic intestinal pseudo-obstruction (CIPO) is a rare, severe disease characterised by the failure of the intestinal tract to propel its contents, which results in a clinical picture mimicking mechanical obstruction in the absence of any lesion occluding the gut.

Affected individuals are often unable to maintain normal body weight and normal oral nutrition. The severity of the clinical picture, generally characterised by disabling digestive symptoms with intervals of subocclusive episodes, contributes to deterioration of quality of life. Furthermore, CIPO often passes unrecognised for a long time so that patients almost invariably undergo repeated, unhelpful and potentially dangerous surgical procedures.

Should the patient develop severe disease, with a very dilated colon, a decompressing caecostomy is the treatment of choice.

Management of CIPO remains extremely challenging and often disappointing. There may be a family history, and, in severe cases, life expectancy is no more than early adulthood. A greater awareness of the clinical features and natural history of CIPO would help to discourage surgical procedures.[12]

INTESTINAL OBSTRUCTION IN THE EARLY POSTOPERATIVE PERIOD

Gastrointestinal ileus or obstruction can occur after any abdominal operation, including gynaecological surgery. The surgeon may also be asked to see patients, often elderly and with co-morbidity, who have undergone orthopaedic or cardiac procedures and have apparent bowel obstruction. This group usually have colonic pseudo-obstruction (see Chapters 11 and 16). Each case must be judged on its merits and the differentiation between true postoperative mechanical obstruction and paralytic ileus can be difficult. In patients with a mechanical obstruction, appropriate surgical intervention is frequently delayed as a result of this diagnostic dilemma. In these patients, the use of either a contrast-enhanced CT or water-soluble contrast study is often helpful and should be considered early.[13]

PERITONITIS

Small-bowel pathology may present as an acute abdomen, with either localised or generalised peritonitis. This may be as a result of perforation or gangrenous bowel at the end stage of any condition causing obstruction. This section considers conditions that present primarily with inflammatory signs.

CROHN'S DISEASE

Crohn's disease is a chronic, relapsing inflammatory disease that can affect any part of the GI tract. A common presentation is inflammation of the terminal ileum, and this occasionally presents as an acute abdomen. The small bowel alone is affected in approximately 30% of patients and the small bowel and colon together in 50%.[14]

Where possible, the management of patients with Crohn's disease should be undertaken by a surgeon with a special interest in this condition and the reader is referred to the much more detailed account of this disease in the *Colorectal Surgery* volume of this *Companion to Specialist Surgical Practice* series. Only first principles for managing an acute episode are discussed here.

PRESENTATION

An acute episode of Crohn's ileitis typically presents with abdominal pain, diarrhoea and fever, and this can be the first presentation of the disease in a patient who was previously well. This acute presentation is more likely in young adults; hence, it is frequently mistaken for AA.

Other clinical presentations occur, although they are less likely to be acute. Resolving Crohn's disease may produce fibrosis in the ileum that can cause obstructive symptoms. These tend to be subacute or chronic, and an acute presentation with small-bowel obstruction is rare.

Entero-enteric or enterocutaneous fistulae occur in Crohn's disease because of the transmural inflammation, sometimes complicated by abscess formation, resulting in local peritonitis.

INVESTIGATION

A young patient who presents with right iliac fossa pain, with symptoms that are more insidious than typical appendicitis, should alert a clinical suspicion of Crohn's disease. Inflammatory markers may be markedly elevated (C-reactive protein, white cell count, platelet count, alkaline phosphatase, erythrocyte sedimentation rate), but these are not specific to Crohn's disease. An ultrasound scan may show thickening of the bowel wall or a mass, but contrast-enhanced CT will provide more detailed information and is the preferred investigation in this setting.[15]

SURGERY FOR ACUTE CROHN'S DISEASE PRESENTING DE NOVO

If a patient with known Crohn's disease presents with an acute flare-up, or Crohn's disease is diagnosed preoperatively at the first presentation, the patient should be referred to a surgeon with a special interest.[16] The unexpected finding of inflammation of the terminal ileum or caecum at laparoscopy or laparotomy for suspected appendicitis or any other condition does not necessarily imply Crohn's disease as it can be difficult to differentiate it from infectious enteritis. Even if it were to be Crohn's ileitis, resection might not be the most appropriate strategy if the dominant symptoms relate to inflammation. No further procedure on the suspected Crohn's disease is required. Further diagnostic investigations are then arranged as appropriate. Only when the patient has obvious small-bowel obstruction, should the area of inflamed bowel be resected.[17]

MESENTERIC ISCHAEMIA

While acute small-bowel ischaemia can be caused by a closed loop obstruction, this section reviews mesenteric ischaemia due to embolism or thrombosis, arterial or venous, which may be acute or chronic. Chronic mesenteric ischaemia is also termed 'mesenteric claudication' and is usually caused by a stenosis in the proximal part of the superior mesenteric artery. Patients develop cramp-like abdominal pains after eating, caused by the increased oxygen requirements to the small intestine, which cannot be met by increased blood flow because of the stenosis. Weight loss is often associated due to 'food fear' as the patient avoids eating due to the associated onset of abdominal pain. The disease is usually associated with atherosclerosis and the investigation of choice is mesenteric angiography (Fig. 15.9a and b). A specialist vascular surgeon should manage these patients.

This condition is discussed in more detail in the *Vascular and Endovascular Surgery* volume of this *Companion to Specialist Surgical Practice* series and is not discussed further here.

Acute mesenteric ischaemia can affect any part of the GI tract but is most common in the small bowel and colon. Acute ischaemia to the small bowel will usually produce infarction, whereas ischaemia to the large bowel presents with bloody diarrhoea and abdominal pain, which will usually

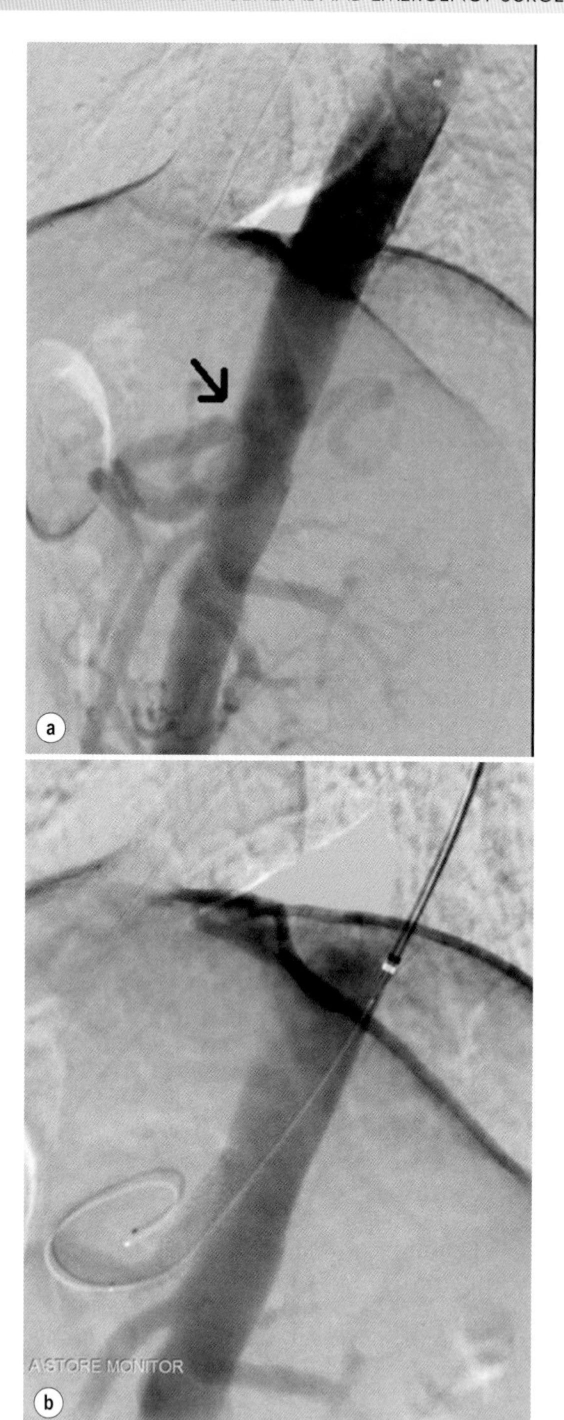

Figure 15.9 **(a)** Angiogram demonstrating focal high-grade ostial stenosis of the coeliac artery (*arrow*) in a patient with chronic mesenteric ischaemia. **(b)** The stenotic region has been managed by endovascular stent placement. (Images courtesy of Dr Bhavesh Natha, Cape Town.)

settle over the course of a few days and is often termed 'ischaemic colitis'. Rarely, delayed strictures may occur.

Thrombosis may occur in the superior mesenteric artery or its branches, usually associated with underlying atherosclerosis. Embolus is often associated with atrial fibrillation when an atrial thrombus dislodges and lodges in the superior mesenteric artery distribution. Venous thrombosis in the distribution of the superior mesenteric vein is a less common cause of acute small-bowel ischaemia but may be related to increased blood coagulability, portal vein thrombosis, dehydration, infection, compression and vasoconstricting drugs.

Early detection of acute mesenteric ischaemia is difficult (see Chapter 11) and is the primary reason for its high morbidity and mortality. It is more common in the elderly patient who gives a history of vague but worsening abdominal pain, but it is by no means confined to this age group and should be considered in any age group, particularly patients with new-onset atrial fibrillation. Further difficulty is added by initial examination findings often being unimpressive, resulting in diagnostic delay.

Where the presentation is a short history with severe pain and tenderness, and there is a high index of suspicion, if possible, early contrast CT should be performed and if a mesenteric thrombus/embolus is identified, a vascular surgeon should be contacted. The patient should then proceed directly to diagnostic laparoscopy or laparotomy. At surgery, a decision must be made as to (a) whether the ischaemic bowel is localised and after resection of frankly gangrenous bowel an adequate length compatible with life will remain; and (b) whether there is an option of vascular reconstruction to salvage the remaining bowel, particularly if it is ischaemic but not yet dead. Exploration of the superior mesenteric artery with removal of an embolus may avoid an extended small-bowel resection and re-vascularise the remaining ischaemic bowel.[18] Bypass for an arterial thrombus with underlying vascular disease is much more complicated and less likely to be successful.

If surgical resection is carried out, primary anastomosis may be performed, provided the blood supply to both proximal and distal margins is adequate. Viability and vascularisation of remaining bowel and anastomoses may be assessed using intraoperative ICG fluorescent dye angiography (which provides intraoperative visual assessment of blood flow to the bowel wall) (Fig. 15.10).[19,20] If embolectomy and vascular reconstruction have been performed, or there is any doubt about the margins, then anastomosis should be deferred. In this situation, the safest option is formation of a double-barrelled stoma, or to staple off distal and proximal bowel ends with re-exploration planned within 48 hours. At re-operation, an anastomosis may be performed, or the proximal limb of bowel exteriorised if anastomosis still appears risky. However, if the patient develops significant postoperative complications, for example cardiac insufficiency, then the planned re-look laparotomy may become life-threatening and untenable. For this reason, in patients with significant cardiac disease, the first option is to be preferred, although management of a high proximal stoma brings with it its own problems of high fluid loss, nutritional supplementation and long-term management.

✔✔ Overall prognosis is better following acute mesenteric venous infarction as compared to acute mesenteric arterial ischaemia, and survival better following arterial embolism as compared to arterial thrombosis.[21]

MECKEL'S DIVERTICULUM

Meckel's diverticulum is a remnant of the omphalomesenteric or vitelline duct. It arises from the anti-mesenteric

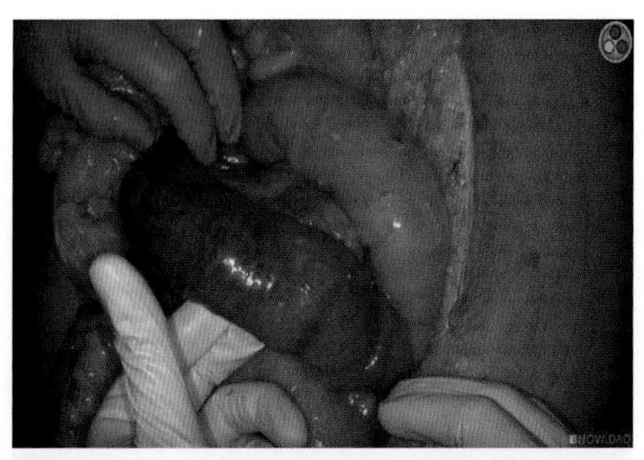

Figure 15.10 Indocyanine green (ICG) angiography of acute mesenteric ischaemia patient at re-look laparotomy. Note vascularised bowel takes up ICG and appears green with near-infrared imaging, whereas the unvascularised bowel does not appear green.

border of the distal ileum, approximately 60 cm from the iliocaecal valve. It may contain ectopic tissue, usually gastric mucosa, and is estimated to be present in approximately 2% of the population. Meckel's diverticulum may remain asymptomatic throughout life, particularly if it has a broad base and does not contain ectopic gastric mucosa. Occasionally, a band may exist between the diverticulum and the umbilicus, which can cause small-bowel obstruction. This should be treated as for a congenital band adhesion, although resection of the diverticulum, which in this setting is usually elongated and appears pathological, should accompany division of the band. Occasionally, the diverticulum may intussuscept, also causing obstruction. Again, this will require reduction and excision. Should reduction not be possible (in which setting the nature of the lead point will not be obvious), the entire intussusception mass should be excised. Other common complications of Meckel's diverticulum are haemorrhage and inflammation when the patient presents with signs and symptoms similar to AA. Unless there has been a preoperative CT, this diagnosis is rarely suspected before surgery and the diagnosis is made on the operating table (Fig. 15.11a) once a normal appendix has been found. The diverticulum should be excised, and the small bowel repaired (Fig. 15.11b). Overt, obscure or occult GI bleeding may occur from a Meckel's diverticulum containing ectopic gastric mucosa and the diagnosis is usually established by CT angiogram. The treatment is surgical resection, and this can be done laparoscopically after delivery of the diverticulum through an extended port site incision. If found incidentally at an unrelated operation, an asymptomatic Meckel's diverticulum should not be excised.

HAEMORRHAGE

Disease of the small intestine is an occasional cause of acute GI haemorrhage.[22] There are no specific clinical features that distinguish the small bowel as the source rather than the colon, except that the blood loss may be less 'fresh' and more like melaena. As discussed in Chapter 13, it is important to exclude bleeding from a gastroduodenal source at an early stage by upper GI endoscopy. The commonest causes are vascular malformation, jejunal diverticula, peptic ulceration in a Meckel's diverticulum, and small-bowel tumour.

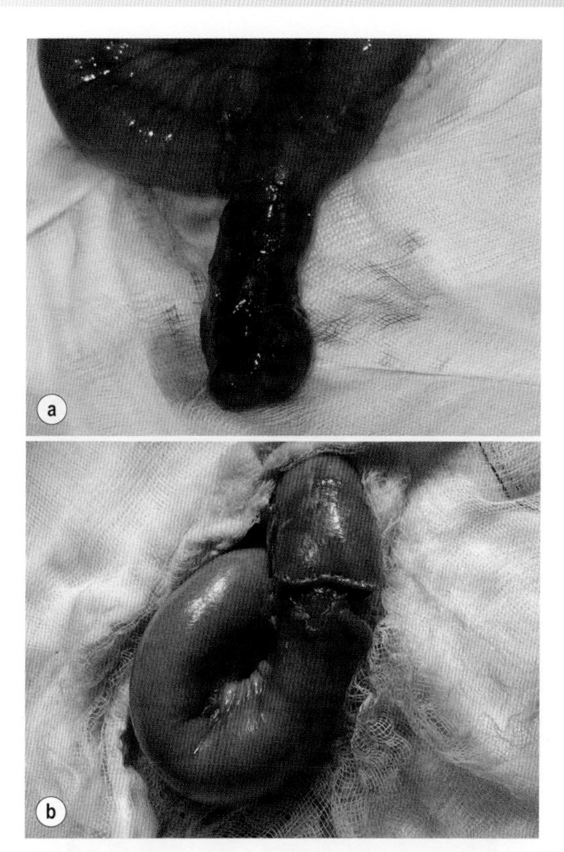

Figure 15.11 **(a)** Acutely inflamed Meckel's diverticulum identified at laparotomy. **(b)** Operative view after resection of the Meckel's diverticulum shown in **(a)**.

Vascular malformations and Dieulafoy's lesions are particularly challenging, as they are frequently not visible except when they are bleeding.

Every attempt should be made to identify the site of bleeding before surgery is contemplated, because at operation a vascular abnormality may produce no external signs. Particularly challenging to identify is bleeding from the biliary tree or distal duodenum beyond the easy reach of the gastroscope. Double balloon and capsule endoscopy have increased the diagnostic yield, the former being both diagnostic and allowing for endoscopic therapies such as argon plasma coagulation (APC) of vascular malformations. If endoscopic management is unsuccessful, the lesion can be tattooed for surgical resection. A limitation of CT angiography results from the mobility and variable anatomical layout of the small bowel, which can make it difficult at laparotomy to pinpoint a radiologically identified bleeding point. CT angiography may identify a bleeding point (Fig. 15.12a), following which formal angiography may allow embolisation of the bleeding vessel (Fig. 15.12b). It must be remembered that a potential complication of this strategy is bowel ischaemia and a low index of suspicion for bowel ischaemia must be maintained post embolisation.

If the previously mentioned interventions have been unsuccessful and surgery is indicated, there are multiple interventions that can help in localisation of the bleeding site, namely: tattoo via double balloon endoscopy, intraoperative endoscopy or, if bleeding appears brisk, segmental soft bowel clamps can be placed throughout the small intestine, resecting the segment that fills up with blood after a period of waiting. Blind

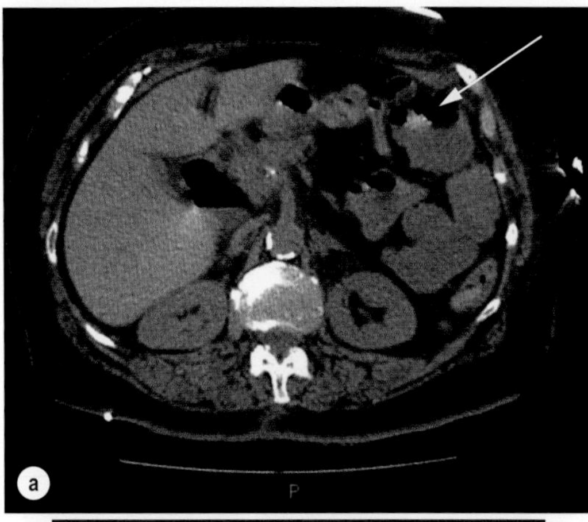

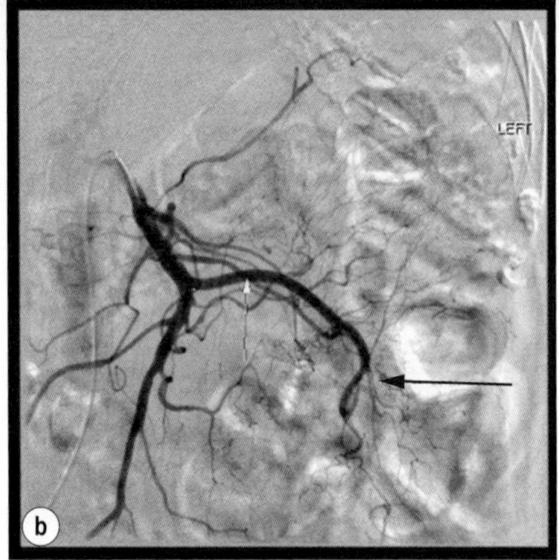

Figure 15.12 **(a)** Computed tomography angiogram with intravenous contrast demonstrating a bleeding point in the jejunum. **(b)** Mesenteric angiogram demonstrating embolisation of the bleeding point shown in **(a)**.

resection is often unrewarding, and the risks of re-bleeding are high. If no bleeding point can be identified, the surgeon can either close the abdomen and await events, hoping that further bleeding does not occur (and this is often the case), or divide the small bowel around its midpoint, bringing out two stomas. Subsequent bleeding can then be identified to one or other side and endoscopy used to localise it further. These techniques are often heard in surgical discussion, but experience of them is extremely rare. Moreover, emergency surgery is usually not necessary, because ongoing, continuous life-threatening haemorrhage is unusual. This allows investigation of these patients between bleeding episodes.

APPENDICITIS

AA is the most common intra-abdominal surgical emergency requiring surgery, with an incidence of 7–12% in the population of the USA and Europe. Although frequently described as a childhood illness, the peak incidence is towards 30 years of age. It is slightly more common in males (1.3–1.6:1), but appendicectomy is more common in women because of other mimicking conditions. The reader is referred to Chapter 11 for description of some of the general features and investigation of patients with acute abdominal pain, many of which relate directly to AA.

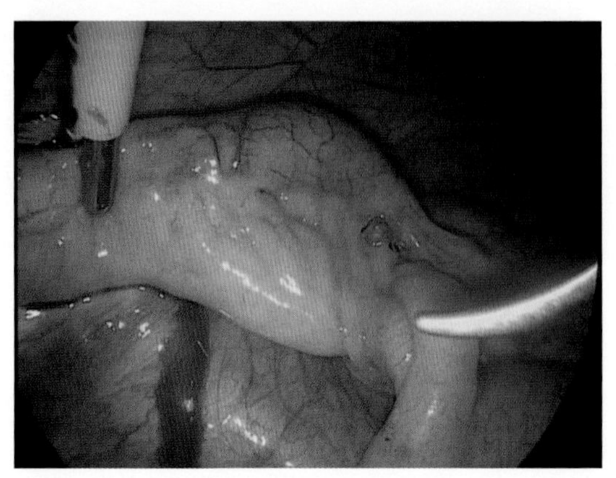

Figure 15.13 Laparoscopic view of acute appendicitis with a faecolith evident in the proximal third.

AETIOLOGY AND PATHOLOGY

There are three common aetiological hypotheses for appendicitis, namely: mechanical, infective and hygiene. The *mechanical hypothesis* draws on the fact that appendicitis has a lower incidence in populations with a high-fibre diet, such as in Eastern and Southern Africa. In groups with a low-fibre diet, the transit time of stool is slower and thereby, it is proposed, a propensity to form faecoliths.[23] Faecoliths are a specific cause of appendicitis in about one-third of specimens and are composed of fats (coprosterols), inorganic salts (calcium phosphate) and organic residue (vegetable fibres) in a proportion of 50%, 25% and 20%, respectively[24,25] (Fig. 15.13). The lumen may also be obstructed by tumours of the caecum or appendix, or by enlargement of lymphoid aggregates within the appendix wall.

The *infective hypothesis* draws on the finding that viruses such as dengue, influenza, Epstein–Barr, rotavirus and cytomegaloviruses, bacteria such as *Campylobacter*, *Brucella* and *Salmonella* as well as parasites like *Entamoeba histolytica*, *Schistosoma mansoni/japonicum* and *Enterobius vermicularis* have been isolated in specimens or indirectly implicated in the pathogenesis of appendicitis. These pathogens are thought to cause appendicitis by invading the lamina propria and initiating oedematous obstruction of the narrow lumen of the appendix.[26,27]

The *hygiene hypothesis* stems from the observation that there was an increase in the incidence of appendicitis in Britain from 1895 through 1930 before declining. It was thought that the increase was due to better housing and sanitation. This resulted in a compromised GI immune system and an abnormal response to gut pathogens and commensals. Unfortunately, none of these hypotheses is completely satisfactory.

The pathology of AA is classically described as suppurative, gangrenous or perforated. Typically, there is full-thickness inflammation of the appendix wall. As the disease progresses, adjacent tissues, particularly the omentum, may also become inflamed. Histologically, haemorrhagic ulceration and necrosis in the wall indicate gangrenous appendicitis, and subsequent perforation may be associated with a localised periappendiceal mass/abscess or generalised peritonitis.[25]

CLINICAL FEATURES

The presentation of AA varies widely, but the classical history and examination findings are described as: central abdominal pain migrating to the right iliac fossa over 4–24 hours; loss of appetite, nausea, sometimes vomiting and fever; diarrhoea is uncommon, but when present should not be confused with gastroenteritis, which is rarely associated with abdominal tenderness (as opposed to pain). In females, the gynaecological history is important, including menses, vaginal discharge or previous endometriosis. On examination, the patient usually exhibits a tachycardia, a low-grade pyrexia and localised peritonitis in the right lower quadrant.

The condition is most difficult to diagnose at the extremes of age: in the very young because of the lack of history and often late presentation; and in the elderly because of a wide list of differential diagnoses and often unimpressive physical signs.

Another factor producing atypical signs is the variation in the position of the appendix. A retrocaecal appendix can give rise to tenderness in the right loin and/or right upper quadrant, whereas a pelvic appendix may be associated with very little abdominal discomfort and a history of diarrhoea, although deep suprapubic pressure and rectal examination may elicit tenderness.[28]

AA is one of a dwindling number of conditions where a decision to operate may be based solely on clinical findings. A classic history and the presence of localised right iliac fossa peritonism in a male are highly predictive of AA. The risk of morbidity and mortality is significantly increased if the appendix perforates, and to err on the side of overdiagnosing, AA remains accepted as best surgical practice. The updated World Society of Emergency Surgery (WSES) Jerusalem guidelines advocates the use of scoring systems such as the Adult Appendicitis Score (AAS), or the Appendicitis Inflammatory Response (AIR) to assist in clinical diagnosis of AA.[29] These scoring systems aid in the objective diagnosis of appendicitis and have been shown to decrease the negative appendicectomy rate.

Laparoscopy offers an alternative to what may turn out to be an unnecessary laparotomy, and this is especially applicable in women of childbearing age where a classic history and the presence of peritonism is less reliable than in males. This allows the exclusion of other causes of abdominal pain such as endometriosis, pelvic inflammatory disease and ovarian pathology.

INVESTIGATIONS

The majority of these investigations are discussed at length in Chapter 11 and will not be repeated here except to emphasise the key points. Urinalysis is essential, particularly in women. Although pus cells and microscopic haematuria can occur in appendicitis, their absence may be useful in excluding significant urinary tract disease. The presence of organisms may confirm the diagnosis of urinary tract infection and if in doubt urgent urine microscopy should be requested. Pyelonephritis or pyonephrosis may be difficult to differentiate clinically from an acutely inflamed retrocaecal appendix and patients with pyuria require urgent investigation of the urinary tract to exclude these diagnoses prior to appendicectomy. Ultrasound may identify gynaecological causes of pain and visualise an inflamed appendix (Fig. 15.14) and has a high specificity when positive. However, it cannot reliably be used to exclude appendicitis.

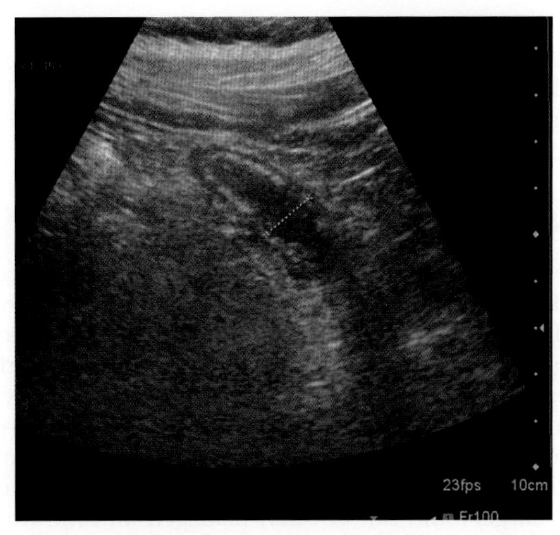

Figure 15.14 Ultrasound scan demonstrating an acutely inflamed appendix.

There has been an increasing trend towards using CT in the assessment of patients with acute lower abdominal pain. A recent meta-analysis concluded that CT utilisation has reduced negative appendicectomy rates and proposed the routine use of CT in adult patients with suspected appendicitis.[30] It remains an appropriate practice to proceed directly to open, or now increasingly, laparoscopic appendicectomy (LA) in young males with a high clinical suspicion of appendicitis, and laparoscopy in women of childbearing years. It is reassuring if a preoperative ultrasound demonstrates a pathological looking thickened appendix. However, there should be a low threshold for CT imaging when there is diagnostic doubt, particularly in older patients, and for those in whom the risks of intervention are increased by comorbidity, previous abdominal surgery, or morbid obesity.

DIFFERENTIAL DIAGNOSIS

Just as appendicitis should be considered in any patient with abdominal pain, many other abdominal emergencies must be considered in the differential diagnosis of AA. Common conditions presenting in similar fashion include gastroenteritis, mesenteric lymphadenitis, gynaecological diseases, right-sided urinary tract disease and disease of the distal small bowel. Gynaecological disorders are probably the most important group as illustrated by the normal appendicectomy rate being highest in young women. The commonest are acute salpingitis, Mittelschmerz (mid-cycle) pain and complications of ovarian cyst. Torsion, or haemorrhage into an ovarian cyst, usually presents with a sudden onset of very severe pain, which may provide a diagnostic clue. To avoid missing a complicated ectopic pregnancy, females of childbearing age should routinely have a pregnancy test (although appendicitis is not uncommon in the first trimester of pregnancy).

The improvement and increased availability of imaging techniques and laparoscopy has provided the opportunity to reduce the stubbornly high proportion of normal appendices removed in the 'open surgery' era, typically up to 20% of patients, and even reaching 29% in women of childbearing age.[31] Although it is clearly advantageous to spare patients unnecessary surgery, the morbidity and mortality of failing to diagnose appendicitis until perforation has occurred is greater than that associated with the removal of a normal appendix. If ultrasound and CT are not readily available, diagnostic laparoscopy is the best option when there is a clinical suspicion of AA.

MANAGEMENT

Once AA has been diagnosed, the options are surgical or NOM with antibiotics. Short delays, even up to 24–36 hours in selected patients, are safe and likely to aid access to imaging and/or laparoscopy and are not associated with an increased rate of infectious complications. However, where optimal surgical systems allow for expeditious surgery, prompt appendicectomy is advocated.[29] As an example, a patient who is systemically well does not require out-of-hours surgery and can be safely managed with intravenous antibiotics, pending surgery in the morning.[32,33]

SURGICAL TREATMENT

Open appendicectomy

The key points for an open appendicectomy (OA) are:

1. A transverse muscle splitting incision over McBurney's point.
2. If the appendix is obviously inflamed, it should be removed taking care to make sure the base of the appendix, where it joins the caecum, is properly identified.
3. Local lavage performed and the wound closed.
4. If the appendix is macroscopically normal, examination should be undertaken of the terminal ileum (for at least 60 cm to exclude an inflamed Meckel's diverticulum) and small-bowel mesentery and pelvis, both by palpation and direct visualisation. Any free peritoneal fluid should be collected for subsequent culture. The presence of bile staining indicates proximal bowel perforation, such as perforated peptic ulcer, and faecal fluid indicates colonic perforation. In both instances, a full laparotomy is indicated. In the former situation, it is best to close the right iliac fossa incision in preference to an upper midline, but in the latter, some surgeons advocate extending the right iliac fossa incision medially as a muscle-cutting lower abdominal transverse incision. If in doubt, a midline incision is best.
5. An alternative technique for evaluating the peritoneal cavity without a laparotomy or wound extension is to close the appendicectomy wound over a laparoscopic port using a strong purse-string suture or through a wound protector with a cap designed for laparoscopic port insertion. Laparoscopy can then be undertaken with insertion of more ports as needed to allow manipulation of abdominal organs. If this is difficult, closure of the appendicectomy wound and a standard subumbilical open laparoscopy incision should be performed.
6. It used to be traditional teaching to bury the appendix stump, but LA has proven that simple ligation of the stump is adequate.[34] If the appendix has perforated at the base, formal repair of the caecal pole is advised. Leaving a long stump should be avoided as this can become ischaemic, leading to complications. Similarly, failing to remove all the appendix will result in recurrent symptoms and appendicitis of the remaining stump. The use of surgical drains remains controversial and will ultimately depend on the extent of local contamination and whether or not there was an abscess cavity.
7. All patients should receive prophylactic broad-spectrum antibiotics to reduce wound infection, which is the commonest complication after appendicectomy.[35,36] A single dose is as effective as three doses for wound prophylaxis. For perforated appendicitis, antibiotics should be continued until signs of sepsis have settled. In complicated appendicitis, provided that there are no ongoing signs of sepsis, postoperative antibiotics should be continued for 3 days.[37] When patients can tolerate diet, completing the course of antibiotics orally will reduce hospital stay without additional complication.[38] Although the risk of deep vein thrombosis (DVT) is relatively low in young patients, prophylaxis is best administered as a routine. Laparoscopy does not preclude the need for DVT prophylaxis.

✔✔ Prophylactic antibiotics should be administered in all patients undergoing appendicectomy for acute appendicitis in order to reduce the risk of wound infection.[29]

Laparoscopic appendicectomy

The advantages of LA have been extensively studied over the last 20 years, although individual studies have produced conflicting results.[39–41]

As skills in laparoscopic technique have become more widespread, LA has become increasingly common.[41] It seems reasonable to proceed with LA for any patient in whom an acutely inflamed appendix is discovered during diagnostic laparoscopy, providing the surgeon has the relevant skills. Obese patients and those of large build will benefit more from the laparoscopic approach by avoiding the larger wound required at open surgery.

✔✔ A Cochrane database systematic review of 85 studies involving 9765 participants compared laparoscopic appendicectomy with open appendicectomy. The main advantages of laparoscopic versus open appendicectomy were reduced postsurgical pain, reduced risk of wound infection, shorter hospital stay and more rapid return to normal activities. Two studies reported that adults who received laparoscopic appendicectomy had better quality of life 2 weeks, 6 weeks and 6 months after surgery. Disadvantages of laparoscopic appendicectomy were a higher rate of intra-abdominal abscesses (in adults, but not in children).[40] The updated Jerusalem guidelines from the WSES recommends laparoscopic appendicectomy as the preferred approach over open appendicectomy for both uncomplicated and complicated acute appendicitis, where laparoscopic equipment and expertise are available.[29]

The key principles for LA are similar to the open approach with the following additions:

1. The pelvis is much easier to examine and the opportunity to examine it and the rest of the peritoneal cavity should be taken.
2. Thorough lavage is easier, but it is important to remove all the effluent. If there has been significant contamination and a large amount of washout has been used, it is advisable to leave a small drain in the pelvis for the first

12 hours or so to allow any residual fluid to drain out after the patient sits up. It can then be removed.

3. While formal ligation and division of the appendix mesentery is standard practice in OA, this is not necessary in the laparoscopic approach. The appendix can be dissected from its mesentery from tip to base with electrocautery without formal division of the mesentery. Occasionally larger vessels may require to be clipped, but this is uncommon.

The appendix can be secured with a pre-formed loop ligature or a Hem-o-Lok®, which has been shown to be both safe and effective[42] (Fig. 15.15). The application of an endoscopic stapling device to the appendix and/or meso-appendix is discouraged due to unnecessary associated cost.

It is important to remove the appendix through the abdominal wall without contaminating the soft tissues. Most appendices can be drawn into the 10-mm laparoscopic port, thus eliminating abdominal wall contamination, particularly if the appendix has been dissected off the mesentery. A large, friable, or perforated appendix should be handled gently and removed in a retrieval bag, taking care to remove all debris, including any loose faecolith.

One of the reported complications of LA is leaving too long a stump and risking recurrent symptoms.[43] Care must therefore be taken to ensure that the entire appendix has been fully mobilised to avoid this complication.

The normal appendix at open surgery

An unexpected normal appendix discovered through a right iliac fossa appendicectomy incision should be removed. While this may be associated with some morbidity, it does avoid future dilemma in patients presenting with recurrent symptoms and a scar that suggests the appendix may have been removed. Postoperative wound infection remains the same as after an OA for an inflamed (but non-perforated) appendix. A late complication which also needs to be considered is ASBO. In a historical cohort study of 245 400 patients who underwent appendicectomy in Sweden with population-based matched controls, the cumulative risk of surgically treated small-bowel obstruction following OA was 1.3% after 30 years compared with 0.21% for non-operated controls.[44]

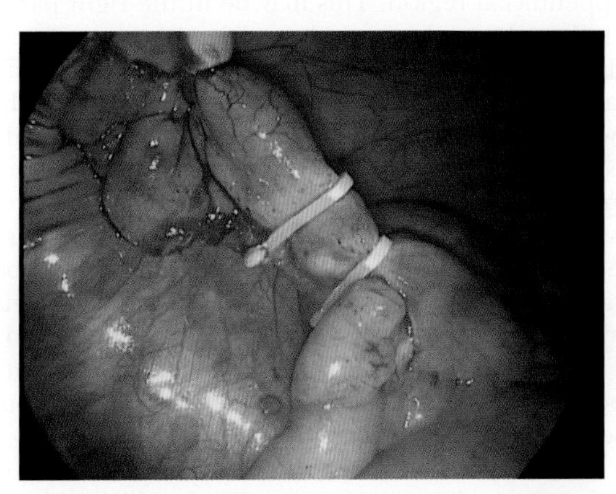

Figure 15.15 Appendix base secured with Hem-o-Lok® at laparoscopic appendicectomy.

The normal appendix at laparoscopy

When the appendix is found to be normal and an alternative diagnosis, such as pelvic inflammatory disease or diverticulitis, is identified at laparoscopy, surgical judgement should be used regarding its removal (Fig. 15.16). Although the evidence is weak, the updated Jerusalem guidelines of the WSES advocates the removal of macroscopically normal appendices in clinically suspected appendicitis, with no other intra-abdominal pathology, as surgeon's judgement of normal appendices is variable and inaccurate. This is backed up by the following data:

1. There is a small incidence of appendicitis on histological examination of a macroscopically normal appendix.[45]
2. A study evaluating the ability of laparoscopy to discriminate between a normal and an inflamed appendix demonstrated a sensitivity of 92% and a specificity of 85% if an appendix with isolated mucosal inflammation was considered to be inflamed.[46]

NON-SURGICAL TREATMENT

It is recognised that simple appendicitis can be successfully managed with antibiotics alone in selected patients. This contentious topic has been reviewed in two recent meta-analyses.

The first compared five studies including 1116 patients.[47] Complications were reported in 5% of patients in the antibiotic and 8% in the appendicectomy group. There was a 23% appendicectomy rate within 1 year in the antibiotic group. The study concluded that there should be a change in practice towards shared decision-making around surgery or NOM in patients with clearly uncomplicated appendicitis.

There are limitations to this meta-analysis, many of which are recognised in the paper. The major morbidity reported in the surgical group is perforation, yet this is part of the

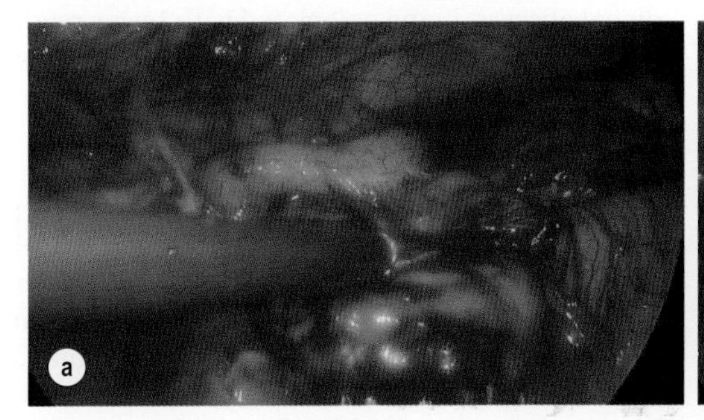

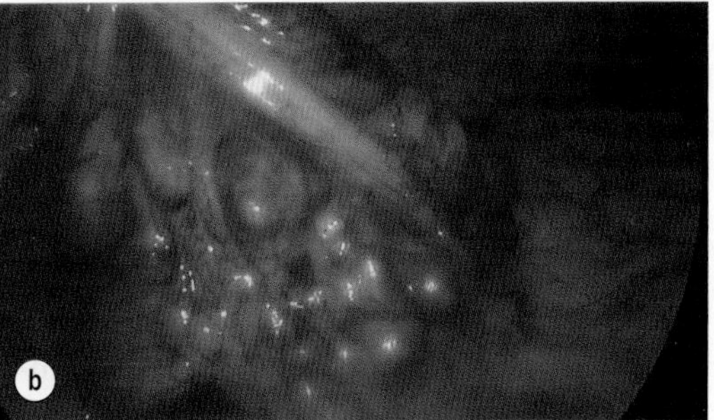

Figure 15.16 Caecal diverticulitis with **(a)** normal appendix in patient presenting with right iliac fossa pain. **(b)** Extensive caecal diverticulitis. (Images courtesy of Dr Simon Paterson-Brown.)

disease spectrum of appendicitis and not a complication of surgery. Exclusion of this single complication reduces the complication rate in the surgical group to 9 of 489 patients, or 1.8%. In none of the studies analysed were the complications classified according to severity. There is also evidence of probable selection bias, with slow recruitment in two of the biggest trials, one of which recruited only 20% of all the patients presenting with uncomplicated appendicitis. This raises concerns that the healthier patients were treated with antibiotics. Furthermore, only 23% of procedures in the surgical group were performed laparoscopically, which is recognised to have a lower wound infection and adhesion rate than open surgery. A final concern is that the recurrence rate of 23% of appendicitis within 1 year has to be seen as a failure of antibiotic therapy.

In the APPAC randomised trial, appendicectomy resulted in an initial success rate of 99.6%. In the antibiotic group, 27.3% of patients underwent appendicectomy within 1 year of initial presentation for AA. Of the 256 patients available for follow-up in the antibiotic group, 72.7% did not require surgery.[48] The 5-year follow-up results of the APPAC trial reported that, among patients who were initially treated with antibiotics, the likelihood of late recurrence was 39.1%. Only 2.3% of patients who had surgery for recurrent AA were diagnosed with complicated forms of the disease. The overall complication rate was significantly reduced in the antibiotic group compared with the appendicectomy group (6.5% vs 24.4%). This long-term follow-up supports the feasibility of NOM with antibiotics as an alternative to surgery for uncomplicated AA.[49] Of note is that the presence of an appendicolith has been identified as an independent prognostic risk factor for treatment failure in NOM of uncomplicated AA. When presenting together with AA, the presence of appendicoliths is associated with increased perforation risk.[50]

✓ While antibiotic treatment will be successful in the short term (up to 1 year), in many patients with uncomplicated appendicitis, the high failure rate (39%) means that laparoscopic appendicectomy remains the authors' treatment of choice in the majority of patients with suspected acute appendicitis. A small subgroup of patients who are well with minimal signs might be considered for antibiotic treatment after full discussion of the risks and benefits, and perhaps considering other circumstances.

TREATMENT OF ATYPICAL PRESENTATION OF ACUTE APPENDICITIS

APPENDIX MASS

The natural history of AA left untreated is that it will either resolve, become gangrenous and perforate, or become walled off by a mass of omentum and small bowel. The latter prevents inflammation spreading to the abdominal cavity. Such a patient usually presents with a longer history, often a week or more, of right lower quadrant abdominal pain, and appears systemically well but has a tender palpable mass in the right iliac fossa. The differential diagnosis includes Crohn's disease in younger patients and carcinoma of the caecum in older patients. Confirmation is obtained from ultrasound or CT. Appendix mass is best managed non-operatively as the risk of perforation has passed and removal of the appendix at this late stage can be difficult and is associated with a significant complication rate. A 2010 meta-analysis reported that the NOM of complicated appendicitis (appendix mass or abscess) is associated with a decrease in complications compared with appendicectomy, with a similar duration of hospital stay.[51] In the systemically well patient, NOM may include percutaneous drainage of any fluid collections.

Following resolution of the symptoms and mass, routine interval appendicectomy (6 weeks to 3 months) was considered essential to prevent recurrent symptoms in the young and to exclude carcinoma in the elderly. However, providing carcinoma can be excluded by other means, such as CT and colonoscopy, routine interval appendicectomy is no longer recommended. In the majority of patients, the appendix has been destroyed and in one study only 9% of patients treated non-operatively for an appendix mass subsequently developed recurrent symptoms within 5 months.[52] If symptoms recur, then it is reasonable to offer these patients surgery.

✓✓ A systematic review has confirmed that non-operative management of an appendix mass will be successful in the majority of patients and recurrence of symptoms is low. As a result, the routine use of interval appendicectomy is no longer justified.[51]

APPENDIX ABSCESS

In some patients, the appendix becomes walled off by omentum but has perforated and an abscess will develop in the periappendiceal region. This may be in the right paracolic gutter, the subcaecal area or the pelvis and can be visualised by either ultrasound or CT (Fig. 15.17). Unlike with a simple 'appendix mass', the patient is usually systemically unwell with abdominal tenderness. As for all abscesses, drainage is the best treatment, either under radiological control or surgically. There is no doubt that surgical drainage can be associated with significant complications, not least because tissues and organs adjacent to the abscess will be friable and must be handled with great care. The alternative of radiologically guided drainage has been reported to produce lower complications and equivalent early operation/re-operation rates.[53,54] It would therefore seem reasonable to use the non-operative approach in any patient in whom overt signs of peritonitis are absent. If surgery is required, then the residual necrotic appendix should be identified and resected. Laparoscopic surgery in experienced hands is a safe and feasible alternative first-line treatment for appendiceal abscess, being associated with fewer readmissions and fewer additional interventions than conservative treatment, with a comparable hospital stay.[4]

CHRONIC APPENDICITIS

As noted already, there is certainly a group of patients who suffer from recurrent appendicitis[55] and who benefit from appendicectomy. CT can help assessment in difficult cases, but for many patients laparoscopy is the best investigation, at which the appendix can be removed. A small, randomised trial has reported improvement in chronic recurrent right lower quadrant pain following LA compared with laparoscopy alone.[56]

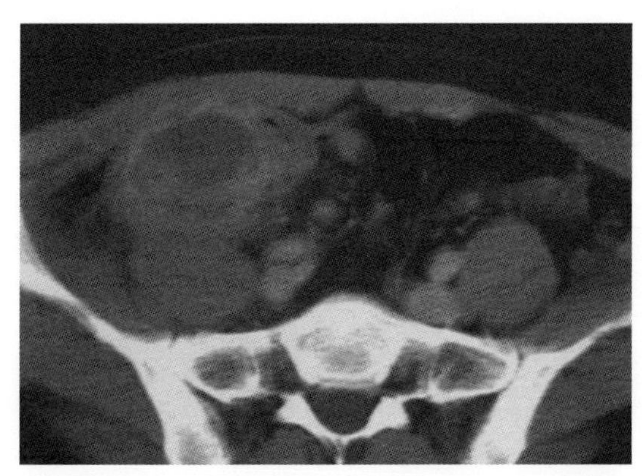

Figure 15.17 Computed tomography demonstrating an appendix abscess.

APPENDICITIS IN PREGNANCY

The rate of appendicitis in pregnancy is similar to that in the non-pregnant female population. Suspected appendicitis is the most common indication for surgery for non-obstetric conditions during pregnancy, and occurs in approximately 1 in 500 pregnancies per year. Appendicitis occurs more frequently in the second trimester than in the first or third.[56] Preoperative diagnosis of AA can be difficult in pregnancy, and a low threshold for surgical intervention has traditionally been recommended, as complicated appendicitis is associated with a higher rate of foetal loss and increased maternal morbidity. A systematic review (SR) reported a negative appendicectomy rate of 12–24%, higher than that in the non-pregnant population, and rates of foetal loss of 3.4%, 12.1% and 7.3% in simple, complicated and negative appendicectomy, respectively.[57] Recognition of the risk associated with negative appendicectomy[58] has led to the American College of Obstetricians and Gynecologists recommending magnetic resonance imaging in patients in whom an ultrasound scan has failed to show AA.[59] Where emergency access to such imaging is not possible and there remains a high suspicion of AA, surgery should not be delayed.

Many reports have demonstrated LA to be a safe and effective procedure during pregnancy. With modification of port positions, the laparoscopic approach has even been reported during the third trimester. Multiple studies on OA versus LA have been published and reviewed, with conflicting results. An overview of SRs on OA versus LA found that four recent SRs do not provide consistent results, with differing findings and conclusions. Foetal loss is arguably the most important obstetric outcome in the consideration of the effect of different approaches to appendicectomy in pregnancy. All four SRs reported a significantly higher rate of foetal loss after LA than after OA; however, the data is heavily influenced by a single study that was published in the early days of LA. Concerns are raised regarding the methodology of this very influential study, and if excluded there is no difference in foetal loss between LA and OA.[60] Currently, the Society of American Gastrointestinal and Endoscopic Surgeons continues to recommend LA as the treatment of choice for pregnant patients regardless of gestation.[61]

A reasonable approach in these patients is to use laparoscopy in the first trimester or when, despite adequate imaging, the diagnosis is in doubt. In later pregnancy, open surgery may be preferred when the diagnosis is confirmed, but the approach will depend upon surgeon expertise. In all cases, there should be a low threshold for conversion to open surgery if difficulties are encountered. In the third trimester, the incision for OA may be high in the right upper quadrant and is not a procedure for unsupervised trainee surgeons.

POSTOPERATIVE COMPLICATIONS AND OUTCOME

HOSPITAL STAY

The duration of hospital stay depends on local resources, policies, the patient's general condition and any co-existing disease. It is now clear that LA is associated with a more rapid return to normal activities, lower morbidity rate and a shorter hospital stay than conventional surgery.[39–41]

WOUND INFECTION

This is the commonest postoperative complication, occurring in around 10–15% of patients following a conventional right iliac fossa incision. In most patients, the inflammation is superficial, responding promptly to antibiotics, but in some there will be abscess formation, sometimes requiring surgical intervention. The use of a wound protector during OA has been shown to decrease wound infection and their use is encouraged.[29] Wound infection is significantly less following LA.[41]

There is no evidence that wound infiltration with local anaesthetic agents is associated with any increase in the incidence of wound infection.[62,63]

OTHER SEPTIC COMPLICATIONS

Pericaecal fluid collections are relatively common and are usually indicated by the presence of abdominal discomfort and a low-grade pyrexia. They can usually be diagnosed by ultrasound, and the initiation of antibiotics with re-laparoscopy and lavage of the right iliac fossa via the previously used port sites results in rapid recovery. An alternative is radiological aspiration. Pelvic abscess is a less common complication that presents with lower abdominal discomfort and swinging pyrexia. The symptoms may be delayed by 10 days or more and a soft tender mass may be palpable on rectal examination, although this is not always the case. Again, ultrasound and often CT is required for diagnosis and, if pus is aspirated, a percutaneous drain should be placed if possible. Occasionally, a pelvic abscess may be difficult to drain percutaneously and, in this situation, early re-look laparoscopy (in preference to re-look laparotomy) and pelvic washout with drain insertion is usually straightforward and immediately effective. An alternative approach is antibiotics or occasionally drainage of the abscess into the rectum if possible. The decision is influenced by the general condition of the patient. Prolonged use of antibiotics should be avoided, and further attempts made for drainage if the collection is not resolving on repeated imaging.

As in any patient who has undergone laparoscopic abdominal surgery, the presence of increased abdominal tenderness or generalised peritonitis in the first 24 hours may indicate an unrecognised iatrogenic injury to the intestine and mandates immediate re-look laparoscopy.

PROGNOSIS

The mortality of appendicitis is associated with the age of the patient and delayed diagnosis (perforated appendix).

In a report on 573 244 appendicectomies in the USA from 2006 to 2008, the mortality rate was 0.31%. This was highest in patients with perforated appendicitis.[64] A further consideration is the incidence of subsequent tubal infertility after appendicectomy. A meta-analysis has shown that appendicitis does not affect fertility in women; it does, however, increase the risk of subsequent ectopic pregnancy.[65]

APPENDICEAL TUMOURS

Neoplasms of the appendix are rare. They are found in approximately 1% of appendicectomy specimens. Neuroendocrine tumours (NETs) are the most common, comprising 30–80% of all appendiceal neoplasms.[66,67]

NEUROENDOCRINE NEOPLASM

Appendiceal NET is a relatively frequent subgroup of neuroendocrine neoplasms with an approximate incidence of 0.15–0.6/100 000/year.[67–73] The majority of appendiceal NETs originate from serotonin-producing enterochromaffin cells. The tumours appear to have a neuroectodermal origin and more benign features than other NETs.[68] Appendiceal NET are prevalent at autopsy and rarely attain clinical significance. Many may perhaps undergo spontaneous involution since the prevalence is reported as higher in children than in adults.[69]

It follows that appendiceal NETs are often an incidental finding at surgery and are expected to occur in 3–5 in 1000 appendicectomies.[68,73] Approximately 70% are located in the tip of the appendix, resulting in them seldom occluding the lumen and causing appendicitis.[68,73] Patients with appendiceal NETs are generally younger than those with other NETs, having a mean age of 40 years, with a slight female predominance. The overall metastasis rate is 3.8%, with distant metastases in 0.7%.[69] Early-stage NETs have an excellent prognosis, with 5-year survival rates of 95–100% for local disease and 85–100% for regional disease.[67,71,73] This is in contrast with metastatic disease, where 5-year survival is less than 25%.[67,72,73]

✓✓ The majority (approximately 90%) of appendiceal NETs are < 1 cm in diameter and have minimal risk of presenting with metastases. These lesions may be cured by simple appendicectomy.[67,70,73] This treatment is also apparently safe for most lesions measuring 1–2 cm, although rare cases in this group have presented with lymph node metastases.[68,73] Right hemicolectomy should be performed for the 1–2 cm NET with high-risk features, namely: positive or unclear margins, deep meso-appendiceal invasion (>3 mm), high proliferation rate (WHO grade 2) or angioinvasion. NET with a diameter > 2 cm should likewise be treated with a right hemicolectomy.[73]

MUCINOUS TUMOURS

Adenomas and low-grade appendiceal mucinous neoplasms (LAMNs) typically occur in patients in their sixth decade. The majority of mucinous neoplasms of the appendix are either asymptomatic, present with chronic right iliac fossa pain or a mass. Some patients may present with pain that mimics AA.[74–76] Diagnosis is usually made with imaging performed for chronic pain, or occasionally at colonoscopy, where a bulging appendiceal orifice may be recognised (Fig. 15.18).

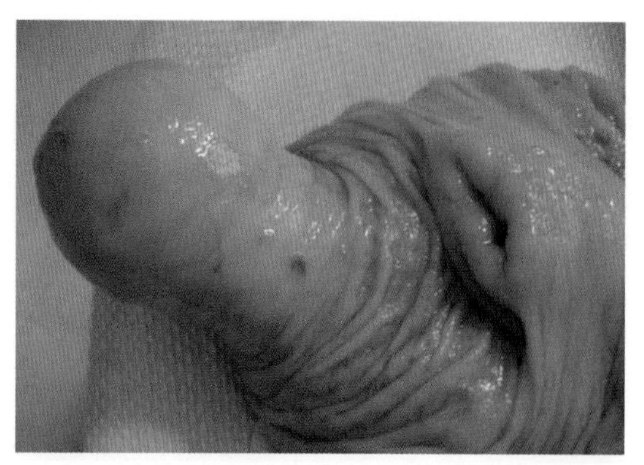

Figure 15.18 Appendiceal mucinous neoplasm specimen demonstrating bulging appendiceal orifice.

Pseudomyxoma peritonei (PMP) is the consequence of a perforated mucinous tumour of the appendix. This mucinous neoplastic epithelium is gradually seeded throughout the peritoneal cavity.[77,78] PMP is commonly diagnosed by gynaecologists in patients presenting with pelvic discomfort or enlarged ovaries secondarily involved by mucinous tumour deposits. Histological studies of many PMP cases presumed to be due to ovarian mucinous tumour peritoneal spread have been found to be of appendiceal origin.[79,80] The very slow accumulation of mucin means the process of distension and gradual perforation may be minimally symptomatic and occur years before the presentation of PMP.[77,78]

There are three histological entities grouped together as mucinous neoplasms of the appendix: adenoma, LAMN and invasive adenocarcinoma.[81] An appendix with an adenoma or LAMN may, on gross examination, appear either unremarkable or dilated with tenacious mucin, although there should be no mucin on the external surface. As the process advances, the wall of an appendix with LAMN frequently becomes fibrotic and hyalinised, and may have extensive calcification creating a 'porcelain appendix'.[76,81] Alternatively, it may become transformed into a fibrotic cyst lined by attenuated neoplastic mucinous epithelium.

Simple appendicectomy is sufficient treatment for adenomas and LAMNs (Fig. 15.19), but if the appendix margin is found to be involved at histology, then an ileocaecectomy is indicated[76,82] (Fig. 15.20). This operation offers no additional benefit over appendicectomy alone for patients with LAMNs that are confined to the appendix.[83,84] Given the possibility of peritoneal recurrence in patients with ruptured tumours, patients with acellular mucin on the appendiceal serosa should have wide excision of the surrounding tissue that has encapsulated the mucin. The peritoneal cavity and omentum should also be copiously washed in an effort to prevent the development of PMP. Some specialist units now offer radical 'peritonectomy' and high-temperature intraperitoneal chemotherapy for patients at high risk of recurrence, and referral to one of these units should be considered in such patients.

ADENOCARCINOMA

In contrast to other appendiceal neoplasms, the majority of patients with adenocarcinoma present with a picture of AA.[85] Other presentations include a palpable mass, obstruction, GI bleeding or symptoms referable to metastases. Appendiceal adenocarcinomas fall into one of three separate histologic

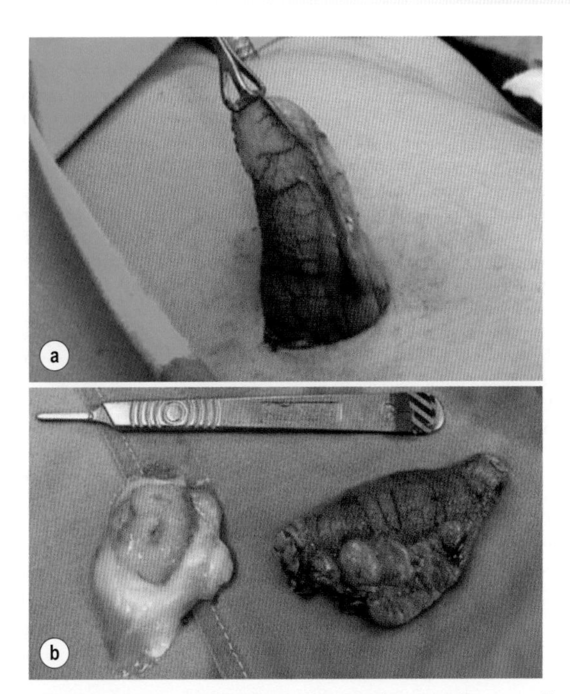

Figure 15.19 **(a)** Appendicectomy for mucinous adenoma discovered in pregnant patient with right iliac fossa pain. **(b)** Appendix specimen demonstrating distal dilatation at adenoma site and mucin from within appendiceal lumen.

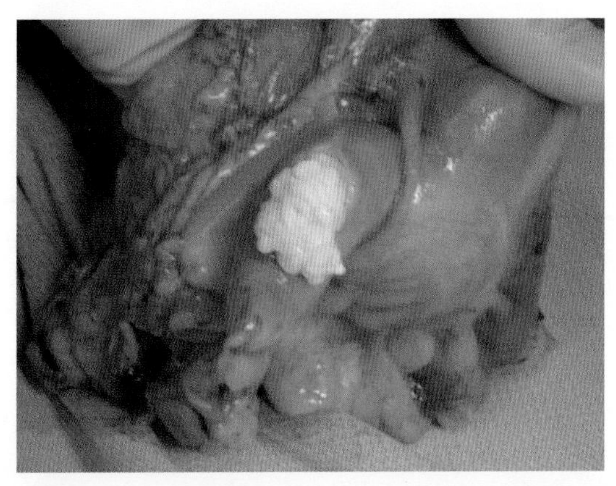

Figure 15.20 Ileocaecectomy for mucinous tumour of appendix involving base of appendix (see Fig. 15.18). Specimen opened to demonstrate appendiceal mucin.

types: (i) the most common is the mucinous type, which produces abundant mucin; (ii) the less common intestinal or colonic type closely mimics adenocarcinomas found in the colon; and (iii) the least common is signet ring cell adenocarcinoma, which is associated with a poor prognosis.[86]

Although controversial, invasive adenocarcinoma of the appendix on histology warrants a subsequent right hemicolectomy both to achieve complete tumour resection and to adequately stage the tumour by examining the right colic lymph nodes.[87–90] Most studies have shown that right hemicolectomy offers improved 5-year survival rates relative to appendicectomy alone; however, the prognosis of appendiceal carcinoma is worse than for adenocarcinoma of the colon.[87,88,90] See also the *Colorectal Surgery* volume of the *Companion to Specialist Practice* series.

Key points

- The most common emergency conditions affecting the small bowel are obstruction, haemorrhage and ischaemia.
- Early management requires adequate clinical and radiological assessment, which might include contrast radiology and CT (see also Chapter 11).
- Surgery for acute appendicitis is superior to antibiotics alone because of the latter's high recurrence rate.
- Laparoscopic appendicectomy results in less pain, fewer wound complications and faster return to normal activities than open appendicectomy.
- A non-operative approach is indicated in the majority of patients with appendix mass or abscess, with radiological drainage as required. Subsequent interval appendicectomy is only indicated in those patients with recurrent symptoms. Care must be taken to ensure that underlying diseases other than appendicitis have been excluded (e.g., caecal carcinoma and Crohn's disease), which usually requires CT and colonoscopy.

 References available at http://ebooks.health.elsevier.com/

RECOMMENDED VIDEOS

- Laparoscopy of ischaemic bowel – https://youtu.be/wyohLCbFTV0
- ICG examination of ischaemic - https://youtu.be/gRHebsuTymc
- Laparoscopic adhesiolysis – https://youtu.be/BKo0mAoog6M
- Open appendicectomy – https://youtu.be/ 8OK-_4Wx3QY
- Laparoscopic appendicectomy – https://youtu.be/GfmicbfAeD0
- Laparoscopic appendicectomy in a pregnant patient – https://youtu.be/mvVOWLh6_vE
- Other useful videos from the authors can be viewed on https://www.youtube.com/channel/UCLSczWba4suPdj6CAD615Q

ACKNOWLEDGEMENT

The fifth edition of this chapter was written by Peter Lamb. We have retained much of the information, revising, and updating it as appropriate. We acknowledge the excellence of his work.

KEY REFERENCES

[21] Schoots IG, Koffeman DA, Levi M, et al. Systematic review of survival after acute mesenteric ischaemia according to disease aetiology. Br J Surg 2004;91:17–27. PMID: 14716789

Data from 45 observational studies including 3692 patients were reviewed. Prognosis after acute mesenteric venous thrombosis is better than for arterial ischaemia, and that for arterial embolism is better than that for arterial thrombosis.

[29] Di Saverio S, Podda M, De Simone B, Ceresoli M, Augustin G, Gori A, et al. Diagnosis and treatment of acute appendicitis: 2020 update of the WSES Jerusalem guidelines. World J Emerg Surg 2020;15(1):1–42

This World Society of Emergency Surgery guideline summarises management of all aspects of acute appendicitis with data review for each recommendation.

[35] Andersen BR, Kallehave FL, Andersen HK. Antibiotics versus placebo for prevention of postoperative infection after appendicectomy: update of Cochrane Database Systematic Review 2003;(2). Cochrane Database Syst Rev 2005;3:CD001439. PMID: 16034862

This systematic review confirmed the advantage of prophylactic antibiotics in reducing wound infection following appendicectomy.

[36] SIGN guideline 104. Antibiotic prophylaxis in surgery. Scottish Intercollegiate Guideline Network; April 2014. www.sign.ac.uk

This guideline demonstrated that prophylactic antibiotics during appendicectomy reduced wound infection with an odds ratio of 0.33 and the number needed to treat to prevent one wound infection being 11.

[39] Masoomi H, Mills S, Dolich MO, et al. Comparison of outcomes of laparoscopic versus open appendectomy in adults: data from the nationwide inpatient sample (NIS), 2006–2008. J Gastrointest Surg 2011;15:2226–31. PMID: 21725700

This nationwide review confirms the decrease in infective morbidity from laparoscopic appendicectomy.

[40] Jaschinski T, Mosch CG, Eikermann M, Neugebauer EA, Sauerland S. Laparoscopic versus open surgery for suspected appendicitis. Cochrane Database Syst Rev 2018;11(11):CD001546. https://doi.org/10.1002/14651858.CD001546.pub4. Published 2018 Nov 28

This Cochrane review recommends laparoscopic appendicectomy for all patients (if the required skills are available).

[42] Lucchi A, Berti P, Grassia M, et al. Laparoscopic appendectomy: Hem-o-lok versus Endoloop in stump closure. Updates Surg 2016. PMID: 28013455

Randomised trial demonstrating no difference between Endoloop and Hem-o-Lok in closure of the appendix stump during laparoscopic appendicectomy, but Hem-o-Lok costs less and is easier to use. See also https://www.sages.org/meetings/annual-meeting/abstracts-archive/application-of-hem-o-lok-clip-in-basic-laparoscopic-procedures-a-single-center-experience-on-856-cases-and-review-of-data-from-food-and-drug-administration/.

[49] Salminen P, Tuominen R, Paajanen H, Rautio T, Nordström P, Aarnio M, et al. Five-year follow-up of antibiotic therapy for uncomplicated acute appendicitis in the APPAC randomized clinical trial. JAMA - J Am Med Assoc 2018;320(12):1259–65

Five-year follow-up data on the APPAC randomised control trial of surgery versus antibiotic therapy for acute uncomplicated appendicitis. Demonstrates a 5-year recurrence rate of 39% in patients treated with antibiotics alone.

[52] Deakin DE, Ahmed I. Interval appendicectomy after resolution of adult inflammatory appendix mass – is it necessary?. Surgeon 2007;5(1):45–50. PMID: 17313128

A systematic review confirming that non-operative management will be successful in the majority of patients and recurrence of symptoms is low.

[73] Pape UF, Niederle B, Costa F, et al. Consensus guidelines for neuroendocrine neoplasms of the appendix (excluding goblet cell carcinomas). Neuroendocrinology 2016;103(2):144–52. PMID: 26730583

ENET consensus guideline.

Colonic emergencies

16

Scott R. Kelley

INTRODUCTION

Colonic emergencies result from obstruction, inflammation/infection, perforation, haemorrhage or ischaemia. Herein we discuss aetiology, pathogenesis, presentation and management. Emergency compared with elective colon surgery is associated with a two- to threefold increase in mortality, hence interventions to convert an emergency into an elective operation should be considered when safe to do so. In addition to a thorough history and physical examination, patients must be resuscitated and optimised as far as practicable prior to proceeding to the operating room. Multidisciplinary approaches to patient care and thorough radiographic and colonoscopic evaluation are often extremely beneficial for planning and treating this complex population. When possible, patients should be preoperatively evaluated, educated and site-marked by stoma therapists. If facilities are inadequate, transfer to a referral centre should be considered.

COLONIC OBSTRUCTION

Colonic obstruction can occur secondary to multiple causes (Table 16.1) and can be partial or complete, intrinsic or extrinsic, and adynamic or mechanical. The most common causes are neoplasia, diverticulitis and volvulus. Treatment for obstruction is dependent on the location, cause, patient presentation and goals of care.

A distal colonic obstruction in the presence of a competent ileocaecal valve hindering retrograde flow of enteric content, or colonic volvulus, will result in a closed loop obstruction. Antegrade flow of enteric content and bacterial overgrowth progressively increase intraluminal pressure, which is followed by venous occlusion, intramural hypoperfusion, arterial occlusion, thrombosis, ischaemia, necrosis and perforation. Consequently, a closed loop obstruction mandates expedited care.

Mild obstruction (stenosis) typically presents with cramping abdominal pain and constipation. Imaging may reveal an area of luminal stenosis. Endoscopic advancement through the stricture is often not possible. Colon proximal to the stricture is not dilated and surgery can be planned in an elective fashion. Severe obstruction presents with proximal bowel dilatation, pronounced abdominal distension, absolute constipation (failure to pass flatus or stool) and varying degrees of tenderness, which in combination with signs of systemic toxicity (elevated heart rate, leucocytosis) necessitate emergency surgery (ES).

NEOPLASTIC OBSTRUCTION

Approximately 20% of patients with colon cancer will present with an obstruction, with the majority being elderly. Nearly 30% will have hepatic metastasis at the time of surgery. Obstruction secondary to colon cancer often presents with a constellation of symptoms including abdominal distension, alteration in bowel habits, weight loss, change in stool calibre and/or consistency, nausea, emesis, obstipation and absence of flatus. Symptoms usually develop slowly and typically reflect the site of obstruction. Right-sided masses typically cause obstructive symptoms (abdominal cramping, pain), whereas left-sided cancers are more commonly associated with a change in stool calibre, consistency and alteration in bowel habits.

Initial management includes bowel rest, analgesia, resuscitation and correction of laboratory abnormalities. Nasogastric tubes do not decompress the colon and are not necessary unless the patient is experiencing nausea/emesis. Plain abdominal radiographs will identify large bowel dilatation, and if the ileocaecal valve is incompetent, small intestine distension may also be noted. Computed tomographic (CT) imaging informs surgical planning and provides staging information which may be key in defining goals of care, and should be obtained unless immediate operative intervention cannot be delayed. If CT is not available, a water-soluble contrast enema will identify the level of obstruction and can be useful in distinguishing pseudo-obstruction (Ogilvie syndrome) from causes of mechanical obstruction. Endoscopy may be both diagnostic and therapeutic.

INTERVENTION: COLONIC STENTS

Colonic self-expandable metal stents (SEMS) may be used as a bridge to surgery for those with partial obstruction or for palliation in patients with inoperable disease.[1] Although technical success is greater than 90%, complications include perforation (up to 13%), stent failure after technically successful positioning (up to 12%), stent migration (1–13%), re-obstruction (4–23%), pain (up to 7%) and bleeding (up to 4%).[1,2] Perforations are more common with intraluminal stents left in place for a prolonged period of time, stents crossing acute angles and in patients receiving antiangiogenic drugs such as bevacizumab.[3,4] Non-palliative stenting ('bridge to surgery') provides the opportunity to decompress the distended proximal colon, medically optimise patients in preparation for surgery, complete a preoperative colonoscopy, and pursue a single-stage operation using a minimally invasive approach. However, clinically silent microperforations associated with stents have been documented at the time of surgery, raising concerns regarding

Table 16.1 Causes of colonic obstruction

Neoplasm
Volvulus
Diverticulitis
Pseudo-obstruction
Hernia
Stricture
Faecal impaction
Inflammatory
Intussusception
Endometriosis
Adhesions
Ischaemia

oncological outcomes. Small et al.[3] at the Mayo Clinic identified five risk factors associated with complications from self-expandable colonic stents, which included male sex, complete colonic occlusion, balloon dilatation prior to stent placement, mid-stent diameter less than 22 mm, and placement by an interventionalist not familiar with pancreaticobiliary procedures. The first randomised prospective study comparing open surgery to SEMS followed by a minimally invasive resection (endolaparoscopic) for left-sided colon cancer was reported in 2009. No stent-related complications were reported, technical and clinical success for stenting was 83%, and only 38% underwent a single-stage operation in the open compared with 67% in the endolaparoscopic arm. All in the stent arm underwent ostomy reversal and six in the open group were left with a permanent stoma.[5] Pirlet et al.[6] in a French multicentre prospective randomised controlled trial compared the outcomes of ES to SEMS as a bridge for surgery. The primary outcome was the need for a stoma (temporary or permanent) for any reason. The secondary endpoints were mortality, morbidity and length of hospital stay. The study was closed early secondary to stent-related perforations. Among the 60 patients accrued, 17 in the open group versus 13 in the SEMS group were left with a stoma. The multi-institutional Dutch Stent-In Study Group evaluated colonic stenting as a bridge to elective surgery versus ES, with the primary outcome of mean global health status during a 6-month follow-up. The study was closed early secondary to increased morbidity in the SEMS group, and specifically six perforations in the SEMS versus none in the operative arm. They concluded that colonic stenting has no decisive clinical advantages to ES.[7] Critics pointed out that centres not highly experienced in SEMS placement were involved in the study, which likely resulted in higher rates of perforation. Increased failures and complications have been described if stenting is performed by endoscopists who have placed less than 40 SEMS.[8] A systematic review and meta-analysis of eight RCTs demonstrated that SEMS as a bridge to surgery, compared with ES, had lower short-term overall morbidity (33.9% in SEMS group vs 51.2% in ES group) and lower rates of temporary colostomy (33.9% in SEMS group and 51.4% in ES group). SEMS also achieved a lower permanent stoma rate (22.2% for SEMS vs 35.2% for ES) and an increased success of primary anastomosis (70% in SEMS group and 54.1% in ES group), with no difference in overall mortality within 60 days after surgery.[9] Foo et al.[10] performed a meta-analysis of seven randomised controlled trials evaluating oncologic outcomes and found that SEMS had a significantly higher overall recurrence rate than ES, although disease-free and overall survival at 3 years were similar. The multicentre randomised controlled ESCO trial recently compared morbidity rates after colonic stenting as a bridge to surgery versus ES in the management of left-sided malignant large-bowel obstruction and found that the two treatment strategies were equivalent. There was no difference in oncologic outcomes at a median follow-up of 36 months, and there was a significantly lower stoma rate noted in the SEMS group.[11] Preliminary results from the UK ColoRectal Endoscopic Stenting Trial (CREST) revealed that 30-day postoperative mortality, length of hospital stay, critical care usage and quality of life were not different between the two treatment groups (SEMS and surgery). Long-term results are still pending.[12] The European Society of Gastrointestinal Endoscopy (ESGE) recently updated their guidelines with recommendations for the use of SEMS.[1]

✔✔ According to the European Society of Gastrointestinal Endoscopy (ESGE):

1. Colonic stenting to be reserved for patients with clinical symptoms and radiological signs of malignant large-bowel obstruction, without signs of perforation.
2. Stenting as a bridge to surgery to be discussed, within a shared decision-making process, as a treatment option in patients with potentially curable left-sided obstructing colon cancer as an alternative to emergency resection.
3. Colonic stenting as the preferred treatment for palliation of malignant colonic obstruction.
4. Consideration of colonic stenting for malignant obstruction of the proximal colon either as a bridge to surgery or in a palliative setting.
5. A time interval of approximately 2 weeks until resection when colonic stenting is performed as a bridge to elective surgery in patients with curable left-sided colon cancer.
6. Colonic stenting should be performed or directly supervised by an operator who can demonstrate competence in both colonoscopy and fluoroscopic techniques and who performs colonic stenting on a regular basis.
7. A decompressing stoma as a bridge to elective surgery is a valid option if the patient is not a candidate for colonic stenting or when stenting expertise is not available.[1]

INTERVENTION: OPERATIVE

Resectable disease can be pursued in an oncological fashion in single or multiple stages. Choice of operative approach is multifactorial and dictated by surgeon experience, clinical condition of the patient and operative factors (tissue quality, contamination, synchronous cancer, proximal dilatation). For those not in extremis, a single-stage primary anastomosis with or without a protective diverting ostomy can be pursued. Morbidity and mortality have been shown to be equivalent between single- and multi-staged procedures in appropriate candidates.[13] Laparoscopic approaches have typically been avoided secondary to lack of visualisation, risk of iatrogenic perforation and increased time to perform the procedure, although in the hands of skilled laparoscopic surgeons these are not absolute contraindications.

Some form of intraoperative colonic decompression is usually required to facilitate handling of the distended colon and visualisation of the intracoelomic cavity. Techniques to decompress through a laparotomy incision include needle aspiration, suction, lavage and endoscopic. However, on-table lavage of faeces has not been noted to decrease anastomotic complications.

For needle decompression, a purse-string suture using a small needle is placed through the tenia of an accessible portion of dilated colon. A large angiocath (14-gauge or larger) is placed through the middle of the purse-string and the needle is removed leaving the soft flexible catheter sheath in the lumen of colon (Fig. 16.1). The sheath is then connected to suction. Needle decompression works well to decompress gas, though it is too small to decompress stool and blood. If unable to decompress adequately, a pool tip suction catheter can be placed through the same defect after making a small colotomy (Fig. 16.2). Once adequate decompression is obtained, the catheter can be removed and the purse-string suture secured.

More thorough lavage can be carried out after placing a large-diameter catheter with multiple distal holes connected to a Y-connector through the ileocaecal valve into the right colon. One limb of the Y-connector is connected to irrigation and the other to suction (Fig. 16.3). If the catheter becomes clogged, it can be readily irrigated. After decompression is achieved, the catheter can be removed and the purse-string secured, or pushed into the ascending colon and removed with the specimen for a right colectomy. Closed systems for retrograde colonic lavage are also available.

Evaluation for synchronous tumours, liver metastasis, local invasion and the presence of peritoneal carcinomatosis should be carried out. A curative resection, including *en bloc* resection of surrounding involved structures, is pursued when possible. Metastasis does not preclude resection and re-establishment of intestinal continuity. For palliation during surgery, a decompressive ostomy is the preferred approach in those with unresectable disease who are operative candidates. If creation of an ostomy is not possible, an intestinal bypass procedure can be considered. In rare instances, a loop ostomy can be performed under local anaesthesia for palliation in decompensated patients unable to tolerate general anaesthesia.

DIVERTICULAR

In Westernised countries, diverticular disease affects around 40% by age 60 and 60% by age 80, and the diagnosis appears to be rising.[14] Acute diverticulitis occurs in 10–25%, and of those 20–25% experience a complicated form (perforation, abscess, stricture, fistula). Recurrent episodes of diverticulitis can result in fibrosis of the colon wall, stricturing and obstructive symptoms. Approximately 10% of colonic obstructions result from diverticular strictures.

Initial management and imaging is as noted above. For obstruction presenting with a concomitant abscess, active inflammation or phlegmon, a trial of conservative treatment including antibiotics, with or without interventional radiology-guided procedures, may allow the obstruction to resolve as inflammation improves.

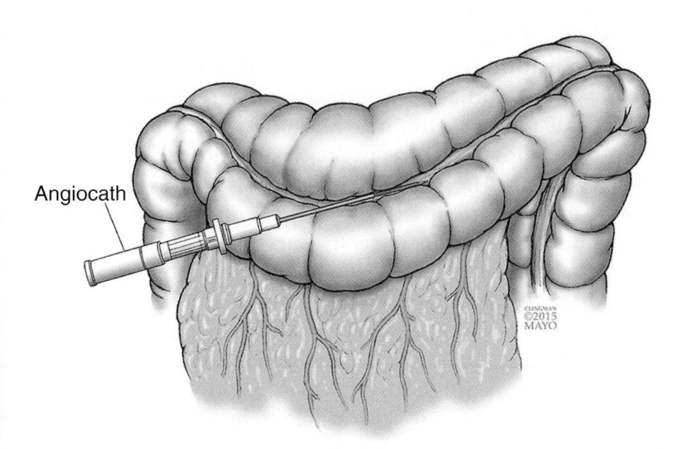

Figure 16.1 Needle decompression of colon. (Used with permission of Mayo Foundation for Medical Education and Research, all rights reserved.)

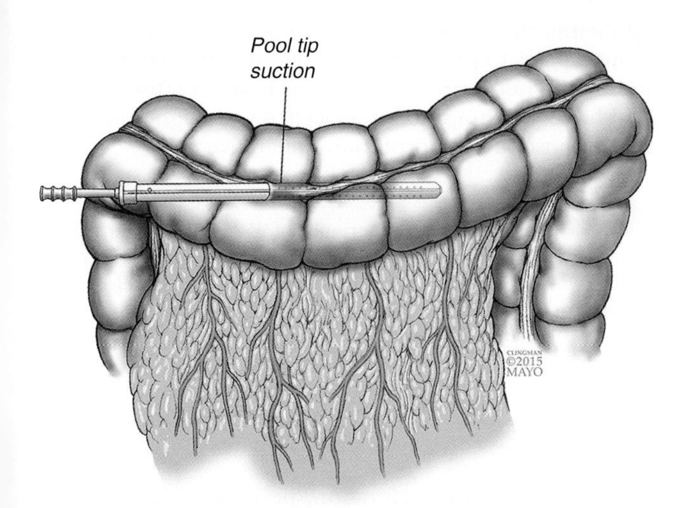

Figure 16.2 Pool suction decompression of colon. (Used with permission of Mayo Foundation for Medical Education and Research, all rights reserved.)

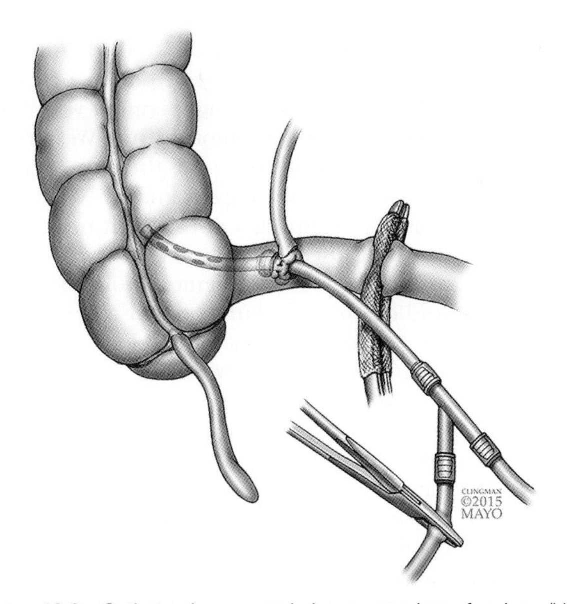

Figure 16.3 Catheter lavage and decompression of colon. (Used with permission of Mayo Foundation for Medical Education and Research, all rights reserved.)

Urgent/ES is rarely performed for colonic strictures secondary to diverticular disease and only in cases of complete obstruction. Partial obstruction solely related to stricturing is pursued in an elective fashion. SEMS can be used as a bridge to surgery allowing for decompression of the distended proximal colon, provide the opportunity to medically optimise patients, complete a preoperative colonoscopy and pursue a single-stage surgery. Few studies describe SEMS for diverticular strictures and most are single-institution experiences. Small et al.[15] described the use of stents in 23 patients, of whom 16 were associated with diverticular disease. Complications included perforation (4), migration (2) and re-obstruction (2), and 87% of the time occurred 7 days after placement. An emergency procedure was converted to an elective surgery for 84%, although the authors recommended that resection should be attempted within 7 days of SEMS placement. Multiple other small studies have also reported high rates of complications; mainly perforation, migration, obstruction and no improvement. Using SEMS for diverticular strictures is unproven at this time and may not represent a valid therapeutic option unless the patient is unfit for surgery.[16]

Operative approaches include open or minimally invasive segmental resection, with or without a protective diverting ostomy, and Hartmann's procedure. It is important to note that in many cases it may not be possible to distinguish diverticular stricture from malignancy preoperatively, in which case resection should follow oncological principles given that malignancy is more frequent. As noted above, the choice of operation and need for ostomy is dependent on the condition of the patient, tissues and the experience of the surgeon. Procedures for decompressing the colon apply as described above.

SIGMOID VOLVULUS

Sigmoid volvulus is for the most part an acquired condition and encompasses 60–80% of all colonic volvulus. In Westernised countries, it is most commonly associated with the elderly, debilitated, neurological conditions, those institutionalised or taking psychiatric medications and laxative abuse. Males and females are equally affected. Although the aetiology is unknown, it is thought to be secondary to constipation and colonic lengthening. Sigmoid volvulus in younger age groups is more common in non-Westernised countries. Worldwide, sigmoid volvulus is the most common cause of bowel obstruction during pregnancy. Congenital anomalies such as Hirschsprung's disease, gut malrotation and parasitic disease caused by *Trypanosoma cruzi* (Chagas disease) are also associated with sigmoid volvulus. Volvulus of the sigmoid colon can occur in either a clockwise or counter-clockwise orientation as the colon elongates and rotates on a narrow pedicled mesenteric base.

Although a few patients describe symptoms of recurrent distension followed by spontaneous detorsion resulting in explosive large-volume bowel movements, the vast majority present as an emergency with abdominal pain, distension and absolute constipation. Diagnosis can be made most of the time with an abdominal X-ray revealing a dilated colon in the shape of a 'coffee bean' or 'omega loop' with its apex pointing toward the right upper quadrant, though only present radiographically in 50–80% (Fig. 16.4).[17] A water-soluble contrast enema reveals a 'bird's beak' appearance in the rectosigmoid region, which is secondary to narrowing at the level of the torsion. CT has become the imaging modality of choice and in addition to a dilated loop of colon often reveals a characteristic 'whirl sign' whereby the mesentery twists around the vasculature.

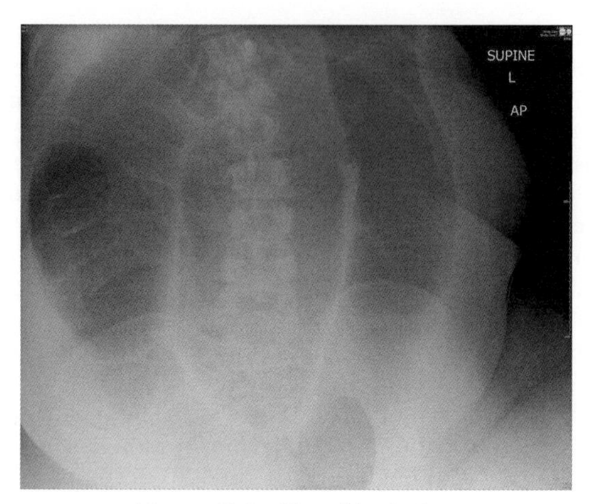

Figure 16.4 Sigmoid volvulus.

Fluid and electrolyte abnormalities, common in patients with sigmoid volvulus, need to be corrected. For patients without perforation or peritonitis, rigid or flexible sigmoidoscopy with minimal air insufflation is performed to detort the volvulus and decompress the proximal colon. Flexible endoscopy allows for direct visual inspection of the colonic mucosa and in those with suspicion of necrosis detorsion should not be attempted and surgery should be pursued. Detorsion alone results in recurrence in the majority of cases. A rectal tube may be placed to decrease the chance of immediate re-volvulisation while the patient is optimised for colonic resection, preferably during the same hospitalisation. Evaluating patients in the United States Veterans Affairs Medical System, Grossmann et al.[18] noted mortality of 24% for ES versus 6% for those able to be treated in an elective fashion following endoscopic decompression. A single-centre experience of 952 patients over a 46-year period noted that morbidity and mortality for ES was 35% and 16% versus 12.5% and 0% for elective.[19] If the patient has not had a recent colonoscopy, and if feasible, a full mechanical bowel preparation and endoscopic colonic evaluation should be pursued prior to proceeding to the operating room. In addition to higher rates of recurrence, non-operative management has been shown to be associated with higher mortality rates in those without prohibitive operative risks.[20]

✔✔ A single-centre experience of 952 patients over a 46-year period noted that morbidity and mortality for emergency surgery was 35% and 16% versus 12.5% and 0% for elective. The principal strategy in the treatment for sigmoid volvulus is early non-surgical detorsion followed by elective surgery in uncomplicated patients, while emergency surgical treatment is performed for patients with bowel gangrene, perforation, or peritonitis, other difficulties with diagnosis, unsuccessful non-surgical detorsion and early recurrence.[19]

ES is pursued for perforation, peritonitis, ischaemia or the inability to endoscopically reduce the volvulus. Unless prohibited at the time of surgery (haemodynamic instability, intraperitoneal contamination, etc.), a segmental resection and primary anastomosis should be pursued. In those with

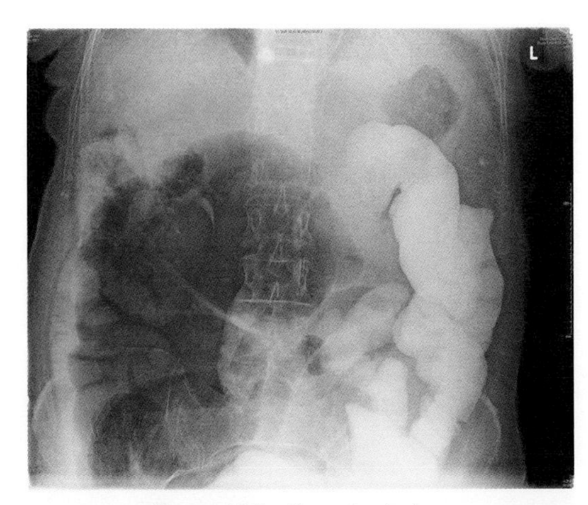

Figure 16.5 Caecal volvulus.

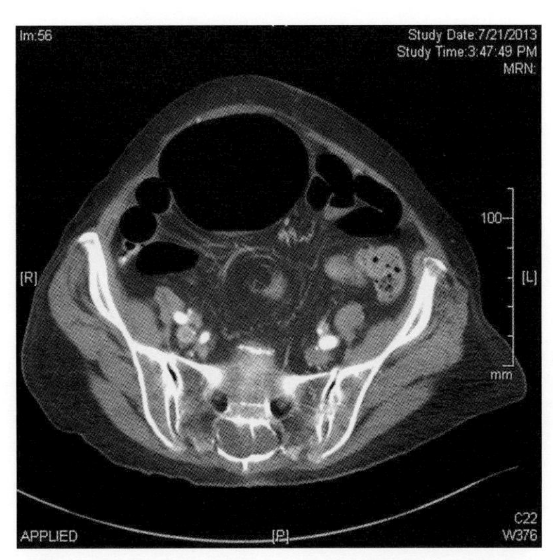

Figure 16.6 Mesenteric swirl on computed tomography of caecal volvulus.

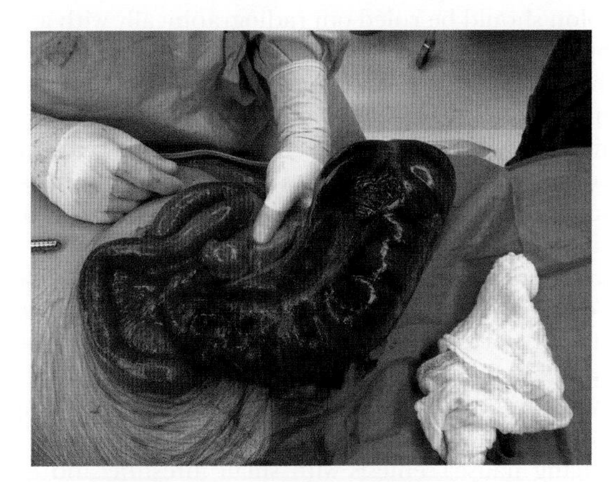

Figure 16.7 Ischaemic caecal volvulus.

uncomplicated sigmoid volvulus, morbidity and mortality have not been shown to differ between primary anastomosis and Hartmann's procedure. Faecal decompression with on-table lavage carries the added risk of spillage and contamination and has not been noted to decrease anastomotic complications. If the volvulus is ischaemic, resection should be pursued without reducing the volvulus to decrease the chance of systemically disseminating toxins. Previously described fixation and plasty procedures (sigmoidopexy, mesenteric fixation, mesosigmoidoplasty, etc.) are associated with high rates of recurrence and should be avoided.

CAECAL VOLVULUS

Caecal volvulus comprises around 15–30% of all colonic volvulus and is more common in those with prior abdominal surgery, women, younger age groups, pregnancy and constipation. Volvulisation most commonly occurs in a clockwise orientation when there is a lack of retroperitoneal fixation and includes the ascending colon and terminal ileum, rather than just the caecum.

Patients often present with sudden onset of abdominal pain, distension, nausea and emesis. Spontaneous detorsion of the volvulus is uncommon. Abdominal X-ray may reveal a large dilated loop of intestine in the shape of a 'coffee bean' or 'comma' extending across the abdomen to the left upper quadrant (Fig. 16.5).[17] CT has become the imaging modality of choice and in addition to a dilated loop of colon often reveals a characteristic 'whirl sign' where the mesentery twists around the vasculature (Fig. 16.6).

Endoscopic decompression should not be attempted and definitive management requires operative intervention. Once resuscitated, and unless prohibited at the time of surgery (haemodynamic instability, severe intraperitoneal contamination, etc.), a segmental resection of the hypermobile segment and primary ileocolonic anastomosis should be pursued. If the volvulus is ischaemic, resection should be undertaken without reducing the volvulus to decrease the chance of systemic dissemination of toxins (Fig. 16.7).

Other surgical procedures described for caecal volvulus include caecostomy and caecopexy. Both are associated with recurrence rates as high as 25% and mortality as high as 33%. Caecostomy is associated with inadequate decompression, clogged tubing, abdominal wall infection, persistent fistulisation, perforation and peritonitis. Unless surgical resection is contraindicated, caecostomy and caecopexy should be avoided.

CAECAL BASCULE

Caecal bascule is a type of caecal volvulus that results from the caecum folding anteriorly onto itself without mesenteric twisting. Patients often present with intermittent and recurrent obstructive symptoms making diagnosis difficult. CT is the most useful imaging modality. Management and operative intervention is the same as for caecal volvulus.

ACUTE COLONIC PSEUDO-OBSTRUCTION

Acute colonic pseudo-obstruction (ACPO), also referred to as Ogilvie's syndrome, results in non-mechanical distension of the colon and is primarily a problem of transiently absent colonic motility. It is most commonly associated with elderly, frail, institutionalised patients but also occurs in hospitalised patients after orthopaedic, gynaecologic and abdominal surgeries as well as those with cardiac and infectious aetiologies. It is has been postulated that parasympathetic inhibition likely plays a key role, though the pathophysiology is unknown.

The clinical presentation is characterised by marked abdominal distension, discomfort, nausea, emesis and constipation. Pain on examination is typically less than expected.

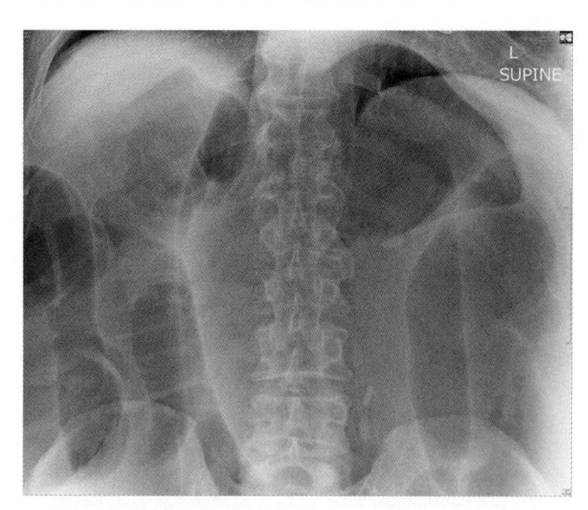

Figure 16.8 Acute colonic pseudo-obstruction.

Abdominal X-rays reveal significant dilatation of the entire large intestine (Fig. 16.8). Mechanical obstruction of the left colon should be ruled out radiographically with a water-soluble contrast enema or CT scan with rectal contrast, which will reveal free flow of contrast through the colon without a point of obstruction. Perforation is rare, but caecal diameter greater than 12 cm is associated with higher rates of spontaneous perforation and mortality doubles with an increase from 12 to 14 cm. Ischaemia and perforation are associated with mortality greater than 40%.[21]

Non-operative supportive care (bowel rest, resuscitation, correction of electrolyte abnormalities) is pursued in the absence of perforation or suspected ischaemia. Suspected precipitating illnesses such as urinary tract infections should be sought and treated. Nasogastric tubes do not decompress the colon and are not necessary unless the patient is experiencing nausea/emesis with small intestine and gastric distension. Medications that inhibit gastrointestinal transit (opiates/narcotics, antidepressants, antipsychotics, calcium channel blockers, antidiarrhoeal agents, anticholinergics) should be discontinued. Medications shown to worsen pseudo-obstruction, such as laxatives and enemas, should also be avoided. In most cases, colonic pseudo-obstruction will resolve spontaneously, though failure to resolve after 6 days is more commonly associated with perforation.

The use of intravenous (IV) neostigmine, a reversible acetylcholinesterase inhibitor, may be considered in selected patients as first-line therapy.[22] However, serious side effects including bradycardia, bronchospasm, hypotension and asystole effectively exclude most patients with the condition in UK practice. Frankel et al.[23] recently published a retrospective review of 30 patients with ACPO who were treated with subcutaneous neostigmine on regular wards and only monitored with standard nursing observations. They noted 93% of patients had clinically successful resolution of ACPO, and no clinically evident serious adverse events occurred.

Endoscopic decompression helps to ease the discomfort of severe colonic distension. Perforation, peritonitis and ischaemia are all contraindications to proceeding. Mechanical bowel preparation and enemas should be avoided. Advancement to the caecum is often difficult to achieve and not necessary. A long colonic decompressive tube positioned at the hepatic flexure can be placed to gravity or low wall suction to help sustain decompression (Fig. 16.9). To maintain

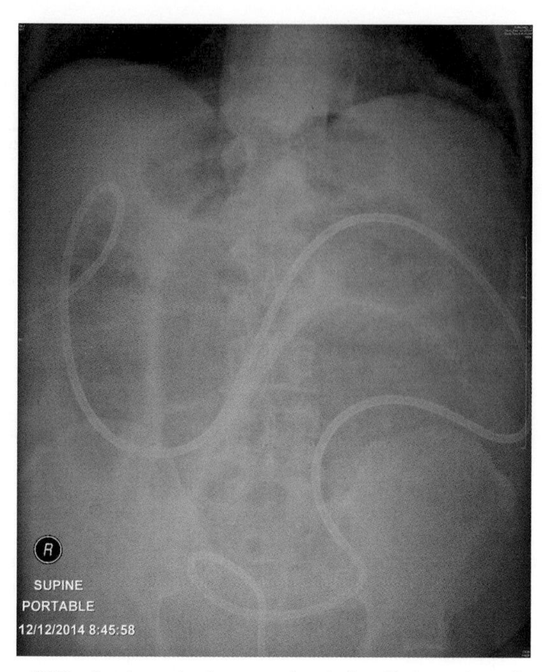

Figure 16.9 Acute colonic pseudo-obstruction post endoscopic decompression.

patency, the tube should be flushed every 4–6 hours. Once the pseudo-obstruction resolves, the decompression tube can be removed. It is not uncommon for patients to undergo multiple colonoscopic decompressions (15–30%) before a sustained response is achieved.[24]

Subcutaneous methylnaltrexone, a peripheral μ-opioid antagonist, can be used in patients receiving chronic opioid therapy, though supporting data are lacking. Low-dose daily polyethylene glycol (PEG) solution has been shown to be effective in preventing recurrence of ACPO.[25] Blocking sympathetic outflow with epidural anaesthesia has been shown to improve pseudo-obstruction in small series.

✔ Administration of polyethylene glycol (PEG) in patients with Ogilvie's syndrome after initial resolution of colonic dilatation may increase the sustained response rate after initial therapeutic intervention.[25]

When all non-operative measures have failed to resolve ACPO, surgical intervention may be considered. However, the inordinately high risk secondary to underlying frailty and comorbidities in this patient population effectively rules out surgery for most.[26] Decompressive ostomies do not prevent recurrence of pseudo-obstruction, increase long-term morbidity and are inadvisable.

Poor surgical candidates can be considered for percutaneous tube caecostomy to vent the colon if they cannot tolerate surgery, fail medical management and endoscopic decompression, and are without perforation, peritonitis or ischaemia.[27] Only case reports and small series have documented the success of tube caecostomy, which can be performed endoscopically, under radiological guidance, or laparoscopically. Issues with the procedure include inadequate decompression, clogged tubing, retraction, dislodgement, skin erosion, abdominal wall infection, leakage, fistulisation, perforation and peritonitis. Morbidity is noted to be around 50% and mortality 20–30%.

Table 16.2 Toxic megacolon diagnostic criteria

Radiographic evidence of colonic dilatation
Classic finding of more than 6 cm in the transverse colon
Any three of the following:
Fever (>38°C/101.5°F)
Tachycardia (>120 beats/min)
Leukocytosis (>10.5 × $10^3/\mu L$)
Anaemia (<60% of normal)
Any one of the following:
Dehydration
Altered mental status
Electrolyte imbalances
Hypotension

Adapted from Jalan KN, Sircus W, Card WI, et al. An experience of ulcerative colitis. I. Toxic dilation in 55 cases. Gastroenterology 1969;57(1):68–82.

Table 16.3 Causes of toxic megacolon

Inflammatory bowel disease
Infectious colitides
Clostridium difficile
Salmonella typhi
Shigella
Campylobacter jejuni
Yersinia enterocolitica
Entamoeba histolytica
Cryptosporidium
Cytomegalovirus
Chronic obstructive pulmonary disease
Diabetes
Immunosuppression
Kidney failure
Chemotherapeutic drugs
Kaposi's sarcoma
Colonoscopic overdistension
Cystic fibrosis

INFLAMMATION/INFECTION

TOXIC COLITIS/MEGACOLON

Toxic megacolon may occur as the initial manifestation of acute colonic inflammation or an acute exacerbation of chronic colitis. It is characterised by acute colitis, ≥ 6 cm non-obstructive segmental or complete dilatation of the colon, and signs of systemic toxicity (Table 16.2). Although multiple rare causes have been described in the literature (Table 16.3), it is most commonly associated with inflammatory bowel disease (IBD; ulcerative colitis, Crohn's, indeterminate colitis) and pseudomembranous (*Clostridium difficile*) colitis. The pathophysiology is thought to be secondary to local inflammatory mediators inhibiting smooth muscle tone causing colonic dysmotility and toxic dilatation.

Patients often present critically ill (fever, tachycardia, leucocytosis) with abdominal distension and tenderness, tympany and diarrhoea. A high index of suspicion is essential since symptoms may be non-specific or masked by medications (steroids, immunosuppressants, narcotics/opioids) or other factors (elderly, debilitated). Opiates/narcotics, antidepressants, antidiarrhoeal agents, anticholinergics, hypokalaemia and barium enemas are known to induce and exacerbate the condition. Systemic toxicity differentiates patients with toxic megacolon from those with colonic dilatation due to other processes.

In confirmed IBD, aggressive medical therapy for a period of 5–7 days can be continued if clinically stable and no deterioration is appreciated. This must be pursued cautiously, ideally with collaborative decision-making by gastroenterologists and surgeons. However, toxic megacolon is a late sign, and surgery should be aggressively pursued in the face of deterioration or a lack of measurable improvement within 24–72 hours given the devastating consequences of colonic perforation: mortality rates leap as high as 20% in cases of colonic perforation in comparison to 4% without.[28]

Aggressive resuscitation and correction of electrolyte derangements should be pursued with the goal of reversing physiological defects and the toxic state. Patients should be closely monitored with serial examinations and resuscitated in a critical/intensive care unit. Serial abdominal X-rays can track the progression of colonic distension, though the diameter of the colon is not as important as the patient's overall clinical picture. Abdominal and pelvic CT may help determine aetiology and evaluate for pneumatosis, subclinical perforation and abscesses. Medications that slow colonic motility and function must be avoided. For significant gastrointestinal bleeding and anaemia, transfusion may be necessary.

Treatment of severe/fulminant colitis secondary to IBD includes the initiation of high-dose IV corticosteroids (methylprednisolone dose equivalent of 40–60 mg/day). Upwards of 20–40% will fail to respond and treatment beyond 7 days adds no benefit in those without a response. Increased rates of colonic perforation have not been documented with high-dose steroids. In hospitalised adult patients with acute severe ulcerative colitis refractory to 3–5 days of IV corticosteroids, the use of either infliximab or cyclosporine has been shown to decrease rates of colectomy within 90 days of hospitalisation. Over a median follow-up of 4.5 years, 1- and 5- year colectomy-free survival rates were 70.9% and 61.5% in patients treated with cyclosporine, and 69.1% and 65.1%, respectively, in patients randomised to infliximab.[29] Empiric broad-spectrum antibiotics, often routinely administered, have not shown benefit in those lacking infection.

Patients presenting with toxic megacolon without a history of IBD should be empirically treated for *C. difficile* colitis until proven otherwise. *C. difficile* colitis has been associated with an increasing prevalence (3%) of toxic megacolon since 2000, which is attributable to a more virulent strain (BI/NAP1/027) with less responsiveness to standard therapies and higher rates of relapse. These patients are more likely to present with an ileus, and therapy should not be delayed since failure to make an early diagnosis will result in worse outcomes.

Limited lower endoscopy with minimal air insufflation by an experienced endoscopist may be helpful in obtaining biopsies, evaluating for pseudomembranes, and therapeutically decompressing the colon. Pseudomembranes are seen in nearly 90% of patients with *C. difficile* colitis (Fig. 16.10), though rectosigmoid sparing is present in up to 20–30%.

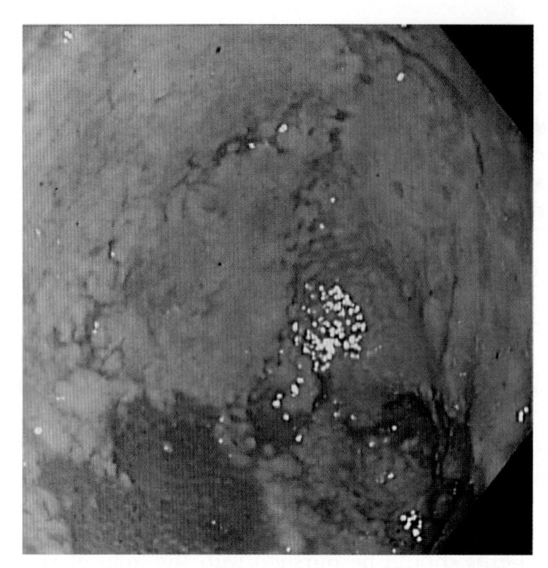

Figure 16.10 *Clostridium difficile* colitis – pseudomembranous colitis.

Continuously diseased mucosa with deep ulcerations and extensive mucosal pseudopolyps may indicate severe ulcerative colitis, whereas intervening normal mucosa, rake ulcers and aphthous ulcers are more suggestive of Crohn's disease.

Indications for ES include diffuse peritonitis, pneumoperitoneum, uncontrolled sepsis and major haemorrhage. Urgent surgery is pursued in those with increasing abdominal pain and/or colonic distension, progressive physiological deterioration, a lack of objective improvement within 24–72 hours and sustained transfusion requirements. Early surgical intervention should be pursued for patients who are immunocompromised, severely debilitated, malnourished or have multiple comorbidities.

Treatment for severe complicated *C. difficile* colitis (WBC $> 15 \times 10^6$/L, Cr > 1.5 mg/dL, hypotension, shock, ileus, megacolon) includes 10 days of vancomycin 500 mg by mouth every 6 hours and metronidazole 500 mg by mouth or IV every 8 hours. For those unable to tolerate oral intake, medications can be administered through a nasogastric tube. Fidaxomicin has not been proven to be more beneficial than vancomycin in cases of complicated *C. difficile* colitis. Patients with an ileus may have vancomycin introduced through a retention enema (500 mg/100 mL normal saline) every 6 hours, or directly instilled colonoscopically since adequate intracolonic concentrations of vancomycin may not be achieved with oral administration.

Other treatments are currently being studied for individuals with *C. difficile* infection, including new agents such as ridinilazole, a nonabsorbable small-molecule antibiotic, immune treatments, live biotherapeutics/probiotics, and treatment with bacteriophages with activity against specific *C. difficile* strains. Of these, only the antitoxin B monoclonal antibody bezlotoxumab has been shown to reduce the risk of recurrent *C. difficile* infection by approximately 40% when prescribed during an initial episode, although the high cost has limited its availability for most patients.[30]

Refractory *C. difficile* infection can be treated with faecal microbiota transplantation. Small studies have shown benefit in treating patients with acute colitis and toxic megacolon with an efficacy rate of > 90%. There is no clear consensus regarding the most appropriate method of delivery (upper endoscopy, nasoenteric tube, colonoscopically, enema), preparation, donated volume, or volume instilled. Some advocate faecal transplant if no improvement with aggressive pharmacotherapy is noted within 48 hours, and more than one transplant may be required to obtain maximal benefit.[31]

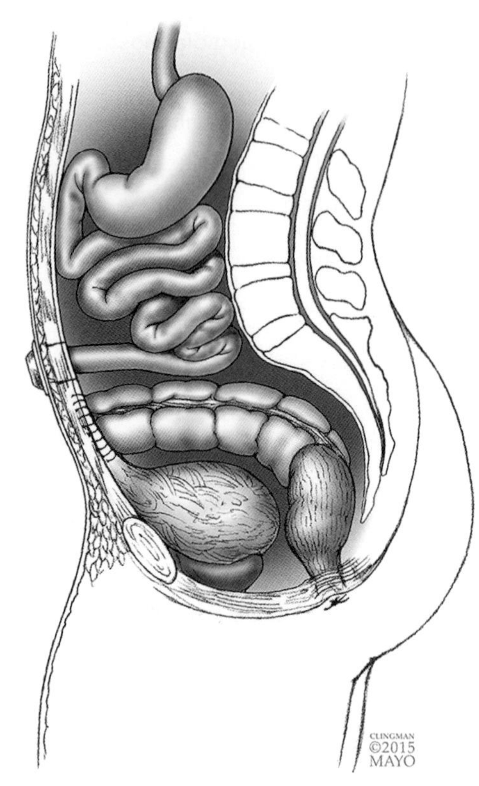

Figure 16.11 End ileostomy with subcutaneously extracorporealised rectosigmoid stump. (Used with permission of Mayo Foundation for Medical Education and Research, all rights reserved.)

Management of toxic megacolon associated with colitides other than *C. difficile* or IBD should follow the same general principles while focusing treatment on the underlying aetiology.

The surgical approach for toxic megacolon, whether performed as an emergency or urgently, most commonly involves an open total or subtotal colectomy with creation of a Brooke ileostomy with preservation of the rectum for a potential future restoration of intestinal continuity. If the rectosigmoid stump is too friable or oedematous to close a sigmoid, mucous fistula or subcutaneously exteriorised proximal rectosigmoid stump is an option (Fig. 16.11). Laparoscopic-assisted approaches are feasible and not a contraindication in the hands of a skilled laparoscopic surgeon. A proctocolectomy with end Brooke ileostomy is very rarely performed and typically only in cases of life-threatening rectal haemorrhage, severe disease preventing creation of a Hartmann's pouch or mucous fistula, rectal perforation, or when re-establishment of continuity or a restorative procedure will not be considered in the future. Re-establishment of intestinal continuity (ileocolonic/rectal anastomosis) or a restorative procedure (ileal pouch anal anastomosis) is not recommended at the time of resection in these patients, as the combination of severe systemic illness, impaired nutrition and high-dose immunosuppression makes anastomotic failure highly likely. Reconstructive options should be deferred until the patient has recovered from colectomy (at least 3 months).

Patients with severe complicated *C. difficile* colitis can be treated with creation of a diverting loop ileostomy followed by colonic lavage with PEG, vancomycin and metronidazole, though robust literature is lacking for this procedure. The initial description by Neal et al.[32] demonstrated lower mortality (19% vs 50%) and higher rates of colonic preservation (39 of 42 patients). A multi-institutional trial comprising 10 centres in the United States operated on 98 patients with *C. difficile* colitis and noted a lower adjusted mortality in the diverting loop ileostomy group (17% vs 39%) and concluded that in patients without contraindications, a loop ileostomy should be considered for the management of *C. difficile* colitis.[33] A more recent study using a National Inpatient Sample database across the United States evaluated trends in diverting loop ileostomy versus total abdominal colectomy as surgical management for *C. difficile* colitis. Of 3021 adult patients who underwent surgery for *C. difficile* colitis, 2408 were subtotal colectomies and 613 loop ileostomies. The annual proportion of patients undergoing only diversion increased from 11% in 2011 to 25% in 2015. Significantly more loop ileostomies were performed within the first day of hospitalisation, in contrast to subtotal colectomies (23% vs 12%). There was no significant difference in in-hospital mortality rates between the two groups (26% vs 31%). Loop ileostomy may represent a viable surgical alternative to total abdominal colectomy, although the grounds for selection of treatment need to be clarified.[34]

NEUTROPENIC ENTEROCOLITIS

Neutropenic enterocolitis, also known as typhlitis, is associated with inflammation and thickening of any portion of the intestine, though most commonly the caecum and terminal ileum. The pathophysiology is unclear and typically seen in patients receiving chemotherapy for neoplastic diseases, but also documented in transplant recipients and those with aplastic anaemia.

Patients present with abdominal pain, diarrhoea with or without haematochezia, nausea, emesis and pyrexia. Neutropenia is a common finding and often resolves as the patient improves. CT is the imaging modality of choice. Most can be treated non-operatively with IV fluids, bowel rest and broad-spectrum antibiotics. ES is pursued for perforation and peritonitis and urgent surgery for a lack of improvement with supportive measures.

PERFORATION

COMPLICATED COLONIC DIVERTICULITIS

Complicated colonic diverticular disease affects 20–25% of those diagnosed with diverticulitis and is associated with abscess formation (15%), stricture (10%), fistulas (<5%) and perforation (1.5%).[35] ES is rarely indicated for stenosis/partial obstruction or fistula, unlike complete obstruction and perforation. Diverticulitis associated with abscess formation (Hinchey I and II) is commonly managed conservatively with bowel rest, broad-spectrum antibiotics and interventional-guided percutaneous drainage. Purulent (Hinchey III) and faeculent (Hinchey IV) peritonitis usually requires urgent/emergency surgical intervention.

Patients with Hinchey III and IV diverticulitis present with systemic signs of sepsis, focal or generalised peritonitis, nausea, pyrexia, rebound tenderness and guarding. Some with purulent peritonitis improve with supportive measures and can be managed non-operatively. CT is the imaging modality of choice. Initial management includes resuscitation and administration of broad-spectrum antibiotics covering anaerobic and Gram-negative bacteria. Careful clinical observation is required in these patients: some improve markedly in the first 24 hours, but any sign of systemic deterioration requires prompt surgical intervention.

After evacuation of faecal matter and/or purulence, the abdomen is irrigated with 6–10 L of warm saline solution. Although of unproven benefit, antibiotic irrigation (gentamicin, polymyxin, etc.) has not been shown to be harmful. Following resection of the diseased sigmoid colon, Hartmann's procedure or primary anastomosis, with or without diversion, may be pursued. Most presenting with Hinchey IV disease undergo a Hartmann's procedure, which removes the septic focus, but future re-establishment of intestinal continuity necessitates a second major operation with resultant morbidity and mortality. Up to 30% of patients never have their end colostomy reversed.[36] In the appropriate population, a primary anastomosis with or without diversion may be pursued. Relative contraindications to creating a primary anastomosis include haemodynamic instability, vascular compromise, severe protein calorie malnutrition, anaemia, bowel oedema, connective tissue disorders and immunosuppression. Primary diversion with a loop ileostomy or colostomy is inadvisable as it leaves the source of sepsis *in situ*.

Touting low morbidity and mortality, small series have proposed laparoscopic lavage as an alternative to resection in selected patients with purulent peritonitis, though a large number of those studies included patients with Hinchey II disease. The studies are heterogeneous, describing different volumes of irrigation, solutions and placement of drains. In order to help define the utility of laparoscopic lavage, large randomised controlled trials have been conducted recently. The Ladies trial was a multicentre (Belgium, Italy, Netherlands) study composed of two arms (LOLA and DIVA) that terminated at 33% of the planned sample size secondary to increased morbidity and mortality in the lavage group. The LaparOscopic LAvage (LOLA) arm compared lavage to Hartmann's procedure and sigmoidectomy with primary anastomosis with or without protective diversion in a 2:1:1 randomisation. Out of 90 patients, 47 were randomised to the lavage group, 21 to a Hartmann's procedure and 22 underwent primary anastomosis. The trial found that lavage was not superior to sigmoidectomy for perforated purulent diverticulitis at 12 months.[37] The DIVerticulitis arm (DIVA) compared sigmoidectomy with or without anastomosis, though the results are still pending. The multicentre DIverticulitis LAparoscopic LAvage (DILALA) trial compared laparoscopic lavage to Hartmann's procedure for Hinchey III diverticulitis and randomised 43 patients to lavage and 40 to the Hartmann's arm. They concluded laparoscopic lavage is a better option for perforated diverticulitis with purulent peritonitis than open resection with colostomy. Two-year data noted that patients in the lavage arm had a 45% reduced risk of undergoing one or more operations within 24 months and had fewer operations than the Hartmann's group. There was no difference in mortality or re-admissions between the two groups. Three patients in the lavage arm and nine in the Hartmann's group had a colostomy at 24 months.[38] Five-year results from the multicentre (Sweden and Norway) randomised Scandinavian Diverticulitis (SCANDIV) trial comparing lavage to Hartmann's procedure found no differences in severe complications or overall mortality. There were more unplanned re-admissions and operations in the lavage group. Recurrence of diverticulitis after laparoscopic lavage was more common (21% vs 4%), often leading to sigmoid resection (30% in the lavage group).[39] The randomised controlled Laparoscopic Lavage for Acute Non-Faeculant Diverticulitis (LapLAND) trial (NCT01019239) from St Vincent's University Hospital, Ireland, concluded in December 2015, and the results are still pending. The French multicentre study (SIGMOIDITE Trial) comparing surgical resection and conservative treatment of purulent peritonitis that originates from diverticulitis concluded in 2017, and the results are still pending (NCT01837342).

✔✔ The DIverticulitis LAparoscopic LAvage (DILALA) and the Scandinavian Diverticulitis (SCANDIV) randomised controlled trials have both demonstrated no difference in severe complication or quality of life, making laparoscopic lavage a feasible option in perforated purulent diverticulitis. Recurrence of diverticulitis after laparoscopic lavage is higher, often leading to sigmoid resection, but without stoma creation, which is usually the case in an emergency setting. Laparoscopic lavage may be used as a bridge to overcome the emergency septic state and lead to an elective sigmoid resection.[38,39]

STERCORAL

Hard inspissated stool (stercus) impacted in the rectum or rectosigmoid region can result in ischaemic necrosis, ulceration and perforation. The true incidence of stercoral perforation is unknown with only around 100 cases reported in the literature. The median age of presentation has been noted to be 60 with an equally reported incidence in men and women. Secondary to increased age, debility and co-morbidities, stercoral perforation is associated with mortality rates close to 50%. Factors noted to be associated with stercoral ulceration and perforation include chronic constipation, debility, megacolon, scleroderma, hypercalcaemia, renal failure and renal transplantation. Medications associated with stercoral perforation include opioids/narcotics, antacids, calcium channel blockers and antidepressants. Maurer and colleagues from the University of Berne, Switzerland, noted that the incidence of stercoral perforation of the colon is likely underestimated secondary to a lack of defined diagnostic criteria.[40] As a result, they proposed the criteria should include: (1) round or ovoid colonic antimesenteric perforation exceeding 1 cm in diameter; (2) faecalomas present within the colon and protruding through the perforation site or lying within the abdominal cavity; (3) microscopic evidence of pressure necrosis or ulcer and chronic inflammatory reaction around the perforation site; and (4) exclusion of other pathological causes of perforation.

Presenting symptoms may include marked abdominal distension, discomfort, peritonitis, nausea, emesis and obstipation. Aggressive resuscitation and correction of electrolyte derangements is carried out in preparation for surgery. Radiological imaging is non-specific and rarely identifies stercoral perforation. Serpell and Nicholls from St Thomas' Hospital, London, UK, noted only 11% were correctly diagnosed prior to surgery.

Management of patients with stercoral perforation is surgical and the diseased segment must be resected. At the time of surgery, multiple ulcers and perforations may be encountered and the entire colon is often filled with inspissated stool. The decision to proceed with resection and stoma versus resection and anastomosis is for the discretion of the surgeon.

COLONOSCOPIC

Perforation during colonoscopy is a rare event occurring in less than 1/1000 procedures with rates in large studies noted to be between 0.012% and 0.016%.[41] Higher rates are associated with biopsy, polypectomy and diseased colons (IBD, diverticular). Mechanisms thought to result in perforation include: (1) mechanical as a result of direct trauma from the scope; (2) barotrauma; and (3) procedural-related (biopsies, polypectomies, use of energy, dilatation, placement of endoluminal stents, etc.). The most common site of perforation is the sigmoid colon, likely secondary to its narrow and tortuous nature. The ascending colon and caecum are most susceptible to barotrauma.

Symptoms include marked abdominal distension, discomfort, peritonitis, nausea, emesis, diarrhoea and constipation. The diagnosis of perforation is not always obvious at the time of colonoscopy and upwards of 50% have delayed presentation.

Initial management includes bowel rest, resuscitation and correction of laboratory abnormalities. Nasogastric tubes do not decompress the colon and are not necessary unless the patient is experiencing nausea/emesis. Flat and upright abdominal radiographs will identify free air. CT with contrast or a water-soluble enema can be used to confirm the diagnosis.

Management depends on both the procedure performed and presentation of the patient. If clinically stable, non-operative management with bowel rest, resuscitation and broad-spectrum IV antibiotics can be pursued. Peritonitis, deterioration or a lack of measurable improvement necessitates surgery or procedural intervention. Placement of endoclips to manage perforations is showing promise in small studies. Trecca et al.[42] presented their own experience in addition to reviewing the literature and found in 78 reported cases, clips were successful in controlling perforations 69–93% of the time. Large defects and peritoneal contamination will require operative intervention whether open or laparoscopic. Depending on the initial colonoscopic procedure performed, segmental resection and anastomosis, primary repair of the colonic defect and resection and creation of a stoma are all options.

Trecca et al.[42] review of the literature and personal experience noted in 78 cases colonoscopically placed endoclips were successful in controlling perforations in 69–93% of cases.

ANASTOMOTIC LEAK/DEHISCENCE

Rates of colonic anastomotic leaks following resection depend on the reporting criteria utilised and have been documented to be as high as 20%, especially for very low anastomoses. Bruce and colleagues from the University of Aberdeen, UK, reviewed 97 anastomotic leak studies and noted 56 different definitions for what constituted a leak. Multiple patient and procedural factors are associated with increased risk of anastomotic leaks (Table 16.4). Mortality rates ranging from 10% to 22% have been documented in association with leaks. Morbidity (long hospitalisation, multiple interventional procedures, wounds, hernias, additional surgical procedures, infection, bowel obstructions, stoma issues, impaired bowel function, DVT/PE, etc.) is significantly increased. Time of diagnosis probably reflects how avidly the complication is sought by the surgeon. Leaks are usually diagnosed during the same in-patient admission but have also been documented beyond 30 days. Patients with an early leak (within 1 week of surgery) often present with relatively subtle signs of sepsis; frank peritonitis is uncommon.

Prompt diagnosis and treatment are imperative to decrease the sequelae of sepsis and prevent mortality. Peritonitis and haemodynamic instability necessitate operative intervention and few, if any, imaging studies are necessary in this population. The difficulty lies in patients presenting with vague (poor appetite, generally not feeling well, etc.) and minimal symptoms, and few clinical signs. There is no one pathognomonic testing modality for identifying an anastomotic leak. As shown by Erb, Hyman and Osler at the University of Vermont,[43] just as many patients without leaks, as those with, experience postoperative tachycardia, tachypnoea, leucocytosis, hypotension and pyrexia. CT and contrast studies are the imaging modalities of choice, although radiological findings can be equivocal and falsely negative, thus necessitating a high index of suspicion. Flat and upright abdominal films can reveal gas under the diaphragm but are of debatable significance in the immediate postoperative period. Localised extraluminal pockets of free air can be seen on CT up to 26 days after surgery, and frank free air up to 9 days. Only air associated with a loculated fluid collection has been shown to be more prevalent in those with an anastomotic leak. Equally, the absence of pneumoperitoneum should not discourage one from pursuing further investigations to evaluate the integrity of the anastomosis.

In addition to the timing of presentation, management also depends on patient and anastomotic factors. Leaks later than 7–10 days make surgical intervention more difficult and indicate higher risk secondary to the desmoplastic peritoneal reaction. For those presenting with peritonitis and haemodynamic instability, aggressive resuscitation and correction of laboratory derangements is pursued while planning for ES.

Peritonitis, deteriorating sepsis or a lack of measurable improvement necessitates surgical intervention. The peritoneal cavity is thoroughly lavaged followed by evaluation of the anastomotic defect, tissue integrity and surrounding structures. Historically, the treatment of choice was resection with creation of a stoma and possibly mucous fistula, and is still a safe option. The reader should take careful note of comments in Chapter 20 regarding ill-advised attempts to repair anastomotic leaks in the presence of sepsis as a leading cause of complex intra-abdominal sepsis and intestinal fistulation.

In clinically stable patients, it is possible to salvage anastomotic leaks by non-operative means with good outcome. Highly selected patients with small contained leaks, whether proximally diverted or not, can be treated conservatively with close observation, bowel rest, parenteral nutrition, broad-spectrum antibiotics and percutaneous interventional-guided procedures. Future restoration of intestinal continuity is difficult for distal leaks and a diverting loop stoma and (transanal) drainage of the area can preserve anastomotic continuity for small leaks.

Other modalities described in the literature for treating low anastomotic leaks include endoscopic (clip, covered stent) and vacuum-assisted devices, though to date these lack robust supporting evidence.

Table 16.4 Risk factors for anastomotic leak

Operative factors
Blood loss
Poor surgical technique
Anastomotic tension
Anastomotic blood supply
Length of surgery
Preoperative mechanical bowel preparation
Left colon/Low anastomosis
Failure to intraoperatively leak test left/low anastomoses
Patient factors
Immunocompromised
Diabetes
Protein calorie malnutrition
Anaemia
Tobacco use
Chronic obstruction pulmonary disease
Obesity
Male
Alcohol abuse
Prior radiation
Emergency surgery
Disease (connective tissue disorders, inflammatory bowel disease, diverticular)
Prior abdominal surgery

HAEMORRHAGE

The colon accounts for approximately 20% of all cases of acute gastrointestinal haemorrhage. Sources, in decreasing frequency, include diverticular disease, neoplastic/polyp, IBD, ischaemic, angioectasias, post polypectomy and post-surgery. The elderly are more commonly affected. For the majority, bleeding stops spontaneously and ES is rarely required. Urgent investigation and control is necessary for unremitting bleeding. Higher rates of bleeding are associated with diverticular disease and vascular ectasias.

Management of colonic haemorrhage depends on the source and includes medical, endoscopic, angiographic and surgical approaches. Depending on the patient's haemodynamic status colonoscopy, radionuclide imaging, selective mesenteric angiography and CT angiography (CTA) can all be utilised to identify the source of bleeding. Selective angiography and colonoscopy have the advantage of being both diagnostic and therapeutic.

Once an upper gastrointestinal source is excluded, colonoscopy may be pursued if the patient is haemodynamically stable. Studies have documented high caecal intubation rates and diagnostic accuracy for emergency colonoscopies performed without bowel preparation, though most describe finding sources associated with lower rates of bleeding (ischaemia, IBD, neoplastic/polyp) that did not require intervention.[44] For haemodynamically stable patients, mechanical bowel preparation should be administered to enhance visualisation of mucosal abnormalities. Treatment of localised sources of bleeding (diverticular, angiodysplastic, polyp) includes injection with epinephrine, coagulation, placement of an endoclip and polypectomy. India ink tattoo should be placed at the site of bleeding to help localise the site in the event repeat endoscopic procedures are required. Risks of sedation and perforation must be taken into consideration when pursuing colonoscopy.

For those who cannot tolerate an endoscopic procedure, or colonoscopic localisation was not possible, imaging modalities are pursued. Radionucleotide imaging with the patient's own red blood cells labelled with technetium-99m (^{99m}Tc-RBC) can identify rates of bleeding as low as 0.1 mL/min. Technetium-99m remains active for up to 48 hours and re-imaging can be pursued for intermittent or recurrent bleeding. A negative scan provides evidence there is no active bleeding, and a blush is indicative of bleeding. Disadvantages to ^{99m}Tc-RBC scanning include the time required to perform the test (several hours), high false localisation rate (25%) and inability to identify the source (25–60%). Patients with haemodynamic instability are not good candidates for radionucleotide imaging.

CTA has largely supplanted ^{99m}Tc-RBC scanning by providing the benefit of fast image acquisition, re-formatted three-dimensional vascular reconstruction, localisation of the site of bleeding and higher resolution imaging. CTA can detect bleeding as low as 0.3 mL/min and when active bleeding is present can localise the region 91–92% of the time.[45] Patients with haemodynamic instability, renal insufficiency and allergy to contrast dye are not candidates for the test.

Selective mesenteric angiography can detect bleeding rates as low as 0.5 mL/min. Unless imaging has already localised the bleeding to a particular region, the superior mesenteric artery is typically visualised first followed by the inferior mesenteric artery. CTA is commonly performed prior to mesenteric angiography. When mesenteric angiography is performed < 150 minutes following a positive CTA, the likelihood of identifying an active source of bleeding is 2.89 times higher,[46] and if within 90 minutes, 8.56 times higher.[47] As shown by Jacovides and colleagues from the University of Pennsylvania, with the precise localisation on CTA, the cumulative contrast load with mesenteric angiography and CTA is no different than mesenteric angiography following ^{99m}Tc-RBC scanning. Sensitivity for identifying a bleeding source ranges from 40% to 95%. For intermittent presentations, provocative measures (administration of heparin, vasodilators, thrombolytics or a combination) utilised to induce bleeding to help identify the source have been described in small studies, with diagnostic yields ranging from 29% to 38%. Caution must be taken secondary to the risks of intracranial and uncontrolled haemorrhage. When bleeding is identified, transcatheter therapeutic intervention is pursued. Superselective embolisation of small vessels through microcatheters with microcoils, gelfoam or polyvinyl alcohol is now the preferred procedure. Cessation of active arterial bleeding is as high as 50–75%, with re-bleeding rates of only 22–24%.[48] Embolisation of larger vessels is no longer performed secondary to high rates of transmural ischaemia, perforation and stricture formation. Risks of mesenteric angiography include vascular injury, thromboembolic events, contrast-induced renal insufficiency/failure and pseudoaneurysm formation.

✔ Two retrospective studies evaluating the timing of selective mesenteric angiography following a positive CT angiography revealed an increase in the probability of detecting the source of bleeding, with a 2.89 times higher likelihood if performed within 150 minutes and 8.56 times higher if performed within 90 minutes.[46,47]

Indications for emergency/urgent surgery include transfusion requirements greater than 6 units during resuscitation, ongoing or recurrent haemorrhage unresponsive to non-operative approaches, and persistent haemodynamic instability. An increase in mortality is directly correlated with the units of blood transfused. It has been documented that those requiring more than 10 units of blood experience mortality as high as 27% versus 7% for those requiring less than 10 units. Transfusion of ≥ 4 units of packed RBCs in the first 24 hours of resuscitation is associated with a 50% operative rate. Every effort should be made to localise the source of bleeding prior to proceeding to the operating room. Segmental resection of a localised area of bleeding carries a mortality rate less than 10% versus 10–30% for a total abdominal colectomy. If the source of bleeding cannot be localised, a thorough exploratory evaluation of the entire intestine is performed. On-table intestinal endoscopy by an experienced endoscopist can be utilised to help localise the source. If unable to localise, a total abdominal colectomy is performed when small intestinal sources have been excluded. An ileosigmoid or ileorectal anastomosis, with or without protective diversion, may be considered in haemodynamically stable patients.

ISCHAEMIA

Colon ischaemia, also known as ischaemic colitis, results from reduced colonic perfusion and is the most common type of mesenteric ischaemia. There are multiple causes (Table 16.5). Ischaemia occurs secondary to a lack of sufficient flow to maintain colonocyte metabolic activity, which results in hypoxia. The most common causes are non-occlusive disease, arterial embolic or thrombotic occlusion, and mesenteric vein thrombosis. The superior and inferior mesenteric arteries supply the colon through certain regions, referred to as watershed areas, which receive only collateral circulation. These low-flow vulnerable areas include the caecum, splenic flexure (Griffiths point) and the rectosigmoid region (Sudeck's point). The most common

Table 16.5 Causes of colon ischaemia

Physiological
Hypotension
Hypovolaemic
Haemorrhage
Cardiovascular
Heart failure
Atherosclerosis
Hypercoagulable
Factor V Leiden
Protein C and S deficiency
Prothrombin G2010A mutation
Antiphospholipid syndrome (Lupus anticoagulant)
Antithrombin III deficiency
Polycythaemia vera
Disseminated intravascular coagulation (DIC)
Heparin-induced thrombocytopenia and thrombosis (HITT)
Tobacco (acquired)
Drugs
Vasopressors
Oral contraceptives
Cocaine
Diuretics
Antiarrhythmics
Antihypertensives
Surgery/procedural
Cardiac
Aortic
Autoimmune disease
Systemic lupus erythematosus
Other
Haemodialysis
Embolic/thrombotic
Long distance running
Trauma (blunt or penetrating)
Connective tissue disorders
Mechanical bowel obstruction

area of inconsistent collateral circulation is Griffiths point. Although all areas of the colon can be affected by non-occlusive disease, the watershed areas are the most prominent. Arterial embolic or thrombotic occlusion and mesenteric vein thrombosis more commonly affect the proximal colon. Colon ischaemia predominantly affects those over 65 years of age, is more common in women, and is estimated to be responsible for 16 out of every 100 000 hospital admissions.[49] Most cases will not require surgical intervention. ES is associated with a mortality rate as high as 50%, and highest for right-sided ischaemia. Baseline mortality ranges from 4% to 12%. Mortality in renal transplant recipients has been documented as high as 70%.

Signs and symptoms are often non-specific, depend on the duration and extent of ischaemia, and can include abdominal pain, distension, haematochezia, an urgent desire to defaecate, nausea, emesis, pyrexia, diarrhoea, constipation, renal failure and sepsis. Any patient presenting with abdominal pain and bloody diarrhoea should be evaluated for colonic ischaemia. Markers of ischaemia such as acidosis and elevated lactate, lactate dehydrogenase, amylase and alkaline phosphatase are often absent until late in the course of severe disease. CT is the imaging modality of choice and will reveal segmental bowel wall thickening and mesocolic

Table 16.6 Endoscopic colon ischaemia findings

Mild ischaemic colitis
Pale-appearing mucosa
Mucosal oedema
Petechial haemorrhages
Ulcerations
Moderate ischaemic colitis
Dusky-appearing mucosa
Submucosal haemorrhage
Haemorrhagic ulcerations
Severe ischaemic colitis
Frank necrosis
Circumferential involvement

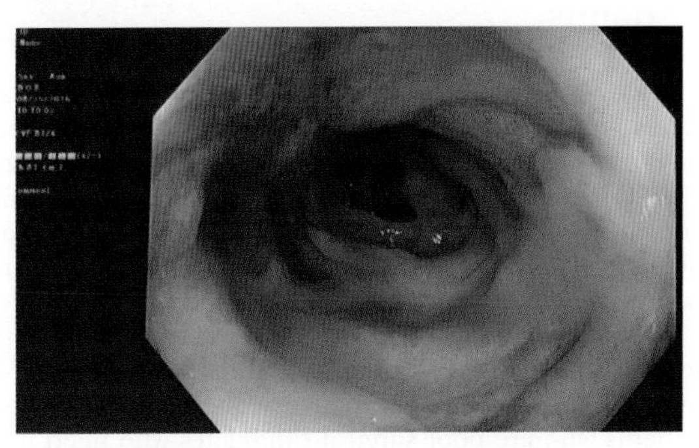

Figure 16.12 Colonic ischaemia.

oedema and stranding. Pneumatosis and portal venous gas suggests transmural ischaemia or infarction and mandates urgent surgical intervention.[50] Since the vast majority of colon ischaemia is secondary to non-occlusive disease (95%), vascular imaging studies are typically not necessary unless acute mesenteric ischaemia is suspected, such as pain out of proportion on examination with a lack of haematochezia. Diagnosis with flexible endoscopy is the gold standard and allows for direct visualisation of the ischaemic segment, which can range from submucosal oedema to full-thickness necrosis (Table 16.6), and the ability to obtain biopsies (Fig. 16.12). To decrease the risk of perforation, endoscopy is typically preformed with minimal air insufflation, in an unprepped bowel, and not advanced proximal to the area of ischaemia. Biopsies of gangrenous areas are avoided. A single inflammatory band of erythema with erosion along the lateral axis of the colon, referred to as the 'single-stripe sign', is highly specific for colon ischaemia. Abdominal X-rays and barium enemas can reveal thumb-printing, a sign of submucosal oedema, though it is non-specific and can be found in multiple inflammatory and infectious colitides.

✔✔ A meta-analysis of three prospective and three retrospective studies revealed that contrast-enhanced multidetector CT correctly identifies the diagnosis of primary acute mesenteric ischaemia with high pooled sensitivity (93.3%) and specificity (95.9%), thus supporting its use as a first-line imaging modality.[50]

Once the diagnosis of colon ischaemia is made, a cause is sought and appropriately treated. Mild disease is noted to be segmental, not isolated to the right colon, and lacking poor prognostic factors observed in moderate disease. Moderate disease includes any three of the following: tachycardia, abdominal pain without rectal bleeding, hypotension, male sex, blood urea nitrogen level greater than 20 mg/dL, serum sodium less than 136 mEq/L, white blood cell count greater than 15×10^9/L, haemoglobin less than 12 g/dL or colonoscopically identified ulceration. Severe disease is defined as more than three of the moderate disease criteria or peritoneal signs, pneumatosis or portal venous gas with CT imaging, gangrene on colonoscopy, and pancolonic or isolated right colon ischaemia on CT or endoscopy. For those presenting with full-thickness necrosis and gangrene, peritonitis, pneumoperitoneum and haemodynamic instability, surgery is immediately pursued. Mild and moderate colon ischaemia is treated supportively with bowel rest, resuscitation, correction of laboratory abnormalities and treatment of the underlying cause of ischaemia. Over 80% respond and avoid surgical intervention. Administration of broad-spectrum empiric antibiotics to decrease the sequel of bacterial translocation may be entertained despite a lack of robust data to support doing so. Nasogastric tubes do not decompress the colon and are not necessary unless the patient is experiencing nausea/emesis. Peritonitis, deterioration or a lack of measurable improvement necessitates surgery intervention.

During surgery, any portion of the colon affected by ischaemia, necrosis and perforation is widely resected and an ileostomy or colostomy created. Taking into consideration the risk of progression of ischaemia, physiological derangements that led to surgery, and tenuous blood flow, a primary anastomosis is not advised. Extensive or patchy involvement can be treated with a temporary abdominal closure and second-look laparotomy to determine the need for further resection.

Key points

- The most common causes of colonic obstruction are neoplasia, diverticulitis and volvulus. Treatment for obstruction is dependent on the location, cause, patient presentation and goals of care.
- The European Society of Gastrointestinal Endoscopy (ESGE) currently recommends self-expanding metal stents for patients with clinical symptoms and radiological signs of malignant large-bowel obstruction without signs of perforation, as a bridge to surgery, with a time interval of 2 weeks until resection, in patients with potentially curable left-sided obstructing colon cancer as an alternative to emergency resection, for patients who are poor surgical candidates who need medical optimisation, and as the preferred treatment for palliation of malignant colonic obstruction.
- CT has become the imaging modality of choice for volvulus. In addition to a dilated loop of colon, a characteristic 'whirl sign', whereby the mesentery twists around the vasculature, is typically seen. Detorsion alone results in recurrence in the majority of cases. Colonic resection should preferably be pursued during the same hospitalisation.
- Acute colonic pseudo-obstruction requires non-operative supportive care (bowel rest, resuscitation, correction of electrolyte abnormalities) and is pursued in the absence of perforation or suspected ischaemia. The use of neostigmine may be considered in selected patients as first-line therapy. Endoscopic decompression can help ease the discomfort of severe colonic distension. When all non-operative measures have failed to resolve acute colonic pseudo-obstruction, surgical intervention may be considered. However, the inordinately high risk secondary to underlying frailty and comorbidities in this patient population precludes pursuing surgery for most.
- Toxic colitis is characterised by acute colitis, ≥ 6 cm non-obstructive segmental or complete dilatation of the colon and signs of systemic toxicity, and is most commonly associated with inflammatory bowel disease and pseudomembranous (*Clostridium difficile*) colitis. Early surgical intervention should be pursued for patients who are immunocompromised, severely debilitated, malnourished or have multiple comorbidities. Urgent surgery is pursued in those with increasing abdominal pain and/or colonic distension, progressive physiological deterioration, a lack of objective improvement within 24–72 hours and sustained transfusion requirements. Indications for emergency surgery include diffuse peritonitis, pneumoperitoneum, uncontrolled sepsis and major haemorrhage.
- Diverticulitis associated with abscess formation (Hinchey I and II) is commonly managed conservatively with bowel rest, broad-spectrum antibiotics and interventional-guided percutaneous drainage. Purulent (Hinchey III) and faeculent (Hinchey IV) peritonitis usually requires urgent/emergency surgical intervention.
- Management of colonoscopic perforation depends on both the procedure performed and presentation of the patient. If clinically stable, non-operative management with bowel rest, resuscitation and broad-spectrum IV antibiotics can be pursued. Peritonitis, deterioration or a lack of measurable improvement necessitates surgery or procedural intervention.
- In clinically stable patients, it is possible to salvage anastomotic leaks by non-operative means with good outcome. Highly selected patients with small contained leaks, whether diverted or not, can be treated conservatively with close observation, bowel rest, parenteral nutrition, broad-spectrum antibiotics and percutaneous interventional-guided procedures. Peritonitis, deteriorating sepsis or a lack of measurable improvement necessitates surgical intervention.
- CT angiography (CTA) has largely supplanted ^{99m}Tc-RBC scanning by providing the benefit of fast image acquisition, reformatted three-dimensional vascular reconstruction, better localisation of the site of bleeding, and higher resolution imaging. CTA can detect bleeding as low as 0.3 mL/min and when active bleeding is present can localise the region 91–92% of the time.
- Mesenteric angiography with superselective embolisation of small vessels through microcatheters with microcoils, gelfoam or polyvinyl alcohol will result in cessation of active arterial bleeding 50–100% of the time, with re-bleeding rates of only 22–24%. Indications for emergency/urgent surgery include transfusion requirements greater than 6 units during resuscitation, ongoing or recurrent haemorrhage unresponsive to non-operative approaches, and persistent haemodynamic instability.
- In acute colonic ischaemia, computed tomography is the imaging modality of choice and will reveal segmental bowel wall thickening and mesocolic oedema and stranding. Pneumatosis and portal venous gas suggest transmural ischaemia or infarction and mandate urgent surgical intervention. Diagnosis with flexible endoscopy is the gold standard and allows for direct visualisation of the ischaemic segment and the ability to obtain biopsies.
- Mild and moderate colon ischaemia is treated supportively with bowel rest, resuscitation, correction of laboratory abnormalities and treatment of the underlying cause of ischaemia, and over 80% respond and avoid surgical intervention.

References available at http://ebooks.health.elsevier.com/

KEY REFERENCES

[9] Arezzo A, Passera R, Lo Secco G, Verra M, Bonino MA, Targarona E, et al. Stent as bridge to surgery for left-sided malignant colonic obstruction reduces adverse events and stoma rate compared with emergency surgery: results of a systematic review and meta-analysis of randomized controlled trials. Gastrointest Endosc 2017;86(3):416–26. PMID: 28392363.

A systematic review and meta-analysis of eight RCTs demonstrated that SEMS as a bridge to surgery, compared with emergency surgery (ES) had lower short-term overall morbidity (33.9% in SEMS group vs 51.2% in ES group), and lower rates of temporary colostomy (33.9% in SEMS group and 51.4% in ES group). SEMS also achieved a lower permanent stoma rate (22.2% for SEMS vs 35.2% for ES) and an increased success of primary anastomosis (70% in SEMS group and 54.1% in ES group), with no difference in overall mortality within 60 days after surgery.

[19] Atamanalp SS. Treatment of sigmoid volvulus: a single-center experience of 952 patients over 46.5 years. Tech Coloproctol 2013;17(5):561–9. PMID: 23636444.

A single-centre experience of 952 patients over a 46-year period noted that morbidity and mortality for emergency surgery was 35% and 16% versus 12.5% and 0% for elective. The principal strategy in the treatment for sigmoid volvulus is early non-surgical detorsion followed by elective surgery in uncomplicated patients, while emergency surgical treatment is performed for patients with bowel gangrene, perforation, or peritonitis, other difficulties with diagnosis, unsuccessful non-surgical detorsion and early recurrence.

[22] Valle RG, Godoy FL. Neostigmine for acute colonic pseudo-obstruction: a meta-analysis. Ann Med Surg (Lond) 2014;3(3):60–4. PMID: 25568788

A meta-analysis of four randomised trials including 127 patients (65 in the neostigmine group and 62 in the control group) revealed neostigmine is a safe and effective option for patients with acute colonic pseudo-obstruction (ACPO) who failed to respond to conservative management. ACPO resolved in 89.2% treated with one dose of neostigmine versus 14.8% in the control group.

[37] Vennix S, Musters GD, Mulder IM, et al. Laparoscopic peritoneal lavage or sigmoidectomy for perforated diverticulitis with purulent peritonitis: a multicentre, parallel-group, randomised, open-label trial. Lancet 2015;386(10000):1269–77. PMID: 26209030.

A multicentre, parallel-group, randomised, open-label trial in 34 teaching hospitals and eight academic hospitals in Belgium, Italy and the Netherlands (the LOLA arm) compared laparoscopic lavage with sigmoidectomy and concluded lavage is not superior to sigmoidectomy for the treatment of purulent perforated diverticulitis. The study was terminated early secondary to an increased event rate in the lavage group. The primary endpoint occurred in 30 (67%) of 45 patients in the lavage group and 25 (60%) of 42 patients in the sigmoidectomy group (odds ratio 1.28, 95% CI 0.54–3.03, P *= 0.58). By 12 months, four patients had died after lavage and six patients had died after sigmoidectomy* (P *= 0.43).*

[38] Kohl A, Rosenberg J, Bock D, et al. Two-year results of the randomized clinical trial DILALA comparing laparoscopic lavage with resection as treatment for perforated diverticulitis. Br J Surg 2018;105(9):1128–34. PMID: 29663316.

A multicentre prospective, randomised, controlled trial (DILALA) comparing laparoscopic lavage and open Hartmann's procedure was conducted in nine surgical departments in Sweden and Denmark. A total of 83 patients were randomised (43 in the lavage and 40 in the Hartmann's group). Follow-up at 24 months revealed no difference in morbidity or re-admission between the two groups. Fewer patients had an end colostomy in the lavage group (3 vs 9), and the lavage group had a 45% reduced risk of underdoing one or more operations and had fewer operations than the Hartmann's group.

[39] Azhar N, Johanssen A, Sundstrom T, et al. Laparoscopic lavage vs primary resection for acute perforated diverticulitis: long-term outcomes from the Scandinavian Diverticulitis (SCANDIV) randomized clinical trial. JAMA Surg 2021;156(2):121–7. PMID: 33355658

A multicentre, randomised clinical superiority trial (SCANDIV) from 21 centres in Sweden and Norway compared the outcomes from laparoscopic lavage (n *= 73) with those for colon resection* (n *= 69) for perforated diverticulitis. Severe complications occurred in 36%* (n *= 26) in the laparoscopic lavage group and 35%* (n *= 24) in the resection group* (P *= 0.92). Overall mortality was 32%* (n *= 23) in the laparoscopic lavage group and 25%* (n *= 17) in the resection group* (P *= 0.36). The stoma prevalence was 8%* (n *= 4) in the laparoscopic lavage group and 33%* (n *= 17;* P *= 0.002) in the resection group among patients who remained alive, and secondary operations, including stoma reversal, were performed in 36%* (n *= 26) versus 35%* (n *= 24;* P *= o.92), respectively. Recurrence of diverticulitis was higher following laparoscopic lavage (21% [n = 15] vs 4% [n = 3];* P *= 0.004). In the laparoscopic lavage group, 30%* (n *= 21) underwent a sigmoid resection.*

[41] Shi X, Shan Y, Yu E, et al. Lower rate of colonoscopic perforation: 110 785 patients of colonoscopy performed by colorectal surgeons in a large teaching hospital in China. Surg Endosc 2014;28(8):2309–16. PMID: 24566747.

A retrospective single-centre study evaluating colonoscopic complications was conducted. A total of 110 785 consecutive patients were evaluated. Two perforations occurred (0.016%). A total of 14 incidents (0.012%) of perforation were reported (7 males and 7 females), of which 9 cases occurred during diagnostic colonoscopy (0.01%) and 5 after therapeutic colonoscopy (3 polypectomy cases, 1 endoscopic mucosal resection and 1 endoscopic mucosal dissection).

[46] Tan KK, Shore T, Strong DH, et al. Factors predictive for a positive invasive mesenteric angiogram following a positive CT angiogram in patients with acute lower gastrointestinal haemorrhage. Int J Colorectal Dis 2013;28(12):1715–9. PMID: 23836115.

Of 30 patients with non-diverticular aetiologies of lower gastrointestinal bleeding, a selective mesenteric angiography within 150 minutes of a positive CT angiography was 2.89 times more likely to identify the source of bleeding.

[47] Koh FH, Soong J, Lieske B, et al. Does the timing of an invasive mesenteric angiography following a positive CT mesenteric angiography make a difference?. Int J Colorectal Dis 2015;30(1):57–61. PMID: 25367183.

Of 48 mesenteric angiographies for lower gastrointestinal bleeding, a selective mesenteric angiography within 90 minutes of a positive CT angiography was 8.56 times more likely to identify the source of bleeding.

[50] Menke J. Diagnostic accuracy of multidetector CT in acute mesenteric ischemia: systematic review and meta-analysis. Radiology 2010;256(1):93–101. PMID: 20574087.

A meta-analysis of three prospective and three retrospective studies revealed that contrast-enhanced multidetector CT correctly identifies the diagnosis of primary acute mesenteric ischaemia with high pooled sensitivity (93.3%) and specificity (95.9%), thus supporting its use as a first-line imaging modality.

17 Anorectal emergencies

Peter G. Vaughan-Shaw | Sarah A. Goodbrand

INTRODUCTION

Acute anorectal pathology constitutes a significant proportion of the general surgeon's workload. The problems encountered range from the acute pain of thrombosed haemorrhoids and perianal sepsis to the management of anorectal bleeding, trauma and irreducible rectal prolapse. Effective management depends upon sound knowledge of anorectal anatomy, accurate classification of the pathology and timely intervention to ensure minimal disruption to normal function. Given its mode of presentation, clinical trials in the management of acute anorectal pathology are infrequent, yet where present are discussed here.

ANORECTAL ANATOMY

The anal canal is a 3–4 cm tube running downwards and backwards from the anorectal angle to the anus. It is divided in half by the dentate line, which demarcates hindgut-derived columnar epithelium above and stratified squamous epithelium below that merges at the anus with the perianal skin. Above the dentate line is the anal transitional zone, lined by cuboidal epithelium for 1–2 cm. The hindgut sensory innervation is supplied by autonomic hypogastric nerves, sensitive only to stretch. Anoderm below the dentate line is innervated from the somatic inferior rectal nerves, making it sensitive to pain, pressure and temperature. However, the dentate line is not a reliable boundary between somatic and autonomic sensation; pain can certainly be felt within the anal transitional zone, which explains why some patients experience severe and immediate pain after rubber band ligation of haemorrhoids despite the band being applied apparently well above the dentate line.

The anorectal sphincter complex can be thought of as a gut tube within a funnel of muscle essential for the maintenance of normal continence. The inner muscle layer is the involuntary internal sphincter, a thickened continuation of the circular muscle of the rectum. Outside this is the funnel of the voluntary external sphincter, formed from striated muscle, continuous at its superior edge with the levator plate. Between these two muscle layers is the intersphincteric space, which contains mucous-secreting anal glands. These glands drain through the internal sphincter via their respective crypts of Morgagni at the level of the dentate line.

Three submucosal anal cushions comprising fibroelastic tissue and arteriovenous anastomoses are found within the anal canal, usually at the 3, 7 and 11 o'clock positions. They normally appose to form a tight seal within the canal, which helps to maintain continence, but in some patients they may enlarge to form troublesome symptomatic haemorrhoids.

ANORECTAL ABSCESSES

Anorectal abscesses, defined as sepsis within the soft tissues that surround the anus, are among the commonest surgical emergencies, with operative treatment being required in about 1 in 5000 of the population in the UK annually. They occur predominantly in adults, frequently in the third and fourth decades of life, with a male preponderance. An anorectal abscess is thought to originate within the intersphincteric space, due to obstruction and suppuration of the anal crypt glands (the cryptoglandular theory). Furthermore, 90% of anorectal abscesses arise as a result of this process and are termed primary anorectal abscesses. The resultant primary infection will produce an intersphincteric abscess which can spread, in a vertical, horizontal or circumferential direction, along several anatomical planes to collect in a number of potential anorectal spaces: perianal, intersphincteric, pelvi-rectal (ischiorectal, or post anal) or supralevator. Circumferential spread results in a horseshoe abscess (Fig. 17.1). The relative frequency with which abscesses occur in the various anatomical locations is shown in Table 17.1.[1]

Both aerobic and anaerobic bacteria are responsible for the abscess formation, with the predominant anaerobic bacteria being *Bacteroides* spp., *Peptostreptococcus* and *Clostridium*; the most commonly isolated aerobic and facultative bacteria are *Staphylococcus aureus*, *Streptococcus*, *Enterobacteriaceae* and *Enterococcus*.[2–4]

Suppurating skin infections, including carbuncles, furuncles and infected apocrine glands, can also cause primary abscesses. The responsible bacterium in these cases is almost invariably staphylococcus and as these abscesses do not communicate with the anal canal they are not associated with fistula formation.[5]

Secondary abscesses are much less common, accounting for just 10% of presentations.[6] They are a manifestation of distinct underlying disease processes, with Crohn's disease, colorectal neoplasia, diabetes mellitus, AIDS and tuberculosis all being potential causes. They can also occur as a complication of anorectal surgery or as a consequence of trauma.

CLINICAL FEATURES

Anorectal abscesses present with signs and symptoms of acute inflammation, with pain being the most common symptom. On examination a perianal abscess can usually be seen as a red, tender, fluctuant swelling near the anal verge; however, ischiorectal abscesses often present as a less distinct brawny swelling on one side of the anus and intersphincteric abscesses usually cannot be seen externally at all. Although

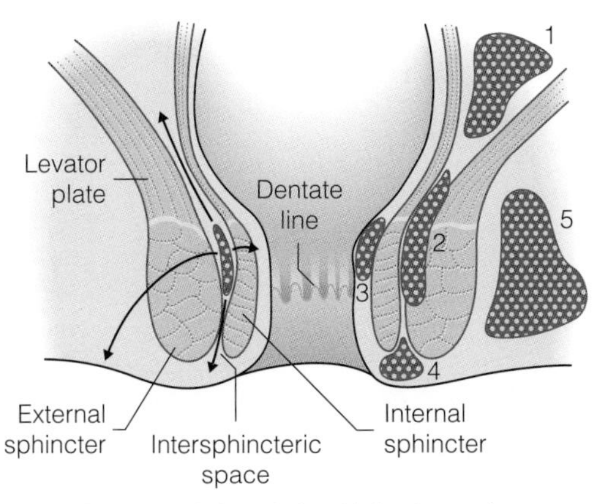

Figure 17.1 The spread of anal gland infection and common sites of anorectal sepsis. Infection of the anal gland within the intersphincteric space can spread in a variety of directions (see left side of diagram), resulting in abscess in a number of classical sites: 1, supralevator; 2, intersphincteric; 3, submucosal; 4, perianal; 5, ischiorectal. Note also the possibility of circumferential extension of sepsis ('horseshoeing') in the intersphincteric, ischiorectal and supralevator planes.

Table 17.1 Location of anorectal sepsis by anatomical site

Anatomical site	Number	Percentage
Perianal abscess	437	42.7
Ischiorectal	233	22.8
Intersphincteric	219	21.4
Supralevator	75	7.3
Submucosal	59	5.8

Data from Ramanujam PS, Prasad MI, Abcarian H, et al. Perianal abscesses and fistulae: a study of 1023 patients. Dis Colon Rectum 1984;27:593–7. With kind permission from Wolters Kluwer Health.

this last type of abscess can be felt through the anal wall as a smooth, tender collection, digital rectal examination is usually excruciatingly painful. This diagnosis should therefore be suspected in patients with severe anal pain and fever. Satisfactory examination is usually only possible under general anaesthesia. In a few patients (particularly those who are immune-compromised or with diabetes mellitus), the perianal sepsis can be associated with cellulitis, which can progress to life-threatening necrotising infection if not treated promptly.[7]

All patients presenting with anorectal sepsis or pain should have an examination of the anorectum, including proctosigmoidoscopy. It is our opinion that this can usually only be performed satisfactorily under general anaesthesia. As the diagnosis is usually obvious, few people would routinely recommend preoperative imaging (although some advocate its use, arguing that by identifying cavities and fistulas there is a reduction in the incidence of recurrence[8]).

RADIOLOGICAL IMAGING

Diagnostic radiology is seldom required to image uncomplicated anorectal sepsis. Its role in the management of acute anorectal sepsis is for investigating complex fistula disease in Crohn's disease or patients with supralevator sepsis to differentiate an intrapelvic source from extension of an intersphincteric or ischiorectal abscess. Imaging is also useful if the diagnosis is unclear, if there is non-resolution of symptoms after operative intervention or in cases of recurrent sepsis. Magnetic resonance imaging (MRI) is a sensitive and specific modality for identifying anorectal abscesses and associated fistula tracts and is the technique of choice in UK practice and beyond.[9,10]

Endoanal ultrasound is an alternative method of determining the origin of the sepsis and delineating fistula anatomy (Fig. 17.2). In experienced hands, it is as accurate as MRI.[11,12]

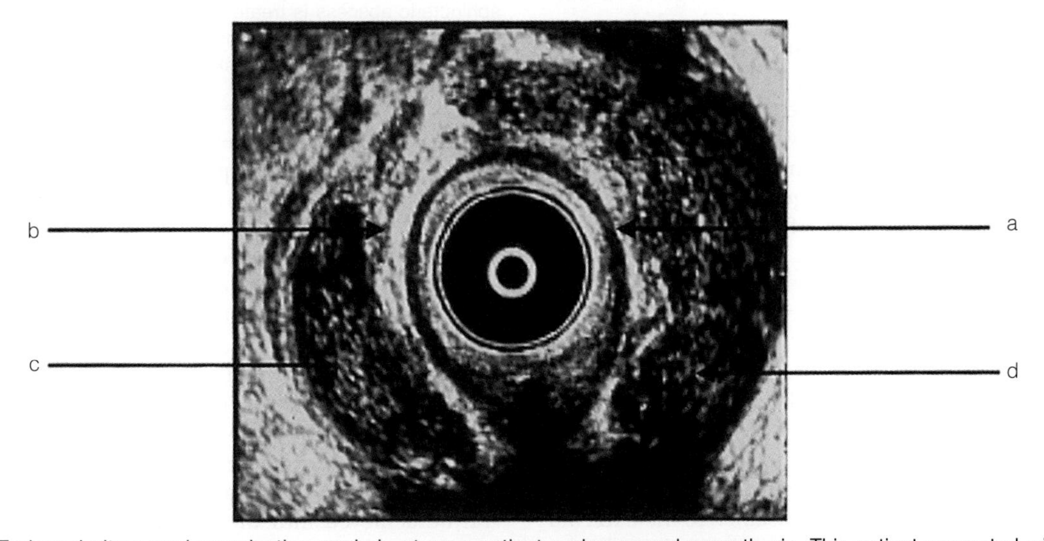

Figure 17.2 Endoanal ultrasound examination carried out on a patient under general anaesthesia. This patient presented with severe anal pain and perianal induration but without any specific area of fluctuance. The ultrasound demonstrates an extensive ischiorectal abscess cavity **(c, d)** extending around the anal canal (**a**, internal sphincter; **b**, external sphincter). (With thanks to Mr Mike Hulme-Moir, previous Clinical Fellow in Colorectal Surgery, Royal Infirmary, Edinburgh.)

TREATMENT

Undrained pus is remarkably destructive and hence sepsis must be drained promptly whilst minimising iatrogenic damage to the sphincter complex and preventing recurrence. In most patients, this involves external drainage via a curvilinear (not radial) incision at the lateral edge of the abscess cavity. This should not be placed too laterally as it will make subsequent fistula management more challenging. Needle aspiration alone is not recommended due to risk of inadequate drainage and abscess recurrence.[13] Adequate drainage should result in prompt resolution of the patient's symptoms; if not, a repeat examination under anaesthetic (EUA) or MRI is recommended to ensure that all sepsis has been completely drained.

Historically, it was suggested that thoroughly 'deroofing' the abscess cavity with a wide cruciate incision was beneficial, but this does little other than giving the patient a larger wound that will take longer to heal. Primary wound closure after incision has been abandoned as it offers little immediate benefit in terms of time to wound healing and probably increases the chance of recurrent sepsis.[14]

If the abscess cavity is very large, an alternative to making a huge incision is to insert a de Pezzer or Malecot catheter via a smaller skin incision. One study showed that using such treatment reduced hospital stay (1.4 vs 4.5 days) and duration of wound management, with no disadvantages seen at long-term follow-up.[15]

Antibiotics are not indicated routinely and should be used only as an adjunct to surgical treatment in immune-compromised patients, or when there is evidence of florid cellulitis or suspicion of necrotising infection.

It is the opinion of the authors that all anorectal abscesses should be drained under general or spinal anaesthetic, although in some centres perianal abscess drainage is commonly performed under local anaesthesia. Drainage of perianal abscesses under general or spinal anaesthetic allows a comprehensive examination to be undertaken and prevents a significant proportion of re-operations. A large retrospective case study of 500 patients treated for perianal abscess at the Mayo Clinic was reported in 2001 and revealed a 7.6% re-operation rate.[16] The reasons for re-operation included incomplete drainage of the abscess cavity at the first operation, missed abscesses (most often posterior collections) and postoperative bleeding. There was no association reported between patient variables (such as age, immune suppression or diabetes), emphasising the need for a thorough primary examination.

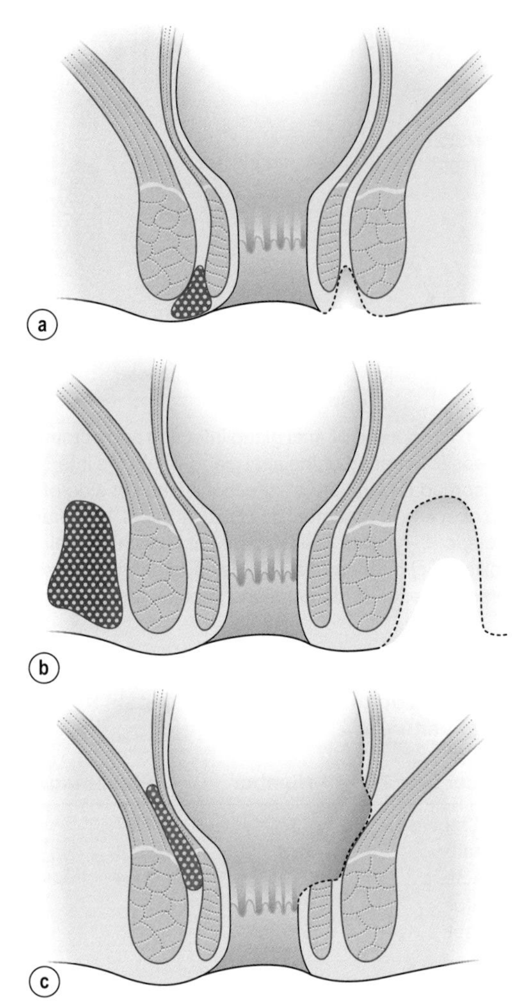

Figure 17.3 Management of specific abscesses. **(a)** Perianal abscess is treated by excision of a small disc of skin and curettage of the cavity. **(b)** Ischiorectal abscess may require excision of a substantial amount of tissue to facilitate drainage. The alternative is to introduce a drainage catheter through a small stab incision. **(c)** Intersphincteric abscess is treated by excision of the mucosa and internal sphincter overlying the abscess. Such an abscess should not be drained through the perineal skin or a high fistula will result.

TECHNICAL TIPS

The management of specific abscesses is shown diagrammatically in Fig. 17.3. Simple perianal abscesses should be drained externally and the cavity gently curetted (Fig. 17.3a). With ischiorectal abscesses, the cavity is often large (Fig. 17.3b) and should be incised as near to the anal verge as possible in order to minimise the distance to the external opening of any subsequent fistula. A large horseshoe abscess in the ischiorectal space is better drained through multiple short incisions than one large circumferential incision. As mentioned earlier, the size of the drainage wound can be minimised if a drainage catheter is used. Intersphincteric abscesses are more challenging and require drainage into the anorectum, which requires excision of part of the internal sphincter (Fig. 17.3c). Submucosal abscesses, although rare, are drained into the anal canal. Supralevator abscesses pose a unique challenge compared with the drainage of other anorectal abscesses. They develop in a space above levator ani, lateral to the rectum. Drainage transrectally is associated with high recurrence rates,[17] whilst concomitant drainage through the ischiorectal fossa results in high fistula-in-ano, which can be difficult to manage. It is therefore recommended that such abscesses be approached radiologically or via an open transabdominal approach. In true pelvic abscesses unrelated to spread from the anal glands, drainage can be achieved into the rectum or vagina. If the abscess is related to pelvic pathology, the primary disease process will need to be resected along with drainage of the pus to prevent recurrence.

Routine bacteriological swabs at the time of abscess drainage do not predict fistula or recurrence rates, and are therefore unnecessary.[18,19] In a recent meta-analysis, an empiric course of postoperative antibiotics following drainage was associated with a reduction in fistula formation in otherwise healthy patients, although quality of the evidence is low.[20]

Internal packing of anorectal abscess cavities has historically been commonly practised within the UK. However, a 2016 Cochrane review concluded that there is a paucity of high-quality evidence to confirm whether packing influences time to healing, recurrence or fistula rates.[21] A recent UK multicentre observational study (2016) demonstrated significant levels of pain, resource utilisation and expense associated with internal postoperative packing and as a result, an ongoing multicentre, phase III randomised control trials was designed to confirm this (PPAC2, currently recruiting).[22] In our opinion, postoperative packing should be omitted as it serves only to cause discomfort, inconvenience and cost, with no clear clinical advantage.

✓ Perianal abscesses are best incised under general anaesthesia with the cavity left open.

✓ Routine bacteriology swabs do not alter management and are unnecessary.[18,19]

✓ There is no evidence that packing the abscess cavity is clinically beneficial.[22]

✓✓ Needle aspiration rather than incision and drainage risks abscess recurrence.[13]

FISTULA-IN-ANO

Perianal abscesses are associated with anal fistulas in about 60% of patients from the outset[23,24]; only 27–37% of these persist after the acute inflammation has resolved.[25–27] Fistula-in-ano increases the likelihood of recurrent anorectal sepsis, a non-healing wound or persistent discharge, and thus the requirement for repeat interventions. For these reasons, many surgeons consider fistula treatment at the primary drainage procedure. However, identifying a fistula when acute inflammation is present can be difficult, especially for the less experienced surgeon. The probing of fistula tracts within friable, oedematous tissue can also lead to the creation of false fistula tracts which can be difficult to manage, and may cause disproportionate damage to the anal sphincter complex.

✓✓ The majority of anorectal abscesses are adequately treated with incision and drainage alone and if a fistula tract is not obvious, it should not be sought.[25–27]

A Cochrane review of six randomised control studies from five different centres from 1987 to 2003 looked at concomitant fistula surgery at the time of abscess drainage in terms of recurrence, need for further surgery and postoperative incontinence.[28,29] The eligibility criteria and treatments offered varied considerably between the trials, making definitive recommendations difficult. Three studies also reported fistula rates of 83–90%,[27] which is higher than would be expected, raising questions about whether iatrogenic tracks may have been created.

The majority of the studies included in the review dealt only with the surgical treatment of low fistulas. In one study, fistulotomy was performed as a second procedure on day 3 of the acute admission.[28] Most studies excluded those with recurrent anorectal sepsis, previous surgery and inflammatory bowel disease (IBD).[30]

All the studies showed that recurrence was less likely after concomitant fistula surgery (risk ratio 0.07–0.24), although follow-up times varied. The overall conclusions of the Cochrane meta-analysis were that synchronous fistulotomy is appropriate for low, uncomplicated fistula tracts. It should not be performed for high fistulas or anterior fistulas in women. It should also be avoided for groups where the risk of incontinence is high (e.g. those who have undergone previous anorectal surgery or have IBD).[28]

✓✓ Synchronous fistulotomy can be performed at the time of abscess drainage for low, uncomplicated fistula tracts to reduce the risk of abscess recurrence and further operations without compromising continence.[28]

MANAGEMENT OF SECONDARY PERIANAL SEPSIS

MALIGNANT DISEASE

These abscesses should be drained like any other anorectal abscess, but definitive treatment will require appropriate management of the malignant lesion. The presence of anorectal sepsis in this context, however, indicates advanced disease either from direct tumour infiltration or perforation, which has implications for further treatment. Consideration should be given to a defunctioning stoma at the time of sepsis drainage in this subset of patients.

INFLAMMATORY BOWEL DISEASE

All abscesses in patients with IBD should be drained promptly and setons inserted into any fistulous tracts as necessary. Management in patients with ulcerative colitis follows the principles outlined above, but the presence of anorectal sepsis and fistulas in IBD should always raise the possibility of the correct diagnosis being Crohn's disease. MRI is often helpful in demonstrating fistula tracts. Recurrent disease is often very hard to treat and an expert opinion should be sought.

NECROTISING INFECTION

Necrotising infection of the perianal tissues is characterised by the rapid progression of synergistic sepsis along fascial planes. The presentation is of a toxic patient with severe perianal pain, though often there may be very little to find on superficial perineal examination at initial presentation. Predisposing factors include poor health, diabetes and immunosuppression. The diagnosis is made clinically. Although blood tests may help distinguish necrotising infections from other severe soft tissue infections,[31] imaging studies should not delay treatment. The condition carries a high mortality (up to 80%) and requires urgent drainage and radical debridement of all involved tissue. A defunctioning stoma or faecal management device[32] may be required to facilitate wound management and several repeat EUAs are often necessary to ensure that only healthy tissue remains. Tissue should be sent for urgent microbiological analysis and antimicrobial advice sought to cover both aerobic and anaerobic organisms. There is little good quality evidence to support any specific medical or surgical treatments,[33] yet the need for radical debridement and broad-spectrum antibiotic cover directed thereafter by cultures and sensitivity is universally accepted.

ANORECTAL SEPSIS IN NEUTROPENIC PATIENTS

The classical features of abscess formation may be absent in neutropenic patients with perianal sepsis. The management of this subset of patients is poorly defined. The largest published study compared operative versus non-operative management and demonstrated comparable mortality.[34] Patients with pathognomonic features of an abscess should be managed operatively, whilst those without should be managed with antibiotics, MRI imaging[35,36] and careful serial clinical examination.[37]

ANORECTAL SEPSIS IN HIV PATIENTS

Improved outcomes in HIV patients presenting with anorectal sepsis reflects optimisation of antiretroviral medical treatment. Wound healing does, however, remain a problem and is correlated with the CD4 count. The best management of HIV patients with anorectal sepsis is identification of specific pathogens, involvement of HIV specialists, liberal drainage and fistulotomies for simple and low fistulas. Invasive procedures should ideally be avoided whenever the $CD4^+$ lymphocyte count is less than 50 cells/μL.

PILONIDAL ABSCESS

Pilonidal sinus disease is an acquired condition that typically occurs in the midline of the natal cleft. The resultant primary skin pits allow debris and loose hairs to penetrate and generate a chronic foreign body reaction in epithelial tracts, which can become acutely infected forming an abscess or cause chronic blood-stained discharge.

Risk factors for pilonidal sinus disease include male sex (twice as many men are affected), hirsutism, obesity, a deep natal cleft and lifestyle factors, particularly prolonged sitting.[38,39] It is rarely seen in patients over 45 years and therefore alternative diagnosis or a secondary cause should be sought in older patients. The causative organism, as with many skin infections, is often *Staphylococcus*, but mixed anaerobes may be cultured.[40]

In the emergency setting, the objective of treatment is simply to drain the abscess to relieve acute symptoms and prevent spreading sepsis. The optimal technique of draining a pilonidal abscess is via a longitudinal lateral (i.e. off-midline) incision.[41] Primary drainage alone has a recurrence rate of approximately 50%.[42]

Excision of the whole sinus tract at the same time as abscess drainage has been attempted but has been associated with recurrence rates of up to 60%.[40] It is therefore advisable to drain the primary abscess only as the initial wound will be much smaller.

A study from Israel assessed 58 patients with acute pilonidal abscess: 29 patients were treated with incision and drainage, the other 29 with wide excision (without closure). The risk of recurrent pilonidal suppuration was similar in the two groups, although those who underwent excision had a longer time off work.[42]

It is therefore recommended that excision of the sinus tract is not undertaken synchronously.[43] It is the authors' usual practice to consider formal excision only after the acute presentation has settled.

Novel techniques for pilonidal abscess drainage are evolving, with several groups suggesting that video-assisted/endoscopic pilonidal abscess treatment (EPAT) provides both adequate drainage and a greater chance of longer-term relief.[44–46] Further well-designed, well-powered studies are required to confirm these small studies.

✔ Pilonidal abscess should be drained by a longitudinal (i.e. off-midline) incision.[41]

✔ Definitive surgery (i.e. excision) should be reserved for those who have recurrent disease and be performed in the elective setting.[40,43]

ACUTE ANAL FISSURE

An anal fissure is a superficial ulcer in the anoderm distal to the dentate line. Anal fissure is common, with an incidence of 1 in 350 people, with acute fissures being significantly more prevalent than chronic anal fissures.[47,48] It can occur at any age but is uncommon in the elderly, and thus if an elderly patient presents with symptoms suggestive of a fissure, serious underlying pathology such as a low rectal or anal cancer must be excluded. Anal fissures can be primary or secondary depending on whether there is a clear causative factor. The pathophysiology of an anal fissure is local trauma, which leads to internal anal sphincter (IAS) spasm, increased resting anal pressure, reduced blood flow and finally ischaemia.[49] Most patients will present via the outpatient clinic but some attend emergently, because of severe pain on defecation, or with a complication of the anal fissure such as bleeding, anorectal fistula, abscess or faecal impaction. The distinction between acute and chronic anal fissures is somewhat arbitrary; an acute fissure is likely if the patient has had symptoms for less than 4 weeks. It is usually a simple diagnosis to make on visual inspection; an acute fissure will present as a small fresh laceration, most commonly in the posterior midline (6 o'clock) position. A chronic anal fissure has additional features, including partially healed edges, visible IAS fibres in its base, hypertrophied anal papilla and sometimes a 'sentinel' skin tag.

The initial treatment of an acute anal fissure is a combination of laxative stool softeners, sitz baths and analgesia. About 50% of acute anal fissures will heal with such measures within 2 weeks.[50]

For those patients with symptoms for more than 2 weeks, topical smooth muscle relaxants such as glycerine trinitrate (GTN)[51] or diltiazem are used to reverse IAS spasm and achieve re-epithelialisation over 6–8 weeks.[52] They are correlated with excellent short-term results, leading to the healing of 90% of acute fissures without the need for surgery.[53]

However, the long-term outlook is less encouraging, with one meta-analysis showing recurrence rates of up to 50%.[54] In this Cochrane review of 15 randomised controlled trials that looked at GTN versus placebo, GTN was found to be significantly better than placebo in healing anal fissures (49% vs 37%, $P < 0.004$). There was no significant difference in efficacy when comparing calcium channel blockers with GTN, although the included studies were heterogeneous. The Cochrane review also found botulinum toxin type A (Botox) injection was no better at healing an anal fissure than placebo or local lidocaine, and no better or worse than topical GTN or a calcium channel blocker. The use of Botox has been assessed mainly for chronic anal fissure, although an Egyptian randomised controlled trial demonstrated good results when used for acute fissures,[55] while another small RCT reported benefit in acute fissure from topical metronidazole.[56]

Lateral internal sphincterotomy (LIS) is much more successful than chemical methods at reducing recurrence rates (approximately 2%), and although some studies have raised concerns about impairment of continence, it appears that a well-planned procedure in selected patients has very little effect on continence.[57,58] However, it has no place in the acute setting and should be reserved for patients with chronic symptoms and hypertonicity.

In those with atypical or intractable symptoms, EUA should be performed to exclude occult sepsis or an alternative aetiology. If a fissure is confirmed at EUA, local anaesthetic and Botox may be infiltrated under the fissure and into the IAS, respectively, to provide symptomatic relief.

✔✔ Most anal fissures will heal with conservative treatment.[51,53]

✔✔ Definitive surgery should be reserved for those with recurrent or non-healing disease.[54,57]

HAEMORRHOIDS

Symptoms relating to haemorrhoidal disease occur in approximately 5% of the population. Haemorrhoids occur because of changes within the vascular, muscular and connective tissue condensations within the anal canal termed the 'anal cushions'. Degeneration of the muscular and fibrous components of these cushions leads to a reduction in the muscle-to-fibre ratio. They can be classified according to their anatomic location relative to the dentate line: internal haemorrhoids arise from the endoderm and are thus covered by columnar epithelium; external haemorrhoids arise below the dentate line and are covered by squamous epithelium (ectoderm). The external parts are innervated by cutaneous nerves from the sacral plexus via the pudendal nerve, and are sensitive to pain.

Most haemorrhoids are asymptomatic or cause minor symptoms only. Patients with complicated haemorrhoidal disease may present as an emergency with anorectal haemorrhage or acute prolapse and thrombosis.

THROMBOSED HAEMORRHOIDS

Thrombosed haemorrhoids occur either as an acutely thrombosed external haemorrhoid (often used interchangeably with perianal varix/haematoma) or thrombosed or strangulated internal haemorrhoids. They can be differentiated by the presence of anoderm overlying a thrombosed external haemorrhoid, which will also usually present as a single 'lump' at the anal margin. Internal haemorrhoids can prolapse chronically but become thrombosed when the tissue becomes fixed outside the sphincter, impeding venous return. Spontaneous thrombosis of the inferior haemorrhoid plexus is the precipitating event in external haemorrhoid thrombosis. There is usually a history of straining and constipation with the onset of acute pain thereafter.

Although acute haemorrhoidal prolapse/thrombosis is immensely painful, it tends to resolve spontaneously within 4–5 days. The mainstays of non-surgical management are good analgesia, laxatives, ice pack/cold compress and topical treatments.[59,60] The main argument for not undertaking emergency haemorrhoidectomy for acutely thrombosed haemorrhoids is firstly that it is painful for about the same amount of time as for natural healing, and secondly the benefits of surgery lessen as the condition resolves. Recent reviews suggest that patients who present after 72 hours of symptoms are best served by non-operative treatment, while those who present before this time may benefit from conventional haemorrhoidectomy.[61] However, the only prospective randomised controlled study comparing operative and non-operative treatment showed that non-operative treatment was associated with shorter hospital stay and less anal sphincter damage.[62]

There is a relative paucity of published literature pertaining to the longer-term consequences of conservative management and the need for subsequent haemorrhoidectomy. A small study from St Mark's Hospital suggested a high incidence of persistent symptoms and requirement for haemorrhoidectomy (54.7%) in these patients.[63]

Definitive emergency haemorrhoidectomy can be difficult, but many retrospective and case-controlled studies suggest similar outcomes to elective haemorrhoidectomy in experienced hands (Table 17.2).[64] If surgery is to be undertaken, several studies have shown that stapled anopexy in the acute setting is associated with shorter hospital stays, reduced pain and earlier return to work compared with conventional open haemorrhoidectomy.[65–67] These findings should be considered against results from the large 'eTHoS trial' which showed better overall quality of life in the traditional excisional surgery group compared with stapled haemorrhoidopexy group in elective practice.[68]

✔✔ Thrombosed haemorrhoids should be treated by conservative management, particularly if presentation is more than 72 hours after onset of symptoms.[61–63]

ANORECTAL HAEMORRHAGE

Rectal bleeding is a common reason for emergency hospital admission. In the majority of cases (>90%), it will cease without intervention. In a major UK audit of lower gastrointestinal (GI) bleeding, haemorrhage from a benign anorectal source accounted for 17% of the cohort[69] and included haemorrhoids, proctitis, rectal varices, rectal prolapse, anal fissures, solitary rectal ulcer syndrome and anal ulceration.

Table 17.2 Results from comparative study on emergency and elective haemorrhoidectomy

	Elective surgery (*n* = 500)	Emergency surgery (*n* = 204)	*P* value
Haemorrhage	27 (5.4)	10 (4.9)	NS
Blood transfusion	10 (2.0)	4 (1.9)	NS
Anal stenosis	15 (3.0)	12 (5.9)	NS
Disturbance of continence	26 (5.2)	9 (4.4)	NS
Sepsis	0	0	NS
Recurrence	38 (7.6)	14 (6.8)	NS

Numbers in parentheses are percentages. *NS*, non-significant.
Data from Eu KW, Seow Choen F, Goh HS. Comparison of emergency and elective haemorrhoidectomy. Br J Surg 1994;81:308–10. © British Journal of Surgery Society Ltd. Reproduced with permission. Permission is granted by John Wiley & Sons Ltd on behalf of the BJSS Ltd.

Performing basic investigations such as digital rectal examination, proctoscopy and rigid sigmoidoscopy during the index admission will readily identify an anorectal source of lower GI bleeding.[70]

If an anorectal source of a lower GI bleed is not clear, unstable patients should undergo urgent CT angiography to localise site of bleeding, while stable patients with a major bleed should be considered for colonoscopy on the same admission.[71]

ANORECTAL TRAUMA

ANAL SPHINCTER INJURIES

Anal sphincter injuries can be divided into obstetric and non-obstetric injuries; the latter include direct anal sphincter disruption and iatrogenic damage during other anorectal procedures.

OBSTETRIC ANAL SPHINCTER INJURIES

Between 4% and 6.6% of all vaginal births are complicated by perineal or pelvic floor trauma, and can occur as a result of vaginal delivery or as an extension to an episiotomy leading to damage of the anal mucosa and/or the anal sphincter complex.[72–75] The severity of sphincter injury can be graded by the degree of disruption of both the IAS and external anal sphincter (EAS). Third-degree tears include complete or partial disruption of the sphincter complex, whilst fourth-degree tears refer to damage of the anal mucosa with complete division of the sphincter complex.

Many obstetric sphincter injuries are not diagnosed in the immediate postpartum period (rates of 26–87% missed injury have been reported[76]) and are the commonest cause of anal incontinence in the longer term.

The repair of recognised sphincter injuries can be delayed for 8–12 hours with no impact on continence.[77] The type of repair (end-to-end approximation or overlapping technique) was evaluated in a 2013 Cochrane review, which found no specific advantage of either technique.[78] The overlapping technique requires more extensive mobilisation of the EAS and is therefore only possible for injuries that involve more than 50% of the EAS. Suture-related morbidity is equivalent for PDS or vicryl.[79] Separate repair of the IAS is recommended, as women with an IAS defect on endoanal ultrasound have higher long-term incontinence rates. The long-term outcomes for primary repair are poor, with rates of faecal incontinence ranging 6–53% depending on duration of follow-up.

NON-OBSTETRIC TRAUMA

Isolated injuries of the sphincter complex are unusual and are normally associated with concomitant injuries to adjacent viscera. The management of such injuries should therefore be directed towards correctly identifying disrupted anatomy and prioritising management. Early treatment comprises debridement of all non-viable tissue and faecal diversion, deferring reconstructive surgery.

RECTAL INJURIES

The management of rectal trauma is dictated by anatomy. Traditional approaches have followed the 'four Ds' (debridement, drainage, diversion, and distal irrigation), but have been refined in recent years. Injury sustained to the intraperitoneal rectum (anterior upper two-thirds of the rectum) can sometimes be primarily repaired, but if there is delay in presentation, significant contamination, major tissue loss, devascularisation or nearby open fractures, resection and formation of anastomosis or stoma should be preferred. Damage to the extraperitoneal rectum (lower one-third) can also be repaired primarily, sometimes via a transanal approach, but again proximal diversion may be needed if injuries are extensive.[80] Sigmoidoscopy should always be performed if blood is seen in the rectal lumen or if an extraperitoneal haematoma is seen adjacent to the rectum at laparotomy. Radiological tests incorporating rectal contrast may also be useful. Traditional principles, including the need to perform pre-sacral drainage and distal washout have been challenged by several recent studies.[81,82] Similarly, diversion is not necessary for non-destructive injuries, whether extra- or intraperitoneal (<25% circumference), where primary repair should be considered.[83] For destructive injuries, resect and perform either stoma (for extraperitoneal) or primary anastomosis (for intraperitoneal injuries in otherwise stable patient). As experience in transanal minimally invasive surgery (TAMIS) increases, such an approach may allow primary transanal repair for non-destructive injuries.

✔ Primary repair of non-destructive rectal injuries should be considered. For destructive injuries, perform resection with primary anastomosis and/or faecal diversion.[83]

FOREIGN BODIES

Rectally inserted foreign objects and the innovative techniques used to remove them are extensively reported in medical literature. A review of these case reports suggests that in many cases removal is possible under conscious sedation, either digitally for low objects or bimanually for those above the rectosigmoid junction.[84] However, the authors' experience is that general anaesthesia is invariably preferable for transanal retrieval of objects of significant size and making an adequate assessment for tissue injury. If transanal extraction measures fail, or there is radiographic evidence of perforation, laparotomy is required. It is recommended that all patients undergo sigmoidoscopy after extraction to ensure no damage to the rectal mucosa has been sustained.

IRREDUCIBLE RECTAL PROLAPSE

Irreducible rectal prolapse presents mainly in elderly patients and is likely to become a more frequent reason for emergency admission in today's ageing population. Firstly, it is essential to distinguish a full-thickness external prolapse from a mucosal prolapse: they are differentiated by the presence of concentric rings of mucosa and a prolapse containing the muscle layers of the rectal wall, rather than mucosa alone. Secondly, it must be ascertained whether the prolapse is ischaemic. In the absence of ischaemia, conservative measures can be undertaken. To reduce the oedema, sugar can be applied (e.g. 50% glucose solution soaked swabs) and manual reduction attempted thereafter with sedation or general anaesthesia, with definitive surgery deferred to a later stage. In the presence of ischaemia, surgical management is the only option. There are no large series to support a surgical procedure of choice, and either a perineal rectosigmoidectomy or laparotomy with resection may be appropriate; the choice is usually dictated primarily by the general fitness/comorbidity of the patient.[85]

FUTURE DEVELOPMENTS

Acute anorectal pathology does not readily lend itself to surgical trials, yet collaborative trial groups (e.g. trainee-led collaboratives) and pragmatic trial designs may improve recruitment to such trials in the future, as exemplified by the PPAC2 trial. Similarly, evolving approaches to elective colorectal surgery (i.e. minimally invasive, robotic) are not immediately applicable to acute anorectal disease. Current management principles for acute anorectal pathology require a robust understanding of anatomy. Where trainee operative exposure and anatomy teaching is diluted by working-time constraints or commitments to service provision, innovative ways to educate and train must be explored, including 3D-printed models, virtual and augmented reality.

RECOMMENDED VIDEOS

- Peri-anal abscess drainage Colorectal YouTube channel at: https://youtu.be/wGCkcQPdO_Q.

Key points

- Anorectal sepsis should be managed by prompt drainage following sound anatomical principles.
- Synchronous fistulotomy can be undertaken with care in low, uncomplicated fistulas but should be avoided in those at high risk of incontinence or when the fistula is not easily distinguished.
- Abscess cavities should not be repeatedly packed following drainage.
- Acute pilonidal abscesses should be treated with off-midline incision and drainage alone.
- Anal fissures should be managed pharmacologically, with surgery reserved for those that fail to heal.
- Acute thrombosed haemorrhoids should almost always be managed non-operatively. Emergency haemorrhoidectomy is recommended only if carried out within 72 hours of symptom onset and by an appropriately skilled surgeon.
- Management of anorectal trauma and retained foreign bodies should be determined by the site of injury and the anorectum should always be re-examined by sigmoidoscopy following foreign-body removal.

 References available at http://ebooks.health.elsevier.com/

FURTHER READINGS

- Recommendations for the Management of Anorectal Abscess, ACPGBI Emergency General Surgery Working Group at https://www.acpgbi.org.uk/content/uploads/2018/11/Anorectal-abscess-pathway.pdf
- ESGAR consensus statement on the imaging of fistula-in-ano and other causes of anal sepsis[86]
- Clinical Practice Guideline for the Management of Anorectal Abscess, Fistula-in-Ano, and Rectovaginal Fistula[87]
- Management of penetrating extraperitoneal rectal injuries[88]
- Rectal Trauma: Evidence-Based Practices[83]

KEY REFERENCES

[13] Sorensen KM, Moller S, Qvist N. Needle aspiration treatment vs. incision of acute simple perianal abscess: randomized controlled study. Int J Colorectal Dis 2021;36:581–8.

A prospective randomised trial of 98 patients with perianal abscess. The recurrence rate was 41% in needle aspiration and 15% in incision drainage, with HR of 3.033 (P = 0.014). Fistula formation was 15% without significant difference between the groups.

[24] Oliver I, Lacueva FJ, Perez V, et al. Randomised clinical trial comparing simple drainage of anorectal abscess with and without fistula track treatment. Int J Colorectal Dis 2003;18(2):107–10. PMID: 12548410.

A prospective, randomised trial of 200 consecutive patients showed recurrence reduced from 29% to 5% in patients in whom definitive treatment of the fistula track was attempted rather than simple drainage. However, due to the higher risk of incontinence, these recommendations were limited to those with low fistulas.

[26] Read DR, Abcarian H. A prospective study of 474 patients with anorectal abscess. Dis Colon Rectum 1979;22:566–8. PMID: 527452.

A large prospective study showing good results for primary fistulotomy along with drainage.

[28] Malik AI, Nelson RL, Tou S. Incision and drainage of perianal abscess with or without treatment of anal fistula. Cochrane Database Syst Rev 2010;7:CD006827. PMID: 20614450.

A review of the current evidence for concurrent fistulotomy at the time of incision and drainage of an acute abscess, showing good results for fistulotomy in low, uncomplicated disease.

[51] Lund JN, Scholefield JH. A randomised, prospective, double-blind, placebo-controlled trial of glyceryltrinitrate ointment in treatment of anal fissure. Lancet 1997;349(9044):11–4. PMID: 8988115.

This study of 80 consecutive patients demonstrated rapid relief of symptoms and after 8 weeks of ongoing treatment 68% demonstrated fissure healing compared with 8% in the placebo group.

[53] Frezza EE, Sandei F, Leoni G, et al. Conservative and surgical treatment in acute and chronic anal fissure: a study on 308 patients. Int J Colorectal Dis 1992;7(4):188–91. PMID: 1293238.

A large study concluding that the condition is self-limiting in the vast majority of patients.

[54] Nelson R. Non surgical therapy for anal fissure. Cochrane Database Syst Rev 2006;4:CD003431. PMID: 17054170.

A review of 53 randomised controlled trials comparing medical and surgical therapy for anal fissure showed some advantage to topical treatments over placebo for acute fissure symptoms, but that surgery was by far the best solution for chronic fissure problems.

[57] Brown CJ, Dubreuil D, Santoro L, et al. Lateral internal sphincterotomy is superior to topical nitroglycerin for healing chronic anal fissure and does not compromise long-term fecal continence: six-year follow-up of a multicenter, randomized, controlled trial. Dis Colon Rectum 2007;50(4):442–8. PMID: 17297553.

A study of 82 patients with chronic anal fissure randomised to GTN treatment or LIS showed better long-term patient satisfaction in the surgical group with no significant compromise to continence.

[61] Rivadeneira DE, Steele SR, Ternent C, et al. Practice parameters for the management of hemorrhoids (revised 2010). Dis Colon Rectum 2011;54:1059–64. PMID: 21825884.

Guidelines issued by the American Society of Colorectal Surgeons reflecting the predominantly office-based practice in North America for these conditions.

[62] Allan A, Samad AJ, Mellon A, et al. Prospective randomised study of urgent haemorrhoidectomy compared with non-operative treatment in the management of prolapsed thrombosed internal haemorrhoids. Colorectal Dis 2006;8(1):41–5. PMID: 16519637.

This study of 50 patients found that conservative treatment was associated with shorter admission duration and less anal sphincter damage as assessed by endoanal ultrasound, with no difference in the number of symptomatic patients at 24-month follow-up.

[64] Eu KW, Seow-Choen F, Goh HS. Comparison of emergency and elective haemorrhoidectomy. Br J Surg 1994;81(2):308–10. PMID: 8156371.

This single centre non-randomised study of > 700 patients concluded that results of Milligan–Morgan haemorrhoidectomy for elective and emergency presentations were comparable.

[65] Wong JC, Chung CC, Yau KK, et al. Stapled technique for acute thrombosed hemorrhoids: a randomized, controlled trial with long-term results. Dis Colon Rectum 2008;51(4):397–403. PMID: 18097723.

This study compared open and stapled haemorrhoidectomy in patients with acute thrombosed haemorrhoids and found reduced pain, faster return to work and greater satisfaction in the stapled haemorrhoidectomy group.

[69] Oakland K, Guy R, Uberoi R, et al. Acute lower GI bleeding in the UK: patient characteristics, interventions and outcomes in the first nationwide audit. Gut 2018;67:654–62.

A major UK snapshot audit of management and transfusion practice in lower GI haemorrhage demonstrating variation in management and over-use of blood products.

Paediatric surgical emergencies 18

Dafydd A. Davies | Jacob C. Langer

INTRODUCTION

While paediatric surgery has increasingly become the domain of the subspecialist paediatric surgeon, adult general surgeons are still often faced with the challenges of assessing and managing children with surgical emergencies. The unique differences between adults and children must be taken into account when addressing every aspect of surgical management, including assessment, diagnosis, resuscitation and operative interventions. Children face a different spectrum of conditions, have different physiological responses to trauma, illness and surgical stress, and have different psychosocial needs.

This chapter will address the common abdominal paediatric surgical emergencies encountered by general surgeons. These will be categorised according to age: (i) neonates (up to 44 weeks post-gestational age), (ii) infants (1 month to 2 years of age) and (iii) children (2 years of age and older).

NEONATAL PERIOD

PRENATAL DIAGNOSIS

Routine prenatal ultrasonography has become the standard of care in many parts of the industrialised world, and has resulted in the detection of many congenital anomalies before birth. Common detectable anomalies relevant to the general surgeon include: abdominal wall defects, congenital diaphragmatic hernia, intestinal obstruction and intra-abdominal masses.

Whenever possible, these patients should be referred for prenatal consultation with obstetrics, neonatology and paediatric general surgery. In most cases, delivery should occur at a hospital with a neonatal intensive care unit and paediatric surgical service. If this is not possible, they should be immediately transferred following delivery and resuscitation.

INTESTINAL OBSTRUCTION

Intestinal obstruction is the most common abdominal emergency in the neonatal period, and is usually due to a congenital, developmental or genetic anomaly.

ASSESSMENT

Assessing neonatal patients for obstruction requires a thorough history, including the nature of any vomiting and the presence or absence of abdominal distension. Since neonates are unable to verbalise, surgeons must gather as many clues as possible from the prenatal, perinatal and family historical details (Table 18.1).

Examination of neonates with suspected intestinal obstruction should start with vital signs and an assessment of the level of resuscitation required. Certain forms of obstruction can cause severe dehydration or sepsis, which will need to be addressed early. Dysmorphic features may give clues to syndromes in which obstruction is common. The abdominal examination should make note of discolouration, distension and signs of peritoneal inflammation such as guarding and rigidity. It is important to look for an incarcerated inguinal hernia as the cause of obstruction (see later). A thorough evaluation of the perineum must also be performed to ensure normal location and patency of the anus.

Routine blood work including electrolytes and complete blood count are helpful in assessing the level of dehydration as well as in determining if electrolyte disturbances or sepsis are contributing to the presentation. It should be kept in mind that serum creatinine in the newborn reflects the mother's levels, and may not be helpful in assessing the neonate's renal function.

Abdominal radiography should be the initial imaging modality for neonates with possible intestinal obstruction. Typically, infants with duodenal obstruction have a 'double-bubble' appearance (Fig. 18.1), whereas those with distal intestinal obstruction will have multiple dilated bowel loops. It is impossible to differentiate distal small-bowel obstruction from colonic obstruction based on the plain abdominal radiograph in neonates, as the haustral markings seen in adults are not visible in this age group.

A contrast study is often required to definitively diagnose the aetiology of intestinal obstruction. If malrotation is suspected, an urgent upper gastrointestinal contrast study should be performed first. Once this has been excluded, a contrast enema can be done to exclude distal pathology if this is indicated. For those infants with distal obstruction on plain radiograph, a contrast enema will help to differentiate the three most common causes of distal obstruction: meconium ileus, jejuno-ileal atresia and Hirschsprung disease (HD; Fig. 18.2). Water-soluble contrast should always be used instead of barium, to avoid the possibility of barium leaking into the abdominal cavity should a perforation occur, and also because water-soluble contrast is more effective in relieving the obstruction in cases of meconium obstruction.

Neonates with suspected intestinal obstruction should be transferred in a temperature-controlled transport isolette to a specialised paediatric surgical unit for evaluation and definitive management. Resuscitation should begin as soon as the patient is assessed and should continue during transport. Nasogastric decompression with a large-calibre nasogastric tube (size 8–10

French) is important to improve ventilation, monitor resuscitation and limit bowel distension and subsequent ischaemia.

SPECIFIC FORMS OF INTESTINAL OBSTRUCTION

Oesophageal atresia

This anomaly is characterised by a gap in the oesophagus, resulting in a blind-ending proximal pouch. In 90% of cases, the distal oesophagus is connected to the back of the trachea as a tracheo-oesophageal fistula. Oesophageal atresia is usually first suspected when the baby has difficulty swallowing saliva and may have coughing or respiratory distress during the first feed.[1] Intubation may be needed if ventilation or respiration is significantly impaired. The diagnosis is confirmed by inability to pass a 10–12 French nasogastric tube. This tube should be left in the proximal oesophageal pouch and placed on continuous suction to reduce aspiration of secretions. Operative repair should only be performed by an experienced paediatric surgeon and involves division of the fistula and end-to-end anastomosis of the proximal and distal oesophagus. Associated cardiac anomalies are common with this condition and should be ruled out prior to the baby receiving a general anaesthetic.

Table 18.1 Important considerations in the neonatal history

Prenatal history	Previous pregnancies (complications and outcomes) Maternal gestational illnesses (e.g. gestational diabetes, pregnancy-induced hypertension) Screening ultrasonography (dates and findings) Other prenatal investigations and outcomes (e.g. maternal alpha-fetoprotein/betaHCG/oestrogen levels, chorionic villous sampling, amniocentesis)
Perinatal history	Weeks of gestation Induced or spontaneous labour Complications of delivery APGAR scores
Neonatal history	Complications Infections Feeding history (initiation, type, rate achieved) Passage of meconium in the first 24 hours of life Other anomalies identified
Family history	Maternal and paternal health Previous congenital anomalies Cystic fibrosis Consanguinity

Meconium ileus

Cystic fibrosis (CF) is the most common autosomal recessive disorder in Caucasian children.[2] The disease alters the regulation of chloride transport in epithelial cells resulting in a variety of clinical manifestations. About 10–15% of children born with CF will develop meconium ileus, in which the meconium becomes sticky and causes intraluminal obstruction. This can further lead to complications of volvulus, atresia or perforation. In addition, meconium ileus may occasionally occur in children without CF. A diagnostic work-up, including both sweat chloride determination and genetic studies, must be done on all children with meconium ileus.

Abdominal radiograph may show distal intestinal obstruction with a bubbly appearance in the right lower quadrant due to gas mixing with the viscous meconium (Fig. 18.2a).[2] There may also be intraperitoneal calcification if *in utero* perforation has occurred.

Following resuscitation and nasogastric decompression, a water-soluble contrast enema will reveal a microcolon (small calibre) and multiple meconium plugs in the terminal ileum (Fig. 18.2a). In approximately 50% of cases, the contrast enema will relieve the obstruction. If progress is made, but the infant remains obstructed after the initial enema and is otherwise stable, the procedure can be repeated. If the contrast enema is unsuccessful in relieving the obstruction and/or no further progress has been made, a laparotomy must be done. If there is no volvulus or perforation, enterotomies are made and mechanical washout is performed. Complications of volvulus, acquired atresia or perforation are managed by intestinal resection with or without a stoma, depending on the condition of the bowel and of the patient.

Intestinal atresia/stenosis

Atresia and stenosis can occur at any point in the alimentary canal. The two prominent aetiological theories are failure of recanalisation of the intestine during foetal development, or an ischaemic event *in utero*.[3] Early resuscitative measures should be initiated and confirmatory diagnosis can usually

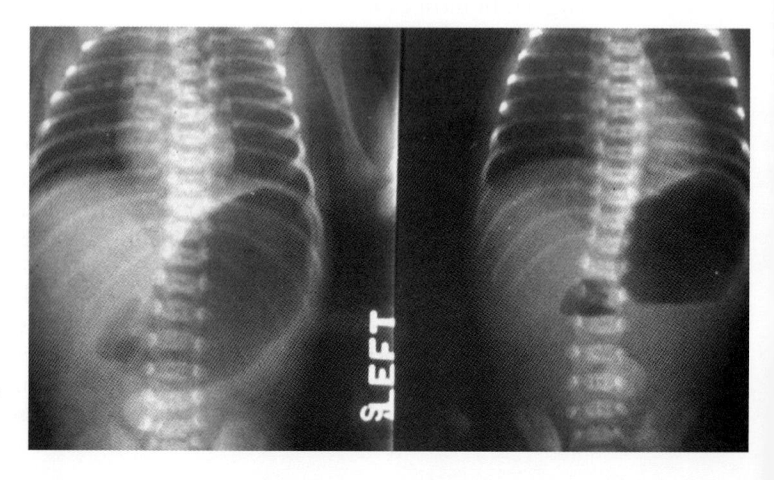

Figure 18.1 Abdominal radiograph of an infant showing the typical 'double-bubble' appearance resulting from duodenal obstruction.

be made with either upper or lower gastrointestinal contrast studies. The presence of a 'double-bubble' sign on abdominal radiograph is considered diagnostic for duodenal atresia (Fig. 18.1), although this finding associated with distal gas may also be due to stenosis, duodenal web or malrotation. Trisomy 21 is present in one-third of children with duodenal atresia. Patients with distal atresia will typically have multiple dilated loops of bowel on the plain abdominal radiograph. Although a diagnosis of proximal obstruction can be confidently made based on plain radiography, those with distal obstruction should always undergo water-soluble contrast enema to differentiate atresia from meconium ileus or HD (Fig. 18.2a–c).

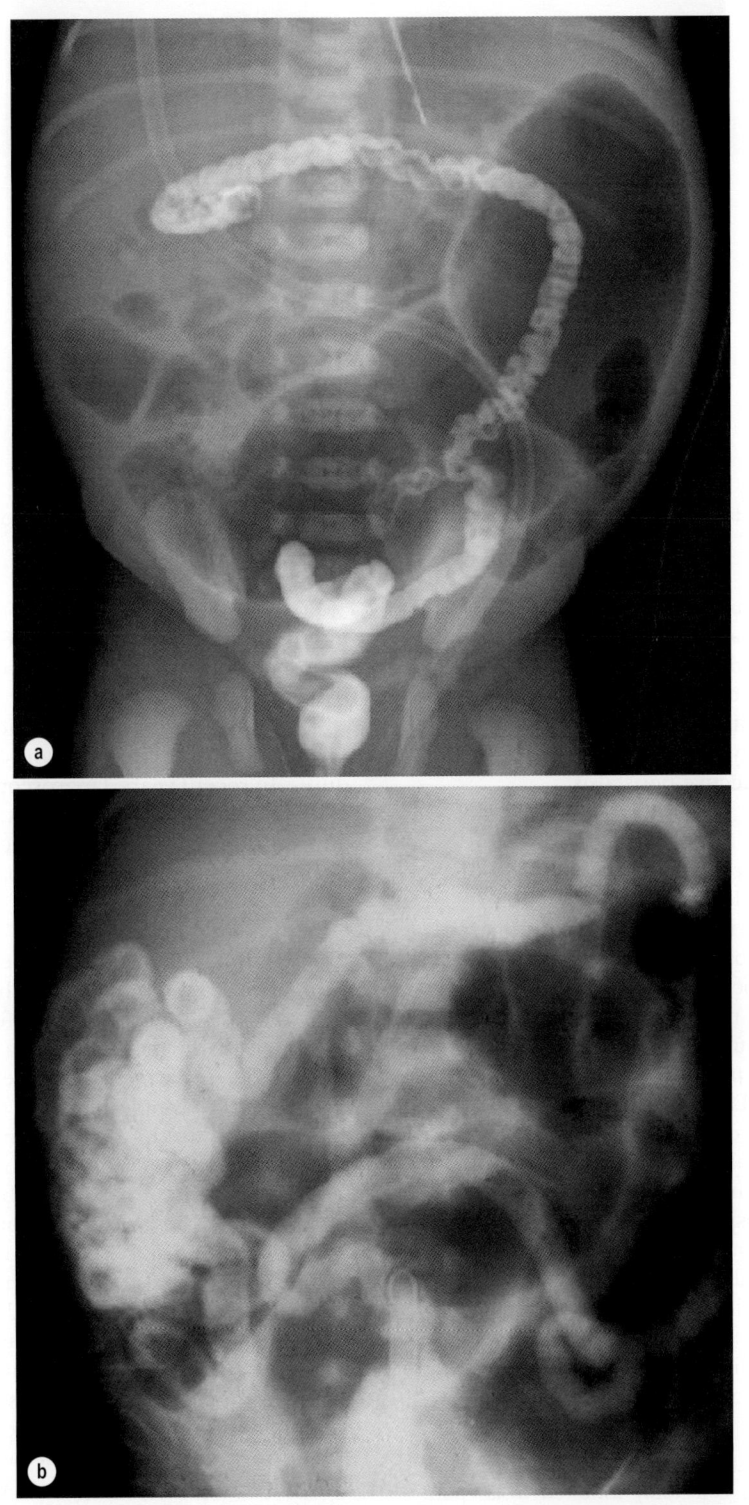

Figure 18.2 Water-soluble contrast enemas of infants with distal bowel obstruction. **(a)** Meconium ileus, showing a microcolon, dilated proximal small bowel and a soap-bubble appearance in the right lower quadrant. **(b)** Ileal atresia, showing a microcolon, contrast entering the distal small bowel but dilated proximal small bowel without contrast.

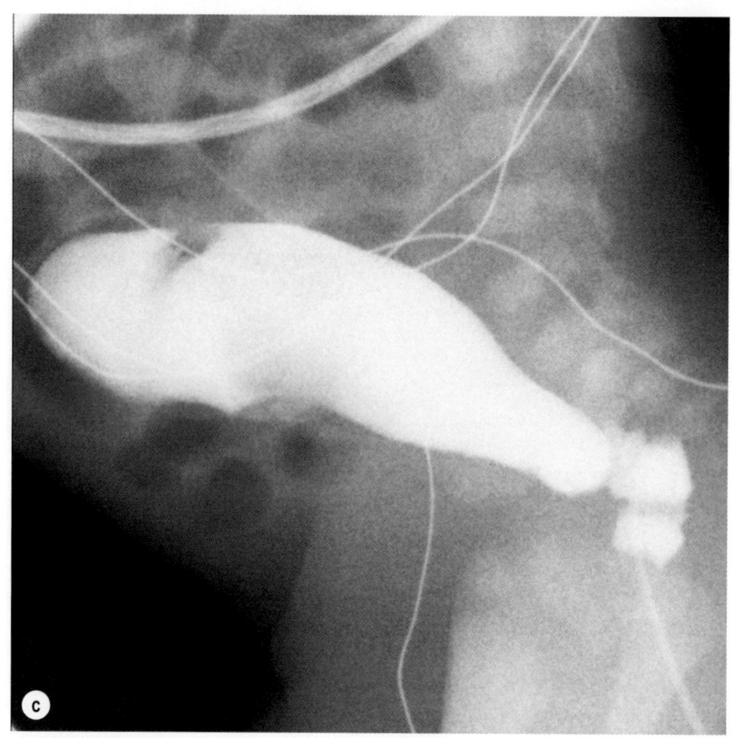

Figure 18.2 **(c)** Hirschsprung disease: lateral film showing a contracted distal rectum with dilated bowel proximally.

Since most infants with intestinal atresia are stable once decompressed and resuscitated, we recommend transfer of such neonates to a facility with paediatric surgical expertise. Most of these anomalies are treated with a primary anastomosis. If there is significant dilatation of the proximal segment, tapering enteroplasty should be done as the dilated bowel tends not to have effective peristalsis.

Hirschsprung disease

HD is a congenital disorder characterised by lack of ganglion cells in the distal bowel. This results in failure of peristalsis and functional obstruction. The 'transition zone' is usually located in the rectosigmoid, but HD can affect the entire colon and in rare occurrences the small bowel. HD most often presents in the neonatal period with distal bowel obstruction and failure to pass meconium in the first 24 hours of life. Patients can present later in life with a history of severe constipation. Early identification and management are important to prevent complications of HD such as enterocolitis and nutritional problems.

Water-soluble contrast enema has a sensitivity and specificity of 70% and 83%, respectively, and may therefore be normal, particularly in the newborn.[4] The gold standard for the diagnosis of HD is rectal biopsy, either by a suction technique at the bedside, or full-thickness biopsy.

Initial management, after resuscitation and nasogastric decompression, includes digital rectal stimulation and/or rectal irrigations (10 mL/kg normal saline).

✔ Although the historical teaching for Hirschsprung disease was routine diverting colostomy followed by a 'pull-through' operation several months later, the current standard of care is primary reconstructive surgery without a routine colostomy in most patients.[5]

Preliminary levelling colostomy should be reserved for infants presenting with severe enterocolitis, colonic perforation or failure to decompress with rectal stimulations and irrigations.

There are a number of options for surgical correction of HD, including the Swenson, Soave and Duhamel procedures. In recent years, laparoscopic and transanal approaches have been described, which have decreased morbidity and shortened hospital stay. These operations should all be performed by an experienced paediatric surgeon.

Anorectal malformations

Anorectal malformations can be divided into low and high anomalies. Low anomalies are characterised by rectoperineal or rectovestibular fistulas in female patients. Most males with high malformations have a fistula from the rectum to the bladder neck or urethra. Females with high anomalies usually have a single channel (cloaca) formed by coalescence of the urethra, vagina and rectum. Less commonly, there may be rectal atresia without a fistula, and some infants present with an anal membrane or anal stenosis.

Infants with these malformations usually present in the first day of life with distal bowel obstruction. Low malformations in girls with large fistulas can permit adequate evacuation of stool, and are occasionally missed. Careful examination of the perineum of all newborns for anal patency and position is important. Many of these patients will suffer from associated anomalies that need to be investigated prior to proceeding with anatomical repair of the anorectal malformation.

The next consideration is to determine if the defect is amenable to primary repair or whether faecal flow should be diverted with a colostomy followed by delayed secondary anatomical repair. Children with a rectoperineal fistula can usually be managed with a local procedure from

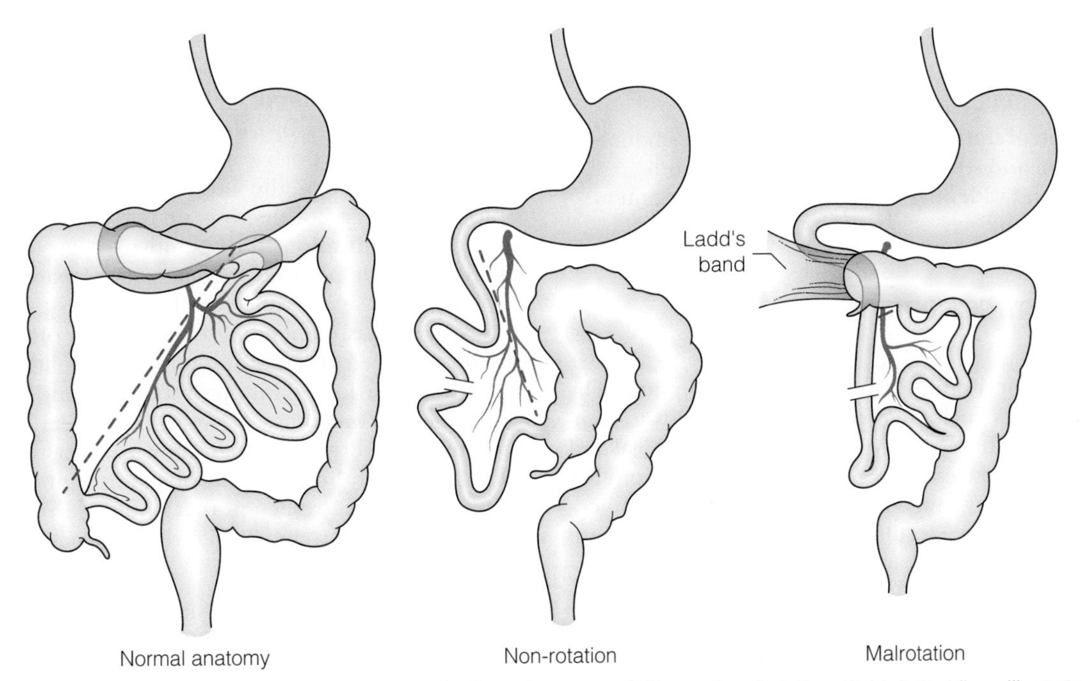

Figure 18.3 Schematic illustrations depicting normal intestinal rotation, non-rotation and malrotation. Bold dotted lines illustrate the width of the mesenteric base in each situation.

below, without a colostomy. Children with high anomalies are usually managed with a preliminary colostomy. The use of a colostomy in females with a rectovestibular fistula is controversial. The colostomy can be made using either the transverse or the sigmoid colon, and can be a loop or divided stoma. The authors agree with Pena and Hong's[6] recommendation for a divided colostomy in the proximal sigmoid colon. Predictors for poor long-term continence in these patients include a rectourinary fistula to the bladder neck or prostatic urethra, tethering of the spinal cord and the presence of an absent or hypoplastic sacrum. Depending on the nature of the anomaly, repair can be carried out using a posterior sagittal approach, a laparoscopic approach, or a combination of posterior and abdominal approaches. Technical expertise is crucial to success, and these procedures should only be performed by experienced paediatric surgeons.

Malrotation

The process of normal rotation and fixation occurs between the 6th and 10th week of development. If no rotation occurs, the patient is left in a position of non-rotation, which has a wide-based mesentery and does not require correction. Classic malrotation occurs when the process is interrupted part way through, leaving the caecum and the duodenal-jejunal junction (ligament of Treitz) close to each other (Fig. 18.3). Because this arrangement results in a narrow-based mesentery, the bowel is prone to midgut volvulus around the superior mesenteric vessels, which may lead to intestinal ischaemia. Malrotation with midgut volvulus is one of the true paediatric surgical emergencies. Failure to recognise this condition early can be catastrophic, leading to loss of large portions of bowel and subsequent short-bowel syndrome or death.

Rotation abnormalities are most often asymptomatic. While volvulus can occur at any time, it is most common in the first week of life.[7] The most common presentation of malrotation is bilious vomiting, which may occur for two reasons: midgut volvulus with kinking of the duodenum, or compression of the duodenum by Ladd's bands. Peritonitis and shock from midgut volvulus are late symptoms and are associated with a worse prognosis. Every attempt should be made to diagnose and correct malrotation before this occurs.[8] For this reason, every infant who presents with bilious vomiting should be considered to have malrotation with midgut volvulus until proven otherwise.

Any patient with suspected malrotation and volvulus needs urgent imaging and surgical consultation. Abdominal radiograph is often non-diagnostic but may show a dilated stomach, a 'double bubble' with distal gas, or a relatively gasless abdomen. Upper gastrointestinal contrast study is the preferred examination. A nasogastric tube placed prior to the exam can not only aid in decompression of the stomach but also the administration of the water-soluble contrast. The chief radiographic signs of malrotation are:

- abnormal position of the duodenojejunal junction
- spiral, 'corkscrew' or Z-shaped course of the distal duodenum and proximal jejunum and
- location of the proximal jejunum in the right abdomen.[8]

Abdominal ultrasound may show abnormal orientation of the superior mesenteric artery and vein, or a 'whirlpool sign'.[9]

The operation to correct malrotation involves a laparotomy (although a laparoscopic approach may be undertaken for children without clinical or radiological evidence of midgut volvulus).[10] If there is volvulus, the bowel is untwisted and checked for viability. If there is ischaemia, the bowel is wrapped with warm towels and re-inspected. Grossly necrotic bowel is resected, and the rest is left in, with a second-look laparotomy planned for 24–48 hours later. In children who have necrosis of the entire midgut, a palliative approach without resection should be considered.

If the intestine is viable, a Ladd procedure should be performed. This operation consists of five stages:

1. Division of Ladd's bands.
2. Mobilisation of the colon to the left side of the abdomen.
3. Mobilisation and straightening of the duodenum.
4. Dissection and widening of the small bowel mesentery.
5. Appendicectomy.

INFLAMMATORY CONDITIONS

ASSESSMENT

The diagnosis of peritonitis in the neonate is complicated by a number of factors, including the patient's inability to communicate with the surgeon, as well as several anatomical and physiological differences between neonates and older children/adults. The very thin abdominal wall may develop oedema and erythema as a result of underlying inflammation. Neonates breathe primarily with their diaphragms, so peritonitis results in rapid, shallow respiration, and ultimately will cause elevation in Pco_2 and respiratory failure. Localised peritoneal signs can be elicited by palpation, but the examiner must be gentle as the signs of involuntary guarding may be very subtle. In addition, the neonate does not have a well-developed omentum, so ability to localise inflammation may be impaired.

Neonates with peritonitis will often develop systemic sepsis, which may differ in its presentation to older children and adults. Signs of sepsis in neonates may include lethargy, temperature instability (either fever or hypothermia), increased ventilation requirements, thrombocytopenia, a high or low white blood cell count, and acidosis.

SPECIFIC FORMS OF ABDOMINAL INFLAMMATION

Meconium peritonitis

This condition occurs when there has been prenatal intestinal perforation, resulting in chemical peritonitis. Prenatally there may be evidence of free fluid or calcification within the abdomen. In some cases, the foetus is able to localise and wall off the perforation, which may result in a meconium cyst. The aetiology of the perforation is often distal obstruction, usually from meconium ileus or intestinal atresia, but in some cases the perforation is idiopathic.

Management of meconium peritonitis involves fluid resuscitation, nasogastric drainage and antibiotics. If there is evidence of associated intestinal obstruction, a contrast enema may be helpful preoperatively. Laparotomy should be carried out with resection of the involved bowel and either stomas or primary anastomosis, depending on the condition of the child and the bowel.

Necrotising enterocolitis

Necrotising enterocolitis (NEC) is most commonly seen in preterm and small-for-gestational-age infants.[11] The aetiology of NEC is unknown, but a combination of bacterial colonisation, intraluminal substrate and intestinal ischaemia/hypoxia all appear to be important.[12]

NEC should be suspected in neonates with sepsis, increased abdominal girth, feeding intolerance, abdominal wall discolouration, or bloody stools. Abdominal radiograph may show pneumatosis intestinalis, portal venous gas or free intra-abdominal air (Fig. 18.4). Ultrasound may show pneumatosis, free fluid, or intestinal hypoperfusion and hypomotility.

Initial management of NEC includes bowel rest, nasogastric decompression, broad-spectrum antibiotics, parenteral nutrition and supportive measures to optimise perfusion and oxygenation of the bowel. Persistent clinical deterioration and signs of necrosis or perforation are generally considered indications for operative intervention. Options include bedside peritoneal drainage, or laparotomy with resection of grossly necrotic bowel and either primary anastomosis or stomas, depending on the status of the child and the bowel.[11,13] A recent randomised controlled trial in neonates less than 1500 g with perforation found no significant difference in outcomes between peritoneal drainage and laparotomy.[14] Prior to laparotomy, parents should always be informed of the possibility of a long segment of necrosis requiring massive resection that would leave the child with short bowel syndrome. Palliative management should be considered in these infants.

Isolated ileal perforation

This condition resembles NEC, in that it primarily affects preterm and small-for-gestational-age infants. However, infants with isolated ileal perforation do not have any abnormalities of the intestine other than localised perforation, usually in the distal ileum. It is unclear whether this represents a very localised form of NEC, or a distinct entity. Clinically, these infants present with sudden deterioration, sepsis and free air without any evidence of pneumatosis seen on the abdominal radiograph. In general, the same principles of treatment are applied to ileal perforation and NEC.

OTHER NEONATAL CONDITIONS

INCARCERATED INGUINAL HERNIA

Inguinal hernias are very common throughout childhood. Hernias in children almost always arise from persistence of the processus vaginalis. If the processus contains only fluid, it is known as a hydrocele; the hydrocele is communicating if the processus remains open, and non-communicating if the processus has become obliterated proximal to the fluid. Communicating hydroceles should be repaired electively if they have not closed by 1 year of age.

In most cases, inguinal hernias are asymptomatic and can be repaired electively. Incarceration of bowel may result in complete bowel obstruction and represents a surgical emergency as both the bowel and the testis may become ischaemic. The risk of incarceration is greatest in newborns and is approximately 30% in the first 2 years of life. Premature infants are at highest risk.

Neonates and infants presenting with an incarcerated hernia should be resuscitated if necessary, and an immediate attempt should be made to reduce the hernia. In contrast to the adult with an incarcerated hernia, testicular ischaemia is far more common than intestinal ischaemia, and it is appropriate to be aggressive about reducing the hernia. Multiple attempts and the use of sedation may be necessary. Ice should not be applied to the hernia, as it may induce hypothermia. Surgical repair of an incarcerated hernia in an infant is a formidable undertaking. The sac is often thin and oedematous, and the risks of injury to the cord structures and recurrence of the hernia are very high. Therefore, if a

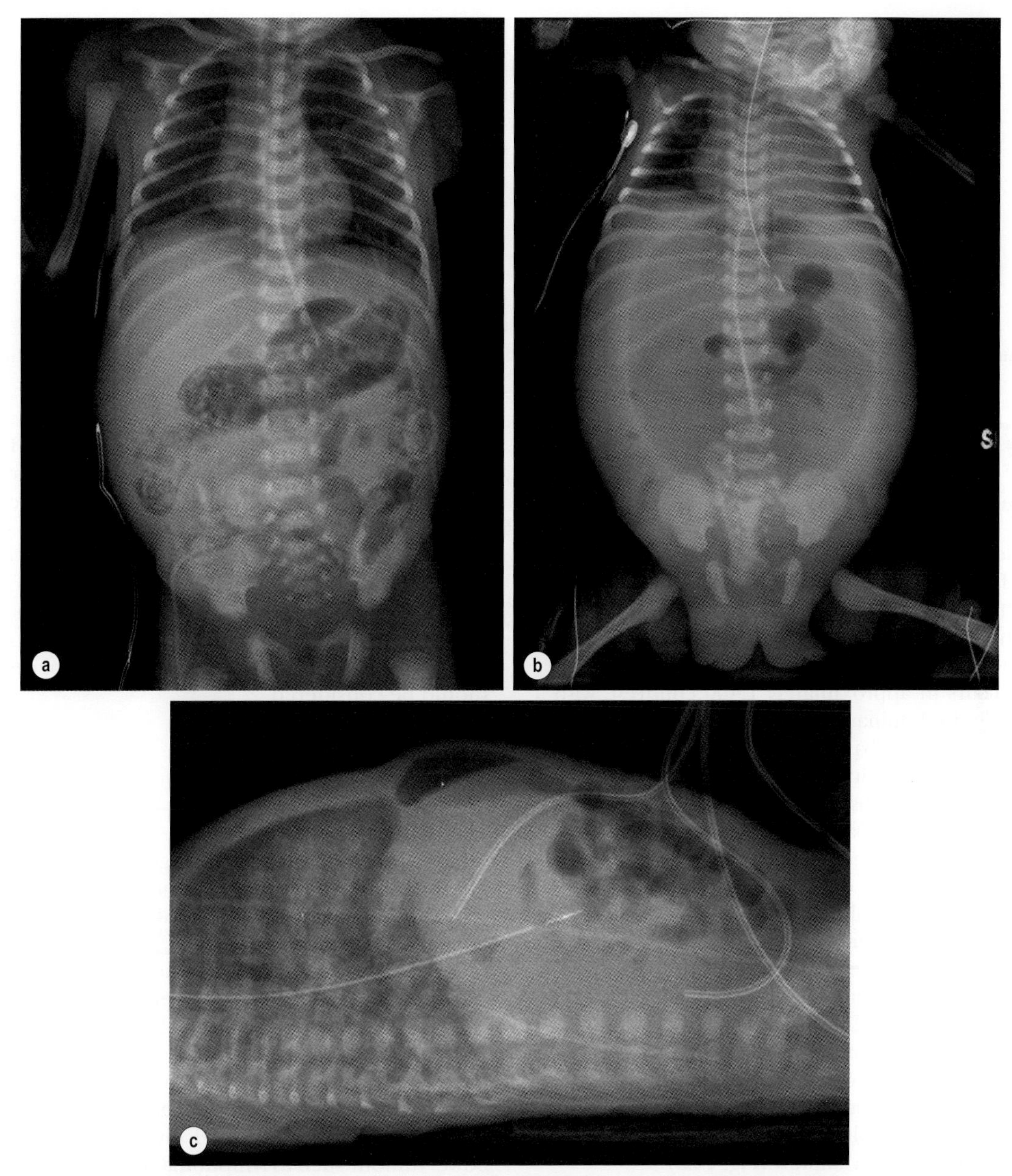

Figure 18.4 Abdominal radiographs of infants with necrotising enterocolitis. **(a)** Pneumatosis intestinalis. **(b)** 'Football sign' on supine film depicting intra-abdominal free air. **(c)** Free intra-abdominal air on lateral film.

general surgeon is unable to reduce the hernia and a paediatric surgeon is accessible, the patient should be referred immediately.

✔ If the hernia is reduced, repair should be undertaken 24–48 hours later, allowing some of the oedema to settle, but hopefully before re-incarceration.[15]

Inguinal hernia repair in infants can be performed using an open or laparoscopic technique.

ABDOMINAL WALL DEFECTS

Gastroschisis is characterised by an abdominal wall defect to the right of the umbilicus, through which most of the intestinal tract protrudes.[16] Omphalocele (also called exomphalos) is characterised by herniation of bowel with or without solid organs into the umbilical cord. Gastroschisis tends to be an isolated anomaly, whereas omphalocele is often associated with chromosomal, cardiac, renal, limb and facial anomalies.

If the diagnosis is made prenatally, delivery should occur at a centre with paediatric surgical support. Resuscitation and nasogastric decompression should begin in the delivery room. The bowel or sac should be wrapped in warm, saline-soaked, sterile gauze and covered with sterile plastic wrap to minimise heat and evaporative fluid loss.

Repair of both conditions should be done by an experienced paediatric surgeon. Options include primary closure, or staged closure using a preformed Silastic® silo that allows the bowel to be reduced gradually into the abdomen over 1–6 days.[17]

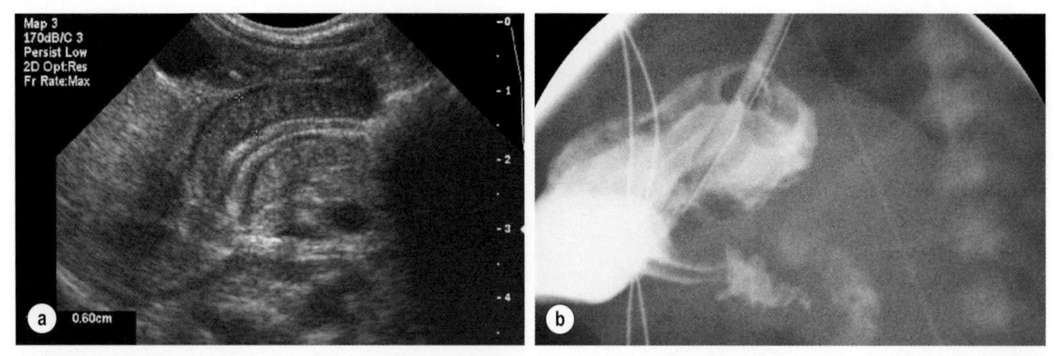

Figure 18.5 Images of hypertrophic pyloric stenosis. **(a)** Abdominal ultrasound. **(b)** Upper gastrointestinal contrast study.

INFANCY

HYPERTROPHIC PYLORIC STENOSIS

Hypertrophic pyloric stenosis (HPS) is an acquired condition in which the pylorus becomes abnormally thickened, causing gastric outlet obstruction. This occurs in infants during the first 2–12 weeks of life and is characterised by projectile, non-bilious vomiting, usually occurring after feeds. HPS occurs in approximately 1:400 children, with a significant male predominance.[18]

Diagnosis is suspected based on a history of progressive, forceful, non-bilious vomiting in a child of the appropriate age. Physical examination usually reveals some level of dehydration. The presence of a palpable 'olive' in the epigastrium has a 99% positive predictive value for the disease.[19] Vomiting of gastric contents leads to depletion of sodium, potassium and hydrochloric acid, resulting in the typical hypochloraemic, hypokalaemic metabolic alkalosis. The kidneys attempt to conserve sodium at the expense of hydrogen ions, often leading to paradoxical aciduria.[20] The level of dehydration can be estimated by clinical examination, urine output and serum chloride and bicarbonate levels. If the pyloric olive is not palpable, the diagnosis can be confirmed by ultrasound (pyloric length > 16 mm and single wall thickness > 3 mm). If an experienced sonographer is not available, the diagnosis can be made using a barium swallow (Fig. 18.5).

Surgery should be deferred until the infant is fully resuscitated. This is accomplished by using normal saline or Ringer's lactate with potassium. Most children should receive a bolus of 20 mL/kg, and then an infusion consisting of 1.5 times the maintenance requirement (i.e. 6 mL/kg/h for this age group) until the urine output and electrolytes have been normalised.

Surgical management of HPS consists of extramucosal longitudinal splitting of the pyloric muscle. The original procedure described by Ramstedt in 1912 was carried out through a transverse right upper quadrant incision.[21] This technique has been modified in many institutions to utilise circum-umbilical incisions or laparoscopic techniques. Following pyloromyotomy, many infants will experience continued vomiting for 24–48 hours, although the majority will eventually tolerate feeds and be discharged. Postoperative complications are rare but include wound infection, duodenal or gastric perforation and incomplete pyloromyotomy.

While intravenous access and fluid resuscitation can occur in most centres, some countries have experienced a centralisation of the surgical management of HPS to paediatric surgical centres only. Some evidence exists that there may be shorter postoperative stays and reduced complications in these centres.[22] We recommend that as long as the paediatric, anaesthetic and surgical teams are experienced and competent, and that as long as patient volumes allow for the maintenance of expertise, these patients can be managed in smaller centres. Otherwise, since the surgical procedure can be delayed, transfer to an experienced centre should be considered.

INTUSSUSCEPTION

Intussusception, or 'telescoping of the bowel', occurs when one portion of bowel invaginates into a more distant portion. This results in venous congestion, bowel wall oedema, intestinal obstruction and ultimately full-thickness necrosis of the intussusceptum. The peak incidence of intussusception is seen at 6–9 months of age.[23] The majority are ileocolic with hyperplastic lymphoid tissue in Peyer patches acting as a lead point.[24] These are often referred to as 'idiopathic'. Asymptomatic small bowel to small bowel intussusception may be seen incidentally on abdominal ultrasound, or sometimes may be associated with Henoch–Schonlein purpura or CF. Less than 5% of intussusceptions are due to a pathological lead point such as a Meckel diverticulum, polyp, or small bowel tumour such as lymphoma or leiomyoma. Intussusception occurring outside of the usual age range or those that recur should raise suspicion for a pathological lead point.

Few children with ileocolic intussusception will demonstrate the classic triad of intermittent severe abdominal pain with drawing up of the legs, palpable abdominal mass and 'red currant jelly' stool. Physicians must have a high index of suspicion due to the variability of symptoms. Patients may present with irritability, lethargy, abdominal pain, vomiting, diarrhoea or constipation, haematochezia, fever, dehydration or shock. Management should initially focus on diagnosis and resuscitation.

Following fluid resuscitation, imaging should be performed to confirm the diagnosis of intussusception. Abdominal radiograph may show air–fluid levels and distension of the small bowel and there may be a characteristic lack of air in the right lower quadrant. Ultrasonography has a high sensitivity and is currently the test of choice.[24]

✔ Traditionally, the treatment of intussusception has been barium enema. More recently, pneumatic reduction using air or CO_2 has been associated with an 80–95% success rate.[24]

If the intussusception is partially but not completely reduced, it is worth trying again a few hours later, since some of the oedema may have been eliminated by the first attempt and a second attempt may be associated with a 50% chance of success.[25] Pneumatic pressures of 60–100 mmHg are recommended.[26]

Surgical intervention is reserved for those patients who fail hydrostatic or pneumatic reduction, or have signs of infarcted or perforated bowel such as peritonitis, or free air on abdominal radiograph at the time of presentation. At laparotomy, the intussusception is manually reduced if possible. If the intussusception is not reducible, the bowel appears necrotic, or a pathological lead point is identified, a segmental resection should be performed with primary anastomosis. Excellent results using a laparoscopic approach to this condition have been documented.[27]

CHILDREN

APPENDICITIS

Appendicitis is the most frequent abdominal surgical emergency in children.[28] As in adults, the classic presentation is mid-abdominal pain moving to the right lower quadrant, anorexia, vomiting, low-grade fever and localised tenderness with peritoneal signs in the right lower quadrant. Presentation in children may be atypical, particularly in those under 5 years of age. Some authors have attempted to quantify the usefulness of specific findings in children using scoring systems. Clinical scoring systems such as the Alvarado Score and the Paediatric Appendicitis Score have been shown to be both sensitive and specific (Table 18.2).[29–31]

Table 18.2 Paediatric appendicitis score

Clinical findings	Points
Percussion/hopping tenderness/coughing	2
Anorexia	1
Pyrexia	1
Nausea or vomiting	1
RLQ tenderness	2
Leukocytosis (WBC > 10 000/μL)	1
Neutrophilia ('left shift')	1
Migration of pain to RLQ	1

A score of 6 or more has been shown to be associated with a high likelihood of the child having acute appendicitis.[30]
RLQ, right lower quadrant; *WBC*, white blood cell count.
Reproduced from Samuel M. Pediatric Appendicitis Score. J Pediatr Surg 2002;37(6):877–81. With permission from Elsevier.

In the otherwise well, stable patient with an equivocal presentation, the diagnostic options include observation with serial examinations, or imaging with ultrasound or computed tomography (CT) (Fig. 18.6). There is a great deal of controversy as to which technique is more appropriate. Ultrasound is clearly more operator-dependent, but the overuse of CT scans in childhood should be avoided due to the risk of radiation-induced malignancy later in life.[32] Both have excellent accuracy.

Increasingly, surgeons are using a laparoscopic approach to appendicectomy in children. As in adults, the benefits of the laparoscopic approach include reduced postoperative pain and length of stay, as well as a decrease in wound infection. There is some evidence that the rate of intra-abdominal abscess may be higher after laparoscopic appendicectomy in children with perforated appendicitis.[33] The laparoscopic approach may also be beneficial in children who are muscular or obese, and in adolescent females, where the incidence of ovarian pathology as a cause for the symptoms is higher.

There is some recent evidence in the adult literature that simple, non-perforated appendicitis may be safely managed with antibiotics alone, avoiding appendicectomy.[34] While there are some preliminary studies in children that suggest similar outcomes,[35–37] further evidence will be necessary before this approach can be recommended. This topic is discussed in more detail in Chapter 15.

Approximately 40% of children present with perforation, and the incidence is over 65% in those aged 0–4 years old.[28] In contrast to non-perforated appendicitis, these children usually present with prolonged symptoms, higher fever, higher white blood cell count and more diffuse peritoneal signs. Some children present with frank sepsis and diffuse peritoneal contamination; these children benefit from resuscitation, followed by immediate appendicectomy and peritoneal washout. Many children with perforated appendicitis present with a prolonged history and a localised abscess or phlegmon on imaging. This condition can be managed either by early operation, or by non-operative management

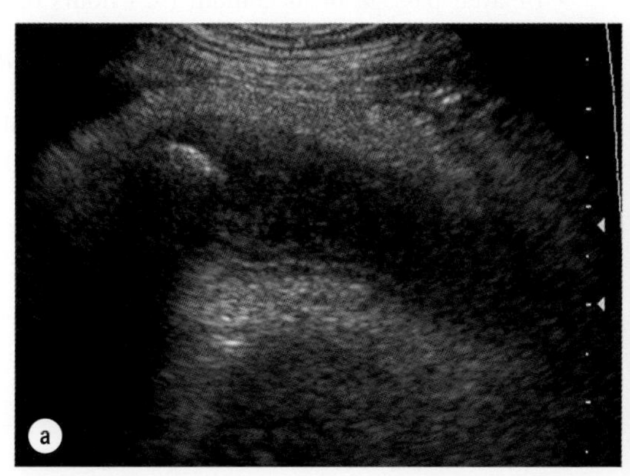

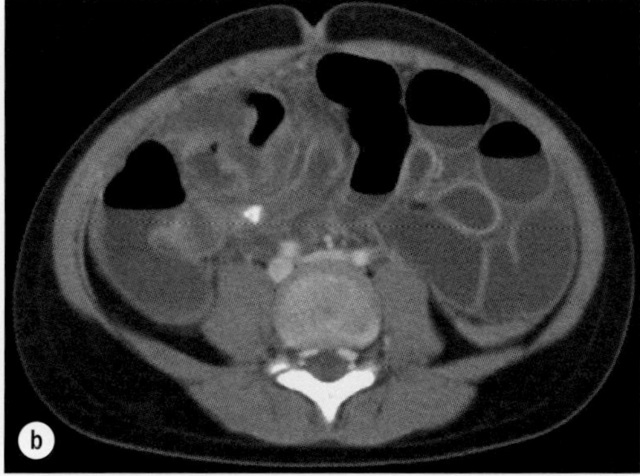

Figure 18.6 Ultrasound **(a)** and computed tomography **(b)** images of children with acute appendicitis. A faecolith is visible at the base of the inflamed appendix in both images.

consisting of broad-spectrum antibiotics and image-guided drainage of any purulent collections. The need for a subsequent interval appendectomy later is controversial. We reserve the use of interval appendicectomy for those with an appendicolith on imaging, since their risk of recurrent appendicitis is over 50%.[38] (See also Chapter 15.)

Evidence-based guidelines have been published to aid surgeons in choosing appropriate antibiotics for appendicitis, whether it is perforated or not.[39] While geographic variations in antimicrobial resistance need to be taken into account, we recommend generally following these guidelines.

FLUID RESUSCITATION OF THE CHILD WITH A SURGICAL EMERGENCY

Fluid and electrolyte management in children are made challenging by differences in total body water and compensatory mechanisms, as well as changes in physiology throughout childhood. Total body water is as high as 80% of body weight in neonates and decreases to the adult level of approximately 60% by 1 year. Degree of dehydration can be estimated from the history and physical examination. Children with mild dehydration (1–5% of body fluid volume) show few clinical signs but frequently have a history of 12–24 hours of vomiting or diarrhoea. Those with moderate dehydration (6–10%) are often lethargic, have low urine output (usually evident as fewer wet nappies), weight loss, loss of skin turgor, sunken eyes or fontanelle, dry mucus membranes and crying without tears. If severe dehydration (11–15%) is reached, the child may develop cardiovascular or neurological instability. Children have very active peripheral vasoconstriction so that blood pressure will be maintained until advanced intravascular volume depletion is reached with onset of hypotension, irritability or coma. However, tachycardia is an early sign that should be recognised and treated.[20]

The urgency of fluid replacement depends on the degree of dehydration and the cause of the fluid loss. The goals of treatment are the restoration and preservation of cardiovascular, neurological and renal perfusion. In the event of dehydration resulting from an inflammatory condition that will require urgent surgical intervention, such as appendicitis, isotonic fluid (normal saline or Ringer's lactate solution) should be given in 20 mL/kg boluses until signs of cardiovascular compromise subside. For situations in which there is no urgency to do an operation, such as pyloric stenosis, the fluid deficit can be replaced more slowly. This has the advantage of avoiding sudden fluid shifts, and the possibility of cerebral oedema and seizures, which are particularly likely in neonates and infants. The commonly used protocol is to calculate the fluid deficit and replace half over the first 8 hours, and the other half over the subsequent 16 hours.

PAEDIATRIC TRAUMA

The principles of trauma management are the same for children as they are for adults. Securing the airway and ensuring adequate ventilation are paramount before treating bleeding and circulatory collapse. Fluid resuscitation is based on the patient's size, keeping in mind the differences in physiological response to hypovolaemia mentioned in the previous section. As with adults, two boluses of crystalloid (20 mL/kg) should be given through large-bore intravenous lines as quickly as possible. If there is still suspicion for ongoing bleeding, blood products are in a balanced fashion with packed red blood cells, platelets and fresh-frozen plasma. Again, 20 mL/kg boluses should be the goal.

The principles of managing penetrating trauma in children are the same as in adults. However, children sustaining blunt abdominal trauma are more prone to solid organ injury due to the low-lying nature of these organs with respect to the paediatric rib cage and the relative laxity of the abdominal wall. In general, injuries to the spleen, liver and kidney can be managed non-operatively regardless of the grade of injury. Operations are rare for blunt abdominal trauma in children. The indications for laparotomy in a child with blunt abdominal trauma include: evidence of peritonitis on abdominal examination, free intra-abdominal air on imaging, inability to normalise haemodynamic status despite resuscitation efforts, rapidly expanding abdomen associated with persistent hypotension, and need for transfusion of more than one-half of the blood volume over 24 hours.

Key points

- Neonatal and complex surgery in children should ideally take place in specialised paediatric surgical units, with subspecialised paediatric surgical, anaesthetic and intensive care unit support.
- Resuscitation is the first step in the management of all children with surgical problems.
- *Beware the child whose vomit is green!* Bilious vomiting in a neonate or child is usually associated with intestinal obstruction, and every child with bilious vomiting should be assumed to have life-threatening malrotation and midgut volvulus until proven otherwise.
- A high index of suspicion for intussusception should be maintained in children in the high-risk age group (3–12 months of age) presenting with intermittent abdominal pain, vomiting and/or bloody stools.
- Delayed passage of meconium (>24 hours of life) should arouse suspicion of Hirschsprung disease.
- Incarcerated inguinal hernias should be reduced if possible, and repaired within 48 hours of reduction.
- Tachycardia is an important sign of intravascular fluid depletion in children; hypotension is a late finding.

References available at http://ebooks.health.elsevier.com/

Management of trauma for the general surgeon

19

Valentin Neuhaus | Pradeep H. Navsaria | Andrew John Nicol

INTRODUCTION

The global burden of disease related to trauma is immense, with more than 1.5 million deaths each year due to violence, 1.25 million deaths in road traffic accidents annually, and nearly 1 million children die each year because of injury.[1] These numbers are expected to increase in the next 20 years and trauma is among the top 10 causes of death globally.[2] The numbers of injured survivors have increased, with up to 1 billion patients seeking medical assistance after an injury annually,[3] and depending on the geographical location every eighth hospital admission now is related to injury. The associated global costs are excessive approaching 2% of a country's gross national product with respect to road accidents[4]; however, it must be emphasised that there are considerable variations between different countries.

The trimodal death distribution, first described by Trunkey in 1983, may have changed in the past years, but it remains a good model to understand the timing and causes of death following injury.[5,6] The first peak relates to patients with non-survivable injuries (e.g. complete aortic rupture). Despite preventive measures (e.g. seat-belts, airbags, helmets, avoiding drunk-driving), which remarkably reduces the first peak and the years of life lost, injuries continue to cause death and morbidity.[3] The majority of patients die within the first 24 hours after an accident,[7] and this second peak comprises patients arriving alive in the emergency department, with head, thoracic and abdominal/pelvic injuries being the predominant lethal injuries. Unrecognised or untreated abdominal injury is one of the most important causes of preventable death.[8] One of the main goals of trauma surgery is to diminish this peak and Advanced Trauma Life Support (ATLS®) with its primary and secondary survey is one way to evaluate and treat severely injured patients in this phase.[9] The third peak comprises patients dying at a later stage due to multiorgan failure and sepsis.

✔✔ The Advanced Trauma Life Support (ATLS®) guidelines are a crucial part of the early evaluation and management of all trauma patients.[8]

Trauma surgery has evolved tremendously over the past 50 years. The traditional dogma of mandatory exploration of all penetrating wounds has changed to selective non-operative management (NOM) in neck and abdominal trauma.[10–12] Damage control surgery and damage control resuscitation have been introduced. Abdominal compartment syndrome and intra-abdominal hypertension have been identified and strategies put in place for prevention. Early institution of blood and lower volumes of crystalloids are seemingly beneficial. There is a far better understanding of coagulopathy in the trauma setting and specific transfusions ratios have been shown to improve survival. A more restrictive transfusion regime is also associated with less infection.[13] Imaging is far more frequently available and the introduction of focused assessment with sonography in trauma (FAST) and extended FAST (eFAST) in the resuscitation room is changing surgical algorithms. There is much to be enthusiastic about in our management of the injured patient, but we also need to be aware of the fact that clinical signs are vital in our assessment and that there should not be an over-reliance on special investigations.

EVALUATION OF THE INJURED PATIENT

PRIMARY AND SECONDARY SURVEY, DAMAGE CONTROL SURGERY, TRANSFER

The goal of the primary survey is to identify and instantaneously treat life-threatening injuries. This early management phase is called the 'golden hour'.[14] Pre-hospital and in-hospital time plays an important role in this resuscitation phase as the mortality is highest within the first 24 hours after the incident.[15] Patients are assessed and resuscitated along the ATLS **ABCDE** algorithm. The following life-threatening injuries must be ruled out:[9]

- **A**irway: airway obstruction (due to foreign bodies, aspiration, facial or laryngeal injuries)
- **B**reathing: tension pneumothorax, open pneumothorax with a sucking wound, massive haemothorax, cardiac tamponade, flail chest
- **C**irculation: shock (mainly caused by haemorrhage)
- **D**isability: severe traumatic brain injury
- **E**xposure: hypothermia

The pathophysiological consequences of these injuries are *hypoxia* (caused by airway or breathing problems), hypotension/*hypoperfusion* (caused by circulation problems) and *hypothermia* (exposure problem). Hypoxia and hypoperfusion result in anaerobic metabolism with accumulation of acidic metabolites, a deficiency of adenosine triphosphate (ATP) and failure of the Na/K-ATPase pump. This failure causes cell swelling and damage, and finally organ dysfunction. Serum lactate, pH and base excess are good parameters to assess the adequacy of organ perfusion and oxygenation. Higher lactate level and the duration of hyperlactatemia correlate with mortality after trauma.[16] Hypoperfusion also leads to increased excretion of stress hormones, which consecutively increases the contractility of the heart, the heart rate as an early sign of relevant blood loos and local vasoconstriction with hypoperfusion of the skin, muscles, kidneys and the intestine (centralisation). Blood pressure drops later with ongoing blood loss and exhausted compensatory mechanisms. Heat loss while lying exposed, cold intravenous fluids and opened body cavities during surgery cause hypothermia. Hypothermia itself negatively influences the coagulation system and myocardial function. The three 'hypo'-problems lead to the well-known deadly triad of *hypothermia, acidosis* and *coagulopathy*.[17]

The treatment in this primary phase is priority-oriented and kept as simple as possible.[9]

All patients are given supplemental oxygen. A definitive airway (intubation or surgical cricothyroidotomy) will clear any airway obstruction. Needle decompression and intercostal drains usually resolve any life-threatening tension or open pneumothoraces. A thoracotomy is required for a massive haemothorax (>1500 mL drainage) or for ongoing bleeding (>200 mL/h for the next 4 hours), patients in profound refractory shock or undergoing cardiopulmonary resuscitation after penetrating trauma. The main goal in circulation problems is to stop the bleeding and restore the volume. Chest (e.g. intercostal arteries), abdomen (mainly spleen, liver, mesentery or kidneys), pelvis or long bones (fractures) and external wounds (with vascular injuries, extensive scalp or torso injuries) are the main sources. Intercostal drains, direct compression, packing, or (partial) resection of bleeding organs, aortic cross-clamping, Pringle manoeuvre, vessel repair or shunting are some basic techniques to stop the bleeding. Unstable pelvic fractures are temporarily stabilised by a pelvic binder, C-clamp or external fixator. Long bone fractures are externally or internally stabilised to reduce bleeding, alleviate pain and enable intensive care. A damage control resuscitation in patients with major haemorrhage can improve outcome: minimised, balanced, volume resuscitation, especially in penetrating injuries, until early successful bleeding control, but an adequate volume substitution and pharmacologic adjuncts (tranexamic acid) have then to be carried out and adequate urine excretion has to be achieved.[18,19] Using the Glasgow Coma Scale (GCS), a patient with a score less than 9 must be intubated and evaluated with a computed tomography (CT) scan of the brain. The CT of the brain should be delayed in the case of a patient who is haemodynamically unstable requiring operative intervention. Warm infusions, blankets or warming devices such as a Bair Hugger 3 M© are used to limit and treat hypothermia.

DAMAGE CONTROL SURGERY

Further relevant injuries can now be sought and treated in the next phase, the 'secondary survey', usually carried out from head to toe. Basically, definitive repair of all relevant injuries is the main target. However, the extent of these therapeutic measures as well as the surgical procedures in the primary survey must be considered. Trauma causes a first hit and a consecutive systemic inflammatory response syndrome (SIRS), which can trigger reduced resistance to infection. Early extensive surgical care of all injuries, acting as a second hit, can lead to a further immune response with resultant multiorgan dysfunction, failure or even death.[20] In addition, if certain criteria are met (e.g., hypotension on admission, abdominal vascular and major liver injuries), only abbreviated operative procedures, so-called *damage control surgery*, should be applied.[21] Damage control surgery is a well-established surgical strategy, mainly in major abdominal trauma, but also in other conditions, and should enable patients not to slip further into an unsalvageable metabolic state of the deadly triad of hypothermia, acidosis and coagulopathy.[22–24] Damage control surgery aims to quickly stop the bleeding and limit contamination without restoration of the anatomy (e.g. to pack or remove solid organs, staple bowel injuries and to temporarily close the abdomen), and to normalise the pathophysiological parameters in the intensive care unit (ICU).[25] No major surgery is carried out during this ICU stage. Oxygen delivery, blood pressure, heart rate, urinary output, body temperature, pH, lactate and coagulation must be normalised in the ICU. Aggressive volume resuscitation, abdominal packing and the accumulation of intra-abdominal blood increase the risk of an abdominal compartment syndrome in some of these patients and the intra-abdominal pressure should therefore be monitored (IAP > 20 mmHg with new organ dysfunction).[26] Reduction in cardiac output, renal failure, impaired ventilation and raised intracranial pressure are several pathophysiological consequences of raised intra-abdominal pressure (see Chapter 20). After normalisation of these parameters, a re-look is performed with definitive surgical care and primary abdominal wall closure without mesh if possible. The timing here is crucial; the possible consequences are re-bleeding if returned too early, and infection and sepsis if returned too late to the theatre to remove abdominal packing.[27] Patients ideally remain intubated, ventilated, under antibiotic cover and return to theatre 24–48 hours after the first operation.

The following pathophysiological parameters, signs and criteria are indicators to proceed with damage control surgery:[22,28]

- Hypothermia < 35°C
- Acidosis pH < 7.2
- Lactate > 5mmol/L
- Coagulopathy INR > 1.5
- Systolic blood pressure < 90 mmHg
- Mass transfusion (10 and more blood units)
- Trauma mechanism (e.g. multiple torso gunshot wounds [GSWs])
- Injury Severity Score (ISS) > 36 points
- Major vascular (e.g. inferior vena cava injury) and visceral or pelvic injuries
- Higher age and comorbidities
- Inability to control bleeding by conventional methods
- Inability to close the abdomen
- Abdominal compartment syndrome during attempted abdominal wall closure
- Need to reassess extent of bowel viability

Referral patterns

Depending on the hospital facilities, some care cannot be provided locally and the patients must be transferred as soon as possible to a trauma centre or another suitable facility. Typical injuries warranting a transfer are:[9]

- Severe or moderate head injury
- Major pulmonary contusions

- Flail chest
- Cardiac or great vessel injury
- Acute spinal cord injury
- Solid organ injuries
- Unstable pelvic ring injury
- Severe open fractures or amputations
- Several long bone fractures
- Polytraumatised patients
- Severe burns
- Older patients (>55 years) or patients with comorbidities

Patients with these injuries are ideally treated in a level I trauma centre which has been associated with better outcomes and improved survival.[29]

REGIONAL INJURIES

INJURY SCORING SCALES

The American Association for the Surgery of Trauma (AAST) publishes the most widely accepted and used injury classification system for neck, chest and abdominal injuries, which is available online at http://www.aast.org/Library/TraumaTools/InjuryScoringScales.aspx. Organ injuries are graded into five increasing severity categories, grade I being minor haematomas or lacerations and grade V completely shattered or devascularised organ injuries.

✔✔ These injury severity scores are important as they help to guide treatment, have a prognostic value and allow the comparison of results in the literature.[30]

BLUNT AND PENETRATING ABDOMINAL TRAUMA

Abdominal organs are less protected than those of the chest. General surgeons are consequently often confronted with intra-abdominal trauma. The timing of assessment and treatment depends on the haemodynamic status of the patient and the clinical evaluation. In the primary survey, a clinical evaluation of the haemodynamic status, the abdomen and a FAST is required, particularly in blunt trauma or suspected haemopericardium. Haemodynamic stability is defined as systolic blood pressure > 90 mmHg, pulse rate < 100/min *and* no more than 1–2 L of crystalloid infusion.[31] Vital signs must be cautiously interpreted, especially in elderly patients, young patients and patients who are under the influence of certain medications and always be correlated with the injuries and metabolic response of the patient.[32] A narrowed pulse pressure in normotensive patients can be a subtle warning sign of haemorrhage.[33]

A thorough clinical evaluation is required in the secondary survey, with inspection, palpation, percussion and auscultation. Repeated examination is the key as physical signs may be delayed or altered in the case of drunk or drugged patients, patients with traumatic brain injuries, acute spinal cord injuries and with distracting injuries. Adjuncts (nasogastric tube, urinary catheter, FAST, CT of the abdomen, diagnostic laparoscopy [DL]) are helpful tools, particularly in these patients to rule in or out a relevant intra-abdominal injury.

The most important method in clinically evaluable patients remains serial clinical examination. In penetrating trauma, the authors do not recommend ultrasound of the abdomen or invasive procedures such as local wound exploration or diagnostic peritoneal lavage.

The further priority of assessment and treatment is dictated by the mechanism of injury, sustained injuries, haemodynamic status of the patient and clinical evaluation. Typical indications to proceed with a laparotomy are:[9]

- Haemodynamic instability due to an intra-abdominal injury (positive ultrasound or clinical evidence of intraperitoneal bleeding)
- Peritonitis (tenderness of the abdomen and abdominal guarding)
- Organ evisceration
- GSWs with a transabdominal trajectory
- Confirmed stomach, rectum or genitourinary system (bladder, ureter, vagina) injuries after penetrating trauma
- Free intra-abdominal air
- Hollow viscus rupture or perforation
- Patient develops peritoneal signs or haemodynamic instability after failed NOM.

A few decades ago, all penetrating wounds mandated a laparotomy. More than 30% of the laparotomies were negative (no intra-abdominal injuries) or non-therapeutic (the intra-abdominal injury does not need any intervention).[34] Short-term morbidity of a trauma laparotomy is high (wound infection, intra-abdominal abscess, pneumonia, urinary tract infection, deep venous thrombosis, pulmonary embolus) and long-term complications (small-bowel obstruction and incisional hernia) are encountered in 15% after trauma laparotomy.[35,36] This is independent of whether the laparotomy was therapeutic or unnecessary. To reduce unnecessary laparotomies and their consequences, selective NOM was developed in asymptomatic and haemodynamically normal patients. Lower transfusion requirements, fewer abdominal infections, shorter hospitalisation, lower mortality and lower costs are positive consequences of NOM.[37,38] The decision to proceed with NOM is crucial. The fear of re-bleeding, missing a hollow viscus injury and the consequences of a delayed laparotomy are still constant companions.[39] The fear may be exaggerated since delayed laparotomies do not increase the risk of adverse events if carried out within 12–24 hours.[40] Serial examinations are mandatory to detect failure of NOM and to act appropriately in a timely fashion, with risk factors for failed NOM being age older than 55, haemodynamic instability, higher specific organ and total injury severity grade, size of haemoperitoneum, contrast blush on CT and use of anticoagulants. Angioembolisation may play an important role in patients with these risk factors and solid organ injuries.[41]

SPECIAL INVESTIGATIONS

Focused assessment with sonography in trauma

FAST is a non-invasive, cheap, easily reproducible, focused examination of the chest and abdomen, which can be performed at the bedside by the treating trauma surgeon. The primary goal of FAST is to detect free fluid (presumably blood in a trauma patient) in the abdomen, chest or the pericardium, as an explanation for the haemodynamic instability of a patient. The goal *is* not to detect distinct organ injuries. FAST can be carried out within 5 minutes, with the specificity to detect free fluid in blunt trauma being 90–100% and sensitivity 60–100%.[42,43] FAST, however, is operator-dependent, despite an easy learning curve.[44] False-negative results are misleading and often seen in patients with obesity or surgical emphysema. The ultrasound can be falsely negative if it is performed too early, as it needs more than 500 mL of blood in Morrison's pouch to be visible.[45,46] FAST performed too early is associated with more interventions.[47] Ideal indications are blunt torso trauma, haemopericardium, children and pregnant patients. The goal of eFAST is to diagnose a pneumothorax, which can be done with a higher sensitivity than a chest X-ray.[42]

Computed tomography

Contrast-enhanced CT is the gold standard to detect and grade torso injuries in stable patients as well as to rule out significant injuries.[48] Contrast blushes can also represent active bleeding spots, which are amenable to angiographic embolisation. It is non-invasive, but it usually requires transport to radiology, time and is expensive.[9] Contrast material can cause allergic reactions and induce nephropathy. The overall accuracy and sensitivity is high except for diaphragmatic, bowel and some pancreatic injuries.[49] A special algorithm is needed for diaphragmatic injuries (see later in this chapter). The index of suspicion of bowel injuries is high in the presence of:

- free fluid and no solid-organ injury,
- free extraluminal gas,
- thickened bowel wall,
- mesenteric stranding and
- haematoma surrounding a hollow viscus.

Ideal indications for CT are stable patients with blunt trauma, penetrating back or flank trauma, penetrating trauma with questionable extraperitoneal tract, right upper quadrant/right-sided thoraco-abdominal trajectory (i.e. to exclude liver injury) and haematuria (i.e. to exclude upper urinary tract injury). In transpelvic penetrating wounds with haematuria, a CT cystogram is helpful to guide further treatment.[9,38] It is currently not clear if routine or selective scanning is recommended in polytraumatised patients, where there is a clear trend to a whole-body CT.[39,50]

Diagnostic and therapeutic laparoscopy

Laparoscopy is a minimally invasive procedure; however, it requires special expensive equipment, surgical skills and usually general anaesthesia. There is as yet no role for DL in the haemodynamically unstable patient, as pneumoperitoneum further compromises the haemodynamic, pulmonary and renal status. In elective trauma situations, it has been successfully used in diagnosis and repair of peritoneal breach, stomach, minor liver, suspected extraperitoneal rectal and, specifically, diaphragmatic injuries. It can help to avoid a laparotomy in a highly selected patient group.[51,52]

BLUNT TRAUMA

The spleen (40–55%), liver (35–45%) and small bowel (5–10%) are the most frequently injured organs in blunt abdominal trauma.[9] Major pelvic or chest injuries are commonly associated with relevant intra-abdominal injuries, and serial clinical examination usually detects these injuries. A seat belt sign or a buckle-handle injury raises the suspicion

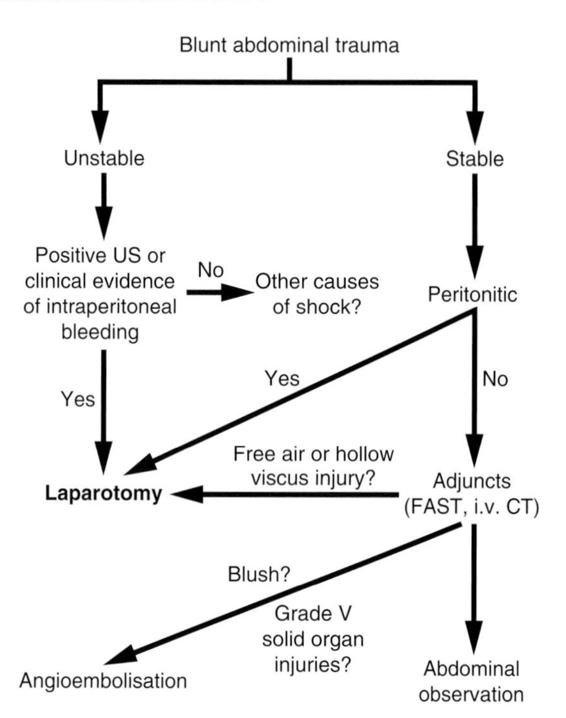

Figure 19.1 Management of blunt abdominal trauma. *CT,* computed tomography; *FAST,* focused assessment with sonography in trauma; *US,* ultrasound.

of a mesenteric, duodenal or pancreatic injury and such patients need admission and further investigations.[9] NOM has become the standard of care in most patients with solid organ injuries with no indications to proceed with laparotomy (predominantly *haemodynamic instability* due to major haemorrhage). FAST or CT are most often used as adjuncts in NOM. *Hollow viscus rupture* and/or *peritonitis* are still clear indications to proceed with operative treatment. Free air or free intra-abdominal fluid without parenchymatous organ injuries must raise the suspicion of a hollow viscus or mesenteric injury and mandates a laparotomy, especially in patients with a severe head injury or complete spinal cord injury due to unreliable physical examination.[53]

Fig. 19.1 presents an algorithm for the management of blunt abdominal trauma.

Spleen

The spleen provides important immunological function by clearing intravascular antigens, hence infectious complications are feared after splenectomy. Demetriades et al.[54] analysed 269 patients with blunt splenic trauma, one-third of whom underwent splenectomy. Wound infection, intra-abdominal abscess, urinary tract infection, pneumonia and septicaemia were complications encountered in 32% of the splenectomy group versus 5.2% in the splenic preservation group, with splenectomy raising the infection risk 10 times. Other relevant risk factors for infections were hypotension on admission, an ISS > 16 and hollow viscus injury. The recommendation is therefore to preserve the spleen if possible.

Splenic preservation, however, is not always feasible. *Haemodynamic instability* and a severely blunt injured spleen remain a clear indication to proceed with laparotomy and probable splenectomy. In a large retrospective case series of the most severe splenic injuries (AAST grade IV and V),

58% of all patients were initially managed non-operatively.[55] NOM failed in 38%, mostly within 48 hours. Risk factors were *grade V splenic injuries, concomitant brain injury and contrast extravasation on CT.* Age (>55 years), anticoagulation drugs, cirrhosis and the need for blood transfusion must also be taken into account.[56] Either surgery should be undertaken in these patients, or angioembolisation if patients are stable but have contrast extravasation.[57] Prophylactic splenic arterial embolisation in patients at high risk for splenectomy (splenic pseudoaneurysm, splenic arteriovenous fistulas, AIS 3 and higher) was not superior to surveillance and embolisation as required in a randomised study.[58] Interestingly, the use of anticoagulation (e.g. warfarin) did not affect the outcome of spleen (and liver) injuries.[59] Patients after angioembolisation of the splenic artery also had higher rates of deep venous thrombosis.[60] Angioembolisation may cause a reactive thrombocytosis and hence a higher risk of deep venous thrombosis. Early prophylaxis should be considered in these patients.

✔✔ Grade V splenic injuries, especially in combination with a head injury, predict failure of non-operative management.[45]

Delayed haemorrhage, splenic artery pseudoaneurysm, splenic abscess or pseudocyst are complications after NOM. However, a 6-hourly serial physical examination and haemoglobin (Hb) estimation in a high-dependency unit (HDU) or ICU with bed rest for 1–2 days seems to be safe to avoid and detect these complications. Mechanical deep venous prophylaxis can be started immediately. Medical prophylaxis can be started after 48 hours without a higher risk of bleeding or NOM failure in isolated blunt splenic injury.[61–64] Length of in-hospital observation remains unclear; however, 5–7 days or even less in isolated minor splenic injuries with unproblematic observation seems acceptable.[65] Activities should be restricted for 6 weeks.

All patients after splenectomy should receive active pneumococcal and meningococcal vaccination within 2–3 weeks after the operation as well as seasonal flu vaccination.[66,67]

LIVER

Patient selection is crucial for NOM of blunt liver trauma. A large study at our institution analysed 134 patients with blunt liver injuries.[37] One in four patients required urgent surgery due to haemodynamic instability (31%), peritonitis (46%) or CT findings mandating surgery other than the liver injury (23%). Systolic blood pressure < 90 mmHg at admission was present in more patients. However, hypotension on arrival was successfully treated in 70% with a fluid bolus of no more than 1–2 L of crystalloid transfusion. These patients did not need surgery for the liver injury. The remaining patients were non-responders and required surgery. Operative management comprising evacuation of haematoma and drainage only was needed in 37% of patients. Liver-related complications were encountered in 20% after surgery: necrosis, haemobilia and biliary fistula. NOM was initiated in three quarters of patients consisting of serial clinical examinations and Hb estimations in HDU or ICU, with no routine follow-up CTs. NOM was successful in 95%. Increasing abdominal pain and tenderness, spiking temperature, drop in blood pressure or a fall in Hb level were typical indicators of NOM failure. Liver-related complications were encountered in 7%: biloma, biliary peritonitis, liver haematoma and abdominal compartment syndrome. We concluded that NOM is safe, feasible and successful in selected patients. Patients for NOM must be *stable, not peritonitic,* and *amenable for clinical evaluation.* A CT scan with intravenous contrast should always be performed for patients managed by NOM.[68]

Similar results were presented by Van der Wilden et al.,[69] who analysed 393 patients with AAST grade IV and V blunt liver injuries. One-third of the patients proceeded to surgery due to haemodynamic instability. The remaining two-thirds of patients were managed non-operatively, which was successful in 91%. Failure of NOM occurred due to recurrent liver bleeding or biliary peritonitis. We concluded that even high-grade liver injuries with haemoperitoneum and contrast extravasation can safely be treated non-operatively, which contrasts with high-grade splenic injuries. Importantly, nearly 70% of all NOM patients had a diffuse haemoperitoneum, 27% demonstrated contrast extravasation on CT and one quarter of all patients in their NOM group had angioembolisation of the liver.

Mechanical thromboprophylaxis, feeding and mobilisation should be started as early as possible in stable patients with NOM and no contraindications.[68,70] Medical thromboprophylaxis can be started after 48(–72) hours in grade 3–5 liver injuries.[62,64]

✔✔ Most blunt liver injuries can be managed non-operatively in the stable patient.[50]

KIDNEYS

Low-grade blunt kidney injuries, such as kidney contusions, are successfully treated non-operatively. The evidence for higher-grade injuries is unclear. Haemodynamic instability and/or urine extravasation are indications to proceed with surgery, which generally means nephrectomy. A study that analysed 206 patients with AAST grade IV and V blunt kidney injuries demonstrated that one in four patients needed an urgent laparotomy due to haemodynamic instability. Nearly 60% of these patients underwent a nephrectomy. In three quarters of patients, NOM was started and successfully accomplished in 92%. Angioembolisation was undertaken in every sixth patient. Haemodynamic instability, peritonitis or abdominal compartment syndrome were the reasons for NOM failure. The authors concluded that even higher-grade blunt kidney injuries with urine extravasation in haemodynamically stable patients can safely be treated non-operatively.[71]

BLADDER

In patients with gross haematuria and possible bladder injury, a CT cystography is recommended to rule out bladder injuries. Intraperitoneal bladder injuries must be repaired, while simple extraperitoneal injuries can be treated non-operatively with a urinary catheter in place for 10 days. However, if the anterior pelvic ring is approached, also an extraperitoneal injury should be repaired. Simple repairs in asymptomatic patients can be followed up clinically, all other injuries need a follow-up cystogram.[72]

ABDOMINAL STAB AND LOW-VELOCITY GUNSHOT WOUNDS

Penetrating wounds between the nipple line and the knees can potentially cause intra-abdominal injuries. The difficult questions to answer are: (1) has the peritoneum has been penetrated; and (2) an intra-abdominal injury requiring surgery has occurred. Penetrating wounds with solid organ injuries can still be managed non-operatively in many selected cases.[73]

STAB WOUNDS

Stab wounds do not penetrate the peritoneum in one-third of the patients, particularly after being stabbed to the flank or the back due to the thick muscle layers. If penetration of the peritoneum has occurred, only 50–75% of patients have an injury requiring surgery.[74] Intra-abdominal stab wounds most commonly injure the liver (40%), small bowel (30%), diaphragm (20%) and colon (15%).[9] A study of 186 patients with abdominal stab wounds[75] found that 40% of the patients had a laparotomy.[12,76] Indications to proceed with surgery were haemodynamic instability, peritonitis, organ evisceration or a high spinal cord injury in addition to the abdominal stab wound. In 5%, the laparotomy was deemed negative or non-therapeutic and overall mortality rate was 1%. Furthermore, 60% of patients were treated non-operatively, which was successful in 90% of cases. The remaining 10% developed positive abdominal signs and subsequently underwent a laparotomy. In 33% of these patients, the laparotomy was unnecessary. The authors concluded that *unstable* patients, patients with an *acute abdomen* or *organ evisceration* need urgent surgery. Asymptomatic and haemodynamically stable patients can however selectively and safely be treated with 4-hourly serial physical abdominal examination, recording of vital signs (blood pressure, heart rate, respiratory rate and temperature) and Hb estimation over a 24-hour period. CT of the abdomen was only recommended in patients with haematuria, since the main indications for operation are reliably detected by serial clinical examination and the tract of the stab wound is hard to visualise on a CT scan.[77]

✔✔ Selective non-operative management for abdominal stab injuries in stable patients is safe and effective.[30,54]

Organ evisceration mandated provisional closure of any apparent perforations and extension of the stab wound under local anaesthesia to reduce entrapped and congested bowel to avoid strangulation in the emergency room. In mildly symptomatic, haemodynamically stable patients, *omentum eviscerating* through the wound was successfully ligated, resected, pushed back into the abdomen, and the fascia closed in the emergency room without laparotomy, as confirmed in another study.[78] *Haematuria* in unstable, peritonitic or patients with organ evisceration was an indication for a single-shot intravenous pyelogram (IVP) with an iodinated contrast medium (e.g. 100 mL of Ultravist 300 [Bayer, Germany]) to demonstrate both kidneys are functioning in case a nephrectomy is required. In the NOM group, haematuria was further investigated with an abdominal CT scan with intravenous contrast to assess the severity of the kidney injury. Only AAST grade V kidney injuries (completely shattered kidney or avulsion of renal hilum that devascularises the kidney) were an indication for surgery.[75]

Penetrating *retroperitoneal injuries* of the colon, duodenum or urinary tract are difficult to detect clinically. However, according to a large prospective study, stab wounds to the flank or back should be managed the same way as anterior stab wounds.[79] Because of these clinical difficulties, some trauma surgeons ask for a triple-contrast CT to rule out retroperitoneal injures in stable asymptomatic patients with penetrating back or flank trauma. CT findings mandating a laparotomy are:[74]

- Contrast extravasation from colon
- Major urine extravasation from kidney
- Haematoma adjacent to major retroperitoneal vessel
- Free air in retroperitoneum, not attributed to wounding object
- Evidence of injury above and below diaphragm
- Free fluid in peritoneal cavity

Fig. 19.2 presents an algorithm for management of abdominal stab wounds. Based on clinical resources and preferences local wound exploration or diagnostic imaging are alternatives to serial clinical exams.[80]

GUNSHOT WOUNDS

GSWs transmit a higher energy and are more destructive than stab injuries. If the peritoneum is breached, the likelihood of having an intra-abdominal injury is nearly 100%. Small bowel (50%), colon (40%), liver (30%) and abdominal vessels (25%) are most commonly injured.[9] Some algorithms require prompt laparotomy for abdominal GSWs regardless of the clinical situation. This approach, however, results in 5–30% of unnecessary laparotomies, especially in GSW to the flank or the back, with complication rates up to 40%. On the other hand, the major concern of NOM is missing a hollow viscus injury. The decision to proceed with NOM is critical.

A large prospective study of 1106 patients with an abdominal GSW from our hospital[38] showed that three out of four patients needed an urgent laparotomy—in a similar study, we found a laparotomy rate of 71% (therapeutic in 92%).[12] *Peritonitis, haemodynamic instability* or *ongoing blood loss* (more than 4 units of packed red blood cells within 24 hours) were clear indications to proceed with an operation. Only 3.5% were unnecessary laparotomies and the mortality was nearly 7%. On the other hand, one in four patients were treated non-operatively, with a success rate of 95% and no GSW-related death. The indication for NOM was a haemodynamically normal patient without signs of peritonitis and an intact level of consciousness. Most patients with NOM had a CT, and to continue with NOM the CT must show no active extravasation and the tract of the bullet must be away from the stomach, duodenum, small and large bowel. NOM consisted of 4-hourly serial physical abdominal examinations, recording of vital signs (blood pressure, heart rate, respiratory rate and temperature) and Hb estimation over a 24-hour period in HDU with continuous haemodynamic monitoring. We concluded that NOM is safe and feasible in selected patients with abdominal GSW, and serial clinical examination and selective use of CT scanning is essential. This is confirmed in studies from New England, California and in a meta-analysis.[81–83] NOM is even safe in hemodynamically stable, not peritonitic patients with liver GSW.[84] Unstable patients and patients with peritonitis remain clear indications

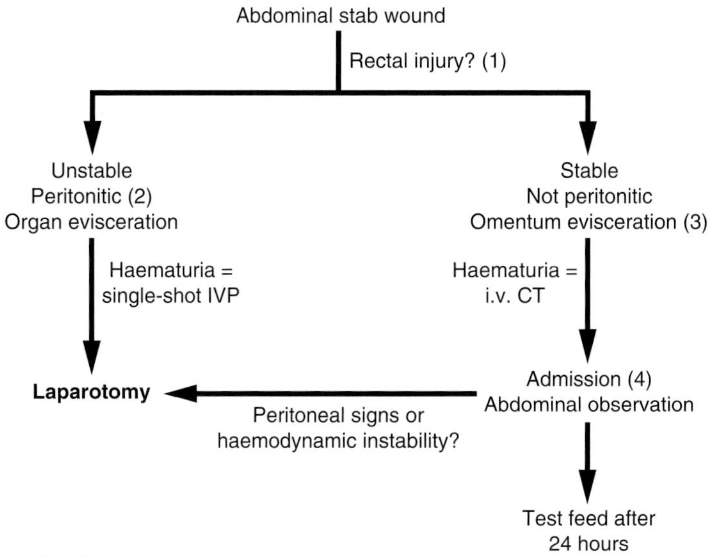
Abdominal stab wound
Rectal injury? (1)
Unstable
Peritonitic (2)
Organ evisceration
Stable
Not peritonitic
Omentum evisceration (3)
Haematuria =
single-shot IVP
Haematuria =
i.v. CT
Laparotomy
Admission (4)
Abdominal observation
Peritoneal signs or
haemodynamic instability?
Test feed after
24 hours
(1) See 'Rectal injury algorithm'
(2) Low threshold to proceed with laparotomy in patients with a high spinal cord injury or severe head injury in addition to the abdominal stab wound, or intoxicated patients
(3) Diagnostic laparoscopy in left thoraco-abdominal omental evisceration or persistent left upper quadrant tenderness – after 24 hours' observation
(4) No local wound exploration or diagnostic peritoneal lavage recommended

Figure 19.2 Management of abdominal stab wounds. *CT,* computed tomography; *IVP,* intravenous pyelogram.

for operative management. Furthermore, patients with disabilities (severe head injury or acute spinal cord injuries) or intoxicated patients must undergo an urgent operation due to the unreliable physical examinations.

Fig. 19.3 presents an algorithm for the management of abdominal GSWs.

Small bowel, colon and rectum

Such injuries can usually be primarily repaired if less than 50% of the bowel wall is involved. If more than 50% of the bowel wall is involved or devascularisation of the bowel segment has occurred, resection and primary anastomosis is still possible in haemodynamically stable patients, with an ISS < 25, without peritonitis and no significant underlying diseases.[85] According to a meta-analysis of the Eastern Association for the Surgery of Trauma, a colostomy is not recommended in these circumstances.[86]

Rectal surgery is technically more demanding and repair not always feasible. Penetrating rectum injuries have a still higher morbidity and mortality and therefore need special considerations. Debridement, distal wash-out, diverting colostomy and presacral drainage were the mainstays of rectal injuries in the past. This has however changed to a simpler approach as reported in an analysis of 118 rectal injuries from our institution.[87] Digital rectal and proctosigmoidoscopic examinations were standard assessments in patients with a missile trajectory near the pelvis and a possible rectal injury. The examinations were positive in 73%, and respectively 89% for intraluminal blood. The goal of these examinations was not to visualise the injury but to verify intraluminal blood. All intraperitoneal rectal injuries were successfully primarily repaired with or without diversion. Extraperitoneal injuries remained untouched and only a sigmoid loop colostomy protected the rectum for 3 months. All patients received triple antibiotic treatment for 24 hours (penicillin, gentamicin and metronidazole) or until they were afebrile for a period of 24 hours. One-third of patients also had a concomitant penetrating bladder injury. Due to the high risk of rectovesical fistula, all intra- as well as extraperitoneal bladder injuries were repaired in this series, with any extraperitoneal rectal injury unrepaired. Only one rectovesical fistula developed, but healed spontaneously with prolonged urinary catheterisation. Rectal injuries with a purely extraperitoneal trajectory were verified with DL (no peritoneal violation and no intraperitoneal blood) and a loop colostomy was performed.[52,88]

Fig. 19.4 presents an algorithm for the management of rectal injury.

Kidneys

Haematuria in penetrating abdominal trauma is associated with a renal injury in 80% and requires further investigations,[89] with a single-shot IVP being mandatory in unstable patients to demonstrate both kidneys are functioning. In stable patients, an abdominal CT with intravenous contrast is required to assess the severity grade of the kidney injury. We analysed 95 patients with a kidney GSW,[31] and the following indicators were used to proceed with operative management:

- Haemodynamic instability due to the kidney trauma
- Vascular pedicle, renal pelvis or ureteric injuries (AAST grade V kidney injuries)
- Renal exploration for all suspected kidney injuries without complete preoperative imaging

Of these 95 patients, 65% underwent urgent laparotomy. Operative management consisted of nephrectomy in 66%

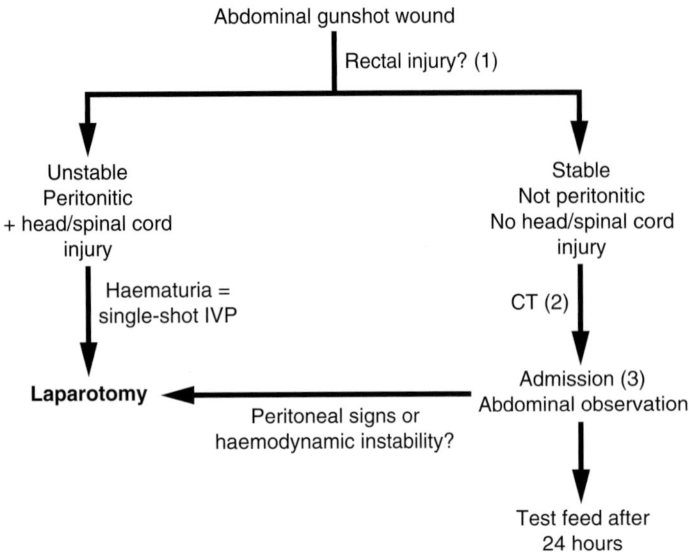

(1) See 'Rectal injury algorithm'

(2) Absolute CT indications: trajectory concerns; right upper quadrant/right-sided thoraco-abdominal trajectory; transpelvic trajectory (inclusive CT-cystogram); haematuria (if vascular pedicle, renal pelvis or ureteral injuries are present proceed with laparotomy)

(3) Failure usually implicates a repeat CT-scan +/- percutaneous intervention in solid organ injuries

Figure 19.3 Management of abdominal gunshot wounds. *CT*, computed tomography; *IVP*, intravenous pyelogram.

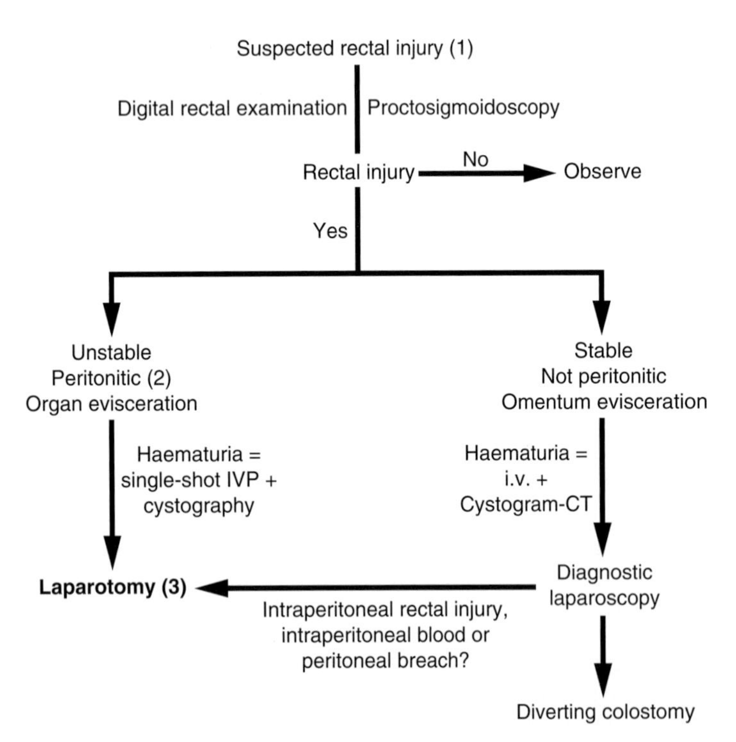

(1) Suspicion: transpelvic, gluteal, upper thigh gunshot or stab wound; blood per rectum

(2) Low threshold to proceed with laparotomy in patients with a high spinal cord injury or severe head injury in addition to the penetrating trauma

(3)
- *Intraperitoneal rectal injury:* repair
- *Extraperitoneal rectal injury:* no touch, but diverting colostomy
- Intra- or extraperitoneal *bladder injury in combination* with a rectal injury: *bladder* repair and prolonged catheter drainage

Figure 19.4 Management of rectal injury. *CT*, computed tomography; *IVP*, intravenous pyelogram.

due to hilar injuries or severe irreparable parenchymal disruption. NOM entailed serial physical examination for 48 hours and bed rest until macroscopic haematuria had resolved. Haematuria for more than 72 hours mandated renal angiography to diagnose and treat false aneurysms or arteriovenous fistulas.[89] The success rate of NOM was 91%, with the remainder (9%, three patients) undergoing laparotomy, in two cases without exploration of the kidneys. There were no kidney-related complications. Ideal candidates for NOM were stable patients amenable to reliable clinical examination with a right-sided thoracoabdominal or extraperitoneal GSW.

Some authors have suggested that there is a higher nephrectomy rate after routine surgical exploration; however, no higher risk of nephrectomy despite routine exploration was found in a previous prospective study.[90] NOM was in contrary associated with lower need for nephrectomy and less complications.[91]

Duodenum and pancreas

The location and proximity of these organs to other vital structures make injuries complex, difficult to detect and challenging to treat. In addition, they nearly always have concomitant intra-abdominal injuries. Simple surgical management algorithms should be applied to such complex injuries. In a retrospective review of 75 patients with a GSW to the duodenum, the authors showed that most duodenal injuries can be primarily repaired if less than half of the circumference is involved. The injured area may need to be debrided or even resected with a primary end-to-end anastomosis performed. In such circumstances, a feeding jejunostomy (14G Foley catheter used in Witzel-type technique) should be considered to support enteral nutrition.[92] All repairs were drained with a Penrose-type drain and no pyloric exclusion procedures were required. Pancreaticoduodenectomy was only performed for a devascularised duodenum or head of pancreas, ampullary injury and/or distal bile duct injuries. In another large review of 219 patients with a GSW to the pancreas from our Trauma Centre, treatment was kept as simple as possible.[93] All patients had a laparotomy, 77% had minor pancreatic injuries without major ductal injury and treatment consisted of control of haemostasis and drainage of the pancreas; 27% had a major ductal injury left of the superior mesenteric vein and underwent distal pancreaticoduodenectomy; and only 5% had a pancreaticoduodenectomy. On average, there was one emergency pancreatoduodenectomy per year, usually after a damage control procedure.[94] There is no need for complex enteric diversions or pancreaticoenteric anastomoses. The overall complication and mortality rates were high (up to 69%), especially in patients with higher-grade pancreatic and additional vascular injuries. Haemorrhagic shock and blood loss were the main factors predicting mortality, and they were mostly unrelated to the pancreatic injury.[95] Age (>55), severity of the pancreatic injury and additional vascular injury were also independent factors predicting mortality.[96,97] Nearly 18% developed a pancreatic fistula, which resolved with NOM (65%) or with endoscopic sphincterotomy and pancreatic stenting (33%). In a large study with 130 patients with major pancreatic resection (mainly distal pancreatectomies), the intra-abdominal infection rate was 32%, 19% had respiratory failure and 18% developed fistulas.[98] Trauma and pancreatic surgeons working together improves the outcome.[99,100]

Abdominal vena cava

Occasionally the general surgeon may encounter an inferior vena cava injury. Its prevalence is reported as 2.3% of all trauma laparotomies, nearly always after a GSW.[101] Mortality is high (31%) and no complex venous reconstructions were performed in this study. The authors recommend the following procedure: right-sided medial visceral rotation (Cattell-Braasch manoeuvre), temporary control by digital compression of the vena cava against the spine, a Foley catheter may be inserted into the lumen and inflated. Assessment of the injury:

- if simple and accessible, repair should be performed
- if difficult, the vena cava can be ligated in infrarenal injuries

COMPLICATIONS

In general, trauma patients have a considerable risk for ongoing bleeding or re-bleeding, disseminated intravascular coagulopathy, deep venous thrombosis, pulmonary embolism, atelectasis, pneumonia, pleural effusion, urinary tract or wound infection, and sepsis. The best and cheapest way to avoid many of these complications is early mobilisation of the patient. In abdominal trauma, intra-abdominal collections, anastomotic leak, enterocutaneous fistula, bowel obstruction, incisional hernia and abdominal compartment syndrome are feared complications. There are also some organ-specific complications and treatment modalities:[31,38,39,75,84,102]

Liver
- Abscess
- Biloma
- Bile ascites/haemoperitoneum
- Bleeding
- Haemobilia
- Necrosis

Kidney
- Increased perinephric haematoma
- Persistent haematuria due to a false aneurysm or arteriovenous fistula
- Persistent urinary leak
- Infected perinephric fluid collection

Pancreas
- Bleeding
- Peripancreatic fluid collections (pseudocysts and abscesses)
- Pancreatic fistula

Typical warning signs for complications are:
- Airway/Breathing: Increased respiratory rate, low oxygen saturation
- Circulation: Drop in blood pressure or significant fall in Hb level (>3 g/dL)
- Disability: Diminished consciousness, increasing abdominal pain
- Environment: Fever, elevated white blood cell counts, jaundice

These signs warrant a thorough clinical examination and potentially a repeat CT scan.

Fortunately, most complications can be successfully treated non-operatively or with interventional procedures:

- CT- or ultrasound-guided percutaneous drainage of biliary or purulent collections
- Angioembolisation in case of bleeding, haemobilia, haematuria, false aneurysm or an arteriovenous fistula
- Endoscopic sphincterotomy and stenting for biliary leaks
- Endoscopic placement of double J ureteric stents for urinary leaks

In a large review of 412 patients with liver injuries, 12% developed a biliary fistula with the risk factors being operative management, higher-grade liver injuries and liver packing.[103] A minor biliary leak (less than 400 mL/day) was present in 65% of this group and successfully treated without surgery. All drains were removed within 2 weeks. A major leak (more than 400 mL/day) was apparent in 35% of patients and successfully treated with endoscopic sphincterotomy and stenting, with the stent removed after 6 weeks. Major biliary collections should be drained either percutaneously under ultrasound guidance or laparoscopically.

Interestingly, HIV had no negative impact on complications in penetrating abdominal trauma.[104]

PELVIC FRACTURES

The severity of pelvic fracture ranges from insignificant to major and frequently fatal. With increasing trauma force, the likelihood of having an unstable pelvic fracture, i.e. open book or vertical shear fracture, is increased. In addition, an unstable pelvic fracture is often associated with intra-abdominal (16.5%), chest (i.e. aortic rupture in 1.4%) and diaphragmatic injuries (2.1%).[105] Intra- and/or extra-pelvic bleeding sources can cause haemodynamic instability, often due to associated solid organ injuries. Intra-pelvic sources are either the fractured bone itself, venous plexus or arterial vessels, but an arterial source is only present in around 10% of pelvic fractures. Unstable patients with a severe pelvic fracture must be assessed clinically quickly and early, with a chest and pelvic X-ray and with ultrasound (FAST) in blunt trauma.[106] If FAST is positive, patients need urgent laparotomy, some sort of pelvic stabilisation (most easily with a pelvic binder) to tamponade the pelvic haematoma, and extraperitoneal pelvic packing if bleeding/pelvic fracture related hemodynamic instability persists after any intra-abdominal bleeding has been controlled.[107] Packing usually does not stop arterial bleeding and in such patients with persistent haemodynamic instability, postoperative angiography with embolisation of arterial bleeding points must be carried out without undue delay.[108] Packing seems superior to resuscitative endovascular balloon occlusion of the aorta (REBOA; see later in this chapter); however, (partial/intermittent) REBOA in zone III should be considered in haemodynamically unstable patients with suspected pelvic bleeding.[109] Stable patients are usually assessed with a contrast CT to identify an active bleeding site and to determine the extent of skeletal injury. Angioembolisation can be performed where there is evidence of active bleeding. Definitive internal pelvic fixation can be carried out within 24 hours in stable patients but is usually delayed for 4 or more days in unstable patients.[106]

Early medical thromboprophylaxis (within 48 hours) in isolated pelvic fracture is associated with lower mortality and lower thromboembolism.[110,111] The use of vena cava filter did not lower the pulmonary embolism rate or mortality in severely injured patients with a contraindication for prophylactic anticoagulation.[112]

A STEP-BY-STEP GUIDE TO THE TRAUMA LAPAROTOMY

In a trauma laparotomy, some steps are mandatory and some procedures depend on the injuries.

- Inform the anaesthetist and the scrub nurse.
- Prepare the theatre: warm theatre and fluids.
- Prepare the patient: supine, low lithotomy position if an extraperitoneal rectal injury is suspected or in the case of a transpelvic GSW with bleeding as this will allow access into the pelvis if required.
- Give preoperative broad-spectrum antibiotics to cover gut bacteria.
- Drape from nipple to the pubic symphysis.
  - from chin to groin if sternotomy/thoracotomy/saphenous vein graft harvesting needed.
- Preoperative WHO-checklist.
- Full midline incision.
- **First step** = control the bleeding, evaluate the use of intraoperative blood salvage devices.
  - Remove blood with dry packs and pack all quadrants of the abdomen, try to restore the anatomy of the solid organs with packs.
  - Remove packs systematically.
  - Source of major bleeding: spleen, small bowel mesentery, liver, retroperitoneum.
    - Spleen: mobilise and bring the spleen into the operation field, open the lesser sac and occlude manually the splenic artery, decide on splenectomy.
    - Small bowel mesentery: apply digital pressure, clamping and suturing.
    - Liver:
      - Manual compression and packing (ideally six packs), restore the anatomy; most injuries will have stopped bleeding. Do not pack into the liver wound.
      - Get better access to the liver by mobilisation of the liver by taking down the ligamentous attachments.
      - Minor lacerations: use diathermy, argon beam coagulation, fibrin glue.
      - Moderate lacerations: apply Pringle manoeuvre for 20 minutes and suture selectively bleeding vessels and large bile leaks. Remember that packing will not stop arterial bleeding and this needs to be controlled with a polypropylene figure-of-eight suture.
      - Major lacerations: rarely resection or total hepatic vascular isolation is needed, better perform damage control surgery (pack and temporary close the abdomen, transfer to ICU).
      - Drain all liver injuries.
    - Retroperitoneal haematoma: central and/or expanding haematomas must be explored, consider

inflow control by aortic cross-clamping; supra-colic haematoma = medial visceral rotation from the left/ infra-colic haematoma = medial visceral rotation from the right.
- Pelvic haematoma: if haemodynamically stable and not expanding = only external control of the pelvic fracture; if haemodynamic instability or expanding haematoma in penetrating wounds or in open book or vertical shear fractures = extraperitoneal packing. This will not stop arterial bleeding; rather pack and proceed with angioembolisation if haemodynamic status does not improve.
- Stomach: can bleed considerably; close the injury with a running all-layers suture.

Second step = control the contamination.

- Systemic approach: inspect all hollow viscera; a single-layer interrupted suture with 3/0 polypropylene (Prolene®) is a good repair technique.
- Duodenum: Kocher manoeuvre if a duodenal injury is suspected, duodenal repair, drainage.
  - Pancreas: haemostasis and drainage is adequate most of the time.
- Small bowel: debride wound edges, suture any bowel perforations, resection and anastomosis in destructive injuries (>50% of the bowel wall).
- Colon: mobilisation along the white line of Toldt, primary repair or resection and anastomosis (>50% of the bowel wall).
- Rectum: sigmoidoscopy to look for fresh blood as an indicator for a rectal injury; if intraperitoneal = primary repair; if extraperitoneal = diverting colostomy and no direct repair.

Inspect the peritoneum:

- Diaphragm: all injuries should be repaired. If there is a stomach or bowel injury, then the defect in the diaphragm should be opened and the pleural cavity washed out with 4–5 L of irrigation so as to prevent the development of an empyema. Repair with a 1 non-absorbable, monofilament, continuous, full-thickness suture.
- Bladder: intraperitoneal bladder rupture must be repaired in a double-layer technique.
- Closure of penetrating peritoneal wounds.

Irrigation of the abdomen with warmed isotonic saline.

No drains routinely.[113]

Abdominal closure with a continuous 0 nylon or selective temporary abdominal closure for 48 hours if:[27,114]

- in shock
- under tension due to visceral oedema or tissue loss
- abdominal compartment
- abdominal packing
- need for second look.

BLUNT AND PENETRATING CHEST INJURIES

General surgeons often encounter patients with chest trauma and it is therefore worthwhile understanding some of the main injuries and their immediate management. Serial clinical examination and selective NOM is the mainstay in chest trauma.[115] Most of these conditions can easily be managed with simple procedures such as intubation and ventilation, needle decompression, intercostal drainage and volume restoration. Surgical repair is seldom needed.

The first goal is to detect and immediately treat life-threatening injuries in the primary survey:[9]

- Tension pneumothorax
- Open pneumothorax
- Massive haemothorax
- Cardiac tamponade
- Flail chest and pulmonary contusion

Potentially life-threatening injuries must be identified in the secondary survey:[9]

- Simple pneumothorax
- Haemothorax
- Pulmonary contusion
- Tracheobronchial tree injury
- Cardiac injury
- Traumatic aortic disruption
- Oesophageal rupture
- Traumatic diaphragmatic injury

RIB FRACTURES, PNEUMOTHORAX, HAEMOTHORAX AND PULMONARY CONTUSIONS

Rib fracture

Rib fracture is a clinical diagnosis. It can be diagnosed on chest X-ray; however, the main goal of the chest X-ray is to look for relevant concomitant injuries, such as a haemothorax or pneumothorax. Rib fractures may be associated with potentially life-threatening injuries and fractures of the first to third ribs are sometimes a marker for major vascular injuries—as seen in blunt aortic injuries, or an indicator of a liver or splenic injury in lower rib fractures. In elderly patients and in patients with multiple injuries, rib fractures are related to a higher risk of morbidity, particularly pneumonia, and mortality.[116] The Western Trauma Association recommends admitting elderly patients with more than two rib fractures to the ICU. The main treatment consists of adequate *analgesia* (including morphine) to enable the patient to cough. Intercostal nerve blocks or thoracic epidurals are very effective ways to ameliorate the pain level in selected patients. All patients should get chest physiotherapy and supplemental oxygen if needed. In some circumstances, particularly flail chest (three and more ribs are fractured in two places causing a mobile thoracic wall segment) or severely displaced rib fractures, osteosynthesis of ribs can significantly improve thoracic cage stability and hasten recovery.[117–119]

Pneumothorax and haemothorax

These are both frequently seen after blunt or penetrating trauma. Definitive treatment of pneumo- or haemothoraces usually consists of chest tube insertion and subsequently a chest X-ray to document chest drain position, lung expansion and persistent opacities. In haemodynamic instability, need for positive pressure ventilation, in tension or open pneumothorax, obvious haemothorax, or flail chest, the indication to insert a chest drain is clear and urgent. In one study of 635 patients with a haemothorax,[120] two-thirds of the haemothoraces were drained and one-third were treated conservatively. The study went on to say that an *ipsilateral flail chest, pneumothorax* and the *size of the haemothorax* were independent predictors for chest tube insertion. A *massive haemothorax* (>1500 mL of bloody pleural effusion or >200 mL/h for the next 4 hours) is an indication for a thoracotomy. Different chest tube sizes have been compared in patients with traumatic haemothoraces, and it would appear that size does not change the efficacy of drainage and does not affect the rate of complications: 28–32 French chest tubes are therefore probably sufficient.[121]

Some pneumo- or haemothoraces however can safely be treated without drainage with a shorter length of stay, fewer infectious complications and no increase in mortality.[120] An *asymptomatic pneumothorax* less than 1.5–2 cm in size, measured on a chest X-ray, can be treated without chest tube, under certain circumstances even in case of positive pressure ventilation.[122,123] An *occult pneumothorax*, found on CT but not visible on a supine chest X-ray, needs careful monitoring but no chest tube insertion, except for patients requiring positive pressure ventilation, in respiratory distress, proved progression of the pneumothorax or development of a haemothorax.[124] *Asymptomatic or also retained haemothoraces* with less than *300 mL* or 1.5 cm on a CT scan and no other indication for tube insertion can safely be managed with observation.[125] In the case of conservative treatment, a radiological follow-up is recommended after 6–12 hours.

Pulmonary contusions

Pulmonary contusions represent bleeding into lung parenchyma and result in abnormal gas exchange in the affected segment and an arterial blood gas analysis should be carried out to evaluate the pulmonary dysfunction. The chest X-ray changes are often delayed and initially underestimated, whereas CT of the chest can clearly visualise the affected segments and predict the need for mechanical ventilation.[126] Treatment usually consists of analgesia, chest physiotherapy and supplemental oxygen. Not surprisingly, pulmonary contusions are risk factors for pneumonia and acute respiratory distress syndrome.

Intrathoracic complications

Persistent opacities mandate a chest CT to differentiate atelectasis, consolidation, pulmonary contusion, retained haemothorax, other pleural effusions and their exact location. Empyema (4.4%), pneumonia (4.7%) and retained haemothorax (11.3%) are typical complications in patients with drained haemo- or pneumothorax.[121]

The incidence of *empyema* among patients with a retained haemothorax was 27% in a prospective, multicentre study in the USA.[127] Risk factors were ISS > 24, the presence of rib fractures and the number of interventions to evacuate the retained blood. Chest tube insertion significantly increased the length of stay and the risk of empyema.[120] Presumptive antibiotics do not appear to decrease the incidence of empyema, but once present the treatment consists of antibiotics and (CT-guided) drainage.[128] An empyema not responding to non-operative treatment may be approached using video-assisted thoracoscopic surgery with a conversion to a thoracotomy if required.

Pneumonia significantly increases length of stay and mortality. Blunt trauma and ISS > 24, but not a retained haemothorax, were significant predictors for pneumonia. Use of periprocedural antibiotics on chest tube insertion does significantly decrease the pneumonia rate.[129]

Fibrothorax and empyema are feared complications after a *retained haemothorax*. Small (<300 mL) retained haemothoraces eventually resolve over time. Some liquefied retained haemothoraces can safely be treated with a second chest tube. However, some retained haemothoraces are clotted and loculated and need more aggressive treatment. Some surgeons advocate the use of local thrombolysis via the chest drain. Video-assisted thoracoscopic surgery is a safe method to successfully treat a retained haemothorax in up to 80%.[130] The earlier the treatment, the better is the outcome with less mortality and reduced requirement for thoracotomy.

CARDIAC INJURIES

Up to 90% of all penetrating heart injuries are already fatal in the prehospital phase. The remainder are those patients arriving alive in the hospital. They may present as:

- lifeless with signs of life present in the last 5–10 minutes—these patients need an emergency department thoracotomy (EDT) to relieve a tension haemo- or pneumopericardium, stop any exsanguinating haemorrhage, repair of the cardiac injury and massage the heart;
- in persistent haemorrhagic shock despite resuscitation, these patients need urgent exploration either via sternotomy or thoracotomy, depending on the clinical situation, in the operating theatre;
- symptomatic with cardiac tamponade, three quarters of them showing the Beck's triad (hypotension, muffled heart sounds and elevated jugular venous pressure)—these patients need a sternotomy in the operating theatre;
- or stable and relatively asymptomatic—there is a high likelihood of a cardiac injury with stab or GSW in penetrating chest trauma or trajectories crossing the heart area, and it must aggressively be ruled out.[131]

While the first three situations are clear clinical situations and clear indications to proceed with surgery, the last situation poses some difficulties for the trauma surgeon. The clinical examination reveals little except for the penetrating skin wound. A penetrating wound in the 'cardiac zone' (Fig. 19.5) as well as GSWs to the neck, chest, abdomen and back depict a high risk of a cardiac injury.[132] A history of prehospital hypotension alerts the general surgeon. A pericardial rub or a cardiac murmur (i.e. traumatic septal defects or valve injuries) can be a guide. Cardiac ultrasound, chest X-ray, ECG and central venous pressure of greater than 15 cm H_2O can also help in diagnosing cardiac injuries.

Ultrasound identifies a haemopericardium; however, the sensitivity is 87% and limited by the presence of a pneumopericardium or a haemothorax.[132] Ultrasound can be falsely negative if the haemopericardium is draining into the pleural cavity (presenting as a haemothorax) through the penetration in the pericardial sac. These false-negative results can have a catastrophic outcome and must be avoided. False-positive results are encountered in patients and may be related to differing amounts of pericardial fluid in normal individuals and a haemothorax. Pericardiocentesis has no role in the diagnosis of penetrating cardiac injuries and is more likely to cause an injury to the heart.

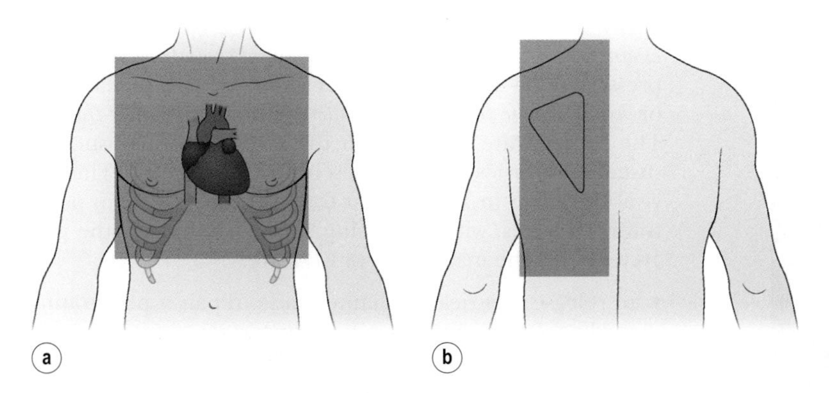

Figure 19.5 The cardiac zone. (a) View from anterior and (b) from posterior.

Chest X-ray can raise the suspicion of an occult heart injury. A pneumopericardium or an enlarged heart shadow are possible signs. Up to 10% of patients with a pneumopericardium become unstable and need urgent decompression. Since the pericardium is poorly distensible, little amount of blood in the pericardium can cause straightening out of the sac at the pulmonary artery concavity. The straight left heart border was examined on erect chest X-ray in 162 patients with a cardiac injury[133] (Fig. 19.6). While there are some differential diagnoses (status post left lower lobectomy, mitral valve diseases, pectus excavatum), the sensitivity of this radiological sign correlating with an operatively confirmed haemopericardium was 40%, with a specificity of 84% and a positive predictive value of 89%. Hence, the straight left heart border sign was a useful sign in predicting the presence of a haemopericardium.

A J-wave, a small positive reflection on the R-ST junction on a standard *ECG*, can also be a sign of a possible cardiac injury (Fig. 19.7). An analysis of the ECGs of 174 patients with a cardiac injury,[134] demonstrated the sensitivity of the J-wave was 44%, specificity 85% and positive predictive value 91%. The authors concluded that a J-wave is a significant sign of an occult cardiac injury if present.

If a haemopericardium is diagnosed, the question remains whether a stable patient needs a sternotomy to treat the cardiac injury or has the cardiac wound already sealed? Many of these cardiac injuries were already found to have sealed or needed no special intervention in view of partial-thickness or tangential wounds if a sternotomy is performed in stable patients with a haemopericardium.[131] A randomised controlled trail in 111 patients comparing sternotomy versus subxyphoidal window with drainage determined that a stable patient with a haemopericardium can be managed with a subxyphoid pericardial window. If there is no active bleeding, the patient can then be managed without a sternotomy, with lower morbidity and mortality.[135] In summary, stable patients with a haemo- or pneumopericardium need a subxyphoid pericardial window to rule out active bleeding, with a sternotomy only mandatory in the case of active bleeding.[136] Electrocardiogram and echographic follow-up is recommended.

✔✔ Subxyphoidal window and drainage is effective and safe in stable patients with a haemopericardium after penetrating trauma. No sternotomy is mandatory.[90]

Fig. 19.8 summarises the management of penetrating cardiac injury.

AORTIC INJURIES

Aortic injuries are more likely to result in death than haemodynamic instability. Typical trauma mechanisms are fall from a height or excessive deceleration causing a rupture usually just distal to the left subclavian artery at the isthmus. Penetrating aortic injuries are usually fatal. A widened mediastinum (>8 cm) on a supine chest X-ray can be a sign of an aortic injury. However, the chest X-ray has a high false-positive and false-negative rate and further investigation is required. Over a period of 10 years, there has been a major shift in the diagnosis of blunt aortic injuries. The AAST compared the results of two observational studies from 1997 and 2007. They concluded that aorto- and echography are no longer regularly used, and contrast CT represents the current gold standard. Treatment also changed tremendously from open repair to endovascular procedures. Consequently, mortality rate as well as procedure-related paraplegia decreased significantly to 13% and 1.6%, respectively. However, early graft-related complications significantly increased to 13.5%. Timing of repair remains controversial and there is a shift to delayed (>12–16 hours) repair—when it can be performed under better or even normalised physiological conditions. This is the current standard in patients with major concomitant injuries if maintaining a low systolic blood pressure to prevent free rupture is possible.[137]

OESOPHAGEAL INJURIES

Oesophageal injuries, either in the neck or in the chest, are rare. The frequency is less than 10 patients per year even in large trauma centres. In a study of 52 patients with penetrating oesophageal injures over an 8-year period,[138] unstable patients with massive bleeding or an expanding haematoma underwent surgery and had endoscopy during the operation to diagnose the oesophageal injury. Stable patients were further assessed. Subcutaneous emphysema and/or prevertebral air were each present in nearly 50% of patients and are the most frequent radiological findings in oesophageal injuries. These patients as well as symptomatic patients (dysphagia, odynophagia, haematemesis or blood in the nasogastric tube, leakage of saliva or gastrointestinal contents from the wound or the intercostal drain) require a water-soluble contrast swallow study to detect an oesophageal injury. About 73% of the oesophageal injuries can be primary repaired and widely drained even if the delay to surgery is more than 12 hours. The authors found a delay to diagnose and treat an oesophageal injury as the most important risk factor for oesophageal-related complications.

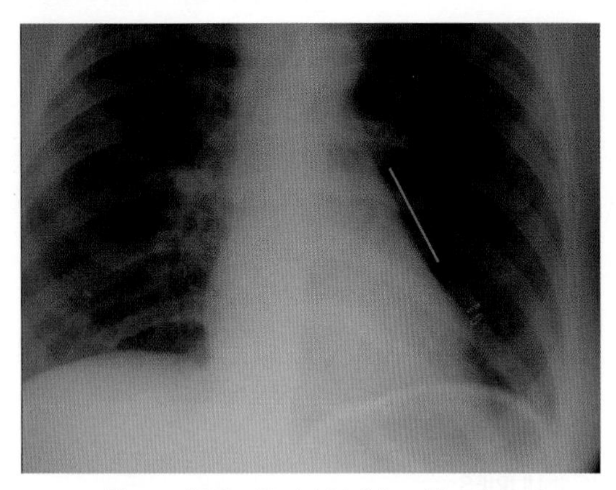

Figure 19.6 Straight left heart border.

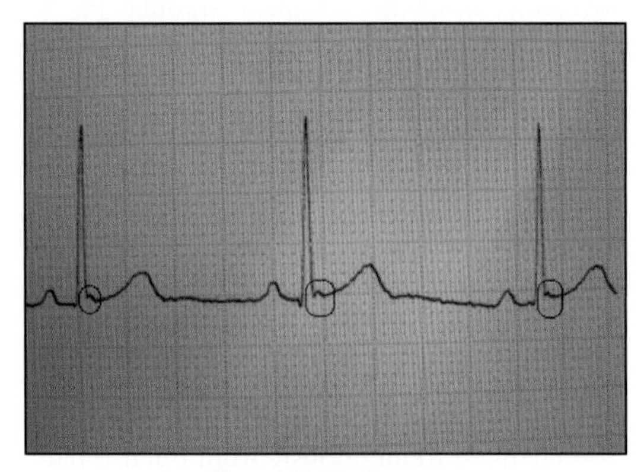

Figure 19.7 J-wave.

Therefore, an expeditious assessment is of paramount importance. For patients presenting late in septic shock, a damage control approach is more suitable with stapling of the injury with drainage and the later formation of an oesophagostomy, gastrostomy and feeding jejunostomy. At a later stage, an oesophagectomy will be required with a gastric pull-up.

TRANSMEDIASTINAL GUNSHOT WOUNDS

Transmediastinal GSWs are associated with a high pre- and early in-hospital mortality due to cardiac and major vascular injuries. Of 133 such patients reported, 87% were unstable or had no vital signs at arrival and 11% arrived dead at the hospital.[139] The reported injuries were: 71% cardiac, 24% thoracic aorta, 35% liver and 29% splenic injuries. Of all the patients in this study, 73% underwent EDT because of loss or imminent loss of vital signs and only 8% of them were discharged alive. In comparison, all patients arriving stable in the emergency department were discharged home. Stable patients may yet have occult cardiovascular or aerodigestive tract injuries and therefore an intravenous contrast-enhanced CT of the chest in stable patients delineates the suspicious tract and predicts injuries. Mediastinal haematoma or air warrants further testing such as bronchoscopy, contrast swallow or endoscopy in theatre in the intubated patient. CT has reduced the need for potentially harmful investigations.[140]

EMERGENCY DEPARTMENT THORACOTOMY

An EDT is rarely indicated, but can be life-saving. Accepted indications are *life-threatening pericardial tamponade* or *exsanguinating haemorrhage with profound shock* (systolic blood pressure < 60–70 mmHg not responding to resuscitation) or *hypovolaemic cardiac arrest after penetrating thoracic trauma.* The success rate depends on the trauma mechanism, the sustained injuries and the presence of signs of life. The survival rate is up to 7% in blunt trauma and 26–35% in penetrating injuries, with increasing survival rates over the past 10 years.[141] The main goals of EDT are:[142]

- to release a pericardial tamponade, repair a penetrating cardiac wound, and open heart massage;
- to control major intrathoracic bleeding (either thoracic wall, lung or great vessel injury);
- cross-clamping of the lung hilum in cases of massive exsanguination from the lung;
- cross-clamping of the descending aorta to improve blood flow to the brain and the heart and limit possible intra-abdominal haemorrhage.

EDT must therefore provide fast access to the pericardium, the pleura, the lung hilum, and the descending aorta. Standard access is via a left anterior thoracotomy. The EDT can further be continued to a clamshell incision providing fast and excellent access to nearly all thoracic structures.[143]

The limits for EDT are:[144]

- prehospital CPR 10 minutes after blunt trauma without response;
- prehospital CPR 15 minutes after penetrating injury without response;
- asystole is the presenting rhythm, and there is no pericardial tamponade.

The Western Trauma Association multicentre group had no survivor after EDT in all these situations. The survival rate was also 0% with patients arriving with no signs of life after blunt trauma in a nationwide analysis from USA.[141]

EDT technique[145]

Patient is intubated and ventilated in supine position.
A thoracotomy set should be available in the emergency department.
Morphine 10 mg and midazolam 10 mg intravenously
Rapidly clean and drape the chest.
Long incision from the edge of the costal cartilage to the left midaxillary line in the fifth intercostal space with the line of incision passing just below the nipple line.

- Consider a right thoracotomy if the penetrating wound is on the right side.

Incise the pleura and divide all layers towards the sternum using a Mayo scissors while avoiding injury to the lung and the internal mammary artery.
Insert a rib spreader to its full extent.
Evacuate any blood.

a. *Incise the inferior pulmonary ligament if possible to mobilise the lung.*
b. *Heart*

Apply an Allis clamp to the pericardial sac and make a long midline incision of the pericardium; avoid injuring the phrenic nerve running anterior to the hilum of the lung. Remove blood clots if applicable and inspect the heart. Unoxygenated blood is dark and indicates a right-sided heart injury. Apply digital pressure to the wound. Close

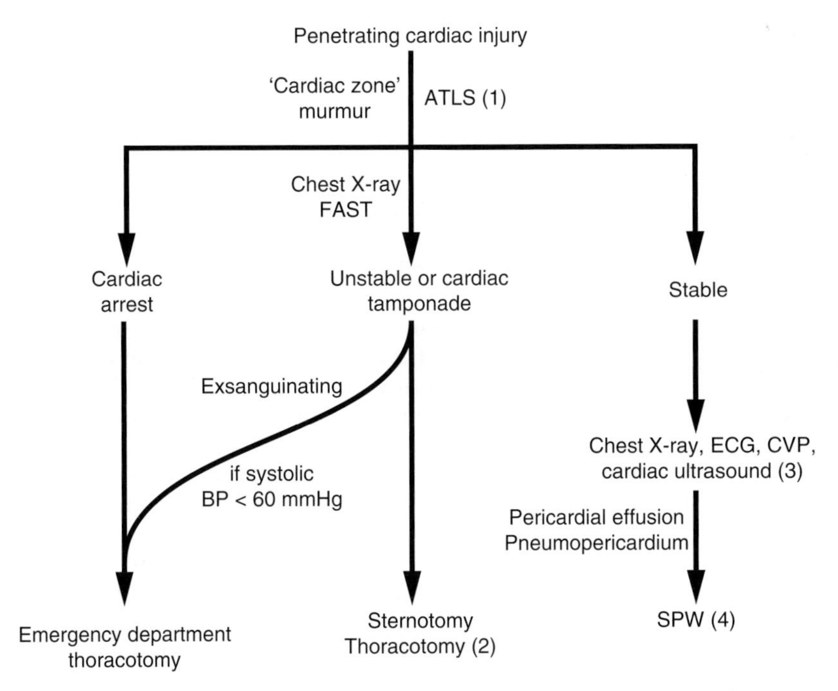
Penetrating cardiac injury
'Cardiac zone' murmur
ATLS (1)
Chest X-ray
FAST
Cardiac arrest
Unstable or cardiac tamponade
Stable
Exsanguinating
if systolic BP < 60 mmHg
Chest X-ray, ECG, CVP, cardiac ultrasound (3)
Pericardial effusion
Pneumopericardium
Emergency department thoracotomy
Sternotomy
Thoracotomy (2)
SPW (4)
(1) Look for airway obstruction, tension pneumothorax, open pneumothorax, massive haemothorax, cardiac tamponade
(2) Penetrating wound medial to the midclavicular line mandates a sternotomy/lateral thoracotomy on the side of the penetrating wound
(3) A haemothorax or a high index of suspicion despite a negative ultrasound mandates a second ultrasound 24 hours later or a CT scan
(4) Blood (clots) in the pericardial sac is a positive SPW, active bleeding mandates a sternotomy

Figure 19.8 Management of penetrating cardiac injury. *ATLS,* Advanced Trauma Life Support; *BP,* blood pressure; *FAST,* focused assessment with sonography in trauma; *SPW,* subxiphoid pericardial window.

the wound with an interrupted monofilament 2/0 polypropylene (Prolene®), if necessary with pledgets (Teflon® or pericardial tissue) (Fig. 19.9). A Foley catheter (ventricle) or a Satinsky clamp (atria) can be of some help. An injury near a coronary artery is best sutured with a mattress stitch to avoid narrowing of the coronary artery.

- Consider internal heart massage and defibrillation with an initial energy level of 10–50 J in cardiac arrest.

c. *Major bleeding chest, lung or thoracic wall*

Inspect the chest wall (light red blood indicating intercostal artery injury), lung (air-mixed blood for lung and dark blood for hilar injuries) and mediastinum for active bleeding.

Stop the bleeding with local compression, swab-on-a-stick, suture or hilar cross-clamping (from cranial).

d. In case of *air embolism* consider hilar cross-clamping.

e. In case of *extrathoracic haemorrhage,* consider aortic cross-clamping a few centimetres above the diaphragm to improve blood flow to brain and heart and decrease haemorrhage into the abdomen or pelvis.

f. Consider division of the sternum and a contralateral thoracotomy (clamshell) to get better exposure.

Temporary closure of the chest and transfer to the theatre for definitive repair and wash-out.

RETAINED KNIFE BLADE

This is a very dramatic injury (Fig. 19.10). Resist removing the blade as it may be tamponading a major vessel. We reviewed our experience with this injury.[146] In 40% of the patients the entry site was the chest, in 21% each it was the neck and back, but rarely the abdomen. All patients were clinically and radiologically evaluated, and all but one patient was haemodynamically stable. X-rays (AP and lateral) were helpful to define the tract and CT angiography was very useful to determine the proximity of the blade to vital structures. After excluding solid organ, hollow viscus or neurovascular injuries, the blade could be extracted in the operating room in nearly 60%. In 5% post-extraction bleeding needed to be addressed. About 40% patients needed either wound exploration or an open operation (thoracotomy, thoracoscopy or laparotomy) and extraction of the knife under direct vision after gaining proximal and distal control of major vessels. All operations were performed under general (94%) or local anaesthesia (6%) in the theatre. Postoperative sepsis was a significant complication after retained thoracic blades.

THORACO-ABDOMINAL TRAUMA

Thoraco-abdominal injuries may cause diagnostic and therapeutic problems, and they are often associated with multiple injuries that require surgery. Depending on the trajectory, cardiac injuries are quite often seen in thoracoabdominal injuries,[147] with diaphragmatic injuries present in up to 60%.[148] Furthermore, there is a high rate of negative thoracotomies (22%) or laparotomies (11%), and inappropriate sequencing was found in 44% undergoing thoracotomy and laparotomy.[149]

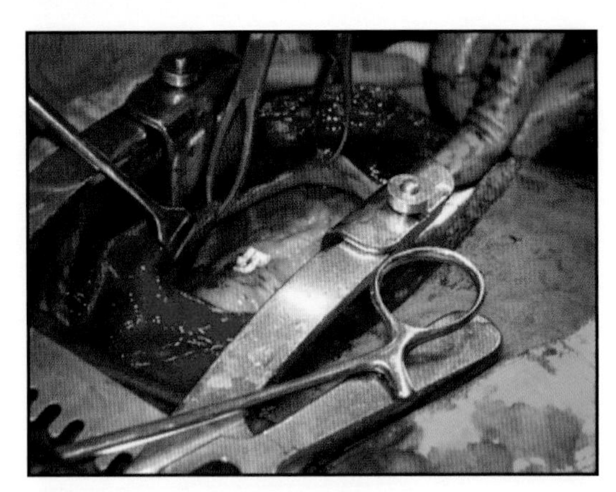

Figure 19.9 Suture of a cardiac injury with pledgets.

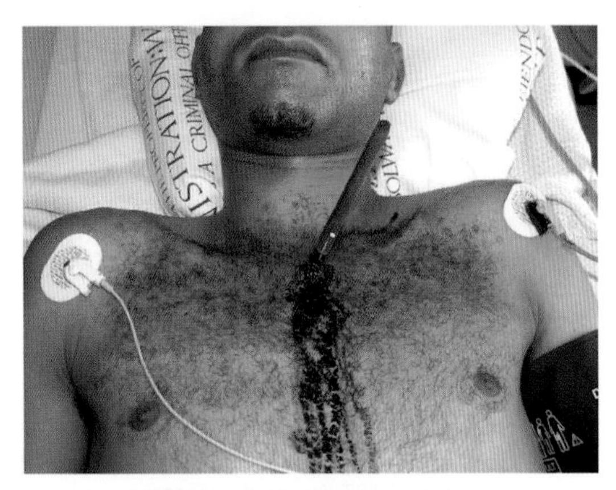

Figure 19.10 Retained blade.

Cardiac injuries with arrest, hypovolaemic shock, or cardiac tamponade, chest drain output (massive haemothorax: > 1500 mL or > 200 mL per hour), peritonitis, or haemodynamic instability due to an intra-abdominal haemorrhage are clear indications to proceed with surgery. Which injury is bleeding more and needs to be addressed first is not always clear: the chest drain output may be from an abdominal bleed through the diaphragmatic injury.[149] Ultrasound can be of some benefit especially to search for a haemopericardium or haemoperitoneum.[150] However, as already mentioned, ultrasound of the heart can be false negative with a haemothorax. In addition, a negative FAST cannot exclude a bleeding source in the abdomen. The burden of both, a thoracotomy and laparotomy, is furthermore immense for the patient, and unnecessary surgery must be avoided as mortality is doubled in these patients.

In a cohort of patients with *thoraco-abdominal stab injuries*,[151] half of all patients (53%) needed only a laparotomy, the indications being either a hollow viscus perforation, a diaphragm injury or a bleeding solid organ injury. No surgery was needed in 40%. The remainder had a thoracotomy/sternotomy, nearly always because of a cardiac injury. The authors in this study concluded that in an unstable patient with a thoraco-abdominal stab wound, a relevant cardiac injury must be ruled out first, followed by abdominal exploration. If clear signs of cardiac injuries are absent, the best approach is to start with a laparotomy and if there remains concern regarding a cardiac injury, then a diagnostic transdiaphragmatic pericardial window can be made. If this window is positive (results in blood), the chest should be opened in the acute phase.

GSWs producing *thoraco-abdominal gunshot injuries* are more complex and most of these patients (66%) need a laparotomy, with 14% requiring a laparotomy and thoracotomy/sternotomy.[152] In this series, 14% had no surgery. In total, one-third needed a thoracotomy; however, most of these patients were in cardiac arrest or agonal and had an EDT with a very poor outcome. The authors summarised that patients either have clear signs of cardiac or major thoracic vascular injuries requiring EDT or have haemodynamic instability requiring a laparotomy. If patients have a clear indication to proceed with a laparotomy but no clear indication to proceed with a thoracotomy, these patients ideally have a transdiaphragmatic pericardial window first to rule out a cardiac injury if the trajectory is close to the heart. Some authors recommend a subxyphoidal approach instead. A subxyphoid pericardial window has a lower risk of pericardial contamination with gastrointestinal contents and can diminish the rate of negative sternotomies and mortality.[147]

Blunt thoraco-abdominal trauma is quite often seen, but rarely needs surgery of one or both cavities. Most of the chest trauma can be managed with supplemental oxygen, chest physiotherapy, analgesia and occasionally with an intercostal drain. Some of the intra-abdominal injuries will require a laparotomy.

In thoraco-abdominal injuries, there is a general increased risk of pleural empyema due to the spillage of gastrointestinal contents through the diaphragmatic injury into the chest. One safe way to lower the risk of intrathoracic septic complications is to enlarge the diaphragmatic injury, to wash-out and drain the thorax and consecutively to close the injury[153] (Fig. 19.11).

DIAPHRAGMATIC INJURIES

Up to two-thirds of patients with a penetrating thoraco-abdominal trajectory have a diaphragmatic injury, which usually does not heal spontaneously.[148] Complications include herniation, incarceration and strangulation of bowel into the chest due to the intrathoracic negative pressure with a high morbidity of 30% and a mortality of 10%.[154] Delayed or missed diagnosis must be avoided and left-sided diaphragmatic injuries particularly should be addressed as these have a much higher rate of subsequent hernia formation. Some patients present with a clear indication, other than the diaphragmatic injury, to proceed with a laparotomy, at which a thorough examination of the diaphragm must be carried out and an injury repaired. In stable and asymptomatic patients, the algorithm is more ambiguous. Clinical examination cannot clearly establish the diagnosis. Haemo- and/or pneumothorax are most often seen on a chest X-ray; however, one-third have a normal chest X-ray.[155] The overall CT accuracy and sensitivity is low. Although thoracoscopy or laparoscopy have a high accuracy, they are however invasive. In a report of 24 highly selected patients with possible diaphragmatic injuries,[155] the patients underwent diagnostic and therapeutic laparoscopy *after* 24–36 hours of

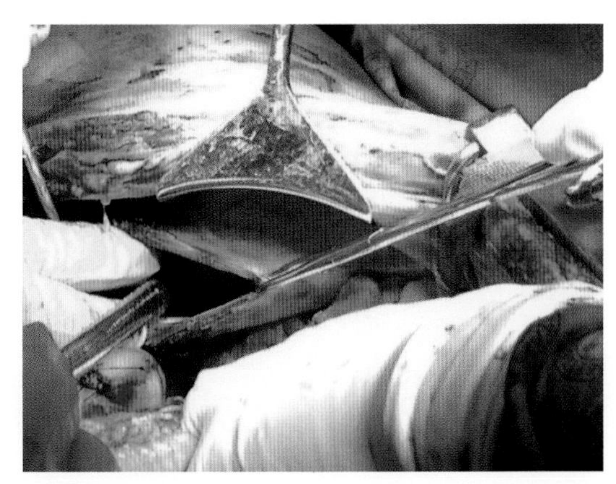

Figure 19.11 Enlarging the diaphragmatic injury to wash out the chest.

uneventful clinical observation (hence no hollow viscus injury). Prevailing indications were:

- omentum herniation through the chest wall;
- persistent left upper quadrant tenderness following abdominal observation;
- free air under the diaphragm despite benign abdominal signs.

Initial observation of the asymptomatic stable patient is advised with a view to performing an interval laparoscopy on all patients with lower left thoraco-abdominal stab wounds. An early laparoscopy tends to be associated with a high conversion rate to a laparotomy.

Blunt diaphragmatic injuries are usually located on the left side and concomitant with major thoraco-abdominal or pelvic trauma. They are often missed as sensitivity of chest X-ray and CT is low. Acute diaphragmatic injuries are best approached via a laparotomy since most patients have relevant abdominal injuries. Chronic diaphragmatic injuries can be repaired via a laparotomy, laparoscopically or by thoracotomy depending on the expertise available.

New guidelines recommend:

- DL (instead of CT) in haemodynamically stable patients with a left thoracoabdominal stab wound (thoracoscopy is an alternative in case of a co-existent haemothorax[80])
- non-operative approach for hemodynamically stable patients with a right-sided penetrating injury
- abdominal approach for acute injuries (usually via a laparotomy, however in certain circumstances also laparoscopic)
- either abdominal or thoracic approaches in chronic injuries.[156]

NECK TRAUMA

PENETRATING NECK INJURIES

Penetrating neck injuries are common in urban trauma centres, can be life-threatening and difficult to treat due to complex anatomy and concentration of vital structures.[157,158] As with penetrating abdominal trauma, there is a clear shift from categorical exploration to selective NOM. Nowadays, nearly 80% of all patients with penetrating neck injuries can be safely and successfully treated without surgery.[158] Only about 10% of patients with hard signs (explained below) need immediate surgery.[159]

Penetrating neck injuries are generally anatomically divided into anterior and posterior triangle injuries. The anterior triangle is further divided into three zones (Fig. 19.12), which helps to appraise possibly injured structures, and guide further diagnostic and therapeutic approaches.

Penetrating neck injuries can be life-threatening. An ABC approach according to ATLS guidelines is recommended.[9,158]

✔✔ The algorithm for penetrating neck injuries is a very useful method of assessing and managing penetrating neck injuries.[110]

All penetrating neck injuries can cause airway compromise due to a local haematoma, secretions, direct laryngeal, or tracheal injuries, surgical emphysema, or decreased level of consciousness with a GCS of less than 9. Air bubbling through the wound is also a hard sign.[159] In all these cases, the airway must be secured either via intubation or cricothyroidotomy. Occasionally, a tracheal tube can be inserted via the open tracheal wound. A cervical (C-) spine injury must be assumed, the C-spine accordingly immobilised and a lateral C-spine X-ray ordered. A thoracic injury must be ruled out clinically and by means of a chest X-ray in every patient with a penetrating neck injury. Next, any fatal bleeding must be assessed and stopped. An unstable patient or a patient with a severely bleeding neck wound, an expanding, or a pulsatile neck haematoma (hard signs) must be treated immediately either with surgery or (easier) with a 20-FG Foley catheter balloon tamponade.[160] Balloon tamponade significantly reduces the need for immediate and late operative exploration (Fig. 19.13). A Foley balloon tamponade can definitively control haemorrhage from venous and minor arterial injuries.[161] Stable patients must be thoroughly examined (i.e. hard and soft signs for neck injuries, including neurological signs), are admitted to a high-care trauma ward and observed with haemodynamic monitoring, airway and neck examination. Certain symptoms warrant further work-up in a timely fashion:[138,157,158]

- CT angiography for possible *vascular injuries* in case of a moderate to large neck haematoma, pulsatile but stable haematoma, pulse deficit, bruit, Foley catheter balloon tamponade, any mediastinal widening on chest X-ray and a retained knife blade.
- Laryngoscopy and bronchoscopy for *laryngeal or tracheobronchial injuries* if dysphonia, hoarseness, tension pneumothorax, severe surgical emphysema, or persistent air leak from chest drain are present.
- Contrast oesophagography and endoscopy in patients with odynophagia, dysphagia, haemoptysis and haematemesis, or signs of subcutaneous emphysema, blood in the nasogastric tube, leakage of saliva or gastrointestinal content from the wound, prevertebral air on lateral neck radiography or a pneumomediastinum to rule out *pharyngeal or oesophageal injuries.*
- *Transmidline GSWs* need routine CT angiography.

Fig. 19.14 presents an algorithm for the management of penetrating neck injury.

Vascular injuries

An arterial injury found on CT angiography needs to be addressed, either surgically (i.e. common carotid artery) or endovascularly. A common or internal carotid injury needs

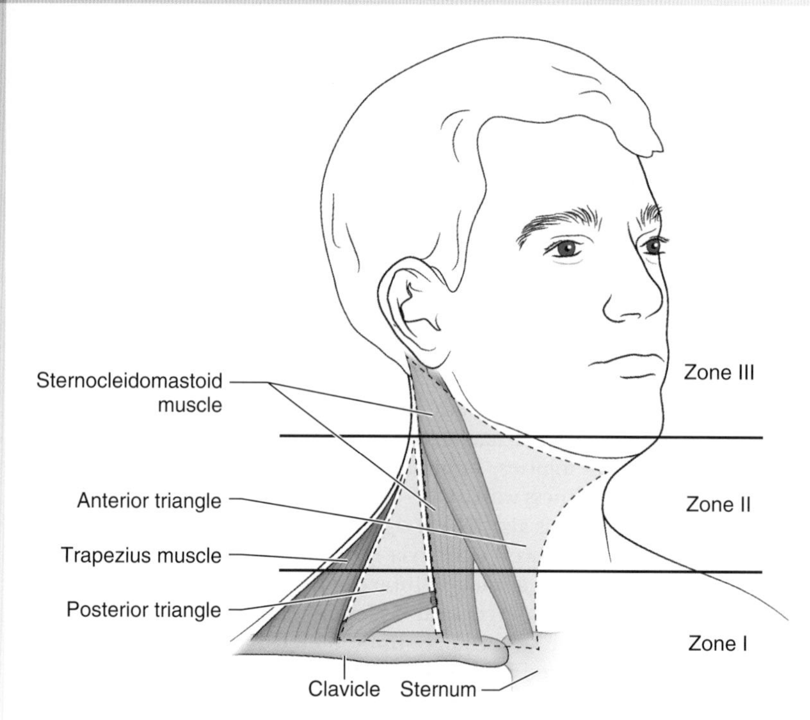

Figure 19.12 Neck zones.

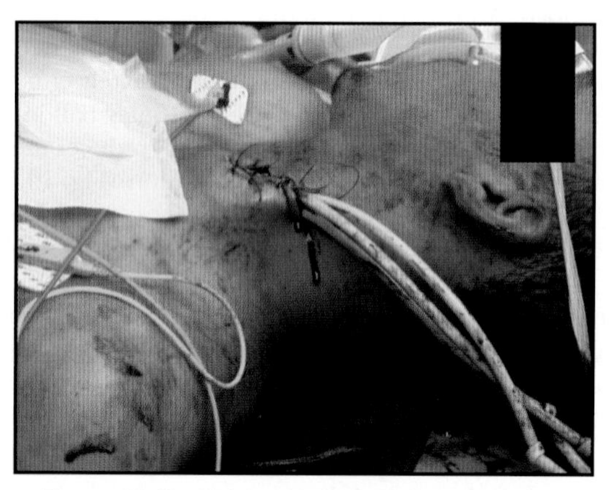

Figure 19.13 Foley catheter balloon tamponade.

to be repaired as soon as possible. Primary repair, end-to-end anastomosis, saphenous vein or synthetic patching/grafting (e.g. polytetrafluoroethylene grafts) are possible repair techniques. Carotid ligation is reserved for comatose patients, patients with CT-proved cerebral infarction or no backflow at surgery. Occluded or dissected vertebral arteries can be treated conservatively. A normal CT angiography after Foley catheter tamponade suggests venous injury. The catheter can be removed in the operating room after 48 hours and the patient observed for another 24 hours in the hospital. In the rare case of re-bleeding, the patient needs to undergo surgical exploration.[157,162]

Oesophageal injuries

Morbidity and mortality are high in oesophageal injuries, especially in delayed diagnosis or presentation. Therefore, the presence of an oesophageal injury must be eliminated in a timely fashion and with a high suspicion. Any air, either cervical or mediastinal, can be a hint for an oesophageal injury and warrants further work-up. Oesophageal injuries must be repaired with a single-layer suture and widely drained.[138,163]

Pharyngeal injuries

Pharyngeal injuries usually heal without surgery.[164] They are treated with antibiotics and nasogastric tube feed. A neck wound must not be sutured for drainage purposes. After a period of 7 days, a contrast swallow is repeated to demonstrate healing.

BLUNT PHARYNGOESOPHAGEAL INJURIES

Blunt pharyngoesophageal injuries are rare. Only 0.02% of patients in a National Trauma Databank were identified with such an injury. Dependent on the injury severity, three of four patients were safely treated non-operatively with antibiotics, nasogastric tube and nil per mouth.[165]

FUTURE DEVELOPMENTS

RESUSCITATIVE ENDOVASCULAR BALLOON OCCLUSION OF THE AORTA

REBOA is a new technique currently under assessment. This technique can provisionally stop a life-threatening haemorrhage, mainly into the abdomen or pelvis, to gain some time to transfer a patient to theatre or to an angiography suite. A catheter is placed into the aorta and a balloon temporarily inflated to interrupt any blood flow distal to it. Some indications are currently being evaluated. Patient selection is challenging but crucial.[166]

HUMAN FACTORS

Trauma management is a team event. Clinical scenarios are often chaotic, time-pressured and emotionally stressful. Optimising team performance and equipping team members with non-technical skills are increasingly recognised as essential skills for effective team-working and vital to ensure favourable outcomes.[167]

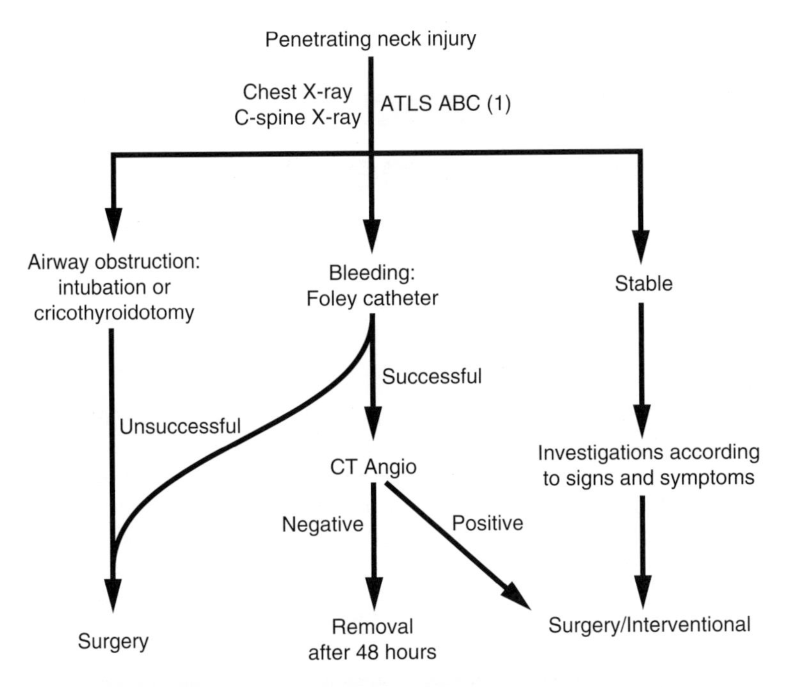

Figure 19.14 Penetrating neck injury. *ATLS,* Advanced Trauma Life Support;

Key points

- Head, chest and abdominal injuries are the main injuries associated with death.
- Abdominal injury is one of the most important causes of preventable death.
- Advanced Trauma Life Support (ATLS) is one way to evaluate and treat severely injured patients in the acute phase.
- The traditional dogma of mandatory exploration of all penetrating wounds has changed to selective non-operative management.
- A laparotomy is mandatory in the event of an acute abdomen, or in the haemodynamically unstable patient with a penetrating wound or in the case of blunt trauma where there is a positive FAST and an unstable patient.
- Life-threatening chest injuries are tension pneumothorax, open pneumothorax, massive haemothorax, cardiac tamponade and flail chest.
- A haemopericardium on ultrasound, a straight left heart border on a chest X-ray, a J-wave in the ECG or an elevated central venous pressure raise the suspicion of an occult cardiac injury and require further investigation.
- An emergency department thoracotomy (EDT) is indicated in life-threatening pericardial tamponade, exsanguinating haemorrhage with profound shock (systolic blood pressure < 60–70 mmHg not responding to resuscitation) or hypovolaemic cardiac arrest after penetrating thoracic trauma.
- Hypoxia, hypoperfusion and hypothermia lead to the well-known deadly triad of hypothermia, acidosis and coagulopathy, which mandates damage control surgery.

References available at http://ebooks.health.elsevier.com/

KEY REFERENCES

[9] American College of Surgeons Committee on Trauma. Advanced trauma life support ATLS student course manual. 9th ed. Chicago, Ill: American College of Surgeons; 2012. p. 366. S. p.

This manual contains all the important knowledge needed for the trauma ABCDE algorithm.

[30] Moore EE, Moore FA. American Association for the Surgery of Trauma Organ Injury Scaling: 50th anniversary review article of the journal of trauma. J Trauma 2010;69(6):1600–1.

This is the most widely accepted and used injury classification system for neck, chest and abdominal injuries.

[38] Navsaria PH, Nicol AJ, Edu S, Gandhi R, Ball CG. Selective non-operative management in 1106 patients with abdominal gunshot wounds: conclusions on safety, efficacy, and the role of selective CT imaging in a prospective single-center study. Ann Surg 2015;261(4):760–4.

This large study showed that non-operative management of selected patients with abdominal gunshot wounds is safe and effective.

[55] Velmahos GC, Zacharias N, Emhoff TA, Feeney JM, Hurst JM, Crookes BA, et al. Management of the most severely injured spleen: a multicenter study of the Research Consortium of New England Centers for Trauma (ReCONECT). Arch Surg 2010;145(5):456–60.

This multicentre study revealed that grade V splenic injuries, especially in combination with a head injury, predict failure of non-operative management.

[69] van der Wilden GM, Velmahos GC, Emhoff T, Brancato S, Adams C, Georgakis G, et al. Successful nonoperative management of the most severe blunt liver injuries: a multicenter study of the research consortium of new England centers for trauma. Arch Surg 2012;147(5):423–8

Even higher-grade liver injuries can be treated non-operatively, as shown by this multicentre study.

[75] Navsaria PH, JU B, Edu S, Nicol AJ. Non-operative management of abdominal stab wounds–an analysis of 186 patients. S Afr J Surg 2007;45(4):128–30. 32

Non-operative management in selected patients is safe. Serial examination in these patients significantly reduced unnecessary laparotomies.

[135] Nicol AJ, Navsaria PH, Hommes M, Ball CG, Edu S, Kahn D. Sternotomy or drainage for a hemopericardium after penetrating trauma: a randomized controlled trial. Ann Surg 2014;259(3):438–42.

This randomised study showed that subxyphoidal window and drainage is effective and safe in stable patients with a haemopericardium after penetrating trauma. No sternotomy is mandatory.

[158] Thoma M, Navsaria PH, Edu S, Nicol AJ. Analysis of 203 patients with penetrating neck injuries. World J Surg 2008;32(12):2716–23.

This prospective observational study presents an algorithm for penetrating neck injuries.

20 Abdominal sepsis and abdominal compartment syndrome

Jonathan C. Epstein | Iain D. Anderson

INTRODUCTION

The diagnosis and management of abdominal sepsis is one of the great challenges the general surgeon faces. Optimal patient outcome requires considered decision-making and prompt action. However, even complex cases of abdominal sepsis can be managed confidently and competently by the application of basic principles. Up to 90% of general surgical mortality follows emergency admission with sepsis,[1] yet there are few units where 90% of resource is targeted at non-elective work. Delay to definitive treatment is the single most common reason for adverse outcomes and anastomotic leak the single commonest complication in fatal cases. Given its frequency and severity, a sound understanding of abdominal sepsis should be integral to every general surgeon's professional practice.

This chapter will address the diagnosis and management of abdominal sepsis, including patients treated in the intensive care unit, where management of abdominal compartment syndrome (ACS), the open abdomen and enterocutaneous fistulas (ECFs) can be particularly challenging. Intra-abdominal compartment syndrome is where intra-abdominal hypertension (IAH) leads to a spectrum of life-threatening pathophysiological changes and is often associated with sepsis. The reader is referred to Chapter 5 for a description of the intensive care management of the surgical patient, and to Chapter 6 for a discussion of surgical nutrition.

DEFINITION OF SEPSIS

Sepsis is defined as life-threatening organ dysfunction caused by dysregulated host response to infection.[2] This definition moves away from previous focus on the systemic inflammatory response syndrome (SIRS), which emphasised inflammation but is widely found in hospitalised patients who never develop infection. In the more recent definition, organ dysfunction is defined by the Sequential (Sepsis-specific) Organ Failure Assessment (SOFA) score: an increase by 2 or more points is associated with in-hospital mortality greater than 10%.[2] An abbreviated score (quick-SOFA) identifies patients with suspected infection at risk of poor outcomes typical of sepsis based on the presence of any two of the following:

- respiratory rate ≥ 22 breaths/min;
- altered mentation;
- systolic blood pressure ≤ 100 mmHg.

Septic shock is defined as a subset of sepsis in which underlying circulatory and cellular metabolism abnormalities are profound enough to substantially increase mortality. Septic shock is identified by the requirement of vasopressors to maintain mean arterial pressure above 65 mmHg and a serum lactate greater than 2 mmol/L (18 mg/dL) in the absence of hypovolaemia. Septic shock is associated with hospital mortality of over 40%.

PATHOPHYSIOLOGY OF SEPSIS

The healthy host response to bacterial invasion includes neutrophil- and macrophage-mediated release of proinflammatory mediators including cytokines, chemokines and nitric oxide at the site of infection (documented in standard texts). If this inflammatory response becomes generalised, systemic vasodilatation, increased vascular permeability and microcirculatory dysfunction with decreased capillary flow lead to hypotension, fluid transudation and ultimately tissue hypoxia. The resulting multiorgan dysfunction syndrome (MODS) is associated with high mortality. Once established, this downward spiral can become independent of the precipitating infective insult and is similar in conditions without initiating infection, such as major trauma, burns and pancreatitis.

The hypothesis that septic shock and MODS may be ameliorated by damping the exaggerated, uncontrolled inflammatory response has not been supported by clinical studies to date. Probably due to the complexity and redundancy of the many pathways involved, targeting a single mediator or even single pathway has had limited clinical success. The predominant current theories can be summarised as follows:

1. **Uncontrolled systemic cytokine release.** Uncontrolled or exaggerated release of cytokines from macrophages in response to cellular injury is proposed to initiate further mediator cascades resulting in neutrophil and platelet activation. There has been particular focus on the role of mediators believed to play a central role, including tumour necrosis factor alpha (TNF-α) and interleukins 1 and 6 (IL-1 and IL-6).[3] However, the measured circulating levels of cytokines vary widely between studies and indeed within study populations.[4] Clinical trials of drugs that inhibit the inflammatory cascade (corticosteroids, TNF-α antagonists and specific monoclonal antibodies) have failed to demonstrate a survival advantage.[3] Individual randomised trials examining the clinical effectiveness of activated protein C in severe sepsis showed promising

initial results, but a recent Cochrane review concluded no survival advantage,[4] and this intervention has now been withdrawn.

2. **Disturbances to coagulation.** Activation of vascular endothelial cells by inflammatory mediators leads to a prothrombotic state, by alteration of both the coagulation and fibrinolytic systems. This can result in haematological failure with a consumptive coagulopathy resulting in disseminated intravascular coagulation (DIC).[4,5]
3. **Immunosuppression.** Septic patients display features of immunosuppression including reduced capacity to clear primary infection and predisposition towards secondary infection with nosocomial pathogens.[4] A number of mechanisms have been mooted—for example, reduced secretion of proinflammatory cytokines such as TNF-α, IL-1 and IL-6 in exchange for increased release of the anti-inflammatory cytokines IL-4 and IL-10 by T-helper cells may play a central role.[6] This pattern of cytokine release has been observed in septic patients in the intensive care setting.[7,8] However, the possibility of immunotherapy to modify this host response has not yielded a therapeutic target to date.

There is an increasing awareness that chronic critical illness develops in a proportion of patients who survive the initial insult that led to the need for intensive care support but remain dependent on long-term organ support. This is characterised by prolonged need for ventilation and may be associated with polyneuropathy, myopathy, catabolism and prolonged delirium. Care for such patients is challenging and living with this condition may not be many patients' choice.

THE SLIPPERY SLOPE OF SEPSIS

Some degree of physiological derangement is common amongst surgical patients on the ward, although this is usually resolved by appropriate treatment of the underlying problem. When significant physiological derangement persists beyond 48 hours, progression to organ dysfunction is much more likely, an event associated with a mortality rate of up to 40%.[9] Mortality, in general, increases with the number of organ systems affected and with the severity of physiological disturbance at onset.[8] Early recognition of deterioration at a time when prompt intervention may yet avert catastrophe is essential.[10] By the time the patient with abdominal sepsis has developed shock, mortality increases from less than 10% to over 50%.[11,12]

It is critical to appreciate that deterioration can often start insidiously, and that early detection is vital as intervention is most successful at this stage. While there are objective criteria that define organ dysfunction as described above, clinical findings are helpful pointers. Hypoxia, oliguria, hypotension, deranged liver function tests or clotting, thrombocytopenia, acidosis and confusion are some of the features that indicate the beginning of a potentially severe systemic derangement.

The benefits of managing such high-risk surgical patients with early critical care input are well recognised.[13,14]

✔✔ The importance of detecting the subtle signs of abdominal sepsis at an early stage cannot be overemphasised and while the rate with which organ dysfunction develops in individual patients will vary, the requirement for rapid identification and treatment is key.

THE SURVIVING SEPSIS CAMPAIGN

In 2008, informed by the results of a number of clinical trials, an international campaign was launched with the intention of improving outcomes in sepsis by standardising care.[15] The emphasis of the campaign was timely identification and treatment of patients with severe sepsis, using goal-directed strategies. Evidence-based guidelines were published in 2004, split into 'bundles' of care to be accomplished within certain time frames (Box 20.1). A total of 165 sites submitted bundle compliance and outcome data on 15 022 patients with severe sepsis. Despite incomplete compliance, a significant reduction in unadjusted hospital mortality (from 37% to 31% over the 2-year study period) was achieved in participating centres.[16] The Surviving Sepsis Campaign (SSC) has continued to reissue guidelines and remains active.

✔✔ The goal-directed treatment bundles developed by the Surviving Sepsis Campaign are a recommended standard of care. Their use in the timely identification and management of patients with severe sepsis has been shown to reduce mortality.[16]

SYSTEMATIC ASSESSMENT

Although effective management of patients with severe sepsis may entail complex investigations and procedures, the results of these manoeuvres are often suboptimal or even lethal without adequate prior resuscitation. A systematic approach such as that described in the Care of the Critically

Box 20.1 Surviving sepsis campaign bundles[15]

Sepsis resuscitation bundle

To be accomplished within the first 6 hours of identification of severe sepsis:

1. Measure serum lactate
2. Obtain blood cultures prior to antibiotic administration
3. Administer broad-spectrum antibiotic, within 3 hours of A&E admission and within 1 hour for current inpatients
4. In the event of hypotension and/or a serum lactate > 4 mmol/L:
   a. Deliver an initial minimum of 20 mL/kg of crystalloid or an equivalent
   b. Apply vasopressors for hypotension not responding to initial fluid resuscitation to maintain mean arterial pressure (MAP) > 65 mmHg
5. In the event of persistent hypotension despite fluid resuscitation (septic shock) and/or lactate > 4 mmol/L:
   a. Achieve a central venous pressure (CVP) of > 8 mmHg
   b. Achieve a central venous oxygen saturation (Scvo2) > 70% or mixed venous oxygen saturation (Svo_2) > 65%

Sepsis management bundle

To be accomplished within the first 24 hours of identification of severe sepsis:

1. Administer low-dose steroids for septic shock in accordance with a standardised ICU policy
2. Maintain glucose control > 70 but < 150 mg/dL
3. Maintain a median inspiratory plateau pressure (IPP) < 30 cmH_2O for mechanically ventilated patients

Ill Surgical Patient (CCrISP) course[17] is recommended as it provides a common management structure for problems of any type or severity (Fig. 20.1). Having a structured approach in times of crisis facilitates speed and reduces the likelihood of management errors. It certainly provides a common language and transparency that lets other health professionals understand the role of interventions, given that an integrated team approach involving diagnostic and interventional radiology, anaesthesia and intensive care is often required.

Patients with abdominal sepsis will inevitably have some degree of physiological instability. The CCrISP course advocates rapid immediate resuscitation following ABC principles of assessment with simultaneous correction of life-threatening conditions and initiation of high-flow oxygen therapy, intravenous fluids and monitoring as required. Some patients will deteriorate catastrophically and require intensive care support, but relatively simple interventions will commonly buy sufficient time for a comprehensive assessment. This assessment aims to determine the cause and severity of any problem and to exclude or optimise other conditions. A thorough review of the patient's notes and charts is essential.

Complications can often be anticipated from the surgical condition in question, knowledge of any recent operative intervention and understanding of comorbidities (Box 20.2). The range of possible diagnoses is often large (Box 20.3) and the initial diagnostic net must be cast widely before drawing it in with the assistance of selective investigations. Reaching a provisional diagnosis and management plan rapidly is important as outcome worsens with delay.

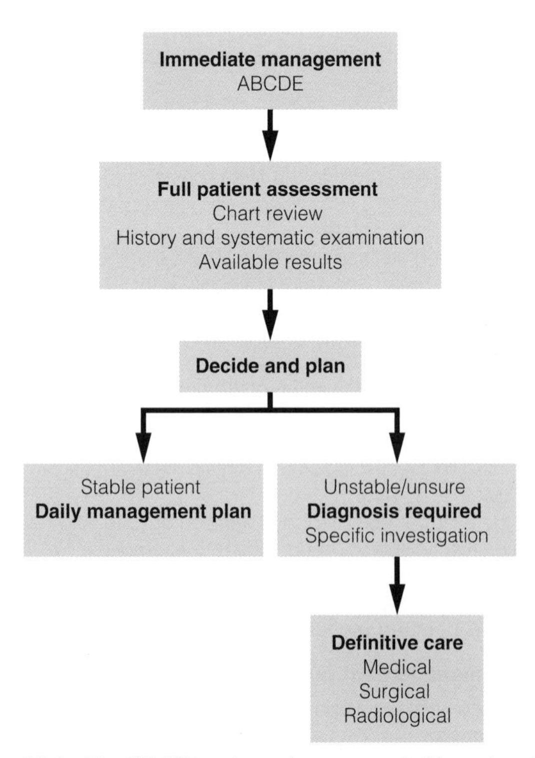

Figure 20.1 The CCrISP system of assessment. (Reproduced from Anderson ID. Assessing the critically ill surgical patient. In: Anderson ID, editor. Care of the critically ill surgical patient. London: Arnold; 1999. p. 7–15. © Hodder Arnold. Reproduced by permission of Hodder Education.)

Patients should improve after clinical interventions. Failure to improve or signs of deterioration suggest a new problem or an incompletely treated initial one. The same systematic CCrISP approach forms the basis of ongoing assessment of the critically ill or at-risk patient on the critical care unit or ward. As repeated complications and setbacks are sadly common in complex cases, the surgeon must anticipate a long campaign rather than a single skirmish and be prepared to take a leading role in ongoing management.

ANTIMICROBIAL THERAPY IN ABDOMINAL SEPSIS

Definitive management of abdominal sepsis requires eradication of the source of infection. However, antimicrobial therapy is also vital.[18] Where sepsis is suspected, blood, vascular access sites, urine, wound and sputum should be sampled for urgent Gram staining and culture. Cultures from the main source of sepsis are several times more likely to be positive (75% vs 18%)[19] than blood cultures, but both are important in the critically ill patient. Once samples for culture have been taken, broad-spectrum antibiotic therapy should begin immediately as delay may negatively influence the outcome.[16] The role of cultures is to enable antibiotics to be changed selectively if the patient fails to respond to initial therapy. The choice

Box 20.2 General manifestations of abdominal sepsis in the ward or HDU patient

- Pyrexia or hypothermia
- Tachycardia
- Tachypnoea
- Confusion
- Oedema
- Metabolic acidosis
- Hypoalbuminaemia
- Thrombocytopenia
- Ileus
- Poor peripheral perfusion
- Hypotension
- Hypoxia
- Lethargy
- Oliguria
- Raised lactate
- Hyponatraemia
- Leucocytosis or neutropenia

Box 20.3 Differential diagnoses to consider in ward patients presenting with apparent abdominal sepsis

Sepsis of other origin (urine, line, chest, etc.)
Cardiac (ischaemia, infarction, dysrhythmias, failure)
Cerebral (toxic confusion, ischaemia)
Pulmonary (atelectasis, collapse, infection, pulmonary embolism)
Fluid imbalance
Other non-septic abdominal complications (e.g. ileus, bleeding)

of antibiotic will be influenced by the clinical circumstances and the expected range of infecting organisms. Early combination antibiotic therapy yields significantly improved survival compared with single-agent use in septic shock.[20] The route of administration must ensure adequate plasma levels and the drugs should penetrate adequately into the tissues. Intravenous infusion is usually necessary. Whenever there is doubt concerning the optimal choice of antibiotics, the advice of a medical microbiologist should be sought. For most abdominal sepsis, coverage of Gram-negative and anaerobic bacteria will be necessary. With biliary sepsis, approximately 15% of cases will involve streptococci species that are resistant to cephalosporins, so the addition of a penicillin is a common approach. With hospital-acquired infection, cover against a broader and more resistant spectrum of organisms will be needed.[18] Fungal infection (usually *Candida* species) is not uncommon in complex abdominal sepsis requiring ICU care and additional antifungal therapy will often be required and is something to be considered in a patient who is not responding to treatment.

✓✓ When severe sepsis is identified, blood cultures should be taken, and broad-spectrum antibiotics administered within 1 hour. This has been shown to reduce mortality as part of a management strategy in sepsis.[16]

✓✓ Combination antibiotic therapy should be used in preference to monotherapy in septic shock as it is associated with a reduction in mortality.[20]

IMAGING IN ABDOMINAL SEPSIS

A range of imaging techniques may be employed to localise an infective focus but computed tomography (CT) with intravenous contrast enhancement provides excellent information in thoracic, abdominal and pelvic sepsis. Consideration should be given to gastrointestinal contrast administration via mouth, nasogastric tube, drain, stoma or rectum. The vast majority of surgical patients can be stabilised sufficiently for scanning to take place safely and the guidance that CT provides in diagnosis and therapeutic intervention should not be underestimated. CT is excellent at primary diagnosis particularly in the complex or postoperative patient where clinical examination is more difficult.[21] Comparison with previous scans is important and the input of an experienced, specialist radiologist is priceless. Modern hospital IT systems allow surgeons to look at scans themselves and routinely reviewing these images permits the surgeon to have more informed discussions. In emergency cases, the surgeon should ideally be present so that decisions about interventional radiological procedures may be made jointly.

Nevertheless, CT (or indeed any diagnostic test) is not perfect. Artefact from drains and metallic prostheses may reduce image quality. Intravenous contrast use is relatively contraindicated in acute kidney injury, although gastrointestinal contrast can still be used to advantage. Even in expert hands, there is a small rate of missed diagnoses and this is amplified in the interpretation of out-of-hours scans in complex postoperative patients.

The chest radiograph still plays a role in patient assessment and ultrasound has the advantage of being portable, harmless and repeatable. The greatest utility of ultrasound probably lies in assessment of biliary and renal pathology and monitoring identified collections. However, it is operator-dependent, and a negative scan will offer little reassurance when the clinical picture is concerning. When a focus of persistent sepsis cannot be identified on primary imaging, investigations such as magnetic resonance imaging particularly for biliary or pelvic pathologies or nuclear medicine modalities such as labelled white cell scanning may help identify occult sources of sepsis.

EARLY SOURCE CONTROL IN ABDOMINAL SEPSIS

Source control describes the physical measures taken to eradicate an infective focus. This includes the percutaneous or operative drainage of collections, debridement of necrotic tissue and definitive surgical procedures to correct an anatomical abnormality. It is intuitive that early source control should improve outcomes in abdominal sepsis and there is evidence for this from studies of perforated peptic ulcer.[22] Delay to source control has been shown to significantly increase mortality in septic shock[23] and expedient source control before progression to septic shock is clearly beneficial.[16,24]

In a complex system such as a hospital it is easy for multiple small individual delays to add up. Managing the multidisciplinary team to achieve prompt and timely intervention is a considerable skill, which requires active and continued leadership from the surgeon. There is often a period of time before being transferred to theatre during which a patient may be resuscitated, but there should be awareness that the sickest patients will require resuscitation in theatre in parallel with source control being obtained. The Royal College of Surgeons of England and the Department of Health have issued timelines regarding the urgency of source control in sepsis (Box 20.4), which are commended as a standard of care.

✓ Expedient control of the septic focus is of utmost importance in the management of severe sepsis. Neither overly prolonged resuscitation nor observation should delay this.[13]

Box 20.4 Timelines for source control in sepsis[14]

Patients with sepsis require immediate broad-spectrum antibiotics with fluid resuscitation and source control.

Septic shock

Control of the source of sepsis by surgery or other means should be immediate and under way **within 3 hours.**

Severe sepsis

Control of the source of sepsis should be performed **within 6 hours** of the onset of deterioration.

Sepsis

Control of the source of sepsis should be performed **within 18 hours.**

AIMS OF TREATMENT IN ABDOMINAL SEPSIS

The management of abdominal sepsis in the emergency surgical admission is relevant to a range of pathology, as covered elsewhere in this volume. Pus should be drained, necrotic tissue excised and specimens submitted for urgent microbiology. While localised collections can be drained percutaneously, generalised peritonitis remains an indication for laparotomy. Spontaneous primary bacterial peritonitis and acute pancreatitis may be considered as exceptions to this rule. Laparoscopy is increasingly used in the management of specific surgical conditions causing abdominal sepsis. It is important to remember that the laparoscopic approach may not always allow adequate debridement and drainage and that the physiological sequelae of a pneumoperitoneum may be poorly tolerated in patients with septic shock.

Whether treatment is radiological or surgical, adequate patient preparation is essential. Coagulopathy must be identified and corrected, and blood should be available if required. Although drainage may be essential to resolve sepsis, not infrequently bacteraemia precipitated by the intervention may cause a temporary deterioration in the patient's condition. Indeed, a bacteraemia may represent the 'second hit' that precipitates deterioration. Such circumstances should be anticipated and an appropriate level of post-procedure care arranged.

In complex cases, particularly in older and sicker patients, a compromise treatment pathway may need to be devised, striking a balance between optimum source control and magnitude of intervention. The opinion of senior colleagues and specialist centres can be invaluable as inadequate treatment will condemn the patient to ongoing sepsis and higher risk of a poor outcome.

Image-guided percutaneous drainage of both spontaneous and postoperative intra-abdominal collections has reported success rates of 70–90%.[25,26] Percutaneous procedures will only be effective if good drainage is achieved. Many percutaneous drains are narrow and inadequate when infected fluid is viscous or contains necrotic tissue. Larger or multiple drains may be more effective and daily flushing can be useful. When radiological drains are placed for abdominal sepsis, the responsibility lies with the surgical team to ensure that the patient's condition improves as expected. On occasions when the patient is not improving after percutaneous drainage, careful thought needs to be given to switching strategy and performing a laparotomy, particularly if there is a possibility of multiple loculated collections or necrotic tissue.

When surgery is performed for sepsis, the procedure will vary according to the underlying pathology. In general, the most straightforward adequate procedure is preferable to a complex and time-consuming operation. There is a current trend towards primary bowel resection and anastomosis in the acute setting, but this should be avoided in unstable patients, in the presence of significant comorbidity or nutritional depletion, or when there is extensive contamination. Generous saline lavage is recommended on completion of the procedure. Delayed skin wound closure may be preferable to primary suture, or wounds may be left to close by secondary intention if sepsis is substantial. In unstable patients a 'damage-control approach' leaving the abdomen open with a return to theatre arranged for definitive treatment may be required.

Obtaining informed consent for treatment may involve both patient and relatives. The potential severity of the situation should not be understated and the possibility of death, stoma creation, the need for intensive care treatment and the potential for further surgery should be discussed explicitly. The average mortality for an emergency laparotomy is around 15%, and increases with age and physiological disturbance.[13] Complementing clinical assessment with an objective determinant of risk from a scoring system (such as P-POSSUM or NELA, see Chapter 4) is valuable in helping to focus efforts appropriately.[13,27]

Postoperative care will almost always be delivered on the surgical high-dependency unit (HDU) or ICU. The surgeon is a key member of the multidisciplinary team, and close cooperation between the surgeon and intensivist is essential (Box 20.5).

✔ Intraperitoneal abscesses with safe access routes should be drained percutaneously under radiological guidance. This intervention carries high success and low recurrence rates.[26]

ABDOMINAL SEPSIS IN THE ICU

The surgeon will be consulted in the assessment and management of patients already in the ICU who develop primary or recurrent abdominal sepsis. The outcome of patients with abdominal sepsis who require ICU treatment depends on age, comorbidities, source of sepsis and degree of organ dysfunction. Control of the source of sepsis is critical for survival of patients with MODS. Survival is greater than 60% when sepsis is eradicated successfully, whereas survival is close to zero if significant abdominal sepsis continues.[28]

The principal causes of recurrent abdominal sepsis in the ICU are shown in Box 20.6. Anastomotic or enteric leakage remains the commonest single cause and should be actively suspected in all 'at-risk' patients who are critically ill or deteriorating. Inadvertent enterotomy during difficult surgery may occur in up to 20% of patients,[29] and the repair is a potential site of weakness that can leak. Gastrostomy and feeding jejunostomy tubes inserted into the gut may also leak and this is more likely when tissue healing is poor.

Box 20.5 The surgeon's role in the ICU

Daily surgical input to:

- Wound and stoma care
- Tubes and drains
- Nutrition
- Ongoing management of sepsis
- Further operations
- Compartment syndrome
- Postoperative bleeding
- Preparation for HDU/ward
- Treatment/advice regarding the underlying surgical disease

Box 20.6 The principal causes of recurrent abdominal sepsis in the ICU

Leaked anastomosis or enterotomy
Leaking gastrostomies and other tubes
Abscesses or collections
Dead or ischaemic gut
Acalculous cholecystitis
Clostridium difficile-associated pseudomembranous colitis
Acute massive gastric dilatation
Neutropenic enterocolitis
Continuing sepsis from 'common' peritonitis sources (perforation of peptic stress ulcer or diverticulum)

Postoperative small-bowel ileus usually resolves within days regardless of the extent of bowel handling.[30] Opiate analgesia and electrolyte abnormalities (hypokalaemia, uraemia) may delay resolution, but failure to progress should prompt consideration of ongoing retroperitoneal or abdominal pathology. Ileus may be difficult to distinguish from adhesive obstruction, and contrast studies help to clarify the situation. Adhesive obstruction frequently resolves, but refractory cases occasionally require laparotomy. However, in a hostile abdomen, such as that found in abdominal sepsis, considerable caution should be exercised in subjecting the patient to further surgery.[31] Whereas a 3-day period of non-operative treatment might be acceptable in the presence of straightforward adhesional obstruction, one should be prepared to wait for considerably longer when faced with a hostile abdomen, provided nutrition can be delivered safely and the patient is regularly assessed. Most cases will resolve, but indications for intervention include evidence of bowel ischaemia, closed loop obstruction and recurrent abdominal sepsis. Recognition of these indications requires regular re-assessment, CT imaging and clinical experience.

ASSESSMENT IN THE ICU

Assessing patients in the ICU is difficult for several reasons. First, the patients are often complex yet unfamiliar if they have been treated previously by other surgeons. Second, sedated, postoperative patients in organ failure display abdominal sepsis differently to new emergency admissions with peritonitis. Abdominal signs are unlikely to be evident unless gross (e.g. flank cellulitis, bowel contents in a drain, necrotic stoma), and the diagnosis of recurrent abdominal sepsis is often made from deterioration in vital organ function and suspicion based on previous treatment and imaging. Contrast-enhanced CT is of great value, but some patients will be too unwell to transfer to the scanner. For this group, exploratory laparotomy may be required. The interpretation of CT images in the recently operated abdomen is not straightforward. Expert reporting will not only confirm the diagnosis but can also potentially identify areas where there is no evidence of inflammation. In a difficult re-operative procedure with dense adhesions, that roadmap can save time and reduce the risk of surgical damage to other organs. Percutaneous drainage has a similar role here as in primary inflammation and the same caveats apply.

The importance of surgeons making their own thorough assessment cannot be overestimated. The surgeon should be satisfied that the diagnosis is secure and that surgery is the best course of action. Part of that process will be engaging in detailed discussion with the intensivist to weigh up alternative diagnoses and sources of sepsis, and to clarify the risks and benefits of intervention at any given point in time. Often this is not clear-cut as patients may have multiple potential sources (e.g. simultaneous pneumonia and abdominal sepsis) or other complicating factors in the context of comorbidities and other ICU treatments.

Whilst the risks of surgery in the ICU population are often self-evident, conservative management has complications too—patients can sometimes be described as being 'too sick *not* to have an operation'. Clear indications for life-saving surgery include generalised peritonitis, inaccessible or multiple collections and presence of dead tissue. Patients with deteriorating organ function and a strong suspicion of abdominal pathology remain a significant group in whom laparotomy may be unavoidable. In some patients, it will be clear that there is no realistic prospect of survival, either from the required operation or, more commonly, the inevitably prolonged ICU course thereafter. It is important that both intensivist and surgeon counsel the family if care is to be limited.

RE-OPERATING IN ABDOMINAL SEPSIS

Re-operating in abdominal sepsis is challenging. From 72 hours after the last operation, dense adhesions make surgery significantly more difficult and the risk of bowel damage increases. Entry to the abdomen can be awkward and an extension of the previous midline incision may help to reach virgin territory. Adhesions are generally most dense around any site of inflammation, as well as around incisions. A preoperative CT scan provides a roadmap to guide the surgeon to the correct location. While a full laparotomy may be desirable, prolonged dissection of adhesions in an area not thought from CT to contain inflammation or a collection may be harmful. The surgeon must deal with the sepsis as thoroughly as possible but balance this with the need for simplicity and speed. Prolonged and complex procedures are likely to lead to systemic deterioration. The prospect of bowel anastomoses healing under such adverse circumstances is not as high as one would like and exteriorisation of bowel ends may be safest. The ability of the patient to withstand further surgery for further complications is very much lower next time around,[28] and the surgeon should see the present operation as the best opportunity for salvaging the patient. Intestinal reconstruction can be attempted when the patient is well and recovered, some months later.

Generally, the simplest and safest procedure will be best, especially in the patient who already has incipient or established organ failure. The principles of damage control defined in the trauma situation apply: drain sepsis, debride necrotic tissue and exteriorise any leaking bowel or anastomoses. Controversy relates to the management of enteric and colorectal anastomotic leaks. While in a well patient, with a small leak and minimal contamination, preservation of a repaired anastomosis with proximal defunctioning and local drainage may be appropriate, this strategy is unlikely to succeed in the critically ill. A first salvage operation in an

ICU patient will successfully eradicate sepsis more than 40% of the time, but a second operation carries a success rate of only 25% and a third operation, only 7%.[28]

In difficult cases, the surgeon must be flexible and have a range of strategies available. In the hostile septic abdomen it may not be possible to take down and exteriorise the primary source of sepsis because of dense adhesions or the anatomical location (oesophagus, duodenum). For inaccessible pelvic sepsis arising from distal small bowel or colon, it may be possible to identify and exteriorise a proximal loop of jejunum without entering and damaging the matted pelvic loops other than to achieve necessary drainage. This will usually relieve the sepsis but at the price of a high-output stoma and prolonged intravenous feeding. For oesophagogastric or duodenal sepsis, all that may be possible is to drain collections and leave large tube or sump drains beside the leaking anastomosis or other septic focus. Placing a T-tube in the defect to create a controlled fistula is also of potential merit. Proximal intestinal contents can sometimes be diverted by way of a surgical gastrostomy. In really difficult situations, it may only be possible to gain entry to pockets of pus or enteric content and leave the abdomen open as a laparostomy. Further pus or enteric content will usually find its way to the surface, assisted by subsequent manual lavage on the ICU or in theatre as necessary. In addition to their role in draining proximal gut secretions, gastrostomy and enterostomy tubes can be placed to facilitate future enteral feeding.

As these laparotomies are often bloody, prolonged and take place in contaminated fields many surgeons leave large drains (24 Ch tube or sump) in the subphrenic spaces and pelvis at the end of the procedure. This may be particularly useful for certain deep cavities (e.g. psoas abscess) or when further leakage is likely or indeed certain. Large Foley catheters can be used to intubate inaccessible bowel to create a controlled fistula (typically the duodenum), and it is often advisable to place an additional large drain just outside the bowel. There can be a particular role for local lavage in pancreatic necrosis but, otherwise, continuing lavage via abdominal drains in the postoperative period is of no proven benefit.

Outcome from surgery for abdominal sepsis in the ICU patient depends on multiple factors. The importance of satisfactory source control has been discussed, but the number of supported organ systems, comorbid conditions, age, frailty and the underlying surgical pathology are also relevant. A further factor associated with survival is the early response to the first operation in the ICU. If there is clinical improvement within 48 hours, then survival is as high as 80%; however, if the patient does not respond in this early phase, survival is reduced to approximately 10%.[28] Given the cost of intensive care, attempts have been made to define those patients with negligible chance of survival. However, due to the heterogeneity of the patient group and the nature of scoring systems in general, it is not possible to use them for decision-making in individual patients. Clinical judgement takes primacy and the scoring systems remain primarily tools for audit and research.

DAMAGE CONTROL LAPAROTOMY

Damage control laparotomy (DCL) is a concept that has expanded from its initial role in trauma surgery (see Chapter 19). Trauma patients can rapidly develop the unholy triad of hypothermia, acidosis and coagulopathy such that surgery becomes un-survivable. Decisive, immediately life-saving manoeuvres are carried out ('staple, pack and go') and the patient returned to ICU for warming and resuscitation, with more definitive surgery deferred for 24–48 hours once coagulopathy has been corrected and homeostasis returned towards normal. Whilst in abdominal sepsis the first laparotomy carries the best chance for salvage,[32] in unstable patients it can be better to make an active decision to quickly drain pus, remove dead tissue, stop bleeding by packing and close overtly leaking bowel with staples (without resection) before terminating the operation. Physiological instability, massive haemorrhage, coagulopathy, ACS and acute mesenteric ischaemia are relative indications for this approach.[32] Packs should generally be removed as early as possible once clotting is restored, and this is usually the next day. The small bowel becomes adherent remarkably quickly and can be damaged as packs are removed. Packs should be removed cautiously under direct vision with saline irrigation and gentle finger separation.

SECOND-LOOK (PLANNED) RE-LAPAROTOMY

These terms refer to scheduled re-exploration of the abdomen, planned at the initial procedure. The term distinguishes it from 'laparotomy on demand', in which the abdomen is explored only when a new problem is identified. After a damage control procedure, a second look is obviously required to complete the necessary definitive procedures but the term is now more commonly applied to 'looking again' after laparotomy for intestinal ischaemia. The extent of intestinal ischaemia may not be fully evident at the first operation and particularly if the bowel has been re-anastomosed, looking again at 48–72 hours can identify further ischaemia before the patient deteriorates. In cases where there is doubt as to the extent of intestinal ischaemia, it may be preferable to resect and staple off the bowel ends and re-assess 48 hours later rather than gamble on anastomosing bowel that might be subclinically ischaemic and doomed to anastomotic failure.

Repeated planned re-laparotomies have been used aggressively for abdominal sepsis with MODS in both Europe and North America for some years. In this method of treatment, the abdomen is typically re-operated upon every 24–48 hours for several days to wash out the peritoneal cavity and remove any ongoing sepsis. A recent randomised trial has shown that this approach is associated with significantly more laparotomies and prolonged ICU stay compared with a 're-laparotomy on demand' approach.[33] There may be a case for a single planned second-look laparotomy in patients with severe faecal peritonitis, but this is debatable. This philosophical approach must not divert the surgeon from maintaining a low threshold for early laparotomy on demand when indicated, as delaying necessary surgery worsens outcome.[28]

✔✔ In patients undergoing surgery for severe secondary peritonitis, re-laparotomy on demand is preferable to 'planned re-laparotomy'.[33]

LEAVING THE ABDOMEN OPEN (LAPAROSTOMY)

As outlined above, the hostile abdomen may be left open to allow pus and enteric contents to drain. It may also be left open when the alternative is closure with undue tension. In appropriate circumstances, this approach can reduce the rate of recurrent sepsis, minimise wound complications and avoid IAH (as discussed further below). It may also allow improved organ function, faster weaning from the ventilator and can facilitate early enteral nutrition. However, this is at the cost of increased fluid loss through evaporation, exposure of the bowel to potential fistulation and considerable psychological distress for the patient. The open abdomen is particularly challenging to nurse as comfortable, secure wound care may be difficult to achieve.[34] Healing is slow and unless the fascia is closed later hernia formation is inevitable. It is undoubtedly a valuable and life-saving technique when needed, but it is also a significant future burden to the patient in its own right and is not to be recommended routinely.[18]

In closing the abdomen during laparotomy for abdominal sepsis, the surgeon should close the fascia conventionally but avoid tension. Tension sutures have little to recommend them and their continued use is not supported. If bowel distension, oedema, haemorrhage (or packing to control it) or the potential for IAH make closure impossible, there are several options open to the surgeon.

A double-sandwich dressing of semipermeable adhesive dressing with moist gauze between the layers of dressing protects the bowel with less adhesion formation than with standard gauze packs. There are various commercial products that can be used and they allow rapid application in comparison with 'home-made' approaches. Alternatively, if other techniques are simply not available, a version of the Bogota bag can be used. In this technique, a sterile 3-L intravenous fluid bag is slit open and sutured to the fascia, covering and protecting the bowel and providing it with a clean, moist environment. Again, as the oedema subsides, usually within 72 hours or so, the Bogota bag or double-sandwich dressing can be removed and the abdomen either closed or a longer-term technique instituted.

In recurrent sepsis, where recovery is likely to be slow, prosthetic mesh can be used to restrain the viscera. Absorbable polyglactin meshes are preferred to non-absorbable polypropylene meshes, as there is less likelihood of disastrous chronic mesh infection and fistulation to underlying bowel.[35] Caution is required in the use of biological implants in this scenario as they are extremely expensive and without proven benefit.

Use of commercial negative-pressure dressings has become widespread as they make wound management considerably more straightforward. Early cohort studies suggested that vacuum-assisted closure was well tolerated in the open abdomen, with intestinal fistulation rates of only 5%.[36] The only randomised trial on vacuum-assisted closure in the open abdomen, which compared it with polyglactin absorbable mesh, did not show benefit and the rate of fistulation in the vacuum-assisted closure arm was 21%.[37] Controversy regarding the rate of intestinal fistulation after application of negative-pressure dressings continues although it should be noted that the most comprehensive case series showed no increased fistula incidence.[38] However, caution is required before contemplating using vacuum dressings in the presence of suture or staple lines, repaired serosal tears or enterotomies.

Many cases of open abdomen management described in the surgical literature relate to cases of trauma or major haemorrhage. These laparostomies can usually be closed within 7 days by conventional techniques. Laparostomy in abdominal sepsis is a different matter and usually runs a much longer course, resulting in retraction of the rectus muscles laterally. The above-described techniques have been combined in expert units to use temporary and protected polypropylene mesh traction with vacuum in the septic open abdomen to prevent muscle retraction and to steadily reduce the size of the abdominal wall defect. However, the techniques are complex, timing-specific and carry very significant risks in non-expert hands.[39] Currently, for the general surgeon forced to create a laparostomy for abdominal sepsis, placement of a polyglactin mesh within the muscular defect remains a safe option.

THE NATIONAL EMERGENCY LAPAROTOMY AUDIT

The National Emergency Laparotomy Audit (NELA) audit is a mandatory joint anaesthetic and surgical national audit of emergency laparotomy in the UK. It measures care in every UK hospital against defined standards including timeliness of assessment and intervention, seniority of decision-makers, facilities, critical care use and seniority of surgical and anaesthetic input. Since 2014, the audit has provided high-quality comparative data which has driven local and national improvements in mortality, length of stay and several other markers of quality of care.[40] Mortality (30-day) has improved from 12% to 9% and length of stay has reduced from 19 days to 15 days. The audit data has provided insights into many of the processes and outcomes of care and stimulated the creation of better patient pathways in many UK hospitals. Specific scientific publications have addressed timing of source control[41], effect of surgical sub-specialisation[42], bowel obstruction[43] and impact of trainee operating[44], for example.

ABDOMINAL COMPARTMENT SYNDROME

Normally, intra-abdominal pressure (IAP) is low (<10 mmHg), but can rise in abdominal sepsis (and other acute abdominal conditions, including trauma and pancreatitis) to the significant detriment of the patient. The condition is probably not as rare as previously thought.[45,46] As abdominal pressure rises, venous return is impaired and cardiac output falls. The tense abdomen can cause pulmonary compromise, oliguria, mesenteric ischaemia and even raised intracranial pressure. These features, similar in some ways to a tension pneumothorax, constitute ACS.[47]

ACS most frequently occurs after laparotomy for peritonitis, abdominal aortic aneurysm repair and trauma, particularly if surgery is prolonged. Tissue oedema results from the combined effects of tissue injury, intravenous fluid infusion and leaky capillaries, bowel distension and haematomas. ACS can even occur in the abdomen that has been left open and packed, especially if there is ongoing haemorrhage. ACS is not restricted to emergency surgery; prolonged elective surgery with a scarred and rigid abdominal wall may also lead to this condition. The anaesthetist may signal an unacceptable rise in the ventilatory pressure as the abdomen is closed but more commonly ACS develops 12–36 hours after surgery on the critical care unit. Oligo/anuria and raised ventilatory pressures are the usual presenting features.

The IAP is measured via the bladder following instillation of 25 mL of normal saline. It is measured through the aspiration port of the catheter tubing using a transducer. The transducer should be zeroed at the level of the mid-axillary line, and IAP measured in the supine position at end expiration.[48] Standardised definitions for ACS were developed in 2006 by an international consensus group[48] (Box 20.7).

A number of medical treatment options are of benefit in reducing IAP.[49] Abdominal wall compliance can be improved with adequate sedation, analgesia and neuromuscular blockade. Intraluminal contents should be evacuated with nasogastric and rectal decompression and the use of pro-kinetic agents. Abdominal fluid collections should be aspirated. Positive fluid balance can be corrected with fluid restriction, diuretics or dialysis/ultrafiltration. However, if pressures above 20 mmHg persist despite these measures, or organ dysfunction worsens, then the abdomen will need to be decompressed and left open using the laparostomy management techniques discussed above.

ENTEROCUTANEOUS FISTULAS

Intestinal fistulas pose a particular set of challenges and require complex management. They contribute to sepsis, malnutrition, fluid and electrolyte imbalances, difficulties in wound care, as well as posing an enormous psychological challenge to the patient.

A fistula is defined as an abnormal communication between two epithelial surfaces. The overwhelming majority occurring in the context of abdominal sepsis result from anastomotic leakage or an inadvertent enterotomy, either overlooked or unsuccessfully repaired. Fistulation from somewhere in the intestinal tract to the laparotomy wound will occur occasionally in every gastrointestinal surgeon's practice. Severe early sepsis may result but more typically there is a period of intestinal ileus, wound infection and clinical stagnation. When the laparotomy wound ruptures or is opened to treat apparent wound infection, the enteric or faecal nature of the content becomes apparent. This may not be convincing to begin with as the enteric flow is usually preceded by a volume of pus and blood mimicking simple postoperative wound infections. Postoperative fistulas may also occur through drains or along recent drain sites, to the vaginal vault in those who have undergone previous hysterectomy and occasionally to the rectum or other parts of the gut.

An ECF is most likely to occur after emergency surgery for another postoperative complication, i.e. sepsis, obstruction or bleeding. In these re-laparotomies, the inherent difficulty of the procedure, brought about by adhesions, bowel distension and friable tissues, makes further bowel damage a real possibility. If that damage is not, or cannot, be repaired effectively and if there is postoperative obstruction, inflammatory phlegmon or an open abdomen, then the likelihood of fistulation increases considerably. The combination of small-bowel obstruction and an undrained abscess is also likely to result in a fistula as the obstructed bowel eventually softens and gives way at or into the collection. Thus, it should be self-evident that repairing a leaking anastomosis when the patient is septic and local tissues oedematous and friable is all too often doomed to failure. Bowel exposed in an open abdomen will also inevitably be subject to some degree of trauma even when the dressings or appliances are handled and changed expertly. In the order of 10–20% of 'laparostomies' will fistulate even with expert care.

A proportion of intestinal fistulas heal spontaneously, although they will cause misery and morbidity while they do so. The factors that contribute to persistence of a fistula are shown in Box 20.8.

Box 20.7 Definitions of abdominal compartment syndrome[48]

Intra-abdominal pressure (IAP)

- Steady-state pressure in the abdominal cavity
- Between 5 and 7 mmHg in critically unwell adults

Abdominal perfusion pressure (APP)

APP = MAP – IAP

Intra-abdominal hypertension (IAH)

Sustained or repeated pathological elevation in IAP ≥ 12 mmHg

Abdominal compartment syndrome (ACS)

Sustained IAP > 20 mmHg (with or without an APP < 60 mmHg) that is associated with new organ dysfunction or failure

Box 20.8 Factors contributing to the occurrence and persistence of postoperative fistulas

Occurrence

Repaired anastomosis
Inadvertent enterotomy (repaired or missed)
New anastomosis in unfavourable circumstances
Persisting abscess or phlegmon causing obstruction
Fistulating disease
Open abdomen

Persistence

Distal obstruction (including constipation)
Open abdomen
Disconnected bowel ends
Local abscess
High output from fistula
Complex fistula
Mucocutaneous continuity
Self-assessment questions

The best-known approach to fistula care is that described at the National Intestinal Failure Unit in Salford (UK), defined by the acronym SNAP (Sepsis, Nutrition, Anatomy, Procedure). The first priority is the expedited treatment of sepsis. Once the necessary resuscitation is in hand, an early CT scan of the abdomen, preferably with both enteric and intravenous contrast, is obtained to identify undrained intra-abdominal sepsis. The frequency of intra-abdominal abscess formation is high, in the region of 66%[50] and this may not be clinically obvious. Without diagnosis and control of the sepsis, the prognosis is bleak. As described earlier, sepsis must be eradicated and the same principles of antibiosis, percutaneous drainage if amenable, surgical drainage if not and diversion if the sepsis is inaccessible apply.

An integral part of early management is wound care and control of the fistula effluent. When there is a small fistula orifice in a drain site or through part of a wound, a stoma bag will suffice. When bowel contents are leaking into a laparostomy, management may be very difficult. Large fistula bags are available. Reducing fistula output by avoiding enteral feed, and administering proton-pump inhibitors, codeine and loperamide, can help. Octreotide can reduce intestinal secretions in some patients, but in our practice its role is relatively limited as it is expensive, unpleasant for the patient and adds little to the steps already described. It is perhaps most useful in pancreatic fistulas.

Immediate fluid management will have to be considered as the patient was resuscitated, but attention will have to turn rapidly to the optimal means of nutrition. Parenteral nutrition (PN) is the mainstay of nutritional support in intestinal fistulation with abdominal sepsis. The potentially negative effect that enteral nutrition often has on output and wound care, particularly in the early stages, should be self-evident. Enteral feeding may also 'feed' the abdominal sepsis if there is complexity to the fistula or a further unrecognised proximal hole in the bowel. There is often partial obstruction associated with the sepsis and in the vast majority of ECF cases it is more reliable to administer PN while the patient stabilises and the situation with regard to sepsis, wound care and anatomy is clarified. In some circumstances, enteral nutrition can take over some, or even all, of the role, but this will usually take time and is only possible in selected patients.

ECF can be categorised as high- or low-output (output above or below 500 mL/24 hours). High-output fistulas are likely to have a significant effect on fluid balance and nutrition. Some proximal fistulas produce several litres of electrolyte-rich fluid per day and maintaining fluid balance can be challenging. Senior surgical staff will need to commit to adequate supervision of the recording of the various inputs and outputs, particularly in the initial phase before steady state is reached. Fistula output will often reduce with time. Many fistulas arising from anastomotic dehiscence will be a side hole anatomically and if there is free distal flow, no sepsis, no bowel disease and no distal obstruction (which may be simple constipation), then spontaneous closure may occur. It is uncertain whether restricted oral intake helps, but it is intuitive to minimise flow to encourage healing. If the fistula has not closed by 6 weeks and there is no apparently reversible factor (e.g. abscess, constipation), spontaneous closure is unlikely and introduction of more liberal oral intake may be reasonable.

In the ICU setting, once sepsis is excluded or controlled and any laparostomy is starting to granulate, oral or enteral feeding can be introduced cautiously, maintaining a careful watch for recurrent sepsis. The nutritional benefit of this will depend on the length and condition of gut available for absorption and it will often take time for enteral feeding to be established. During this phase, combined enteral and parenteral feeding is used.

Early surgery is required for abdominal sepsis not amenable to non-operative intervention where washout, exteriorisation and formation of a laparostomy may be necessary. Attempts at re-operation on an unstable patient to try to correct the fistula are likely to cause more harm than good. Surgery for fistulas is best deferred until the patient is well physically, nutritionally and emotionally, and only after the anatomy has been defined radiologically. This is often many months later and in complex cases is a highly specialist undertaking. The appropriate time to operate is a matter of judgement—prolapse of fistulas/stomas is a useful indication that adhesions have softened as is the ability to pinch to re-epithelialised laparostomy skin. It is axiomatic that 'it is impossible to operate too late—only too early'. Careful planning is required for both the intestinal components of surgery and the abdominal wall reconstruction. In the UK central funding is provided to specialist units where established teams experienced in wound management, skin care, nutrition, central venous catheter care, radiological assessment and definitive surgery are based.

Key points

- Abdominal sepsis is associated with high mortality.
- A systematic approach, based on sound understanding of pathophysiology, is fundamental to successful sepsis management. Adequate resuscitation, early diagnosis, rapid definitive treatment, and accurate and ongoing reassessment are essential if the progression to organ dysfunction and failure is to be avoided.
- Identifying and rapidly treating the underlying cause of sepsis ('source control') is fundamental.
- Radiological intervention for localised sepsis is often key and a logistical challenge for health services to provide on a round-the-clock basis.
- Indications for laparotomy include generalised peritonitis, tissue necrosis, multifocal abscesses and failure of radiological intervention.
- Re-laparotomy is often difficult and advanced techniques may be required.
- Intra-abdominal hypertension and abdominal compartment syndrome are probably under-recognised. Medical management has a role, but in refractory cases surgical abdominal decompression will be required.
- Intestinal fistulas can occur following any abdominal intervention, but are more common after emergency surgery. Prompt eradication of sepsis and attention to nutrition is key. Definitive surgery to correct the fistula should be deferred until the patient is well and the anatomy has been clearly defined.
- Abdominal sepsis often runs a prolonged course and the surgeon must play a central role in coordinating management.

References available at http://ebooks.health.elsevier.com/

KEY REFERENCES

[1] Scottish audit of surgical mortality. 2010. http://www.sasm.org.uk/Publications/SASM_Annual_Report_2010.pdf.

This report reviews all inpatient deaths under the care of surgical teams and highlights the high mortality rate associated with emergency abdominal surgery.

[2] Singer M, Deutschman CS, Seymour CW, et al. The third international consensus definitions for sepsis and septic shock (Sepsis-3). JAMA 2016;315(8):801–10. PMID: 26903338.

Updated definitions of sepsis and septic shock.

[15] Dellinger RP, Levy MM, Carlet JM, et al. Surviving Sepsis Campaign: international guidelines for management of severe sepsis and septic shock: 2008. Crit Care Med 2008;36(1):296–327. PMID: 18158437.

Evidence-based guidelines for diagnosis and treatment of patients with sepsis.

[22] Buck DL, Vester-Andersen M, Møller MH, et al. Surgical delay is a critical determinant of survival in perforated peptic ulcer. Br J Surg 2013;100(8):1045–9. PMID: 23754645.

This Danish cohort study reported increased mortality with every extra hour of delay to reaching theatre.

[28] Anderson ID, Fearon KC, Grant IS. Laparotomy for abdominal sepsis in the critically ill. Br J Surg 1996;83(4):535–9. PMID: 8665253.

This study of repeat laparotomies on patients on ICU reported increased complications and diminishing benefits to subsequent surgery.

[45] Teubner A, Anderson ID, Scott NA, et al. Intra-abdominal hypertension and the abdominal compartment syndrome. (Br J Surg 2004;91:1102–10) Br J Surg 2004;91(11):1527. PMID: 15499645.

Describes the problem of abdominal compartment syndrome, how to recognise it and how to treat it.

[50] Harris C, Nicholson DA, Anderson ID. Computed tomography: a vital adjunct in the management of complex postoperative sepsis. Br J Surg 1998;85:861–2.

Radiological diagnosis and treatment of sepsis in patients with an enterocutaneous fistula is key to optimal outcome.

21 Complications of bariatric surgery presenting to the general surgeon and considerations for the general surgeon when operating on the obese patient

Bruce R. Tulloh | Andrew C. de Beaux

INTRODUCTION

Obesity is now a global health problem, placing an enormous health burden on our society because of the medical comorbidities that are associated with it, including type II diabetes, hypertension, dyslipidaemia, steatohepatitis, obstructive sleep apnoea, arthritis of the weight-bearing joints, gastro-oesophageal reflux, depression and infertility. In general, these medical problems improve or even resolve in parallel with weight loss. Surgery specifically aimed at weight loss ('bariatric' surgery, from the Greek word *baros* = weight, *iatrikos* = medical) has been developing since the 1950s and in the last 30 years, in the wake of advances in laparoscopy, bariatric surgery has become increasingly popular. Surgery remains the only way to produce significant, sustainable weight loss and improvement/resolution of comorbidities in the morbidly obese and indeed improve life expectancy in this group.[1–3] Most bariatric surgery is now performed in centres staffed by surgeons with a specific bariatric interest, usually as part of a multidisciplinary team.

✔✔ Bariatric surgery is the only method of producing long-term, reliable and significant weight loss with resolution of the associated morbidities of morbid obesity.[2]

Although the number of hospitals providing a bariatric service in the UK is undoubtedly growing, as in many other countries, many patients still have to travel long distances for their surgery, some even going overseas to other countries. Procedures are generally performed using laparoscopic techniques and lengths of stay are short. In the event of postoperative complications, patients can therefore present back to their local hospital or clinic, perhaps far from the hospital where the surgery was performed, where there may be no specialist knowledge or expertise in the field. The aim of this chapter is to inform general surgeons of the disease processes underlying obesity, the current bariatric procedures which are commonly performed, to outline the common complications that may arise from these operations and to provide management guidance for those patients that present in an emergency setting.[4–6] As the incidence of obesity in most countries is rising and such patients will present for other general surgical procedures, specific considerations that help such operations will also be discussed.

CAUSES OF OBESITY

While obesity is the result of a chronic energy imbalance when food (calorie) intake exceeds energy expenditure, such an explanation on its own is too simplistic. Obesity should be considered a multifactorial socio-psycho-endocrine disease process.

It is now clear that there is a complex physiological adipostatic system in place that works to maintain a constant body weight in the face of daily fluctuations in energy balance.[7] The hypothalamus is an important control centre for this process, integrating a variety of both short-term and long-term energy flux signals. The gastrointestinal (GI) tract produces a number of hormones including ghrelin, glucagon-like peptides (GLP)-1 and 2, peptide tyrosine-tyrosine, insulin and cholecystokinin, which not only influence gut motility and exocrine secretions but also exert positive and negative feedback on the hypothalamus to regulate appetite. Ghrelin, the 'hunger hormone', is released from the gastric body and promotes appetite, while leptin, a hormone that circulates in proportion to the body's fat mass, has a negative feedback on the hypothalamus to promote negative energy balance. Neural pathways are also involved via vagally innervated stretch receptors in the stomach wall, which induce satiety (and even nausea) in response to gastric distension.

There are also social and psychological drivers to eat. Eating is a pleasurable activity and, for many, meals are the hub of family and social events. Eating may also provide comfort to address fear, loneliness or anxiety. There is now evidence that such negative emotions increase food consumption and that obese people eat in response to emotions more than normal-weight people.[8]

Dieting is known to be difficult and, for many, is not successful in the long term.[9] Modern human beings have evolved from nomadic hunter-gatherers and our physiology defaults to energy storing in periods of food shortage. Thus, dieting induces a physiological adaptation to starvation. This stimulates appetite, induces the bowel to absorb a greater proportion of food eaten, reduces energy loss by a subtle lowering of body temperature and promotes fat storage.

Surgery is the most effective treatment for severe and complex obesity because it alters the physiological processes at the heart of weight homeostasis. Different procedures do this in different ways.[10]

MECHANISMS OF WEIGHT LOSS SURGERY

Traditionally, weight loss operations have been described as either restrictive or malabsorptive, influencing either the volume of food that can be ingested or the absorption of food at the mucosal level, respectively (or both). However, it is more likely that surgery interacts in a beneficial way with the complex adipostatic system outlined above.[10] Patients with gastric bands, for example, who are restricted in their oral intake by the constricting ring around their upper stomach, do not show the normal hormonal adaptation to starving. Part of the band's action appears to be through feedback to the adipostat, possibly via vagal afferents. Similarly, patients undergoing a so-called malabsorptive operation, such as gastric bypass, do not suffer chronic diarrhoea; their weight loss is mediated by a series of gut hormonal changes that influence appetite, food choices and gut motility, amongst other things.

Even so, iatrogenic manipulations of the adipostat are not the full story. In order to achieve the best outcomes, patients still need to make a series of healthy dietary and lifestyle changes along the lines of eating sensibly and being physically active. Most authorities agree that postoperative weight maintenance is improved by the ongoing encouragement, advice and support obtained from long-term follow-up in a bariatric clinic.[11–13]

While weight control is a complex process, the mechanisms behind the postoperative resolution of obesity-related comorbidities are also complex and, even now, not fully understood. Control of type II diabetes mellitus, for example, is known to improve in parallel with the gradual weight loss that follows gastric band surgery.[14] However, the gastric bypass and duodenal switch operations can normalise glucose tolerance much more quickly, even before there has been any appreciable weight loss.[15,16] Such changes are mediated by gut hormones that are stimulated either by a lack of nutrients in the foregut or by the rapid post-prandial delivery of food to the hindgut, with a resultant improvement in pancreatic function and a reduction in peripheral insulin resistance. These processes are well explained elsewhere[7,15,17] and will not be expanded upon here.

BARIATRIC OPERATIONS

The commonest weight loss procedures performed around the world at present are the gastric band, gastric bypass and sleeve gastrectomy. In very obese patients, an alternative operation is the duodenal switch procedure. The main endoscopic option at present is insertion of a gastric balloon, although endoscopic gastric plication is possible. Implantable neuroregulatory devices (gastric 'pacemakers') represent a new direction for surgical weight control by harnessing neural feedback signals to help control eating.

The reason that so many options exist is because no procedure is perfect. Each brings its own benefits and risks. There is little evidence to indicate which operation suits which patient, although most series demonstrate greater average weight loss from operations with a 'malabsorptive' component over 'restrictive' operations alone.[13,18] In practice, the final choice of operation emerges from a detailed discussion between the patient and their surgeon about the options available and the potential risks and benefits of each one.

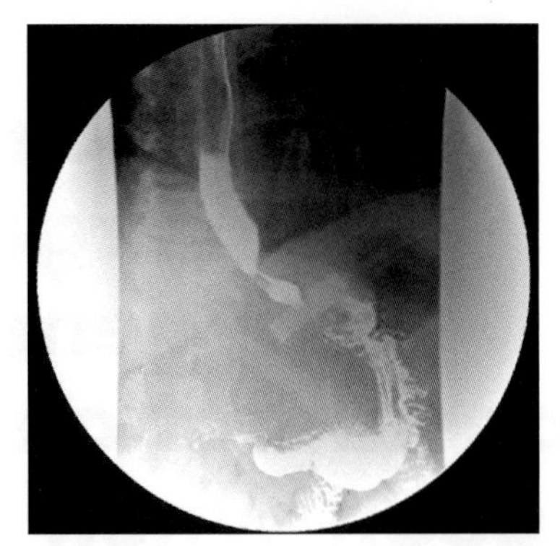

Figure 21.1 Barium meal showing band sitting at a normal angle of approximately 45 degrees, in the 8-to-2 o'clock direction.

GASTRIC BAND

The gastric band is an inflatable silicone ring fixed around the proximal stomach to create a zone of constriction with a small proximal gastric pouch of approximately 30 mL. The band sits around the gastric fundus just below the angle of His, runs along the line of the left crus of the diaphragm and typically lies at about 45 degrees to the horizontal in the 8-to-2 o'clock direction (Fig. 21.1). Many surgeons secure the band in position with a number of gastro-gastric sutures from the fundus below the band up on to the small gastric pouch. The band connects by tubing to an injection port, which is then secured subcutaneously on the anterior abdominal wall. Instillation or aspiration of saline via the subcutaneous injection port adjusts the degree of constriction produced by the band. The amount of saline required in the band varies from patient to patient and often a number of fine adjustments are needed to achieve just the right level of restriction so that patients can manage small portions of normal food.

ROUX-EN-Y GASTRIC BYPASS

This is the most common bariatric operation now performed worldwide. The first step involves using the linear cutting stapler to separate a small proximal gastric pouch, again approximately 30 mL in volume, from the distal stomach, which is left *in situ*. The small bowel is then divided 50–100 cm beyond the duodenojejunal (DJ) flexure and the distal side anastomosed to the gastric pouch, in an antecolic or retrocolic position. The proximal side, representing the biliopancreatic limb of the Roux-en-Y reconstruction, is anastomosed 100–150 cm distal to the gastrojejunostomy (Fig. 21.2). Any mesenteric defects are closed to prevent subsequent internal herniation.

MINI-GASTRIC BYPASS

A more recent modification of the gastric bypass is the mini-gastric bypass, so called because it is quicker and easier to

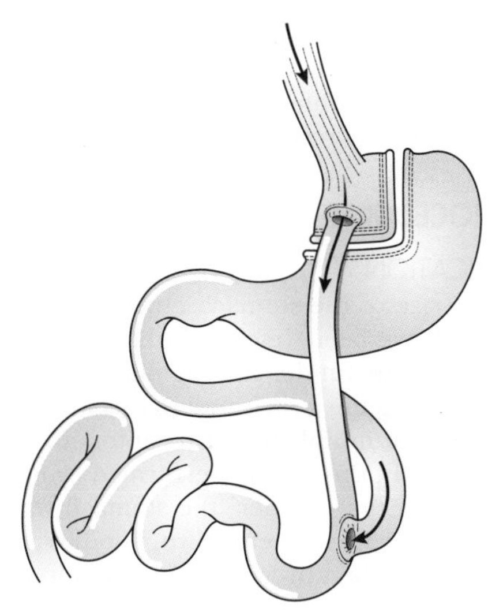

Figure 21.2 Diagram of a gastric bypass.

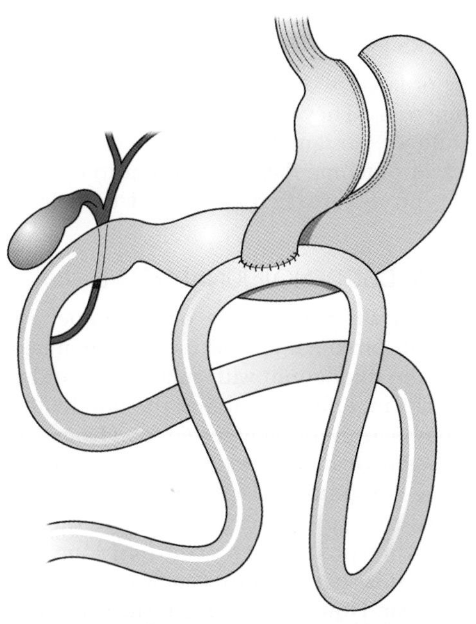

Figure 21.3 Diagram of a mini-gastric bypass.

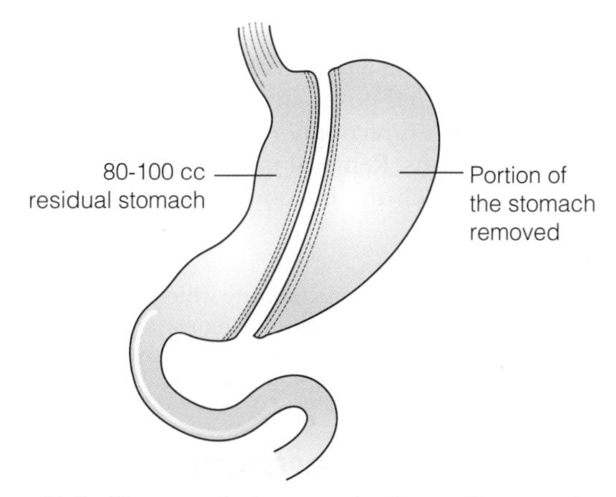

Figure 21.4 Diagram of sleeve gastrectomy. The omentum (not shown) is preserved on the gastro-epiploic arcade.

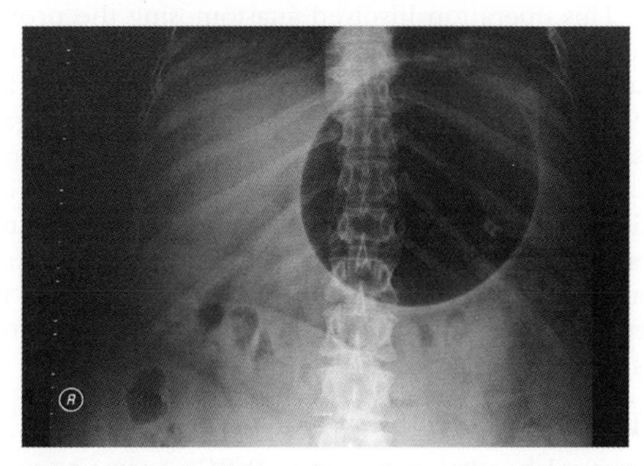

Figure 21.5 Abdominal X-ray of a patient with a gastric balloon *in situ*.

perform. The essential differences between this and a conventional bypass are that a longer gastric pouch is created and a Polya-type antecolic loop gastrojejunostomy, rather than a Roux-en-Y configuration, is constructed (Fig. 21.3). Early results are satisfactory and longer-term outcome data are encouraging.

SLEEVE GASTRECTOMY

This operation was originally developed as the first stage of a duodenal switch operation but soon became a stand-alone procedure when its weight loss outcomes were, at least initially, similar to what was achievable with a gastric bypass.[19] It is also technically easier to perform than any of the Roux-en-Y procedures, particularly in super-obese patients. The greater curve of the stomach is separated from the omentum from the angle of His to a point 5–6 cm proximal to the pylorus. A bougie, commonly around 34 French in size, is inserted down to the antrum and manipulated up against the lesser curve. Using a linear cutting stapler and with the bougie as a guide, the body and fundus of the stomach are excised and removed to produce a narrow, tubular stomach. Note that vagal innervation (and thus pyloric function) is preserved. (Fig. 21.4).

DUODENAL SWITCH

The duodenal switch, or biliopancreatic diversion (BPD) operation, can be performed as a two-stage procedure but is more commonly carried out in one sitting.[20] The first stage is a conventional sleeve gastrectomy. The second stage involves dividing the duodenum just distal to the pylorus and then dividing the small bowel halfway between the DJ flexure and the ileocaecal junction. The distal part of the divided small bowel is then anastomosed to the proximal end of the divided duodenum just beyond the gastric outlet (pylorus). Thus the jejunum is 'switched' for the duodenum. The biliopancreatic (Roux) limb of the divided small bowel is then joined to the ileum 100 cm proximal to the ileocaecal valve. This creates a longer bypassed segment and a much shorter common channel than a standard gastric bypass procedure, resulting in significantly more malabsorption.

INTRAGASTRIC BALLOON

This plastic balloon is inserted endoscopically and inflated with saline under vision to between 500 and 700 mL (Fig. 21.5). This induces a feeling of fullness and thus reduces oral intake. Because the satiety effect wanes after several months, combined with a small risk of leakage/deflation *in situ*, with the associated possibility of distal migration of the collapsed balloon, it is recommended that the balloon is removed after 6 months. Removal involves another endoscopic procedure in which the balloon is punctured, aspirated and withdrawn.

✔ There is little evidence to indicate which operation suits which patient, although most series demonstrate greater average weight loss from operations with a 'malabsorptive' component over 'restrictive' operations alone.[13]

OLDER, MORE OBSOLETE OPERATIONS

JEJUNO-ILEAL BYPASS

It is rare to see patients with an intact jejuno-ileal bypass today. This operation involved anastomosing the proximal jejunum to the terminal ileum less than 100 cm from the ileocaecal valve. It gained popularity between the 1950s and1970s before the emergence of the Roux-en-Y gastric bypass operation. The jejuno-ileal bypass resulted in significant protein malabsorption and vitamin/mineral deficiency, with the long blind jejunal limb commonly leading to bacterial overgrowth. Patients were prone to liver failure as a result of both protein malnutrition and toxaemia from bacterial overgrowth in the blind loop.[11] The majority of patients, if still alive, have had their operations reversed.

VERTICAL BANDED GASTROPLASTY (VBG)

The vertical banded gastroplasty (VBG) operation gained popularity in the 1980s and early 1990s, but its high failure rate and the advent of better procedures have resulted in it being abandoned. Just above the incisura, a short distance in from the lesser curve, the anterior and posterior walls of the stomach were stapled together with a circular stapler. Through the resultant hole made by the stapler, a linear stapler could be applied vertically towards the angle of His. This staple line fixed the anterior and posterior gastric walls together but did not divide the stomach. The outlet of the small gastric pouch thus created was then 'banded' with a 360 degree ring of tape to prevent dilatation (Fig. 21.6). The high failure rate resulted from pouch outlet stenosis and/or pouch dilatation (usually caused by overeating) which was often followed by disruption of the vertical staple line with the consequent loss of restriction to eating.

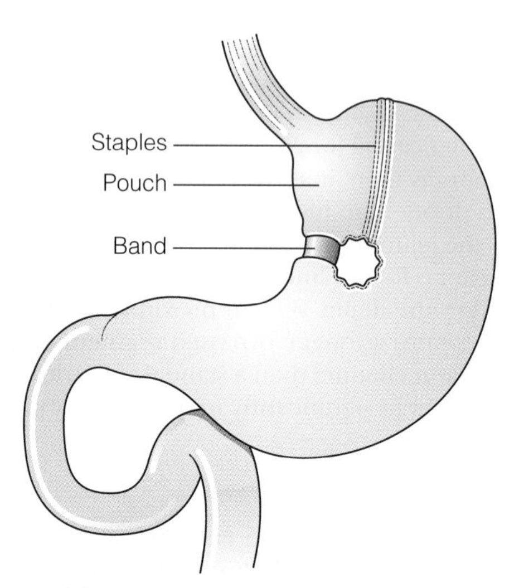

Figure 21.6 Diagram of the vertical banded gastroplasty procedure.

NEWER PROCEDURES

GASTRIC PLICATION

Reducing the size of the stomach either endoscopically or laparoscopically has been described where the greater curve of the stomach at the fundus is invaginated to reduce gastric volume.[21] Infolding the gastric wall in this way may also provide stimulation of mural stretch receptors to reduce hunger. Endoscopically, this can be performed by firing a series of staples or clips that 'gather' the stomach wall from the inside.[22] Outcomes are not yet known, but the same technology has been described previously for plicating the gastro-oesophageal junction for treating reflux where, despite early successes, long-term results have been disappointing.

IMPLANTABLE NEUROREGULATORS (GASTRIC 'PACEMAKERS')

A number of laparoscopically implantable devices are now undergoing trials. They register the presence of food in the stomach and are designed to mediate satiety by vagal feedback. Lack of outcome data in addition to concerns about battery life and cost are currently a block to their more widespread use.

ENDOSCOPIC DUODENOJEJUNAL SLEEVE

This endoscopically inserted tube of thin, impervious plastic material has its proximal end secured to the mucosa of the first part of the duodenum with small barbs and then runs distally for 60 cm, effectively lining the duodenum and upper small bowel, preventing ingested food from making contact with the mucosa until the proximal jejunum is reached. Its effect on the gut hormone milieu mimics that of the gastric bypass and early clinical results have shown a similar improvement in type II diabetes control, along with modest weight loss.[23] It is suggested that such barriers be removed at around 1 year. However, no long-term follow-up information is available regarding the extent of weight regain or the return of glucose intolerance after the barrier is removed and the technique has not gained popularity.

COMPLICATIONS OF BARIATRIC SURGERY

There are *general* complications such as might follow any abdominal operation, and *specific* complications that relate to the procedure performed.

GENERAL COMPLICATIONS

It should be within the capability of any abdominal surgeon to manage the general complications of bariatric surgery, which include pulmonary atelectasis/pneumonia, intra-abdominal bleeding, anastomotic or staple-line leak with or without abscess formation, deep vein thrombosis (DVT)/pulmonary embolism (PE) and superficial wound infections. Patients may be expected to present with malaise, pallor, features of sepsis or obvious wound problems.

However, clinical features may be difficult to recognise owing to body habitus. Abdominal distension, tenderness and guarding may be impossible to determine clinically due to the patient's obesity. Pallor is non-specific and fever and leucocytosis may be absent. Wound collections may also be very deep. These complications in a bariatric patient should be actively sought with appropriate investigations. In particular, it is vital for life-threatening complications such as bleeding, sepsis and bowel obstruction to be recognised promptly and treated appropriately. A persistent tachycardia may be the only sign heralding significant complications and should always be taken seriously.[24]

It is useful to classify complications as 'early', 'medium' and 'late' because, from the receiving clinician's point of view, the differential diagnosis will differ accordingly (Table 21.1). Early complications usually arise within the first few days of surgery but, with ever-advancing laparoscopic surgery and shorter lengths of stay, these may still present to the non-bariatric surgeon after the patient has left the specialist centre.

SPECIFIC COMPLICATIONS

These relate to the procedure performed. Again, they may be grouped into 'early', 'medium' and 'late', although the 'early' complications overlap with the general complications mentioned above. Medium-term complications are likely to arise while the patient is still overweight and thus may be difficult to diagnose. Late complications may develop many years later. Patients at this stage may be of normal weight, and therefore a link to their previous bariatric surgery may not be obvious (Table 21.2).

CLINICAL PRESENTATION

Once the receiving clinician understands the operation that has been performed and the specific complications to look out for, the next step is the interpretation of the presenting clinical features and formulation of a management plan.

Table 21.1 General complications following bariatric surgery (similar to those that may arise following any GI operation)

Early	Medium or late
Bleeding:	Chest infection
Intraluminal (staple/suture line)	DVT/PE
Intraperitoneal (staple/suture line, mesentery, omentum, liver/ spleen injury)	Haematoma or abscess
Subcutaneous (trocar site)	Incisional or port-site hernia
Staple/suture line leak	
Inadvertent GI tract perforation	
Port-site haematoma/infection	
DVT/PE	
Anaesthetic drug reaction, etc.	
Chest infection/atelectasis	
Port-site hernia with or without bowel obstruction	

GI, gastrointestinal; *DVT*, deep venous thrombosis; *PE*, pulmonary embolism.

GASTRIC BAND PATIENTS

VOMITING AND/OR DYSPHAGIA

These are very common and not surprising symptoms, considering that the band works by causing a constriction ring around the upper stomach. Patients with the gastric band are accustomed to a degree of dysphagia and occasional vomiting, so for them to present for medical attention implies that it is 'worse than usual'. These symptoms indicate a degree of obstruction at the level of the band and there are three main causes.

Band too tight

Has the patient had an adjustment recently? Perhaps they have a food bolus obstruction. Once the patient begins to vomit, the gastric wall becomes oedematous within the confines of the band and the apparent obstruction becomes worse. The treatment is urgent band decompression using the subcutaneous injection port (Box 21.1 and Fig. 21.7). Once the patient can drink freely they can be discharged, with arrangement for follow-up by their bariatric specialist team.

Acute band 'slippage'

This is the term commonly used to describe what is really a process of gastric prolapse upwards through the band. It typically occurs months or years after the original operation and is possibly more common when no gastro-gastric tunnelling sutures are used to secure the band in place. The patient usually presents with vomiting, often in association with being able to eat a sizeable meal, as the food accumulates in the large gastric pouch above the band before eventually being regurgitated. Urgent decompression often provides relief but if not, then an urgent contrast swallow should be ordered. Slippage is often evident on a plain abdominal or chest X-rays, with the band lying at an unusual angle (Fig. 21.8), although a contrast swallow provides more conclusive information. The most serious complication of band slippage is ischaemic necrosis of the prolapsed fundus, secondary to distension and/or occlusion of the blood supply to the proximal stomach as it passes through the band. Failure of the symptoms to resolve with percutaneous band decompression is an indication for urgent surgical intervention.

The operation to remove the band is generally by laparoscopy. The tight band must be released. Unclipping it may be difficult, especially laparoscopically, but if possible—and if the stomach is viable—then it may be left *in situ* for an experienced bariatric surgeon to re-position at a later date. An alternative to unclipping the band is simply to cut it in half, after which it should be removed. Once local adhesions have been divided, the band should just slide out. If there is gastric necrosis, then laparotomy and some form of gastrectomy will be required along with complete removal of the band, tubing and injection port.

Band erosion

This is not usually an acute problem but presentation may be precipitated by an aggravation of dysphagia with or without pain and sepsis. Symptoms will not improve after percutaneous band decompression. An urgent contrast swallow may also demonstrate band erosion with leakage of contrast around the band (Fig. 21.9), but the most definitive test

Table 21.2 Specific complications of bariatric surgery: early, medium and late

Procedure	Early	Medium	Late
Band	Gastric perforation Liver/spleen injury with bleeding	Slippage (with or without gastric necrosis) Injection-port migration or infection	Slippage Erosion Injection-port problems Mega-oesophagus
Sleeve	Reflux oesophagitis Staple-line bleed or leak Splenic infarct Omental necrosis	Intra-abdominal abscess or haematoma	Fistula Stenosis of sleeve
Bypass/duodenal switch/BPD	Anastomosis/staple-line bleed or leak Small-bowel enterotomy Early SBO	Intra-abdominal abscess or haematoma Roux limb obstruction Biliopancreatic (blind) loop obstruction	SBO (internal hernia, volvulus, adhesions) Anastomotic ulcer Anastomotic stricture Dumping syndrome Micronutrient malnutrition Gastro-gastric fistula Hypoglycaemia
Mini-gastric bypass	As above	As above	As above plus bile reflux
Intragastric balloon	Nausea/vomiting Gastric ulceration Gastric or oesophageal perforation	Dehydration and electrolyte imbalance Reflux oesophagitis	Bowel obstruction from deflated balloon
VBG		Stomal stenosis	Staple-line disruption
JIB		Bowel obstruction (internal hernia, adhesions)	Malnutrition Blind loop syndrome Liver failure
Duodenal barrier	Duodenal bleeding Duodenal perforation	Dumping syndrome Food bolus obstruction Migration of the device with mechanical bowel obstruction	Unknown
Gastric plication	Bleeding Splenic or liver injury	–	–
Gastric pacing	Nausea/vomiting Infection of subcutaneous implant	–	–

BPD, biliopancreatic diversion; *JIB,* jejunoileal bypass; *SBO,* small-bowel obstruction; *VBG,* vertical banded gastroplasty.

Box 21.1 Urgent percutaneous band decompression

The subcutaneous injection port should be palpable beneath the skin on the abdominal wall, usually close to one of the longer laparoscopic scars. Some surgeons place it over the lower sternum. The patient usually knows where it is. Using a strict aseptic technique, the port is steadied between the fingers of one hand while the other holds an empty 10-mL syringe with needle attached. Ideally a non-coring 'Huber' or spinal needle is used so as not to damage the port, but in an emergency a conventional 23-gauge hypodermic needle works well (although it may not be long enough). Entering at right angles to the skin, the rubber diaphragm of the port is punctured. The needle hits the metal base-plate with a 'clunk' and aspiration can begin. The reservoir is aspirated to dryness; it may contain up to 14 mL. The needle is simply withdrawn when finished and a small dressing applied.

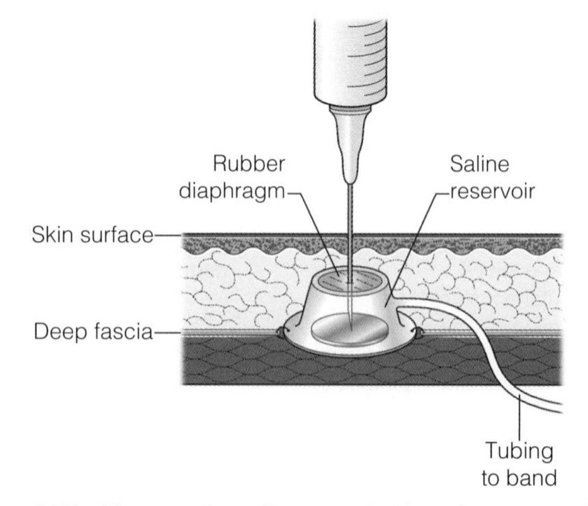

Figure 21.7 Diagram of needle access to the subcutaneous injection port. Strict aseptic technique is important and a non-coring Huber needle should be used.

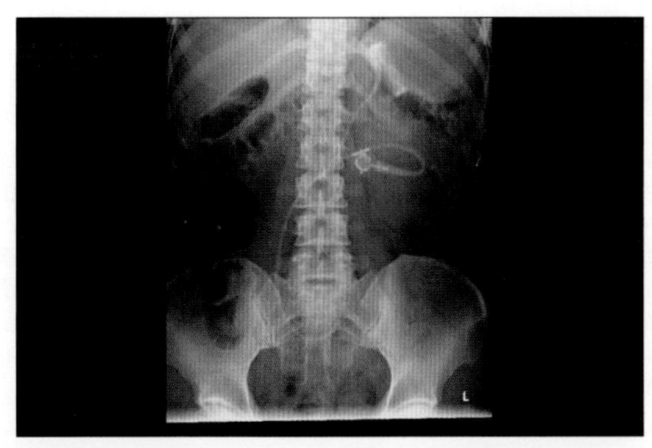

Figure 21.8 Abdominal X-ray of an acute band slip. The band lies 90 degrees out of alignment (compare with Fig. 21.1).

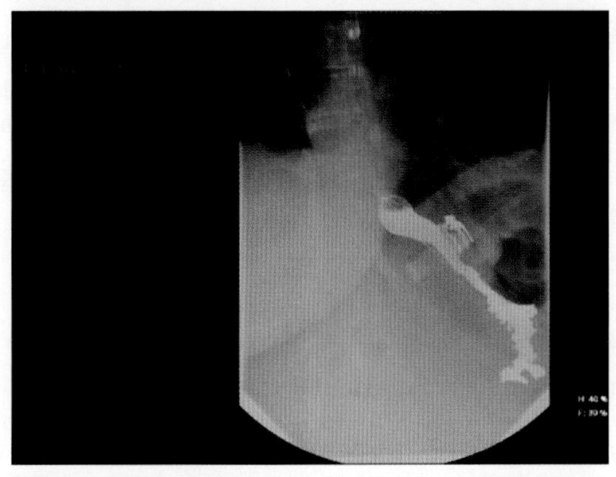

Figure 21.9 Barium swallow demonstrating band erosion. Note the barium leaking out around the band (compare with Fig. 21.1).

for erosion is gastroscopy, where a portion of the white silicone band will be visible from within the lumen. Patients should be referred back to the relevant bariatric team for removal of the band, which is usually possible laparoscopically (see above), leaving a drain to the area. A gastric fistula may result, but this will usually settle with non-operative management.

ABDOMINAL PAIN

This is uncommon in band patients (as a result of the band) and so should alert the clinician to a serious problem such as visceral distension from acute slippage (see above), inflammation related to band erosion (see above), peritonitis from gastric necrosis with or without perforation or postoperative haematoma. If the symptoms are of recent onset (hours) and pain is a prominent feature, necrosis and/or perforation should be suspected and urgent imaging is required, followed by laparoscopy with or without laparotomy if necessary. Peritonitis is an unlikely consequence of band erosion but may occur with gastric necrosis (acute band slippage) or perhaps foreign body perforation of the gastric pouch.

CHEST PAIN

This is a common reason for anyone to present to the hospital emergency department and cardiac causes need to be excluded. In patients with a gastric band, the possibility of band slippage, erosion and reflux oesophagitis (secondary to a tight band) needs to be considered.

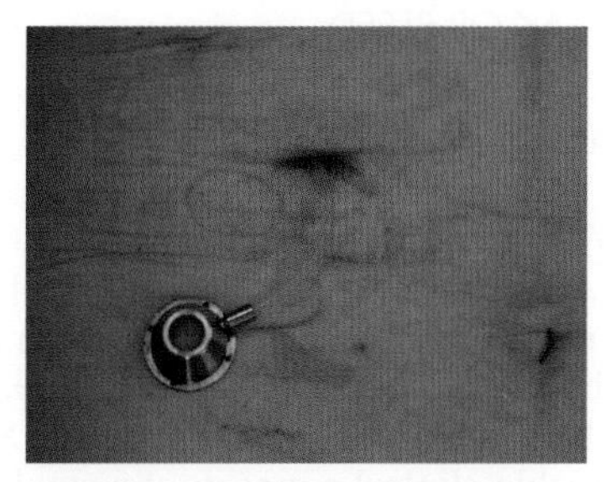

Figure 21.10 Port erosion through the skin.

MEGA-OESOPHAGUS

This is the result of long-standing, excessive restriction and usually follows either a period of excessive band tightness, or chronic malpositioning due to band slippage. If untreated, it can lead to peristaltic failure and risk of aspiration. It is recognised on a contrast swallow. It usually improves over a period of several weeks following band decompression but may necessitate band removal to prevent recurrence.

PORT PROBLEMS

MIGRATION

The subcutaneous injection port may move about within its subcutaneous pocket, depending on how well it has been fixed in position. This makes it difficult to access for percutaneous needle aspiration and if it has flipped over completely, the band will be impossible to decompress.

LEAKAGE

Repeated attempts to needle the subcutaneous reservoir should be avoided as damage to the rubber diaphragm or perforation/rupture of the tubing can produce a slow leak.

INFECTION

The injection port may become infected through breach of sterile technique; this may present as abdominal wall cellulitis or an abscess. An infected port will need to be removed but can be replaced at a later date when the sepsis has completely cleared. Sometimes an infected subcutaneous port may be the first manifestation of band erosion (see above), as the tubing effectively acts as a conduit to convey infected material from the eroded band to the skin surface.

SKIN EROSION

The port may also erode through the skin surface (Fig. 21.10). While not an emergency, this situation may present to the general surgeon. Again, plans will need to be made for removal, then later replacement, of the injection port.

SLEEVE GASTRECTOMY PATIENTS

Early postoperative reflux/vomiting and dysphagia are common as the narrow and oedematous gastric sleeve tends to empty poorly at first. Some degree of reflux oesophagitis is common. Patients are usually discharged from hospital on proton-pump inhibitor (PPI) medication with instructions to adhere to a fluid diet, gradually thickening their intake over several weeks. However, if the problem is severe or associated with early signs of dehydration, then specific complications should be sought.

STAPLE-LINE LEAK OR BLEED

Obvious signs are those of blood loss or sepsis, but disruption of the staple line along the narrow sleeve of remaining stomach may also present with luminal compression, either from oedema or direct pressure such as from a collection or haematoma. A contrast swallow or computed tomography (CT) should demonstrate this, although both imaging modalities may be falsely negative. Furthermore, some obese patients may be too large for the scanner or X-ray table. If there is reasonable clinical concern of a staple-line leak or bleed, perhaps because of grumbling sepsis or worsening anaemia, laparoscopy should be arranged as this is likely to both confirm the diagnosis and allow repair/control/drainage as necessary. A careful gastroscopy could also be considered.

SPLENIC INFARCTION

As the greater omentum is separated from the fundus of the stomach, it is possible to take one or more apical splenic vessels, leading to segmental infarction. This will present as left upper quadrant pain with or without some features of sepsis. A contrast CT should demonstrate this. Non-operative management is usually always successful.

OMENTAL NECROSIS

The blood supply to the omentum may be compromised if the gastro-epiploic arcade is damaged as it is separated from the stomach. Ischaemic necrosis may be the result, presenting with abdominal pain and features of sepsis. Surgical debridement of the necrotic tissue may be required, depending on the extent of infarction, either laparoscopically or by open surgery.

SLEEVE STENOSIS

This is usually a late complication of a staple-line problem but may be evident within the first week postoperatively if an intense local inflammatory reaction is established, usually following an otherwise undetected leak. After imaging as above, rehydration and possibly nutritional support are all that is initially required. At a later date, once any evidence of active perforation or leak has settled, endoscopic dilatation may help, although this brings its own risk of causing further disruption/perforation. Completion sub-total gastrectomy with conversion to a Roux-en-Y bypass may ultimately be required.

GASTRIC BYPASS/DUODENAL SWITCH PATIENTS

STAPLE-LINE LEAK

These operations have several staple lines to consider: the gastric pouch, the gastrojejunal anastomosis, the gastric remnant (in a gastric bypass) and the more distal jejuno-jejunostomy. Only the first two of these can be imaged on a contrast swallow. CT may show the others but the receiving surgeon should have a low threshold for returning the patient to theatre for laparoscopy if a leak is suspected. It should be remembered that a tachycardia or elevated C-reactive protein may be the only evidence of such a problem in obese patients. If more than 48–72 hours have elapsed since the initial operation, then laparoscopic repair is less likely to be feasible and laparotomy may be required. Surgical treatment should address drainage of sepsis, control of any ongoing leakage and provision of nutrition (Box 21.2).

> **Box 21.2 Nutritional support in the bariatric patient**
>
> It is a mistake to assume that obese patients are well nourished: although their diets may have been high in calories, they have often been deficient in protein, vitamins and other micronutrients. As for any patient with an upper GI anastomotic leak, consideration should be given to commencing enteral feeding or total parenteral nutrition. When re-operating on a bariatric patient for complications, it is sensible to place a feeding gastrostomy or jejunostomy at the same time.

> **Box 21.3 Early recognition of complications is essential**
>
> Many of the early complications after gastric bypass and duodenal switch are potentially life-threatening. Prompt recognition is important. CT scanning is useful but delay in the diagnosis will worsen a perilous situation, so urgent return to theatre is often a better strategy.

STAPLE-LINE BLEED

Patients may bleed into the GI tract or into the peritoneal cavity. A bleed into the 'blind' gastric remnant after a bypass will only be evident on CT, or by early return to the operating theatre (Box 21.3). Treatment involves establishing drainage of the collection of the haematoma by gastrotomy and controlling the bleeding point, usually by oversewing the staple line. Placement of a transcutaneous gastrostomy tube is wise, not only to decompress the stomach but also to use for later nutritional support if required. Angiographic embolisation of the bleeding point may be an alternative, but the surgeon must not allow the inherent delays of such intervention to postpone what might be life-saving re-operative surgery.

SMALL-BOWEL ENTEROTOMY

Full-thickness injury to the small bowel can easily be incurred as a result of handling with instruments and perforations may occur 'off-camera', out of the laparoscopic field of view. Missed enterotomies may take several days to become apparent, usually presenting with increasing abdominal pain, tachycardia and fever. Enteric fluid may leak out from one or more of the laparoscopic port sites. CT may demonstrate free intraperitoneal fluid and even intraperitoneal gas, but these findings are non-specific. Return to theatre for laparoscopy or laparotomy and drainage/repair is required.

EARLY SMALL-BOWEL OBSTRUCTION

Early postoperative small-bowel obstruction is uncommon after laparoscopic surgery and should not immediately be attributed to a paralytic ileus. Port-site bowel herniation, often of the Richter type, is always a possibility but after operations involving Roux-en-Y reconstruction one should always consider internal herniation, small-bowel volvulus and iatrogenic jejuno-jejunal anastomotic stricture or distortion. Vomiting will be absent if

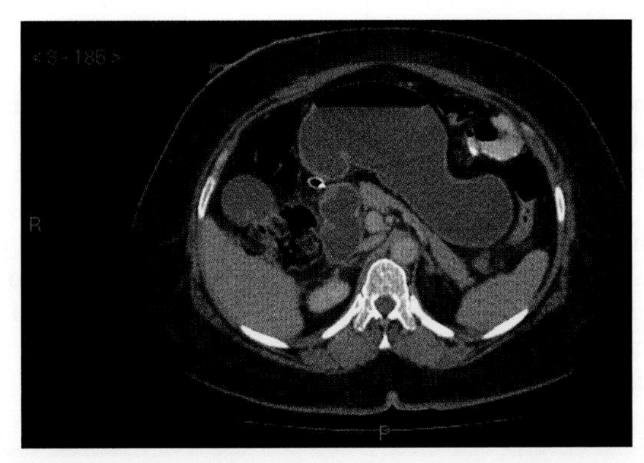

Figure 21.11 CT scan showing 'blind' gastroduodenal biliopancreatic limb obstruction. Note the dilated, fluid-filled stomach and duodenum and the oral contrast in the non-distended alimentary limb.

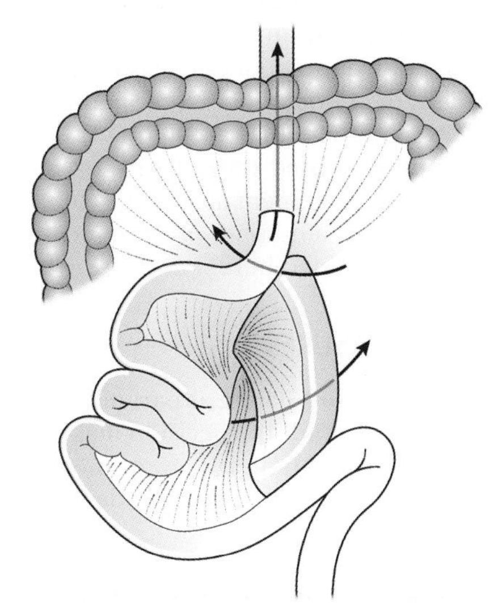

Figure 21.12 The three common sites for internal hernia after Roux-en-Y reconstruction: the mesocolic defect, Petersen's space and the jejunal mesenteric window.

the blind gastroduodenal limb is obstructed and abdominal X-rays may be unreliable, especially in a morbidly obese patient. CT is indicated (Fig. 21.11). The treating surgeon should not delay operating to correct an established obstruction.

LATE SMALL-BOWEL OBSTRUCTION

Small-bowel obstruction arising months or years after laparoscopic gastric bypass is a well-recognised problem. A frequent cause is internal herniation, occurring in up to 5% of cases if the mesenteric defects are not closed.[25] Closure of the defects appears to reduce the risk of internal herniation.[26] Hernias typically develop through the mesocolic defect if the retrocolic route is used, the jejunal mesenteric defect at the site of jejuno-jejunostomy, and Petersen's space between the alimentary limb and the transverse colon (Fig. 21.12). For many patients the presentation is insidious, with post-prandial pain and/or bloating. Imaging may not reveal significant small-bowel dilatation. Laparoscopy is the investigation and treatment of choice, where chyle within the abdominal cavity is a clue to the diagnosis. The ileocaecal junction is identified first and then the small bowel is carefully 'walked' back until the point of internal herniation is seen and reduced. The defect is then closed with non-absorbable material to prevent recurrence.

GASTRO-GASTRIC FISTULA

This is a consideration in the medium to long term if a patient develops weight regain. It may also present with dysphagia or pain on eating. It is often associated with stomal ulcers in the gastric pouch, which prove resistant to acid suppression medication, and likely arises following a staple-line leak with abscess formation that discharges into the gastric remnant. The treatment is surgical to divide the fistula and resect some of the distal stomach. This may be achievable laparoscopically.

Dumping syndrome

A recognised complication of gastric resectional surgery, this syndrome comprises post-prandial cramping abdominal pain, nausea, sweating, light-headedness and sleepiness. It reflects hyperinsulinaemic hypoglycaemia, usually precipitated by a high carbohydrate load in the jejunum from rapid gastric emptying,[27] although it is also described after Nissen fundoplication where vagal injury is the likely cause.[28] Mild forms are common and it is rarely severe enough to present as a surgical emergency, but surgeons should nevertheless be aware of it as a cause of post-bypass malaise. Dietary regulation, medication to slow gut motility and/or somatostatin analogues generally provide relief.

MINI-GASTRIC BYPASS PATIENTS

A similar spectrum of complications can be expected as might follow a Roux-en-Y bypass or duodenal switch. However, because of the loop gastrojejunostomy, bile reflux can be a problem, especially if the efferent limb takes a long time to function.[29] Prolonged nasogastric drainage and nutritional support may be required, with or without the addition of somatostatin analogues or other agents to reduce secretions. If the problem is intractable, conversion to a Roux-en-Y configuration may be necessary.

GASTRIC BALLOON PATIENTS

Nausea and vomiting are almost universal symptoms after balloon insertion but usually subside by the end of the first week. Patients may need intravenous hydration, PPI medication and parenteral anti-emetics over this time. A small minority of patients cannot tolerate oral intake even after several weeks and, in this group, early balloon removal should be offered and will provide instant relief. Although special equipment is required for balloon removal, it can easily be performed by using a standard endoscopic injection needle (to puncture and empty the balloon) and some strong grasping forceps, or a snare, to remove the deflated balloon.

Abdominal or chest pain is uncommon and should raise the possibility of reflux oesophagitis, gastric ulceration or even gastric/oesophageal perforation. If relief is not obtained with hydration, PPI and anti-emetic medication, then gastroscopy is warranted—although urgent CT is the preferred investigation if perforation is a serious consideration.

GASTRIC PLICATION PATIENTS

Whether this is done laparoscopically or endoscopically, the procedure-specific risks include gastric trauma (bleeding or perforation), liver/spleen trauma incurred by traction, direct pressure or injury and perforation of the stomach.[21]

PATIENTS WITH OLDER, NOW OBSOLETE OPERATIONS

As patients will have had their operations many years earlier, only late complications will arise. These include exacerbations of long-standing problems such as blind loop syndrome following a jejunoileal bypass and pouch outlet stenosis after a VBG. Nutritional deficiencies, which may manifest in many ways, are also possible complications (see below).

OTHER POSTOPERATIVE PROBLEMS

GALLSTONES

Dramatic weight loss from any cause promotes gallstone formation owing to mobilisation of cholesterol from peripheral fat stores and changes to the enterohepatic cycle. Patients may present with biliary colic, cholecystitis, pancreatitis or obstructive jaundice and should be managed according to established protocols. Laparoscopic cholecystectomy is generally no more difficult after a bariatric surgical operation than otherwise, but the management of common bile duct stones can be problematic because endoscopic retrograde cholangiopancreatography may be impossible if there has been a previous bypass or duodenal switch/BPD. Intraoperative cholangiography is therefore recommended at the time of cholecystectomy, with concurrent surgical common bile duct exploration if required.

NUTRITIONAL DEFICIENCIES

The common nutritional deficiencies seen in the bariatric surgery population concern thiamine, iron, zinc, vitamin D and vitamin B_{12}. These may have been present preoperatively, in which case replenishment can be difficult, especially if a malabsorptive-type operation has been done. It is common practice for all patients following bariatric surgery to take daily oral vitamin supplements long term. Nevertheless, clinical features of various deficiency syndromes are well documented but, like the neurological manifestations of thiamine deficiency presenting as Wernicke–Korsakoff syndrome, may not be readily recognised by general surgeons. If one deficiency is diagnosed, then others should be sought.[30] These are of particular importance if re-operative surgery is planned because of the possible detrimental effects that nutritional deficiencies might have on wound healing. A good principle is to replenish essential vitamins (especially thiamine) in any patient who is admitted with complications following bariatric surgery which have resulted in a significant reduction in nutritional intake.

FAILURE TO LOSE WEIGHT

Even the best operations do not work for everyone. While most patients do well in the first few months after surgery, and for many the weight loss is maintained indefinitely as they adopt a new and healthy lifestyle, some degree of late weight regain is very common. This rarely means that the operation has been done incorrectly or failed in some way, although this should be excluded first: bands may become too loose, gastric pouches may stretch, staple lines may disrupt, bypassed bowel may adapt. More usually, however, weight regain reflects a re-emergence of underlying poor eating behaviours—in other words, patients tend to slip back into their old eating habits.[31] Ongoing follow-up with the multidisciplinary bariatric team is important to both prevent and manage postoperative weight regain.[11–13]

CONSIDERATIONS WHEN OPERATING ON THE OBESE PATIENT

Obese patients present numerous challenges for surgical as well as anaesthetic and nursing staff, both in the theatre and the wards. For example, obesity has been shown to adversely affect length of operation, intra-operative blood loss, hospital stay and postoperative morbidity.[32] In addition to the comorbidities associated with obesity, obesity itself can influence surgical management at all stages of the perioperative pathway for which a number of extra measures may be helpful and will be outlined here.

PREOPERATIVE MEASURES

Specific preoperative counselling as part of the consent process is required to help with the decision-making for the patient to undergo an operation, in view of the increased risk of complications. Areas to consider include the following.

ANAESTHESIA

Difficult airway access; high airway pressures required (risk of alveolar barotrauma); difficult IV access; tailoring drug doses (especially fat-soluble drugs that may be sequestered in the adipose tissue); positioning and securing on the operating table.[33]

SURGERY

Access/visibility, higher risk of conversion of laparoscopic procedures, larger open wounds, higher risk of wound breakdown and infection. Additional or alternative surgical equipment may be required, for example, long laparoscopic ports or larger retractors.

POSTOPERATIVE CARE

Pain relief, mobility, chest infection, DVT/PE, wound infection and later incisional hernia.

PATIENT OPTIMISATION

This is an important part of the preparation for any elective operation. Patients should be advised to lose weight in preparation for surgery in order to reduce these risks, although this is easier said than done. Referral to a local Weight Management Service is a good start and an achievable timeline and/or target should be given. For example, it is reasonable to expect someone to be able to lose 5% of their total body weight in 3 months, which for a 150 kg person would be 7.5 kg, or about 1 stone. However, it would be much more difficult for them to lose another stone in another 3 months—that is, the steady weight loss cannot be expected to continue at the same rate. Therefore, the urgency of the surgery must be balanced against the feasibility of significant weight loss. In practice, this means that the operation is likely to go ahead with the patient still in an obese state, even though they may have achieved the designated weight loss target. Surgeons need to accept this and not delay surgery indefinitely in the vain hope that the patient will, one day, attain a target which is frankly unrealistic.

Consider a very low-calorie diet (e.g. 1000 calories per day) for 10–14 days leading up to surgery. Such a regime is widely practised in bariatric surgery and is applicable to other upper abdominal procedures, e.g. cholecystectomy, fundoplication or gastrectomy, laparoscopic or open, *where liver retraction is important*. All obese patients have a very 'fatty' liver, which is usually tense and immobile. In such a state, it is difficult to retract and may actually fracture in the attempt. This brief calorie challenge will significantly *reduce liver steatosis* and facilitate its handling during the operation. The diet should be prescribed under the auspices of a dietitian, as a healthy mix of nutrients must be achieved despite the caloric restriction.

Organise appropriate DVT prophylaxis (see Chapter 2). This involves avoiding unnecessary preoperative immobility and using doses of heparin that are appropriately up-scaled according to body mass. Remember also that compression stockings are designed for normal legs and may not fit the obese patient, perhaps digging in, creating a tourniquet effect and negating any potential benefit.

INTRAOPERATIVE MEASURES

Care must be taken in positioning the patient on the operating table, not only to provide optimal access for the surgeon but also to prevent movement (e.g. if the table is tilted) and to protect areas from pressure injury. Table side-extensions, extra padding and/or fixation straps may be required, but these should be positioned carefully to minimise risk to the surgeon (Fig. 21.13). For laparoscopic operations, a number of special techniques are helpful:

1. Significant table tilt. This requires extra patient safety procedures (see above). Table tilt can create extra working space, but be aware that head-up tilt reduces venous return and increases the risk of DVT, while head-down tilt affects diaphragmatic excursion and thus respiratory function.
2. Surgeon stands between the legs (for upper abdominal procedures). With head-up tilt, this provides a comfortable and ergonomic position from which to operate. Measures must be taken to prevent the patient sliding down the table, e.g. foot-plates and fixing the knees straight (Fig 21.13).
3. Extra ports to provide extra retraction. These are often more effective than extreme table tilt. Their use may require an extra assistant.
4. Port angulation is critical: passing through the thick abdominal wall, laparoscopic ports are relatively immobile and thus it becomes important to insert ports in the direction of the operative site. If they are angled incorrectly and cannot 'wiggle' within the abdominal wall, there will be extreme force on the instruments, which is not only uncomfortable for the surgeon but may also lead to instrument malfunction or breakage.
5. Remember that it is where the port emerges on the inside that is important. When correct port angulation is taken into account, the site of skin incision may be some distance from where the surgeon 'usually' places his or her ports. This is especially noticeable in laparoscopic ventral hernia repair, where ports have to be placed more peripherally than usual to maximise working distances inside.
6. Long ports. These are not needed as often as might be expected, but sometimes longer ports are needed to traverse a thick abdominal wall, especially with oblique angulation.

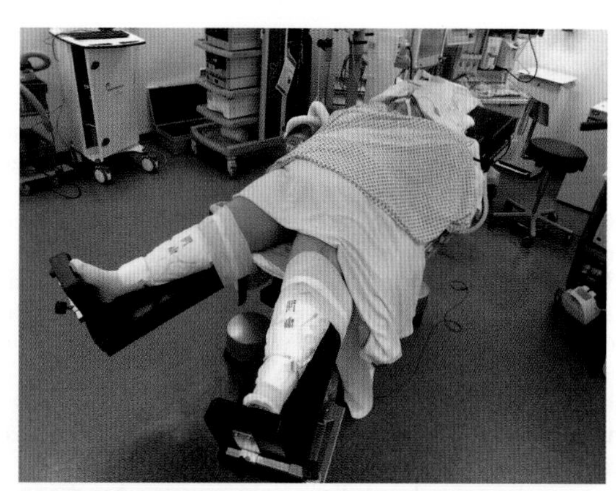

Figure 21.13 Obese patient positioned for a laparoscopic upper GI operation. The legs-apart position and head-up tilt gives comfortable access for the surgeon standing between the legs. Note the padded foot-plates attached to the table and bandages to keep the knees straight in order to prevent the patient sliding down the table when tilted. Anti-embolism stockings and calf compression are also in use. The arms are securely tucked in by the sides.

For open operations, a longer incision is usually required as well as deeper retractors and/or extra assistance. Closure techniques for open incisions may need to be tailored in obese patients. The lateral tension on the skin owing to the sheer weight of subcutaneous skin flaps indicates the use of slowly absorbable, deep dermal sutures to take the tension off the surface closure, e.g. sutures or skin staples. There is mounting evidence that the use of prophylactic mesh during abdominal wall closure reduces wound dehiscence and later incisional hernia formation in obese patients (see Chapter 7).

POSTOPERATIVE MEASURES

Good analgesia is critical to allow deep breathing/coughing and early mobilisation and should be planned in discussion with the anaesthetist preoperatively. Preventive chest physiotherapy is worthwhile and DVT prophylaxis should continue at the appropriate dose. Also do not neglect nutrition: obese patients often have a poor dietary range and may be low in the protein, vitamins and minerals that are needed for good postoperative healing. If an obese patient needs to remain fasting for any length of time postoperatively, provision of nutritional support, including enteral or intravenous feeding, should be considered just as for a normal-weight patient.

Key points

- Weight loss operations are becoming more common, and complications are increasingly likely to present to the general surgeon on call.
- Knowledge of the operation performed will help the receiving surgeon anticipate any problems that might arise.
- It is wise to contact the original bariatric surgical team as they may provide useful advice but, as for all emergency admissions, the prime clinical responsibility for the patient rests initially with the receiving surgeon.
- Physical examination may be difficult and X-rays may be hard to interpret. Look carefully for clinical and biochemical features of dehydration and sepsis.
- Beware the acute band slippage in a gastric band patient. Percutaneous band decompression may provide short-term relief, but definitive operative release/removal/resection may be required.
- Urgent CT to demonstrate a bleed, leak or obstruction in a patient who is unwell following a gastric bypass or duodenal switch procedure can help to make the diagnosis, but immediate return to theatre may be a better strategy.
- Incessant vomiting after gastric balloon insertion may respond to inpatient gut rest and anti-emetic medication, but instant and permanent relief will be obtained by removal of the balloon.
- Tachycardia should never be disregarded as it may be the only clue to an intra-abdominal catastrophe.
- Consider essential vitamin replacement in all patients admitted with complications from bariatric surgery where there may have been a significant reduction in nutritional intake.
- Because complications may arise some years after bariatric surgery, patients may no longer be overweight and thus the link to the initial procedure may not be obvious.
- Preoperative optimisation is an important area to consider, both in general weight loss but also a 2-week very low-calorie diet to reduce liver steatosis.
- Pay close attention to venous thromboembolic prophylaxis.
- Correct and careful positioning on the operating table allows safe movement during surgery, improving access.

References available at http://ebooks.health.elsevier.com/

KEY REFERENCES

[2] Sjöström L, Narbro K, Sjöström CD, Swedish Obese Subjects Study, et al. Effects of bariatric surgery on mortality in Swedish obese subjects. N Engl J Med 2007;357:741–52. PMID: 17715408.

A classic study and the first to show conclusively that bariatric surgery produced lasting health benefits.

[7] Tadross JA, le Roux CW. The mechanisms of weight loss after bariatric surgery. Int J Obes (Lond) 2009;33(Suppl. 1):S28–32. PMID: 19363504.

A fascinating account of the effects of bariatric surgery on the incretin-hypothalamic axis and the brain.

[13] Franco JVA, Ruiz PA, Palermo M, et al. A review of studies comparing three laparoscopic procedures in bariatric surgery: sleeve gastrectomy, Rouxen-Y gastric bypass and adjustable gastric banding. Obes Surg 2011;21:1458–68. PMID: 21455833.

A good review of several series comparing the outcomes of these three popular operations.

[24] Abdemur A, Sucandy I, Szomstein S, et al. Understanding the significance, reasons and patterns of abnormal vital signs after gastric bypass for morbid obesity. Obes Surg 2011;21:707–13. PMID: 20582574.

Beware of tachycardia in the early postoperative period.

Introduction of new technologies into surgical practice

22

Richard J.E. Skipworth

INTRODUCTION

Innovation is a necessity for the art of surgery. It can be defined as the practical implementation of ideas that result in new services or the improvement of existing services. Innovation has been a key driver for continued improvement in patient outcomes over the last decades, and without innovation, the art of surgery might remain fixed, leading to relative stasis in outcomes. In this chapter, the introduction of new surgical technologies (with pertinence to general and vascular surgery) will be discussed. For ease of readability, the chapter has been compartmentalised into different sections. In reality, however, each of these sections actually overlaps, and each type of technology is not mutually exclusive. In fact, combining technologies in novel formats is a central tenet of innovation, leading to disruption of established industries and markets (e.g. development of the smartphone from the mobile phone). Technological combinations with the associated cross-pollination of ideas allows leaps forward in progress. In the future, such overlaps will be accompanied by a blurring of the separation between technology used at work and at home. The COVID-19 pandemic has already seen a dramatic upsurge in the number of medical (including surgical) staff working from home using electronic platforms for collaborative working and patient consultations (e.g. Near Me video consulting service[1]). However, such overlaps can also lead to problems through industrial patent wars and by providing users with an overwhelming choice of solutions for purchase. In this chapter, examples of existing technological solutions will be described, but such lists will be by no means exhaustive, and in the face of an ever-changing modern world, new products will be added daily. Furthermore, the reader should be aware that, in the absence of high-level evidence, product references herein do not represent endorsements.

MINIMALLY INVASIVE AND ROBOTIC-ASSISTED SURGERY

Since the 1990s, laparoscopic surgery has revolutionised the field of general surgery by providing opportunities for earlier postoperative recovery combined with reduced patient morbidity,[2] comparative oncological outcomes[3] and better cosmesis[4]. Recent advances in 3D laparoscopic surgery[5] and ultra-high-definition endoscopic cameras[6] have provided enhanced surgeon vision and depth perception with potential benefits in surgical precision. Laparo-endoscopic single-site surgery (LESS)[7] and single incision laparoscopic surgery (SILS)[8] have now also reduced the number of skin incisions to one for selected laparoscopic procedures, while natural orifice transluminal endoscopic surgery (NOTES) has eradicated the need for skin incisions completely by achieving access to the peritoneal cavity via an incision in the wall of a natural office (e.g. transvaginal cholecystectomy[9]). In some studies, the latter technique has been associated with reduced early postoperative pain and better cosmetic results compared with standard laparoscopic surgery,[9] but it has been slow to be adopted internationally due to theoretical concerns associated with damage to the access orifice and associated bacterial contamination. Instead, robotic-assisted surgery (RAS) has risen to the fore as the next major advance in minimally invasive surgery (MIS), and the global surgical robotics market is anticipated to reach 98 billion USD by the end of 2024.[10] Furthermore, single incision and NOTES-type approaches can still be offered through RAS (e.g. transoral robotic surgery [TORS][11]). The proposed benefits of RAS include:

1. **Increased dexterity and precision**: These are achieved through fully wristed instruments giving 360 degrees of movement with 7 degrees of freedom, alongside motion scaling and eradication of physiological tremor. For these reasons, with regards to abdominal surgery, RAS has gained popularity for procedures focussed on difficult-to-access anatomical areas (e.g. pelvis[12]) or those requiring significant suturing (e.g. ventral wall surgery[13]) in an effort to reduce bleeding, increase rates of intracorporeal anastomoses, accelerate recovery[14] and possibly reduce complications.[14]
2. **Increased magnification**: Can be up to 10–12x.
3. **3D visualisation.**
4. **Elimination of the fulcrum effect at the body wall**: The robotic controls are moved in the same direction as the intended target/action rather than the mirror-image movements required by standard laparoscopy, thus aiding hand-eye coordination.
5. **Improved ergonomics**: The global increase in life expectancy has led to an increase in the retirement age in many countries. Despite this, up to a fifth of surgeons predict that they may need to retire early due to the chronic physical strain of performing standard MIS procedures.[15] Most RAS platforms consist of a master–slave system (Fig. 22.1) that permits enhanced surgeon comfort whereby the surgeon sits at a remote console to control the movements of multiple robotic arms. With increased comfort, it is hoped that such platforms may reduce the rate of chronic work-related injuries in surgeons.

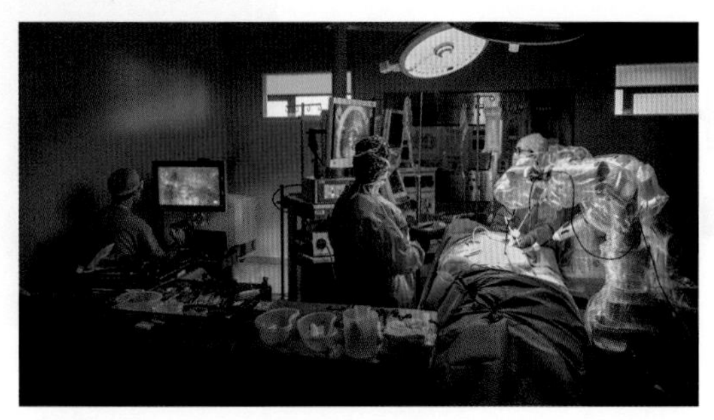

Figure 22.1 The CMR Versius robotic surgical platform in use demonstrating the master-slave arrangement. (Photograph courtesy of CMR Surgical.)

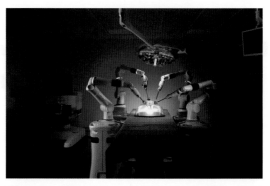

Figure 22.2 The CMR Versius robotic surgical platform demonstrating the separate modular robotic arms. (Image courtesy of CMR Surgical.)

Despite such proposed benefits, in the past, critics of RAS have argued that the expenditure (high costs including purchase, maintenance and disposable instruments), the size, weight and bulk of the platforms; length of operating time[14,16], and the lack of evidence for clinical effectiveness over standard laparoscopic surgery[12,17,18] should limit widespread adoption.

✔✔ Currently, a systematic review of randomised controlled trials indicates that, in most studies, abdominopelvic RAS is not associated with any difference in intraoperative complications, conversion rates or long-term outcomes compared with standard laparoscopic or open surgery.[14] However, RAS is associated with fewer complications in a minority of trials. Overall, RAS is associated with longer operative duration than laparoscopy, but similar to open surgery.

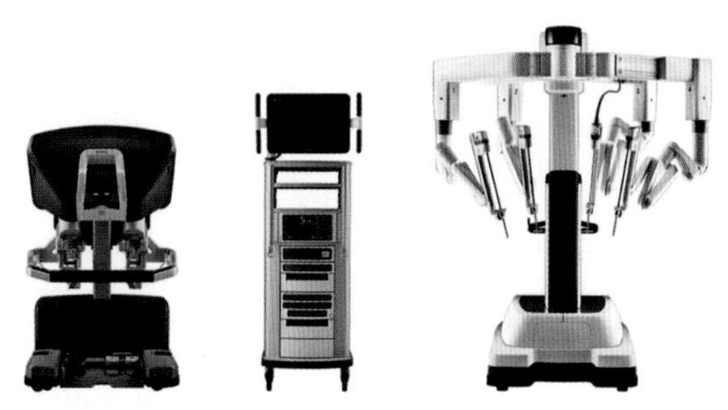

Figure 22.3 The Da Vinci Xi surgical robot. (Image courtesy of Intuitive.)

However, more recently, some of these arguments are showing signs of being overcome. RAS companies are now offering different payment structures without large, upfront costs, and in the future, it is likely that RAS platforms will become more affordable. The recent development of mobile, modular systems (e.g. CMR Surgical Versius[19]; Fig. 22.2) has now also permitted ease of transportation between different theatres and indeed different hospitals, thus allowing the future implementation of RAS in smaller, non-tertiary centres with added potential for progress in telesurgery.

At present, the Da Vinci surgical system from Intuitive (Sunnyvale, CA, USA)[20] remains the market leader. The newer Xi platform has integrated operating table motion (Fig. 22.3), whereas the SP system allows single-port access (Fig. 22.4). However, other robotic platforms are now also commercially available and becoming increasingly popular. Examples include the Versius (CMR Surgical, Cambridge, UK[19]), Senhance (Asensus Surgical US, Durham, NC, USA[21]), Revo-i (Meere Company, Seoul, South Korea[22]) and Dexter (Distalmotion, Switzerland[23]). The market for large surgical robots is likely to become increasingly competitive as major multinational corporations, such as Johnson & Johnson and Medtronic, develop their own platforms (named the Ottava and Hugo[24], respectively).

However, the robotic surgical market is not limited to large devices. There is also interest in smaller and medium-sized devices, and the perspective that robots represent the future of interventional procedures has led to advances in other fields, including NOTES, flexible endoscopy and even nanorobotics (Table 22.1).

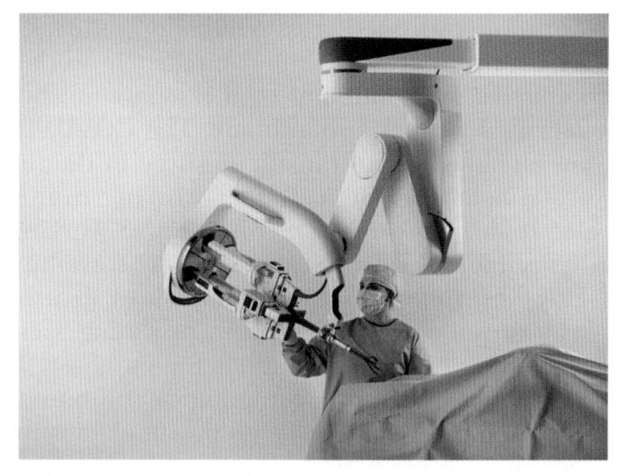

Figure 22.4 The Da Vinci SP surgical robot for single port access. (Image courtesy of Intuitive.)

RAS provides several challenges for surgeons in the future. First, in a multi-platform environment, we will need to ascertain which is the best robot for different surgical specialties and, indeed, different surgical procedures. Second, we will need to ensure that the adoption of such procedures is carried out in a safe and effective fashion, with standardisation of outcomes. The importance of training and validation will be paramount, and training pathways will need to be optimised and of consistent value across platforms. Third, we will need to provide evidence for equity of access within each healthcare system. At present, in developed countries like the USA, over 15% of all surgeries are performed robotically each year.[36] However, low- and middle-income

Table 22.1 Examples of newer forms of surgical robot. Several other platforms are also in development internationally

Mode of Surgery	Example Devices	Manufacturer
Small robots	*MIRA (Miniaturised In Vivo Robotic Assistant) Platform:* investigative single incision device comprising two robotic arms and a camera, focussed on colonic resection[25]	Virtual Incision (Lincoln, NE, USA)
NOTES	*Hominis Surgical System*: for transvaginal benign hysterectomy, salpingo-oophorectomy and ovarian cystectomy[26,27]	Memic Innovative Surgery (Memic) (Fort Lauderdale, FL)
Endoscopic	*Invendoscopy SC210 system:* flexible, self-propelling, singlse colonoscope[28]	Ambu (Ballerup, Denmark)
	Endotics: disposable, self-propelling robotic colonoscope aimed to reduce pain and lateral stretch[29]	Era Endoscopy (Peccioli, Italy)
	Endomina: device used to perform endoluminal full thickness suturing[30,31]	Endo Tools Therapeutics (Brussels, Belgium)
	Flex Robotic System: initially designed for difficult to access anatomical locations, approved for transoral and transanal procedures[32,33]	Medrobotics Corp., Raynham, MA, USA
Nanorobotics	Micro-robots that are ingested or implanted to treat medical problems, enable cell surgery, and target drug delivery, or used in other contexts in innovative devices[34,35]	Experimental

NOTES – Natural Orifice Transluminal Endoscopic Surgery.

countries will have much lower rates than this, and how they will provide future opportunities for RAS remains an unanswered question. Equally, due to its inherent unpredictable and out-of-hours nature, emergency surgery is likely to lag behind elective surgery with regards to the adoption of RAS.

To achieve these various aims, further large-scale randomised clinical trials will be required with an overarching governance framework supported by international surgical institutions and colleges. However, achievement of these aims will also be eased by the next generation of robotic platforms, which will integrate data sources that can be used as audit tools, including video recordings of the entire operations and telemetric data from both the surgeon console and the robotic instruments. Such tools will also allow real-time and retrospective assessments of both technical and non-technical skills, thus refining training pathways and truncating learning curves. Most robotic platforms are linked to the web, and therefore surgeon-specific (and even patient-specific) data will be easily compared and benchmarked internationally. In terms of technological combinations, one can envisage that, in the future, robotic platforms are likely to integrate additional features, such as visual overlay of cross-sectional imaging results or spectrographic/imaging cancer detection systems. Da Vinci systems already offer Iris,[37] which allows a segmented 3D model of patient anatomy (reconstructed from CT scans) to be used in case preparation, and Firefly fluorescence imaging,[38] an integrated fluorescence capability that uses near-infrared technology (see below).

IMAGING, VIRTUAL REALITY AND AUGMENTED REALITY

In section 22.2 and Table 22.1 above, the role of ultra-high-definition stereo-endoscopes as a method of advanced, intra-operative tissue imaging has already been considered. In the future, we are also likely to see further advances in cross-sectional imaging. CT and MRI already permit 3D reconstructions, which in turn can be used for 3D printing of bioprostheses (e.g. maxillofacial/ENT[39]) or pre-operative physical models to enable planning (e.g. endo/vascular[40]). The ability to create 3D reconstructions may even be enabled through smartphone technology.[41] Moving forwards, imaging is likely to cross the line from diagnostics into therapeutics, offering real-time visualisation alongside detailed, potentially cellular-level resolution, with decision-making/algorithmic support. Both PET-CT and PET-MRI scans are standard of care in the staging of multiple cancer types, and such tools already blend the assessment of anatomy with the assessment of dynamic tissue activity and function (e.g. ^{18}fluorodeoxyglucose as a measure of tumour glucose uptake and cellular metabolism). Indocyanine green (ICG), a water-soluble molecule that fluoresces in the near-infrared range (between 790 and 805 nm wavelength), is an example of an advance that allows integrated intra-operative assessment of anatomy and function via the use of specialised infra-red video cameras. Following intravenous injection, ICG is almost completely protein-bound in the circulation before metabolism by the liver and excretion in bile. It has been investigated for multiple uses in the field of general surgery, including the avoidance of common bile duct injury during laparoscopic cholecystectomy[42]). As a relatively cheap and reliable means of assessing real-time bowel perfusion, it has been shown to reduce anastomotic leak rate in colorectal resections.[43] Some robotic platforms are now compatible with ICG utilisation (e.g. Firefly[38]).

One way in which imaging will progress in the future is via the integration of standard imaging, 3D reconstruction techniques, and extended reality formats. Together, these technologies will permit cutting-edge spatial mapping with benefits for pre-operative planning and patient understanding (e.g. Brainlab mixed reality applications, Munich, Germany[44]), and for intra-operative anatomical overlay (e.g. SyncAR, Surgical Theatre, LA, CA, USA[45]). Extended reality (XR) is an umbrella term that refers to all immersive technologies that merge real and virtual environments. XR is composed of augmented reality (AR: an interactive experience in which real world objects are enhanced by digital visual elements, sound, or other sensory stimuli), mixed reality (MR: a merging of real and virtual worlds where physical and computer-generated objects co-exist and interact in real time) and virtual reality (VR: a fully immersive, simulated experience). As simulation becomes an established component of medical undergraduate and surgical postgraduate training, XR tools are currently under investigation as means of delivering effective and high-fidelity simulations,[46] particularly in high-risk situations (e.g. emergency drills[47]) and austere or complex environments (e.g. long duration spaceflight[48]). As such tools become increasingly "lifelike' through enhanced graphics and improved haptics, their role in surgical training and multidisciplinary teamworking will become ever more profound as training on patients will seem ethically unacceptable in comparison. Furthermore, the optimisation of digital simulation will mean that effective and meaningful technical surgical training can take place in the home (e.g. the @HomeVR platform of Fundamental Surgery from FundamentalVR, Boston, MA, USA).

DIGITAL HEALTH, ARTIFICIAL INTELLIGENCE, AND BIG DATA ANALYTICS

Digital health can be considered as mobile health (including mobile applications and wearable devices), health information technology, telehealth and telemedicine, and personalised medicine. Another challenge facing future surgeons will be how to integrate the ever-growing range of digital health applications and "big data" findings into routine clinical care. For example, in England and Wales, the NHS App is now used as a method for patients to access their health records, book medical appointments, check test results, order repeat prescriptions and establish their COVID-19 status.[49] This delegation of personal healthcare responsibility to the patient is an important step to recognise in the rationalisation of surgical service delivery. However, there are inherent risks. Although preliminary data suggest that digital health applications may help to reduce patient anxiety,[50] as the variety of innovative platforms increases in the future, socioeconomic status, internet access, age and other demographic variables may lead to inequalities in patient healthcare literacy. Equally, the volume and transfer of generated data lead to problems and ethical dilemmas regarding system failures, data governance, and cybercrime,[51,52] especially when such digital applications might also be used to connect different patients (e.g. contact tracing during the COVID-19 pandemic[53]).

Digital health offers specific opportunities for surgical patient management. As sensors become smaller, cheaper, and potentially autonomous, and as there remains increasing emphasis on early post-operative discharge in line with enhanced recovery programmes and in the face of ongoing hospital bed pressures, such devices are likely to play an expanding role. For example, in the inpatient setting, wearable sensors allow the continuous monitoring of patient vital signs postoperatively to predict and prevent clinical deterioration (e.g. Vitls, Houston, TX, USA[54]). Following surgery, physical activity accelerometers have been used to objectively measure the return of functional status and global recovery (e.g. ActivPal, PAL Technologies Ltd, Glasgow, UK),[55] and smartphone digital applications have been trialled for the assessment of post-operative wound infection.[56] For outpatients, telemedicine clinic appointments using various digital platforms (e.g. NearMe[1]) have become increasingly common in some countries, particularly during the COVID-19 pandemic. Using web-based platforms (e.g. My Clinical Outcomes[57]) and smartphone applications (e.g. VineHealth[58]), cancer outpatients are being invited to document their symptoms, nutritional status and quality of life online for centralised review during multimodal oncologic therapy, giving clinicians, nurse practitioners and dieticians unique insights into patient life in the free-living environment. In the future, such sensors may also be able to provide a direct link between diagnosis and treatment, similar to other recent developments in medicine (e.g. implantable cardiac defibrillators and continuous glucose monitoring devices). Sensor use in surgery is also not limited to the patient. The collection of objective surgeon physiological data, supported by subjective assessments of non-technical skills, is emerging as a means of measuring operative team performance (so called *surgical sabermetrics*[59]).

Social media platforms (e.g. Twitter) are also being used increasingly by surgeons for educational/research purposes (e.g. #SoMe4Surgery[60]) and to voice political opinions on public health issues.[61] Evidence suggests that such platforms can be used to improve surgical trial recruitment.[62] However, at the present time, there is little governance of these media, and the background consent processes for the online use of patient histories and radiological imaging are often unclear.

Digital health is not confined to utilisation by healthcare professionals, and through the development of smartphones and publicly accessible wearable technologies (e.g. Apple Watch, FitBit, Strava), it has also become an important component of everyday life. Indeed, the use of commercial exercise apps is associated with physical activity level,[63] suggesting that such apps have public health potential for physical activity promotion. There are also publicly accessible mobile applications which cross the barrier into effective healthcare delivery. For example, GoodSAM is an application that has been established as a life-saving method of crowdsourcing CPR-trained bystanders to patients experiencing out-of-hospital cardiac arrest.[64]

The massive expansion of electronic data generated by everyday life has been complemented by the simultaneous expansion in the understanding and statistical analysis of "big data", which can be defined as having volume, variety, velocity, veracity, value and variability.[65] Such datasets can involve pooled data from multiple sources (e.g. clinical, epidemiological, next generation sequencing). The use of massive datasets to solve medical questions is being increasingly employed. Data linkage between primary and secondary care datasets can create powerful insights into the natural history and management of clinical problems (e.g. the relationship between pre-diagnosis haemoglobin levels in primary care and subsequent colorectal cancer diagnosis[66]). Massive international surgical research collaboratives have allowed rapid response to major health threats, resulting in meaningful clinical lessons (e.g. COVIDSurg[67] and GlobalSurg[68]), and facilitated trainee involvement in important clinical research.[69]

The analysis of massive datasets has also stimulated innovation in the fields of artificial intelligence (AI), machine learning (automated analytical model building in which the system learns from the data) and deep learning (an AI function that simulates the working of the human brain). Such techniques have become increasingly used as research tools in disease diagnosis and image analysis (e.g colonic polyps[70]) and in the prediction of patient outcomes (e.g. early recurrence after oesophageal cancer surgery[71]). AI has also been trialled as an adjunct and potential future replacement for human decision-making during cancer multidisciplinary meetings (e.g. Watson for Oncology, IBM, Armonk, NY, USA[72]). In the operating theatre, AI/deep learning analyses of integrated audio-visual data can yield meaningful insights into patient safety and departmental efficiency (e.g. OR Black Box, Surgical Safety Technologies, Toronto, Canada[73]; Touch Surgery Enterprise, Medtronic, Fridley, MN, USA[74]). The future potential for AI technologies in clinical healthcare is effectively limitless.

GENOMICS, REGENERATIVE MEDICINE AND CELL-BASED THERAPEUTICS

Developments in molecular biology have significantly influenced the management of surgical patients (especially cancer patients) in recent years, and are predicted to have further profound impacts in the near future. Advances in cancer screening, oncological therapies (chemotherapy, targeted radiotherapy, proton beam therapy and immunotherapy) and personalised medicine strategies will potentially reduce the need for resectional surgery of locally advanced disease but increase the requirement for risk-reducing surgery in healthy patients with pre-malignant/early conditions. Liquid biopsies of patient blood are emerging as a potentially effective means of both screening for cancer[75] and monitoring for disease recurrence.[76,77] Such biopsies are rapid, non-invasive, and based on the measurement of circulating biomarkers, usually tumour cells, tumour exosomes, or cell-free tumour DNA/RNA, often supported by AI/machine learning analytic algorithms. Some liquid biopsy multi-cancer early detection (MCED) tests (e.g. Galleri by Grail, Menlo Park, CA, USA, which is reported to screen for over 50 different cancer types[78]) have now been clinically validated,[79] and it has been estimated that the potential public health impact of a MCED test as part of routine medical care would result in a 26% reduction of all cancer-related deaths.[80]

Recent trials have suggested the benefit of adjuvant immunotherapies in resected cancer patients (e.g. nivolumab, an agent against programmed cell death protein 1 [PD1] in resected oesophagogastric cancer[81]). In some of these trials, the tumour has been specifically tested for genetic susceptibility to the immunotherapy (e.g. adjuvant trastuzumab for resected breast cancers with HER2 positivity[82]), while in others, no specific genetic tests have been performed and the immunotherapy has been administered empirically.[81] In the future, routine next generation sequencing of biopsied and resected tumours[83] will permit the delivery of targeted immunotherapies within personalised, precision medicine strategies. The FDA has already approved battery tests of cancer-related gene mutations (e.g. MSK-IMPACT: *integrated mutation profiling of actionable cancer targets*, which analyses 505 genes[84,85]) that can be applied to all tumours rather than just the commonly tested ones (e.g. colorectal, melanoma, lung). In some countries, such developments in tumour genomics are supported by government healthcare strategies aimed at simultaneous assessment of patient germline DNA. For example, the 100,000 Genomes Project from NHS England was established to sequence 100,000 genomes from approximately 85,000 patients affected by a rare disease or cancer.[86] The NHS Genomic Medicine Service is planning to extend this project to one million whole genomes sequenced within five years, which when linked to patient health record data, will result in an enormous data repository. Additional developments in the understanding of patient pharmacogenomics (the study of how genetics affects the body's response to drugs) have also influenced the delivery of routine oncology care. For example, it is now recommended routine practice to screen for DPYD polymorphisms (which cause dihydropyrimidine dehydrogenase deficiency) prior to the administration of fluoropyrimidine-based therapies.[87] This expanding characterisation of patient and tumour genetics has led to the rise of ambitious stratified clinical trial programmes (e.g. in pancreatic cancer, PRECISION-Panc funded by CRUK[88] and Precision-Promise by Pancreatic Cancer Action Network[89]). In the future, the step beyond deep sequencing technologies to inform management decisions will be the actual treatment of genetic conditions through in vivo gene editing.[90] Gene editing techniques based on the bacterial CRISPR-Cas9 antiviral defence system have now been used in human trials and have demonstrated clinical efficacy in altering the phenotype of human genetic conditions,[90] thus opening the door to new avenues of treatment for surgical patients with genetic cancer conditions.

Another biological means to influence complex surgical conditions is stem cell therapy. Human trials have been promising with regards to conditions affecting the skin (e.g. burns, ulcers[91]) and eyes[92], and the technique holds promise for neurodegenerative conditions.[93] Regenerative therapy techniques are also of increasing relevance to the field of transplantation. In the future, the indications for transplantation are likely to be extended to include higher risk, obese patients (RAS has been proposed as one method of safely operating on obese patients) and to treat different medical conditions e.g. cancer. An increase in demand will impact further on the major challenge facing modern transplantation, namely the shortage of available organs. Organ perfusion technologies (e.g. OrganOx *metra* for liver transplantation[94,95]), developments in xenotransplantation,[96] and improvements in immunosuppression and the promotion of immune tolerance[97] will help to mitigate the increased demand. Additionally, 3D printing technologies, involving either complete bioengineered organs or composite organs comprising an animal-derived scaffold populated with human cells, also remain viable possibilities for future transplant solutions. Strategies will be required to overcome the cost and time duration of bioprinting techniques and the current difficulties in vascularisation of artificial organs.[98]

IMPLEMENTATION OF NEW SURGICAL TECHNOLOGIES

The goal in surgical innovation is to implement new technologies in a safe and reproducible fashion. Historically, many surgical innovations have occurred during warfare, stemming from the management of battlefield injuries, and such an unpredictable and hazardous environment is not one easily amenable to rigorous clinical research. In the civilian environment, despite the strict existing regulatory approval systems and appropriate guidance from technology companies, many surgical innovations still occur without robust randomised clinical trial data, centralised registries or frameworks of oversight. Even when research opportunities are easily available, the evidence base is not always fully explored. Laparoscopic cholecystectomy is often described anecdotally as one innovation that became widely adopted during 1980s and 90s despite limited evidence at the time. Even when guidelines are widely disseminated, implementation of surgical technology will still be affected by the infrastructure, staffing and patient population of each individual hospital or healthcare setting.

The chief described methodology for the safe adoption of surgical innovation (or other interventional procedures) is the IDEAL framework.[99] This system describes 5 stages of innovation (Idea, Development, Exploration, Assessment, Long-term study) with an emphasis on prospective evaluation, the importance of randomised controlled trials, and the use of centralised registries and rigorous standardised outcome reporting. More recently, a "pre-IDEAL" preclinical stage has also been added.[100]

✔ The safe adoption of surgical innovation should follow the IDEAL framework of Idea, Development, Exploration, Assessment, and Long-term study.[99]

In the future, implementation programmes based around the IDEAL framework, upheld by robust governance and oversight from established surgical institutions, will be required to ensure patient safety and public confidence. In the UK, the respective Royal Colleges of Surgeons have expressed interest and intent in adopting such governance roles, and in 2017, the Royal College of Surgeons of England published their Report on the Future of Surgery,[101] a scoping exercise on the role of future technologies in surgical practice.

CONCLUSION

In the years to come, levels of technology hitherto unknown will become a daily component of surgical practice, all with the unifying aim of improving patient outcomes. All the working environments of surgical life, including the inpatient ward, outpatient clinic, endoscopy facility, interventional radiology suite, and operating theatre, are likely to be affected, and hopefully enhanced. Advanced surgical technologies will be able to diagnose pathologies, recommend therapeutic options, order instruments and drugs, schedule procedures, play a significant role in said procedures, and then monitor the patient for clinical deterioration and postoperative complications. The human surgeon will need to adjust to fundamental changes in their daily roles and to train appropriately (with regular updates) to achieve competence, proficiency and confidence in new innovations.

Key points

- Robotic-assisted surgery (RAS) is the next major development in minimally invasive surgery (MIS) and adoption is increasing across the globe.
- Advances in digital technology, including radiological imaging, virtual reality, digital health, artificial intelligence and big data analytics, are permitting significant progress in the diagnosis and treatment of surgical conditions, and the follow up of surgical patients.
- Genomics, regenerative medicine and cell-based therapeutics offer opportunities for improvements in disease screening, cancer treatment and transplantation.

References available at http://ebooks.health.elsevier.com/

INDEX

Note: Page numbers followed by "*f*" and "*t*" refer to figures and tables, respectively.